The
CLINICAL MEDICINE GUIDE
A Holistic Perspective

DEDICATION

I humbly dedicate this book to Sogyal Rinpoche, a source of supreme inspiration, and to all practitioners working to relieve distress and ill-health.

DR. STEPHEN GASCOIGNE
M.B., Ch.B., C.Ac., Dip.C.H.M.

The
CLINICAL MEDICINE GUIDE
A Holistic Perspective

Clonakilty, Co. Cork, Ireland

Jigme Press

Published in Ireland by

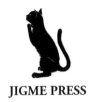

JIGME PRESS

Glebe House, Ardfield, Clonakilty, Co. Cork, Ireland

© Stephen Gascoigne, 2001

ISBN 0-9522189-3-3

First published 1993 as *The Manual of Conventional Medicine for Alternative
Practitioners* in two Volumes ISBN 0 9522189 0 9 & ISBN 0 9522189 1 7
Reprinted in one volume 1995: ISBN 0 9522189 2 5
Reprinted 1996, 1999 (twice)

This Edition 2001

Reprinted 2002

British Library Cataloguing in Publication Data
A catalogue record for this book is available from the British Library.

Printed by Antony Rowe, Chippenham, UK
Cover design and typesetting by Declan O'Donovan
Cat logo and line drawings by Rob Hopkins
Proofreading by Antoinette Walker

Contents

ACKNOWLEDGEMENTS

I owe my thanks to many people during the process of writing this book but especially to:

Mary Aspinwall who edited with great skill and allowed me access to her homoeopathic cases,
Michael Courtney of CityPrint, Cork who gave me invaluable advice and encouragement,
Hilary Gascoigne, a source of unfailing support and encouragement,
Rob Hopkins for his artwork,
Carey Horvath, Dr Maurizio Italiano who kindly allowed me to describe
his homoeopathic treatment of epilepsy (Case two),
Yann Kelly, Declan O'Donovan, Geraldine Petch, Antoinette Walker,
and all those students who have patiently allowed me to develop my ideas.

FOREWORD

Before I arrived in England, I thought that with such an advanced technology and prosperous life-style, the fortunate people who live here would be very peaceful, happy and healthy. Now, the more I treat Western patients, the more I understand that the opposite is true. The society which has everything seems to be splintering and everything has to be approved by the cold eye of science as we forget how to call on our intuitive natures. Our advanced technology does not satisfy the voracious appetite of human desire for progress whilst simultaneously polluting the environment.

The common foundation of the family has been broken because mother and father have little time with their children. The majority of older people are lonely and lack self-esteem whilst many of the younger generation are dissolute. The generation gap widens. Understanding and co-operation between people decline whilst egotism, factionalism, selfishness, indulgence and irresponsibility are rife within our society.

True love and care, the desire for deep understanding and self-awareness have been supplanted by a spiralling consumption of materialism which leads to chronic mental disease and physical illness.

As an Oriental practitioner with a Buddhist perspective, I often ask myself after clinical days, 'Have I done enough to express my gratitude to Great Britain, the country which was kind enough to grant me refuge? How can I best serve all beings that I encounter in this world?'

One fresh morning, Dr Stephen Gascoigne gave me a copy of his book and asked for my opinion.

I feel very touched by this work. In the Philosophy section he writes, 'It depends as much on how medicine is practised as the method of practice.' Yes, it is true that the patient's response depends on the attitude of the practitioner. It is like the relationship between the mother and baby. The old Vietnamese proverb says 'Luong Y nhu tu mau'. It means the good-hearted practitioner looks after their patients like the mother feeding her baby from the beginning of pregnancy throughout their childhood.

A wonderful thing about this book is the emphasis placed on understanding the essence of the relationship between the practitioner and the patient. It is as important as the relationship between mother and child and is called 'the consciousness of the Healing Tao' in the ancient texts. Practitioners should always relate to this and remember Stephen for setting it down in a modern idiom.

Nguyen Tinh Thong
Former Principal and Founder of The London Academy of Oriental Medicine

1 INTRODUCTION

When I trained in conventional medicine, I always had the feeling that something didn't 'sound right' although it was difficult for me to precisely say what that 'something' was. I felt that the fabric of conventional medicine did not hang together in a logical way. I found there were many discrepancies and contradictions that were not addressed and in most situations actively ignored. However, at the time, I thought that this sense of a fruitless struggle with confusion was a problem that was unique to me. Sometimes it is said that to talk to a person who is insane can be very disconcerting since they may appear to be lucid, clear and rational. At the end of the conversation, you may realise that one of you is mad but you are not sure which one. This is how I felt about conventional medicine.

When I was in general medical practice I had a crisis of confidence in that I began to see that many treatments of conventional medicine not only produce little benefit but also can cause harm. This may not have been obvious at first but over months and years I came to see that drug-based treatment leads to effects that are frequently worse than the original problem.

It was only with my subsequent training in Chinese medicine that I came to see conventional medicine in a different light. The information gleaned from conventional medicine may be useful in helping practitioners understand their patients. It is when these ideas are translated into clinical practice that difficulties begin. I remember having a conversation with an acupuncturist and herbalist who grew up and trained in the Orient. He also had been educated in conventional medicine. He said that he had not really understood the connection in conventional medicine between diagnosis and treatment – how one led onto the other. Of course, there *is* no connection between these two things. The use of treatments is based on experience and of 'what works', that is, what seems to remove the symptoms, rather than any sound connection with deeper physiological processes or an attempt to treat the 'dis-ease' that produced the symptoms.

This book is the result of those years of trying to make sense of conventional information. It seeks to transform the information into something that can help our practice of holistic medicine[1]. In many respects it reflects the struggle we all have between the differing philosophies of holistic and conventional medicine. This is especially true for Westerners who have grown up with the belief that conventional medicine is *the* way to treat most disease states. This view is, of course, a minority view as the majority of the world's population subscribe to more holistic views of health and disease and if you live in China, India or most of the so-called Third World you have much more access to holistic methods of treatment.

The main aim of this book is to provide information to those who need access to conventional medical information that is clear and concise. In addition, it serves as a text that supports holistic practitioners not trained in conventional medicine. Since the first edition of 'The Manual of Conventional Medicine for Alternative Practitioners', which this book replaces and updates, it has become the set textbook at many colleges of acupuncture, homoeopathy and herbalism. Its accompanying Study Guide has become a favourite method of study for people training in such therapies.

In this book I have concentrated on describing processes in plain English. Many textbooks are aimed at medical students; hence they are very detailed and written in overly technical language. Whilst they are a useful source of information, they are not always easy to follow or necessarily relevant to the needs of holistic practitioners.

This book mirrors the way in which conventional medicine outlines 'systems' of the body. I have included all diseases that are commonly seen in clinical practice. I have omitted those diseases that are rare and unusual.

In each section I have arranged the information according to principles of *energetic* medicine and although they may appear unusual at first they are more helpful as they apply to the system of medicine we are using. All the references to holistic medicine in the book apply to ideas gleaned mainly from Chinese medicine, my own chosen field of practice, or of homoeopathy.

My other aim is to provide support to holistic practitioners so that the practice of such medicine can be strengthened. I hope in the future that methods of holistic medicine can be made more available. The way forward is to be competent and confident in our practice. Many practitioners I meet feel that they particularly lack confidence when treating serious conditions. They often project this insecurity onto their lack of training in conventional medicine. It is true that my training in conventional medicine has given me experience in seeing and treating more serious disease. However, it is important to emphasise that faith in holistic medicine and its ability to help sickness comes from competence in our chosen field. Therefore, any knowledge of conventional medicine must only be considered as subsidiary to our main practice.

Holistic medicine is our chosen therapy and the one that is most appropriate to the needs of the individual because of its ability to lead towards 'cure'.[2] Conventional medicine is complementary to this and would be better used either for structural problems incapable of any other help, e.g. trauma, or for life-threatening conditions.

Today, we see the opposite situation where holistic medicine is only used after a long period of conventional treatment. We live in a society that gives little weight to ideas of energy and the non-physical. Holistic medicine is criticised by those people who only give importance to material things. This, of course, is at the root of Western thought[3] – a division between mind and body together with the unfortunate association that mind is unimportant or even non-existent. This constant message of division and the undermining of people's belief in the non-physical affect us greatly. We lose faith in our ability to know ourselves and to heal ourselves. We rely on 'experts' who claim to know what is best for us. This disconnection at deep levels is, I think, primarily responsible for the great dissatisfaction and angst that is felt by so many people in the West today. It is no mistake when the sages of India and Tibet say we live in degenerate times.

Today, there is definitely a change in consciousness occurring that is gathering pace. There is increasing interest in holistic medicine, in self-help, in religious faith, in meditation and in matters that formerly were considered non-scientific and of little or no value. Such changes can only develop further, as the momentum for change becomes irresistible. In this climate and that of the future, doctors will find themselves increasingly isolated as people embrace more holistic principles. Major changes in health care practice will come from ourselves as we reclaim those powers we have so carelessly given away to science, dogmatism and the denial of our deeper selves. The role of holistic medicine and holistic practitioners will be increasingly important in the years to come.

This process will not be easy, as there are powerful groups with vested interests in maintaining the status quo. However, the power of the individual cannot be denied and as people become more aware of issues to do with the environment, caring for others, growth and self-development, nothing will be able to stop these changes taking place.

I hope that this book may, in some small way, help in this process.

Layout of the book

There are two assumptions I have made about those using this book. The first is they have a basic knowledge of anatomy and physiology. The second is that they have access to a medical dictionary. I have, as much as possible, written in plain English but there are a limited number of terms which I introduce where necessary.

The Chapter headings correspond roughly to the 'systems' of conventional medicine, e.g. cardiovascular, respiratory and so on. Each Chapter is laid out in similar ways:

- Introduction including energetic view of that system
- Anatomy and physiology – useful to know as a prerequisite to a study of that system
- Diseases
  - Definition
  - Symptoms
  - Complications
  - Investigations
  - Conventional treatment
  - Holistic management
- Symptoms and how to recognise a serious situation.

The section on holistic management includes information from the Chinese medical viewpoint.[4] This will be of use to acupuncturists and shiatsu practitioners but also to anyone with an energetic understanding of the human body. Homoeopaths may see the symptom picture associated with a particular remedy here. I do not intend these sections to be exhaustive as this book is primarily about conventional medical knowledge. I hope it will enable you to see that it is possible to view conventional information from a holistic perspective. This revised and updated edition also includes cases that were treated homoeopathically.

Comparisons between conventional and holistic medical systems need to be drawn with care. Conventional disease labels are fixed entities and apply to people with slightly different clinical pictures and widely different underlying energetic disturbances. Do not fall into the trap of thinking that conventional disease labels always correspond to a particular energetic picture. The whole point of holistic medicine is that it seeks to treat the individual.

The listing of symptoms and how to recognise a serious situation is intended to reassure you that you are not dealing with a potentially dangerous condition and to recognise which situations may require referral to another practitioner.

NOTE: Nothing in this book should be construed as medical advice on an individual basis. I would urge anyone with a health problem that is chronic, severe or not responding to simple, self-help remedies to seek out appropriate advice and help from a competent practitioner – orthodox or holistic. It is your choice.

[1] There is a lot of debate about terminology of non-conventional forms of medicine. There seem to be three main terms employed. Complementary, alternative and holistic all have their advocates. As I explain later in this text, the word complementary (used by people to indicate treatment complementary to conventional medicine) would be more appropriately applied to conventional medicine so that it is only used when other forms of treatment are inapplicable or ineffective. To use the powerful methods of conventional medicine for all and as a first-line of treatment is frequently inappropriate. The term 'alternative' implies something instead of conventional medicine and although it has its value, all too frequently it is perceived as confronting and radical. I prefer to use the term 'holistic' which means whole, the whole person. It can be widely used to include all gentle, non-toxic treatments which seek to see the person as an individual, in a whole way and to provide them the means whereby they can become or remain 'whole'. The word 'healing' means, of course, 'to make whole'. The thrust of this book is to encourage and support the process of 'becoming whole', of 'being healed'.

[2] I use the term 'cure' as it is understood by homoeopathic medicine. The same principle, of course, also applies to any method of healing which is truly holistic. I discuss cure more fully in Chapter 2.

[3] There is a vitalistic tradition to Western philosophy as evidenced by the work of Paracelsus. Homoeopathy belongs to this tradition. When I use the term Western as applied to medicine or philosophy in this book, I am referring to the main strand of science which has become dominant in the Western world, i.e. materialistic, physical.

[4] I have not spent a long time in this book describing the theories of Chinese medicine since this is not my main aim and I do not want to overcomplicate matters. For anyone interested in the basic ideas of Chinese medicine I would recommend two books, *Between Heaven and Earth – A Guide to Chinese Medicine* by Beinfield and Korngold, (Ballantine, 1991) and *The Web Which Has No Weaver* by Kaptchuk (Contemporary Books Inc, 2000).

2 PHILOSOPHY

INTRODUCTION

When I studied medicine there was little mention of philosophy or a discussion of the theories underpinning the practice of conventional medicine. There was mention of a 'medical model'. However, this did not extend to any debate concerning its origin or whether holistic views existed. It was merely stated that this was the way to do it.

I hear holistic practitioners say that there is no philosophy of conventional medicine. There is *always* a philosophical view that drives our actions. We cannot operate without a belief system. In Tibetan Buddhism this sequence of events is described as 'View, meditation and action.' To have an action there must be preceding thought and for this to occur there must be preceding belief. In modern society people think that an action is a spontaneous event. Cause and effect are not seen as being connected.

PHILOSOPHICAL VIEW OF CONVENTIONAL MEDICINE

Conventional medicine, in common with the prevailing scientific view in the West, believes there is only a physical body, which can be measured, weighed and analysed by physical methods. This leads to the available treatments of surgery, radiotherapy and material chemical substances (drugs) that, again, are purely physical in their application. Although there is occasionally mention of mind, indicating an entity other than the physical body, this is seen as being coexistent with the brain. It is not regarded as being non-material in nature. The natural consequence of this belief system is that anything that is not physical is seen as being unimportant. These ideas even enter the language. The word 'immaterial', for instance means 'it does not matter'.

The materialistic ideas behind Western science and conventional medicine have gained ground over the past 2000 years placing a division between spirit and matter, doctor and priest, science and art, man and woman. This separation has pervaded all aspects of society and since medicine reflects the views of the society in which it is practiced we see such a polarisation in conventional medicine. This can be described as a flourishing of the Yang principle[1] (as that term is understood by Chinese medicine). Unfortunately, it has not been balanced or grounded by Yin. Unchecked it leads to aggression rather than assertiveness, Fire which flares up easily and dissipates quickly, a dryness and rigidity which is not balanced by aspects of nurturing and flexibility.

Western society generally separates the spirit from the body. We have people who deal with the body – doctors – who assume the role of mechanics. They 'fix' the physical machine by manipulating physical parts with drugs or inserting 'new' parts. Annual 'health checks' similar to government tests of motor vehicles are advocated fostering the belief that these brief encounters with a qualified 'mechanic' will guarantee health for another year. The spirit is dealt with by priests whose traditional healing role has, over time, been transferred to the realm of doctors.

It is only in recent years that a more holistic view has arisen in science. This is revealed in the new theories of quantum physics whose ideas formerly seemed to be the province of Buddhism or Hinduism.[2] Whilst these are the source of much debate amongst scientists, they have yet to filter through to the practice of medicine. Conventional thought is involved with physicality. Anything else is seen as being non-existent or of no importance.

New specialties such as psychoneuroimmunology try to make some sense of the whole person and bring together ideas from different areas. In the reality of everyday medicine, however, the treatments continue to be those that primarily act on the physical level – surgery, chemicals and radiation.

PHILOSOPHICAL VIEW OF HOLISTIC MEDICINE[3]

Holistic medicine believes there are other aspects to humans (and, indeed all beings) – the non-physical – and that these are at least as important as the physical. These ideas are not new and the acknowledgement of other levels leads to treatments that utilise energetic methods such as homoeopathy, herbal medicine, acupuncture and so on. In recent years there has been a resurgence in healing as people become disillusioned with conventional medicine and seek other methods of help that incorporate ideas of wholeness. At the same time there has been a strong interest in Oriental philosophies and religions that unite body and mind into a single entity.

The essence of holistic medical thought is that there is a vitalistic[4] principle behind and encompassing any physical object.

This means that the physical body is merely the outer manifestation of an inner energetic state. Changes of the inner energies are reflected in the physical body. Symptoms appear when an imbalance of the inner energetic state occurs. As the person is a manifestation of their inner energies, the only way in which true balance can be achieved is by change at the level of those energies. The root must be dealt with. Conventional medicine sees only the outer physical aspect of the person and so can only 'treat' the physical body.

This is not to say there is no benefit in conventional medicine and its methods. In acute life-threatening situations there may be nothing better. However, once the threat of death has passed it would clearly be inappropriate to continue to use such methods. When emergency drugs, e.g. corticosteroids, bronchodilators, antihistamines, antibiotics, etc. are given to people for years or on many separate occasions, this can only lead to severe depletion of the person's energy. With Chinese medicine it would be like using an emergency Rescue Yang formula for years. After 2-3 weeks (once the acute episode has passed) it is clearly appropriate to turn to more gentle, balanced treatments. Since the essence of holistic medicine is vitalistic, many levels of a human being can be recognised. These are not just physical, but emotional, mental and spiritual. The spiritual level is of great importance. Attention to spiritual health can be made by each individual in their own way and there are qualified spiritual teachers who can guide us along our spiritual path. Meditation, ritual, prayer and reading inspiring texts are of inestimable value in achieving increased awareness and moving to higher states of consciousness. One of the reasons why the Western world is so susceptible to mental and emotional anguish and agitation is the loss of contact with these deeper spiritual levels.

Amongst holistic practitioners, the important things to consider in relation to health and disease are the physical, emotional and mental levels. I will consider each in turn and then as a whole to develop a model that we can use to understand disease, its severity and monitor response to treatment. These levels can be ordered into a hierarchy of importance. This can help in assessing the severity of disease, since an imbalance at the deepest level generally indicates more severe disease.

The narrow view of conventional medicine sees health as an absence of symptoms.[5] Whilst it is true that symptoms are a limitation of our function, I prefer to use a more positive definition. I would define health as freedom from limitation of activity. On the physical level, health means no restriction of physical activity. On the emotional level it means the person is happy and well balanced. On the mental level it means that thoughts are clear and awareness is unrestricted. This is clearly a state of perfection but the point is that it is something to aim for. It is a direction, path or process rather than something to be ultimately attained. For example, on the physical level, there are restrictions placed on us by the nature of physical matter and the inescapable fact that our physical body will not last forever.[6]

It is clearly possible for people to achieve more freedom on many levels through medical treatment. This is a laudable aim in itself but we may also consider what we can do with that freedom. Traditionally, it is considered most auspicious to benefit others and to gain greater degrees of self-realisation and self-development. This is the essence of Chinese medicine – that there is no separation between spiritual health and our health in this physical body in this lifetime. Dealing with innermost levels of the spirit, thought and emotions leads to health, attending to the root allows everything to fall into its natural place. This is why in the East mental and emotional levels are given much more weight than the physical. It is only in the West that physical matters assume overwhelming importance.

SYMPTOMS

These may be defined as manifestations of ill health that are reported by the person or observed by the practitioner. Conventionally there is a separation into symptoms that are reported by the person (subjective) and signs that are observed by the doctor (objective). For the purposes of this book I include every manifestation in the term 'symptoms'.

In conventional medicine, symptoms are a manifestation of a physical problem. This may be at a cellular or biochemical level but nevertheless is physical. For the holistic practitioner, a symptom is a manifestation of an imbalance of energy. Depending on the tradition this energy may be referred to as *Qi* (pronounced *chi*), *Ki, Prana,* the vital force but all these terms refer to one and the same thing. Disturbance on this energetic level precedes all symptoms and symptoms often exist before physical changes become manifest.

Symptoms can be differentiated according to the level[7] at which they appear – physical, emotional or mental. By manifestation, I mean at which level in the person does the imbalance appear? I am not referring here to the cause. For example, if a person suffers a bereavement, which could be said to be an emotional factor, the result may be pneumonia (physical) or grief (emotional) or confusion (mental). The particular susceptibility of that person and the strength of their energy determine the level at which the imbalance manifests. The weaker or more imbalanced our energy, then the deeper will the symptom manifest. This is why disease in the West is more serious since our energies are more disturbed at deeper levels.[8]

Symptoms, therefore, mean different things to different practitioners. Conventional doctors see symptoms as being caused by a disease – an inherently existent entity that can be discovered by the doctor. Removal of the disease leads to cessation of the symptoms. The emphasis is on the physical nature of disease and symptoms. They are considered to be negative, unpleasant and to be removed if health is to be achieved. Health is the absence of symptoms and this is a conventional practitioner's definition of cure.[9]

In holistic medicine, symptoms are the result of an internal imbalance. The symptoms are a direct manifestation of the inner energetic state.[10] They point directly to the state of Qi[11] and Blood as understood by Chinese medicine. The holistic practitioner views symptoms as positive and helpful. They are pointing to the inner imbalance and are an opportunity for self-awareness and to regain balance.

In any situation, homeostatic mechanisms try to maintain health – otherwise we would all die from an acute illness such as the common cold or influenza. Symptoms are the body's best attempt at self-healing. They are only severe and deep when there is no other option. If the symptom is removed without balancing the inner energetic disharmony it leads to further imbalance of Qi and Blood. If the symptoms disappear because they were not allowed to be expressed then the energetic imbalance has been suppressed either to a deeper physical level, to the emotional or to the mental level.[12] This is the concept of suppression. This is potentially extremely dangerous and is one of the reasons why conventional medical treatment is often followed by other, more severe disease. Conventionally, these are either seen as unrelated episodes of ill health or called side-effects. From an energetic viewpoint they are the direct results of suppressive treatment.

If the symptoms disappear because the energetic imbalance has been rectified then true cure is the result. This is the aim of holistic methods of treatment. The holistic practitioner views symptoms as positive and helpful. They point to the inner imbalance and provide an opportunity to regain balance and develop greater self-awareness.

You can see why these two contrasting philosophies have such a potential for conflict. If conventional medicine tends to be suppressive and holistic medicine tends to be curative, it is difficult for them to work together to any great extent. They are doing opposite things. Holistic medicine is moving in one direction and conventional medicine is moving in the other – Table 2.1.

Holistic medicine	Conventional medicine
Energetic	Physical
All levels considered	Emphasises physical
Chronic illness but also helpful in acute disease	Crisis intervention, life-threatening situations
Holistic	Separatist
Connectedness	Disconnectedness
Transformative	Eliminative
Labour intensive, natural remedies	Relies on chemicals, technology
Curative	Suppressive
Gives responsibility to the person	Gives responsibility to the disease (and to the doctor)
Not state supported (UK)	State supported
Cheap (distorted by the fact that state support unavailable)	Expensive – in the UK there is often a misunderstanding that health care is free
Disease is merely a term given to a group of symptoms	Disease is an independently existent entity
Disease will change if symptoms change	Disease is fixed state – you have it or you do not
Symptoms – result of energetic imbalance	Symptoms caused by disease
Symptoms – useful, positive, force for change	Symptoms to be got rid of, unpleasant, negative
Health is balanced energies, freedom from limitation	Health is absence of symptoms
Cure is balance of former energetic disharmony	Cure is removal of symptoms

Table 2.1: Comparison of holistic and conventional medical philosophies

Table 2.1 is a comparison of philosophies not practitioners. In the end, the practice of medicine depends upon the view of the practitioner. I know some conventional practitioners whose practice is more in tune with the terms on the left. Some holistic practitioners practice 'conventionally'. It depends as much on how medicine is practiced as the method of practice.

Physical Level

This is the outermost layer of existence and is the one most easily seen. It corresponds to those parts that we can see, touch and perceive with our physical senses. The organs and structures of this level can be ordered according to a hierarchy, i.e. some organs are relatively superficial and some are relatively deep. The organs that are more essential for life are more internal. These tend to be single organs or those with important functions such as the heart, liver and kidneys – Table 2.2.

In Table 2.2, more superficial organs are at the top and the deeper organs at the bottom. If pathology manifests at a particular level, it is possible to reach a conclusion as to its severity. Disease of the heart is clearly more serious than disease of the large intestine; and disease of the stomach is not as serious as disease of the liver. This is usually true although it is also important to take into account each individual symptom picture. Short duration, acute disease is more superficial than long-lasting chronic disease although the acute nature of the symptoms may, in themselves, be hazardous. This distinction between acute and chronic disease is important because they have different meanings regarding the person's energy.

Table 2.3 corresponds to ideas in Chinese medicine that are known as the six stages. Each stage corresponds to a particular organ or organs. Although it is usually used to explain the passage of acute pathogenic influences into the body, there is value in using this with chronic conditions.

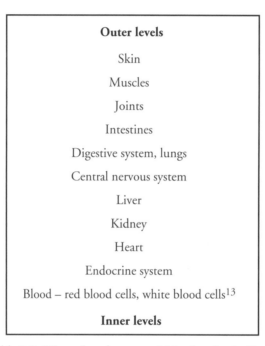

Outer levels

Skin

Muscles

Joints

Intestines

Digestive system, lungs

Central nervous system

Liver

Kidney

Heart

Endocrine system

Blood – red blood cells, white blood cells[13]

Inner levels

Table 2.2: Hierarchy of organs within the physical level

Level[14]	Organs[15]
Taiyang	Exterior level of body, Urinary Bladder, Small Intestine
Yangming	Stomach, Large Intestine
Shaoyang	Gall Bladder, San Jiao – half interior / half exterior
Taiyin	Lung, Spleen – now disease is internal in nature
Shaoyin	Kidney, Heart
Jueyin	Pericardium, Liver

Table 2.3: The six stages of disease according to principles of Chinese medicine

Acute disease may be defined as a disease of rapid onset, short duration that ends in recovery or death and usually has strong symptoms. People who have an acute disease know they are ill! It is clear-cut and indicates that the person is of relatively strong energy. For an acute manifestation to take place there must be strong energy in the system. This is why children tend to have acute illnesses. Subsequently, if the person's energy is somewhat weaker, a chronic illness may result.

Chronic disease can be defined as a disease of slow onset, long duration that ends in gradual deterioration of health. The symptoms are less pronounced than those of an acute disease. This indicates that the person's energy is weaker. This can create difficulties in diagnosis as symptoms may be mild or vague, e.g. elderly people with bronchopneumonia may have a mild or entirely absent cough with no fever. They may only present with breathlessness or perhaps confusion. Chronic disease is generally inexorable in its progress. There are some cases where people recover, perhaps because the cause has subsided or their lifestyle has altered. Treatment needs to be by means of a holistic, energy-based medicine in order for improvement to be lasting and truly curative – see Page13 re: cure, healing and placebo effect.

Superficial, relatively less severe disease

Acute childhood illnesses of measles, mumps, chickenpox, rubella

Common cold

Influenza

Acute upper respiratory tract infections

Tonsillitis

Eczema, psoriasis

Irritable bowel syndrome

Diverticulitis

Ulcerative colitis

Crohn's disease

Asthma

Chronic bronchitis, emphysema

Myalgic encephalomyelitis

Tuberculosis

Sarcoidosis

Cancer

Acquired immune deficiency syndrome

Internal, relatively more severe disease

Table 2.4: Hierarchy of disease according to principles of holistic medicine

There are diseases that do not fit easily into either category and these are the acute manifestations of a chronic illness. Virtually all acute disease is a manifestation of a chronic imbalance and only treating the acute manifestation leads to a worsening of the chronic condition – see suppression on Page13. There are some diseases that are clearly acute in nature, and these are the childhood infectious diseases.

By combining ideas of acute or chronic disease with those of levels it is possible to list diseases according to how deeply they affect the person – Table 2.4. It is important to be aware that conventional medical labels are fixed entities and I have used them as they are *generally* understood. When faced with an individual, we must decide in each case the symptoms presenting rather than the precise name given to them by conventional medicine. The infectious disease listed in Table 2.4 should be considered together with the discussions in Chapter 5 about the nature of infection according to principles of holistic medicine – see Page 46.

The position of a disease in Table 2.4 depends upon the acuteness of the disease and the organ involved. Cancer is at the bottom since it is a serious degenerative condition whilst tonsillitis is placed near the top since it is an acute condition (albeit usually the result of a chronic imbalance). All disease can be considered in this way. This I do throughout the book to give a clear idea as to what is serious, what is not and how to recognise improvement and worsening.

Emotional Level

This is the next level inward and is to do with feeling, emotion or to use the technical word, affect. Mild disturbances on this level manifest as mild irritability or anxiety. More severe imbalance shows as depression and the most severe symptoms are suicidal depression and complete absence of feeling – Table 2.5. The emotional level is discussed in detail in Chapter 16 – Psychological disorders.

Superficial, mild disturbances
Irritability
Anxiety
Sadness
Fear
Depression
Homicidal feelings
Suicidal feelings
Complete absence of feeling
Deep, severe disturbances

Table 2.5: Summary of emotional states listed according to depth

Mental Level

This is even deeper into the person and is the most difficult to see and treat. It is to do with thought and perception – cognition is the technical term. Mild abnormalities may be revealed as lack of concentration or poor memory whilst the most severe appear as hallucinations, confusion or complete disintegration of the personality – Table 2.6. The mental level is discussed in detail in Chapter 16 – Psychological disorders.

Superficial, mild disturbance
Lack of concentration
Poor memory
Thought disorders
Hallucinations
Delusions
Confusion
Disintegration of the personality as in some cases of schizophrenia
Deep, more severe disturbance

Table 2.6: Summary of mental states listed according to depth

Integration of Mental, Emotional and Physical Levels

In an individual person, these three levels are interconnected and you see symptoms on all levels. The main point for the practitioner is to ask, 'Where is the emphasis of the pathology? Where is the main manifestation of the imbalance?' If this is on the physical level it is labelled a physical disease, an emotional disease if on the emotional level, and a mental disease if on the mental level. This explains the common observation that schizophrenics have a much lower rate of cancer than the general population. If most of the energy is focused on the mental level there is not enough to manifest symptoms on the physical. People with cancer tend not to suffer from acute problems such as the common cold or allergic reactions. The pathology is too deep into the physical level for these to occur.

Another aspect to consider is that symptoms change according to the energetic state of the person. In conventional medicine, diseases are perceived as being discrete, fixed entities. In reality the situation is fluid and dynamic. It is important not just to consider the present state but also what preceded this condition. In this way a complete picture may be built up of the person's state of health. Table 2.7 illustrates a person's medical history revealing disease states over a number of years.

Age	Symptoms/disease
6 months	Eczema
2 years	Whooping cough
5 years	Mucus in the middle ear, partial deafness, bowel problems
12 years	Recurrent tonsillitis
19 years	Depression
22 years	Hay fever
25 years	Inflammatory bowel disease diagnosed as ulcerative colitis
35 years	Episodes of indigestion diagnosed as duodenal ulcer
55 years	Onset of tremor, stiffness and rigidity – Parkinson's disease

Table 2.7: Past medical history of a person revealing interconnections of levels

Table 2.7 may seem to illustrate a particularly unfortunate history, but it is in fact a common experience. The main factor determining the next event is whether the treatment given at the time is curative, i.e. the pathology moves to the exterior, or suppressive, i.e. the pathology moves to the inside. Conventional medicine tends to be suppressive since it does not address the underlying energetic imbalance.

When a person with eczema is given corticosteroid creams the rash may well disappear. Some months later a deeper problem, such as asthma, may appear. To a conventional doctor, trained to see people as a collection of separate parts, this is perceived as 'cure' of the eczema and the appearance of asthma. Drugs are given which suppress the asthma and may lead to deeper symptoms perhaps on the mental or emotional levels.

In terms of holistic medicine the pathology is passing into the deeper levels of the person. The person is now more ill than they were previously. Treatment with holistic medicine tends to move the pathology out of the body and treatment of the asthma may lead to reappearance of the eczema. If the eczema is treated appropriately and disappears, this can truly be called cure. The internal levels are balanced and the symptoms have resolved.[16]

Not all people, who have conventional treatment, however, seem to develop a disease worse than the original. It may be useful to discuss the possible consequences of treatment – Table 2.8.

Practitioners are faced with the challenge of deciding why symptoms have disappeared. Was it due to cure or to suppression? With cure, inner levels clear first, as the emphasis of the energetic imbalance moves out of the person. People who receive treatment with holistic medicine report improved energy and feeling better in themselves with improved mental and emotional states before changes in the physical level. In the short term (hours or days) their presenting symptoms may get worse since the treatment is increasing their energy levels. The strength of symptoms is directly related to the strength of the person's energy. Also symptoms that originated on deeper levels (mental or emotional) may move to a more superficial (physical) level. In holistic medicine aggravation is followed by amelioration.

Effect on symptoms	Interpretation
No change	No effect by treatment
Worsen	1. Treatment is curative – short-term aggravation[17] 2. No effect by treatment, condition is worsening 3. Treatment is making the condition worse
Improvement	1. Cure (a) Appropriate treatment – individualised energetic remedy (b) 'Placebo' effect – healing (c) Would have improved anyway – natural movement towards cure or removal of exciting cause 2. Suppression – inappropriate treatment. Superficially may look like an improvement.

Table 2.8: Interpretation of the effect of treatment on symptoms

Suppressive treatment also means that the symptoms disappear but the key here is that internal levels are more disordered. The person may feel tired, lethargic, depressed or anxious and symptoms may now be present on deeper physical levels. This is common after antibiotic treatment. The person has a sore throat, for example, and the administration of antibiotics leads to disappearance of the main complaint. Now the person may complain of tiredness, depression, diarrhoea, 'thrush' symptoms and so on. The problem has been suppressed into the interior. In conventional medicine there is amelioration followed by aggravation.

A practitioner can attain cure in two ways. The first is the application of the appropriate energetic remedy that must be given according to the principles of the therapy practiced. In terms of Chinese medicine this is by diagnosing the condition of the Qi and Blood and treating to balance these two substances. In terms of homoeopathic medicine where 'like is cured by like ' it is by deciding upon the simillimum – the most similar remedy.

The energetic remedy is the key. Conventional medicine may occasionally give the appropriate energetic remedy and examples of this would be the use of platinum[18] for ovarian tumours, digitalis[19] for heart failure, carbenoxolone[20] for peptic ulcers, aspirin[21] for acute fevers. There are very few other examples and the refining of substances together with the administration of large doses leads to toxicity. In Chinese medicine and homoeopathy these substances are used as the result of careful observation, enquiry and the application of a self-consistent theoretical base. In conventional medicine they are used as the result of chance.

I have put 'placebo' effect and healing together because they are essentially the same phenomena. The term placebo is used pejoratively by the medical profession today but it has a long and honourable history. The word[22] is generally applied to a substance that has no known (conventional) medical effect. It has always been known that the mere suggestion that something has healing powers is enough to lead to health in some cases and in some people. The power of placebo is increased by ritual, suggestion and by the perceived ability of the person giving the placebo. Do not underestimate the power of placebo in conventional medicine. This is the reason most heart tablets are red and tranquillisers are green or blue – they are more effective. The ability of doctors to suggest that people can and will get better is known to be a powerful factor in recovery. It may not be much to do with the treatment but with the relationship people have with the doctor. This is true healing and is very effective. People get better *despite* the treatment they receive rather than *because* of it. Many conventional treatments have no proven efficacy or are effective for no known reason. The power of a doctor to heal is an important factor to be considered particularly where strong faith is present.

Of course, this power may have a negative effect when people are told they have no hope, e.g. people with multiple sclerosis may be told that they have a degenerative condition which will lead in a short time to inability to walk and reliance on a wheelchair. Such statements, made by someone in authority, can often act as a highly destructive self-fulfilling prophesy even in people with no disease.

As to suppression, it is possible to do this by any method of treatment. It is commonly stated that holistic medicine is safe and cannot do harm. This is not true and it is possible to suppress disease and symptoms by means of Chinese medicine, homoeopathy and so on. It is not easy and suggests a failure to reach a correct interpretation and treatment. The most powerful suppressant today is conventional medicine, however, and causes many difficulties for holistic practitioners. This, combined with pollution of water, air, food and increased levels of stress and worry are responsible for the increasing rates of chronic disease. The hope for the future is to offer people a holistic to heavily suppressive forms of treatment with information about how to live as healthy a life as possible.

HOW TO RECOGNISE SERIOUS SYMPTOMS

A recurring concern for all practitioners is how to recognise a situation that is serious or life-threatening. For holistic practitioners, this may lead to an undue reliance on conventional sources of help such as investigations or referral to a conventional practitioner. However, in most cases, it is possible to determine clinically which symptoms indicate 'serious' disease[23]? What is serious in conventional medicine is serious in holistic medicine – after all the person is the same! Anyone can understand illness based upon an understanding of symptoms and symptom pictures. It is not necessary for a conventional medical diagnosis to be made.

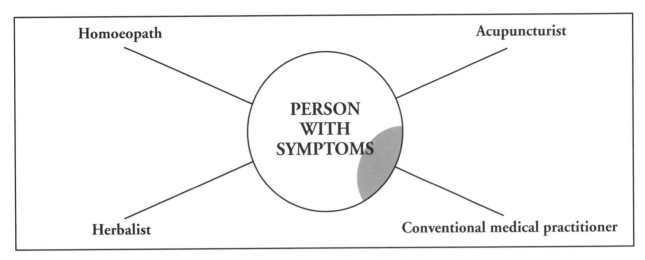

Figure 2.1: Practitioners and their view of the person

Figure 2.1 is a diagrammatic representation of how different practitioners view the same person. Conventional practitioners tend not to see the whole person – they only see the physical. This is why conventional medical terms are relatively restrictive and cannot be directly translated into the terms used by holistic practitioners. There is some correlation but they are not the same things. Holistic practitioners make their own analysis of the case and treatment in the context of their particular therapy since that, by definition, encompasses the whole person. It is important, in addition, to be able to recognise symptoms indicating a serious situation. Some people need closer observation or they may require emergency treatment. It is possible to determine this by close attention to the person and their symptoms.

The seriousness of a symptom is dependent upon the degree of limitation of the person's activity or functioning. If health can be defined as freedom from limitation then disease or a symptom is a limiting factor.

The indicators of a serious situation would be:

- severe symptom
- life-threatening situation (the ultimate limitation in this life being death)
- moving into deeper levels – either physical or into the emotional/mental levels
- acute – this indicates sudden change
- progressive – more symptoms appearing indicating a worsening situation.

Throughout this book I summarise the symptoms that indicate serious situations. A summary is included at the end of each Chapter.

CONVENTIONAL RESEARCH

There is an emphasis in conventional medicine on gathering information and trying to decide if certain treatments are effective or not. The criteria for effectiveness are those I have already discussed, namely, removal of the primary physical symptom. The placebo response has always been recognised as having great power yet conventional medicine seeks to negate or neutralise it in order to determine the 'real' action of the medicine or treatment applied. This is an attempt to discover objective truth by removing the subjective element.

The gold standard of conventional research is the 'controlled clinical trial' (CCT) or 'randomised clinical trial (RCT)[24] which has been in increasingly common use since the 1960s. Prior to that time, the effectiveness of treatments was mainly determined by recommendations from a small number of doctors. In controlled clinical trials neither the person nor the doctor knows whether a 'real' or a 'sham' treatment is being applied. For example, if a drug is being studied, some people will be given the drug and others will be given tablets containing no active substance. In this way, differences in the outcome of the two groups can be attributed to the effects of the drug.

The basic problem of such trials begins with trying to define a particular illness. There are so many variations within 'normal' and these variations become even more numerous when people start to develop symptoms. It is notoriously difficult for conventional doctors to agree on definitions of disease let alone agreeing on what is an effective treatment. This is not a fault of the medical profession but rather it is a natural function of the complexity of human beings and their individuality. It is nigh impossible to catergorise people into rational and easily definable groups. There are general comments that can be made, of course, but any 'generalisation' must ignore significant aspects of the rich variety of human experience. If it is difficult to define a disease clearly, how much more difficult is it to state whether a particular treatment is effective or not? Yet, this is what controlled clinical trials seek to do.

In such a trial, people are allocated to treatment groups and to test groups (control groups) that receive no active treatment. It is intended that such groups are homogenous, in that they have sufficient similarity to enable conclusions to be drawn about the effectiveness or otherwise of the treatment. Human beings though are not homogenous. It is one of the most basic observations, that humans are remarkably diverse. It is impossible to gather together a sufficiently homogenous group to enable such trials to be meaningful. One key example is the previous medical history. One would think that this would be of over-riding importance when considering individual variation. However, no clinical trial has ever considered the importance of prior medical history!

The whole *raison d'etre* of controlled clinical trials is to use groups of people who are representative of the population as a whole. This is both philosophically and practically impossible. In addition, the results will be further tainted by the particular bias of the statistician conducting the survey. I am reminded of when I was teaching a group of students about infertility. I made the statement that it is well known that when a couple go on holiday or adopt a child, they can become pregnant. A student took me to task saying that a clinical trial had determined that this did not in fact occur. It was merely a chance occurrence and there was no connection between the two events. The point here is that although a particular group may lead a statistician to a certain conclusion this does not in any way negate the experience of the individual.

Is it possible for the subjective element to be removed completely? Perhaps the outcome of the trial can be affected merely by mental attitude. A consultant rheumatologist I know was always being asked to perform clinical trials for new anti-arthritis medication but became interested in acupuncture for the treatment of arthritis. His senior registrar was in charge of the day-to-day conduct of the drug trials and many pieces of research were done. As the consultant became more and more involved in acupuncture, he became more and more disillusioned with the efficacy of the conventional medication. The results of the trials became less and less favourable for the drugs until eventually the pharmaceutical companies stopped using his unit for research. It was as if his mental attitude were affecting the trials even though he was not personally involved in them.

It is not possible to eliminate subjective truth and detach it from objective truth. Yin and Yang are inseparable. This only occurs at death. There must be both aspects in life to achieve movement. For holistic medicine, it means that these conventional methods of research are of little help since the subjective element is the very factor we aim to utilise in our treatments. It is the unseen, the vitalistic principle[25] that pervades us all. It is possible to analyse cases and treatments people have received but double blind trials[26] are not applicable.

It is our view that changes results. We create our own reality and this is the essence of treatment. How can people change their mind so that they change their symptom picture? If we believe something to be true, it becomes true and this principle is behind methods of visualisation and meditation used in spiritual practice and medical treatments.[27]

Sadly, the search for more information in conventional medicine may lead to practices that may not be helpful or beneficial. If the person does not know whether they are receiving treatment or not, this does not allow them to make a decision based on information. The principle of informed consent is an essential part of medical practice. Everyone must decide for themselves whether to accept a particular form of treatment and this process is particularly hazardous if they lack information about that treatment.

Animal experimentation is all too often used in conventional medical research. In my opinion this is unethical since it involves inducing suffering to a sentient being. There has never been a case of a medical advance that has resulted from the use of animals and I would hope that the practice will soon cease. Unfortunately, some groups in holistic medicine such as research carried out in China with regard to acupuncture and herbs, use animals in their experiments. As concerned practitioners, it is important to consider these aspects and oppose them. It is our responsibility to relieve suffering, not to inflict it.

DOCTORS AND PATIENTS

It is not my intention to increase conflict between a patient and their conventional medical advisor. In my dealings with people, I try not to place them in the middle of a philosophical discussion between conventional and holistic medicine. As holistic practitioners, we definitely have a role to play in giving people information[28] about medical procedures and treatments. The information in this book will help you do this.

The following advice may be useful for anyone who has dealings with conventional practitioners[29]:

- go with a friend or advocate who can support you – never go alone.
- ask about effects, side-effects and other options available.
- ask why a particular investigation is being performed and how the information will be used.
- remember that your body is your property and no one has the right to do anything without your full, informed consent.
- search out other choices particularly if holistic in their view.
- whatever you decide – be happy!
- seek out sympathetic sources of conventional advice. There are some doctors now who are moving over to holistic views and can offer support and help to people searching for treatment appropriate to their needs.

SUMMARY

Conventional medicine only sees the physical and applies physical treatments.

Holistic medicine is vitalistic in nature and accepts the existence of energies.

Treatment needs to encompass all levels of the individual to ensure cure.

Treatment of only the outer, physical level may lead to suppression and the appearance of more serious disease later.

Symptoms manifest strongly as an acute picture in those with strong energy. They tend to be in less important organs and relatively superficial.

Symptoms manifest weakly as a chronic picture in those with weak energy. They tend to be in more important organs and relatively deep.

The most important things to remember are:

- where is the pathology – at which level?
- where is it going – into the interior or to the exterior?
- is the condition worsening or improving?

---

[1] Yang, in Chinese medicine, is applied to aspects which are active, going upwards and outward, external, hot, masculine, intellectual and so forth. Yin, in Chinese medicine, is applied to aspects which are passive, going downwards and inwards, internal, cold, feminine, intuitive and so forth.

[2] *The Tao of Physics* by Fritjof Capra (Flamingo, 1992), *The Turning Point* by Fritjof Capra (Flamingo, 1983).

[3] Throughout this book I make reference to the term 'holistic medicine'. I know that this is used in many situations to mean widely differing things. When I use this term I am referring primarily to the philosophical views as espoused by Chinese medicine and homoeopathy. They are exceedingly similar in their beliefs despite differences in use of language.

[4] Vitalism is the term which is applied to energetic systems of thought. Its use indicates that there are existent objects which are non-physical in part or whole.

[5] It is difficult to find a formal definition of health which is used by conventional medicine. There is a significant absence of such terms in medical dictionaries. However, in general usage a person would be considered healthy if they had no symptoms.

[6] From the time of conception we are ageing which leads to our eventual death so there is only so much that is achievable with our physical bodies. There is a completely different situation with our mental and emotional health and there are no limitations to the states we can achieve with motivation and the use of meditation and other techniques to purify the mind. This is the realm of spiritual teachers and teachings but it is clear that our health on a mundane level cannot be separated from our health on a spiritual level.

[7] An excellent account of holistic medicine principles, in this case homoeopathy, and theories of levels can be found in *The Science of Homoeopathy* by George Vithoulkas (Grove, 1980).

[8] Chronic degenerative disease is more common in the West as our immune systems become weaker. There are real increases each year in the incidence of diseases such as cancer, heart disease, stroke and so forth. According to the US National Cancer Institute, the incidence of cancer has risen by 11 per cent in the last 40 years. In traditional cultures disease manifests more superficially. This changes as 'civilisation' develops. Homoeopaths use more remedies now which are indicated to treat mental and emotional disease than were used in the last century. Disease has passed into the interior.

[9] The World Health Organisation definition of health is somewhat more positive – 'Health is a state of complete physical, mental and social well-being and not merely the absence of disease or infirmity.'

[10] It may be helpful to consider symptoms as metaphors. Why does a person place a certain pathology in a particular place? What is the meaning of symptoms? For example, the person who is 'pissed off' may get cystitis, the person who has too much of a load to bear may get back pain, the person with a difficult relationship may get a pain in the neck. I shall explore such ideas as I discuss disease states in this book.

[11] Qi in Chinese medicine is difficult to translate but corresponds to vital force or energy of the Western vitalistic tradition of homoeopathy.

[12] *The Chronic Diseases* by Samuel Hahnemann (Homoeopathic Book Service, 1998) contains many accounts of the results of suppressive treatment.

[13] In conventional medicine, this level is to do with immune system components of antibodies and white blood cells. I use the term immune system throughout this book in a wider sense to include all levels from the most superficial energetic layers to the deepest internal organs. Conventional medicine manipulates the blood by means of corticosteroids which reduce lymphocyte levels and cancer chemotherapy which reduces numbers of all cells in the blood. Vaccination is another procedure which markedly affects blood and the immune system.

[14] These terms refer to the stages of Yin and Yang in the body. I mention them here to allow a connection to be made with books on Chinese medical theory.

[15] The names of organs here refer to organ systems as they are understood by Chinese medicine. They include energetic functions and are not the merely physical organs of conventional medicine. By common usage these are always referred to by using an initial capital letter. For example, the spleen in conventional medicine is an organ of the lymphatic system which has a function in red blood cell destruction and the manufacture of lymphocytes. By contrast, the Spleen of Chinese medicine is concerned with transformation and transportation of food amongst other functions.

[16] This is one of the basic tenets of Hering's Law of Cure as stated in homoeopathic philosophy. Cure is the movement of pathology from inside to out, from above to down, from most important organs to least important and symptoms disappear in reverse order of their appearance.

[17] An aggravation is a short-lasting exacerbation of the presenting symptoms. It is due to a resonance between the energy of the person and the energy of the applied treatment. It can be recognised by its short duration (hours or days) and the clearing of internal levels first to be followed by improvement of the physical. It is distinguished from a 'healing crisis' which occurs during the course of treatment. This takes place when the person's energy is strong enough to throw out more symptoms. A healing crisis, particularly in the case of serious disease such as cancer, can be difficult to distinguish from a worsening of the illness. Again you have to pay attention to inner levels and assess according to the treatment applied and its results over a length of time.

[18] Platina is the homoeopathic remedy derived from platinum. Tumours of the ovary are included in the *Materia Medica* entry of platina.

[19] Digitalis was originally extracted from foxglove which is a herbal remedy for dropsy (heart failure).

[20] A derivative of licorice which strengthens Stomach energy and is commonly used in herbalism.

[21] Originally extracted from willow bark, this has the effect of relieving acute fevers by releasing the exterior energy of the body and causing a sweat. Its energy is warm and dispersing in nature.

[22] The root is the Latin, 'I please'.

[23] 'Serious' in this context indicates a situation which is potentially life-threatening. This may due to the immediate situation or a progressive underlying process. This latter case would include cancer.

[24] See *The Controlled Clinical Trial: An Analysis* by Harris L Coulter (Centre for Empirical Medicine and Project Cure, 1991). This is a clear and comprehensive critique of their usefulness and is especially relevant to the needs of holistic practitioners who are increasingly under pressure to 'prove' that their treatments are effective.

[25] *The Presence of the Past: Morphic Resonance and the Habits of Nature* by Rupert Sheldrake (Inner Traditions International, 1998). The vitalistic principle here is called morphic resonance by Sheldrake. It explains the observation that if a rat in one part of the world learns how to get through a maze then very soon all the rats in the world, despite no physical connection with this rat, will know how to get through the same maze. There is an energetic field effect behind the physical events and this explains how connections can occur and effects experienced without any physical contact.

[26] Some people receive no treatment although they do not know this. As a practitioner, I feel it is unethical to provide no treatment to people when I have skills and information which may be helpful. I often think that such trials are for the benefit of the researcher rather than the person.

[27] These are outlined in Chapter 6 with regard to holistic treatments of cancer.

[28] *How To Survive Medical Treatment* by Stephen Fulder (C.W. Daniel, 1995) is an excellent account of the issues around people receiving conventional treatment.

[29] It is wise to check out all practitioners and in the end it is the practitioner we have to feel comfortable with, whether they are holistic or conventional.

3 PATHOLOGICAL PROCESSES

INTRODUCTION

Clinical medicine, of whatever tradition, can be understood by considering symptoms. In conventional medicine there is an increasing understanding of pathological changes that are considered to either underlie or cause disease. There is a reliance on physical processes and the investigations described in Chapter 4 have the intention of discovering their nature. The implicit tenet of conventional thought is that physical abnormality is the cause of disease. In those diseases where an abnormality is absent or difficult to find such as schizophrenia, anxiety or depression the assumption is that one day a physical cause will be discovered.

In conventional medicine the process of inflammation is of primary importance, since it is seen as the basis of many diseases. Other processes include thrombosis, embolism, haemorrhage and the demyelination of nervous tissue. I shall deal only with those that are clinically important.

INFLAMMATION

Inflammation is the result of a wide range of different causative factors yet these factors tend to be ignored. In clinical medicine the approach is that the inflammation itself has to be treated.

The key symptoms of inflammation are:
- redness
- swelling
- pain
- heat
- loss of function.

These are the result of an increased local blood supply providing nutrients and immunological defences in the affected area. Inflammation is a natural response of the body and is the first stage of tissue healing. Suppression of inflammation is often harmful. There are many commonly used drugs that suppress. These include antibiotics, anti-inflammatory agents, corticosteroids and anti-histamines.

The labelling of disease reflects the emphasis on inflammation. The suffix '-itis' indicates that inflammation is present. The majority of conventional disease labels can be seen to be inflammatory – for example tonsillitis, gastritis, vaginitis, bronchitis, colitis, dermatitis. The Latin term for an organ is attached to the -itis to form a label – they are merely descriptive terms. People are reassured by such diagnoses although they are merely labels used to describe the symptoms of the person.

Inflammation has several causes according to conventional medicine – Figure 3.1.

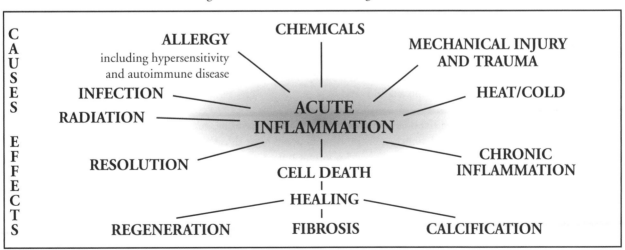

Figure 3.1: Causes and effects of inflammation

Figure 3.1 shows that damage to the cell results in acute inflammation. The causes of cell damage are recognised by conventional medicine as being physical in nature. There is no room for mental or emotional factors. Anyone who has a child will know that psychological factors are a potent producer of fevers and inflammation. This observation is more easily made in children due to their strong energy and its tendency to flare up into heat. I remember one occasion when my son was disturbed at the thought of having to eat something he did not like. Within a few minutes he was hot, flushed and feverish. On being told that he did not have to eat the offending item he settled down and the fever disappeared as rapidly as it had appeared. This was a graphic illustration of the effect of emotional factors and the speed with which symptoms may change.

In general, the causes of inflammation can be divided into two types – those due to infection and those not due to infection. Inflammation due to infection is treated with antibiotics or other drugs to combat organisms. People may also be given antibiotics frequently for inflammation because an infective cause is assumed. In situations not associated with infection, anti-inflammatory drugs of varying kinds will be prescribed. These vary from fairly simple remedies such as aspirin through to powerful drugs such as corticosteroids. The underlying aim is the same – to reduce inflammation.

This practice is potentially harmful as inflammation serves a protective function – as indeed does all symptoms. Removal of the inflammation leads to a worsened state since the original cause is allowed to continue unhindered. This is why problems develop after a suppressed inflammation.

In conventional medicine it is realised that the use of corticosteroids in inflammation associated with infection is harmful. Removal or reduction of the inflammation leads to rapid spread of infection.

The appropriate way to deal with inflammation is to consider the total picture including any exciting or maintaining cause. Then, and only then, deal with the totality. This may mean that an emergency treatment has to be used in occasional life-threatening situations with severe inflammation. However, to treat the vast majority of minor inflammatory symptoms with powerful anti-inflammatory drugs, and antibiotics are included in this category, is not only excessive but hazardous.

ATHEROMA

Atherosclerosis is the development of atheroma that builds up in layers on the interior of arteries and gradually obstructs the flow of blood. The main constituent of atheroma is cholesterol and theories have developed attempting to connect the intake of cholesterol with an increase of atherosclerosis. The American Heart Association say in their literature: 'Exactly how atheroslerosis begins or what causes it isn't known but some theories have been proposed'. Conventionally, it is believed that damage to the lining of the artery is followed by atherosclerosis. This damage, it is suggested, may be possibly caused by increased levels of cholesterol and triglycerides in the blood, high blood pressure and smoking tobacco.

The development of such deposits in arteries is clinically related in some people with ischaemic heart disease – angina pectoris and heart attack. However, there is not a consistent relationship between the development of atheroma and symptoms. Some people have arteries which are so blocked it is difficult to see how any blood reaches the heart yet have few or no symptoms. Others who have little obstruction by atheroma may have a severe heart attack. The key is the function of the heart and this is related to its energy not its structure. As a consequence, holistic medicine may produce improvements in symptoms despite apparently severe obstructive disease.

The factors leading to the development of atheroma are low physical activity, smoking, excessive intake of fatty food and emotional stress. The conventional response to raised cholesterol levels is to restrict fat in the diet and to prescribe drugs that lower these levels. This may not always be healthy and increased rates of cancer may be connected with over vigorous efforts to control cholesterol levels.[1] Cholesterol has had a bad press of late, yet is a vital precursor of many steroid hormones such as cortico*steroids*, oe*strogen*, proge*sterone*, testo*sterone* and so on. The connection is revealed by the similarity in names. Fat is also essential for the absorption of Vitamins A, D, E and K.

Cholesterol is manufactured in the liver and it is this organ that is responsible for high cholesterol levels as well as the digestive system in general. There is definitely a relationship between heart disease and the intake of refined carbohydrates[2] and merely to restrict fat intake is insufficient. Diet is important but so too are emotional states.[3] The best way of reducing cholesterol levels is to deal with reactions to stress and to strengthen the function of the liver and digestion. If the amount of fat in the diet is reduced and cholesterol-lowering drugs[4] given, there is a reduction in serum cholesterol for about 6-9 months and then it has a tendency to begin to rise again. In any event there is no evidence that changing cholesterol levels actually helps heart disease. The manufacturer of atorvastatin, a commonly used lipid-lowering agent, states: 'The effect of atorvastatin on cardiovascular mortality and morbidity has not been established.' In plain English this means that although this drug lowers cholesterol levels, it is not known what, if any, effect this has on disease.

In terms of Chinese medicine, raised cholesterol levels usually correspond to Phlegm in the Blood. It is important to consider particularly the function of the Spleen and the Blood and its related organs – Heart, Liver and Kidney.

Case one

A man aged 52 years came for treatment. He had a past history of a heart attack some 2 years earlier followed by heart bypass surgery. He subsequently had a deep venous thrombosis in his left leg from which the vein for the bypass had been removed. His main complaints were persistent pain and swelling in the left leg. At times the swelling was so severe that water would leak out. He worked in a stressful job with a lot of pressure and worry. His cholesterol level had originally been 9.7 mmol/1 (normal 3.5 – 6.5 mmol/1) and had reduced to 7.9 mmol/1 with drug treatment. He stopped drug treatment because he was not happy with the side-effects and his cholesterol increased to 9.4 mmol/1.

I treated him with acupuncture and herbs, which resulted in an improvement in his general mental and emotional state. He felt happier and calmer. His leg improved and the swelling reduced in size. He had little in the way of pain and started to practice Tai Chi exercises. His cholesterol level over a period of 4 months reduced to 4.7 mmol/1. His Chinese medical diagnosis was Kidney and Spleen Yang deficiency with Phlegm and Damp accumulation.

This case shows that one problem is frequently stacked on top of another until people have several conditions at the same time. The main issue here was his reaction to stressful and worrying work situations and there seems little point in treating the surface – the high cholesterol level – without paying any attention to deeper issues that were causing the levels to rise.

Atheroma is a generalised disease and some people present with heart problems whilst others may have cerebral symptoms or develop renal disease. Several manifestations may be seen in the same person. Once the arterial wall has been damaged by the deposition of atheroma, there may be consequences other than obstruction. These include thrombosis, embolism and haemorrhage. The main distinction between these processes is that the manifestations of atheroma and ischaemia are gradual whilst the others are sudden. Ischaemia, a gradual process, leads to syndromes such as angina pectoris, dementia, transient ischaemic attacks, renal damage and so forth. The sudden processes of thrombosis, haemorrhage and embolism lead to syndromes such as heart attack, 'stroke', pulmonary embolism, deep venous thrombosis and so forth.

HAEMORRHAGE

Haemorrhage is bleeding and may occur in different sites and due to different underlying conditions. It must always be taken seriously although by no means every situation is severe. There are five situations to consider:
- trauma (injury)
- inflammatory disease
- tumours
- degenerative processes
- disorders of clotting.

Injury is self-evident either from the appearance or the history. The treatment required will depend upon the severity of the injury. The more serious situations will have to be dealt with in hospital although there are holistic treatments available which can help to minimise further damage and aid recovery. In an ideal situation these should be employed along with conventional reparative techniques.

Inflammatory disease is the commonest situation in outpatient practice. Disorders such as acute bronchitis, ulcerative colitis, peptic ulceration and so forth may all be associated with bleeding. In these situations, the severity of the situation will be reflected by the amount of bleeding. If it were recurrent, persistent or severe then this would indicate a greater degree of seriousness. It is important in every situation to assess the symptom of bleeding together with the complete symptom picture.

Tumours may cause bleeding and are the thing that most people worry about. Once again, it is important to consider the symptom in the context of the complete clinical picture. If, for example, coughing of blood occurs on one occasion in a person of 20 years with an acute chest problem – cough, sputum of yellow colour and malaise – perhaps there is no need for worry. If however there is coughing of blood over several weeks in a 55-year-old man who smokes, this is a completely different situation and may require further investigation and consideration.

Degenerative processes that lead to haemorrhage are primarily to do with atherosclerosis. Arteries become weakened as the fat deposits build up in their walls. They may rupture and cause haemorrhage. The symptom picture will depend upon the organ affected. Stroke occurs if there is haemorrhage into the brain and this is a relatively common situation in the Western world.

Disorders of clotting are unusual and certainly so in clinics of holistic medicine. The two main causes of these are conventionally considered to be capillary damage and thrombocytopenia.

Capillary damage is the commonest situation and may be due to old age, vitamin C deficiency[5] and treatment with corticosteroids, penicillin and sulphonamide antibiotics.

Thrombocytopenia, a low platelet count, is uncommon. Some cases of thrombocytopenia remain a mystery conventionally and these are labelled idiopathic thrombocytopenic purpura. Others may be due to drugs of many kinds such as quinine, cancer chemotherapy, sulphonamide antibiotics, thiazide diuretics, corticosteroids and others. Bone marrow disease can interfere with platelet manufacture. Some people have antibodies to platelets and this is an example of autoimmune disease.

The conventional treatment of haemorrhage depends upon the cause, and the original disease will also be dealt with in the usual way. Thrombocytopenia is treated either with corticosteroids or by means of removal of the spleen – splenectomy. The spleen has various functions but one is to remove old platelets and red blood cells from the circulation. It follows that if the spleen is removed then the platelets present will survive for longer. The other function of the spleen is in the manufacture and maturation of lymphocytes and so splenectomy has a profound effect on the condition of the immune system. People become more susceptible to developing severe infections and may be given long-term antibiotic therapy, which further undermines their natural immunity.

In terms of Chinese medicine, bleeding may be due to Spleen Deficiency not Holding Blood, Heat leading to Reckless Blood or Stagnation of Blood.

THROMBOSIS

This is clotting. There are complex mechanisms in health to ensure there is balance so that neither extreme of haemorrhage nor thrombosis can occur. Various situations may lead to thrombosis in the blood vessels and some of these are discussed in relation to deep venous thrombosis. In the context of degenerative disease and atheroma, as the arteries become progressively more blocked clotting becomes more likely. This is due to several factors including reduced flow of blood, roughened arterial surface providing places for a clot to adhere to and alterations in the thickness of blood. This situation can lead to thrombosis in an artery and the clinical picture will reflect the site of the clot. If it occurs in the brain it leads to stroke, whilst in the heart it leads to heart attack.

EMBOLISM

An embolus is usually,[6] part of a clot, which detaches and circulates around the blood system. It becomes lodged in a small blood vessel and produces symptoms due to obstructed blood flow. The main clinical situations are stroke (where an embolus breaks off from perhaps an atheromatous carotid artery) or pulmonary embolism, which is secondary to a deep venous thrombosis. Emboli from systemic veins will become lodged in the lungs, whereas emboli from systemic arteries become lodged in the organs, e.g. brain, kidneys, or the extremities (see Figure 7.1 on Page 90).

OEDEMA

Oedema is excess fluid in the tissues and arises because fluid leaks out of the circulation. There are several mechanisms of oedema production in conventional thought.

Fluid is normally present in the intercellular spaces to provide nutrients to cells and remove waste products. When this is increased, oedema becomes evident. There are factors which allow fluid into these spaces and which drain it away. In health these are in balance.

The factors that allow fluid to escape from the circulation and enter the intercellular spaces are:
- arterial pressure greater than osmotic[7] pressure
- capillary permeability
- balance of sodium (extra cellular) and potassium (intracellular)
- volume of water in the body.

The factors that drain fluid away from the intercellular spaces are:
- osmotic pressure greater than venous pressure
- capillary permeability
- patency of veins and lymphatics.

These factors are summarised in Figure 3.2. Any changes in the relative balances of the factors mentioned above may lead to the collection of fluid around the cells.

Figure 3.2: Formation of intercellular fluid

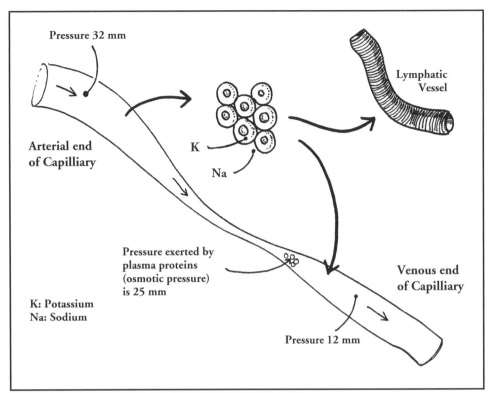

Causes of oedema

Increased capillary permeability

- Allergy – may be general or localised. If general then it tends to be in the upper part of body. There may be other symptoms of allergic reaction such as runny nose, sneezing, wheezing, diarrhoea, and urticaria.
- Inflammatory processes of any type.

Increased sodium levels in the extracellular spaces

- Dietary sodium in food or prescribed drugs, e.g. commonly available formulations of paracetamol and Vitamin C contain large amounts of sodium.
- Disturbed sodium–potassium balance in some kidney disorders.

Increased fluid volume

- Clinically, this is usually secondary to increased sodium levels.
- Retention of water due to kidney disease perhaps with scanty urination or no urine, e.g. nephritic syndrome causing oedema in the face.
- Hormonal imbalances leading to oedema related to changes in the menstrual cycle (e.g. fluid retention pre-menstrually or when taking oral contraception or hormone replacement therapy).

Decreased plasma osmotic pressure due to reduced protein in the blood

- Kidney diseases such as nephrotic syndrome or chronic glomerulonephritis lead to the loss of protein in urine. Such oedema tends to be generalised, worse in the morning and associated with urinary symptoms such as haematuria and loin pain.
- Liver disease interferes with the production of protein and so levels in the blood fall as a result. There will be abdominal distension, right hypochondriac pain, jaundice and possibly a history of drug or alcohol abuse.
- Malnutrition is an inadequate intake of protein. There will be other evidence of inadequate nutrition such as muscle wasting and a distended abdomen.
- Malabsorption is a disturbance of absorption despite normal diet and metabolic activity. Diseases of this type include coeliac disease.

Reduced flow in lymphatic and venous systems

- Venous blockage due to thrombosis or a tumour will tend to give rise to unilateral oedema. In the case of thrombosis the affected limb is painful and swollen.
- Varicose veins are due to defective valve action. They are bilateral and have the typical blue, distended appearance of varicosities. There may be discoloured skin over the ankles.
- Lymphatic system blockage due to tumour or parasitic infestation (elephantiasis). The oedema tends to be non-pitting and there may be evidence of lymphatic gland enlargement. If due to a tumour, the oedema is one sided.

In terms of Chinese medicine, oedema is differentiated into Yang oedema and Yin oedema. Yang oedema is characterised by an absence of pitting on pressure and is due to Wind-water Invasion, Fire-Poison, Damp or Damp-heat. Yin oedema is pitting in type and due to Deficiency of Spleen or Kidney Yang. Its site can help differentiate also as upper body oedema is often due to a Lung imbalance, middle body oedema due to a Spleen[8] imbalance and lower body oedema due to a Kidney imbalance. In Chinese medicine, the allergic oedema (described above) would be seen as a Lung disorder, malabsorption diseases as a Spleen disorder and nephrotic syndrome as a Kidney disorder.

Such holistic views do serve to explain conditions where conventional medicine cannot. There is a condition called idiopathic oedema of women. This rather grandiose terminology means that oedema occurs in some women due to an unknown cause. It tends to appear or become worse either at the end of the day or before a period. There may be associated symptoms such as those that occur in pre-menstrual tension, abdominal bloating and sudden weight changes. There is no explanation in conventional medicine other than an assumption of 'hormonal imbalance'. Such women are given diuretics as a symptomatic measure. They come to rely on this medication until such time as it ceases to work and the oedema, which is never completely controlled, starts to worsen.

In Chinese medicine, it is often due to Spleen imbalance and explains why there is an association with craving for sweet food as well as being worse pre-menstrually. It is a problem on the energetic level and cannot be diagnosed by the physical means of conventional medicine. Holistic medical treatment is very effective. It is not enough, however, just to try to cleanse fluid out of the system. The energy of the digestion needs to be strengthened and then the fluid is controlled. Many women enter a vicious cycle of dieting, excessive exercise and measures such as slimming aids or diuretics. These will serve only to further deplete the digestive energy and lead eventually to more oedema.

GENETICS

This is the 'science of inheritance'. It is an attempt to explain how certain characteristics are passed from one generation to the next. When applied to humans, it seeks to understand the inherited basis to disease. It is an area of medicine that has undergone rapid change in recent years. The application of human or medical genetics is considered to be one of the most promising areas of medicine in the forthcoming years. It is helpful for all of us, practitioners or not, to know and understand the basic principles of genetics as many parts of our lives will be touched by these developments. Textbooks of physiology are good sources of information.

The basic unit of genetic material is the gene which is carried on a chromosome. It is made up of deoxyribonucleic acid (DNA) or (ribonucleic acid) RNA. These are complex molecules consisting of sequences of compounds (nucleotides) that provide the 'code' for the generation of amino acids and thereafter proteins. If there are errors in this code either through inherited defects or due to changes after birth (somatic changes), disease may appear.

More than 200 genetic disorders are now recognised. Many of these are the result of a single gene or chromosome abnormality. The understanding of the influence of genetic changes on diseases such as cancer, rheumatology and so forth is still limited. Such so-called multifactorial diseases are much more complex to understand as they are the result of an interaction between genetic and environmental factors. Currently, there seems to be an increasing belief that the study of genetics will lead to great advances in the understanding and treatment of such diseases. This is unlikely because of the many factors involved in their causation. Such beliefs lead to great pressures on all of us, patients, practitioners and the general public to embrace the new genetic technologies as they offer the hope of a world free from hunger and disease. This hope may be realistic or not depending upon your viewpoint. What is certain is that there are great ethical and moral issues that need to be debated. Hopefully, such a discussion can take place before manipulations are made to our own genetic material and that of the natural environment with unknown and unpredictable outcomes.

Genetic disorders are classified conventionally according to the way in which they are inherited. Essentially, they are of two types:

- Inherited or congenital – these are due to inherited genetic characteristics and their pattern can be more or less analysed and predicted in some and not in others
- Environmental – due to a mutation of the genetic material after birth. Chemicals, ultraviolet light and radiation are considered to be the main causes of such mutations.

Interaction between these factors, genetic inheritance and the environment, are the most common clinical situation. Clinically important examples of these different groups are listed in Table 3.1.

Type	Example
Inherited or congenital	Chromosomal disorder, e.g. Down's syndrome, myopathies, neuropathies
	Gene disorder, e.g. Huntington's chorea, achondroplasia, familial hypercholesterolaemia, familial Alzheimer's disease, cystic fibrosis, phenylketonuria, haemophilia A, red-green colour blindness
Environmental	Mutations of genes after birth generally considered to be due to ultraviolet light, radiation and chemicals
Combined factors	Almost any disease can be slotted into this category but those that are placed here conventionally include high blood pressure, asthma, schizophrenia, ankylosing spondylitis, diabetes mellitus, heart disease, cancer

Table 3.1: Clinically important examples of genetic disorders

The exact appearance of a disease is not completely or invariably dependent upon the underlying genetic changes. There may be 'incomplete penetrance' where a genetic disorder does not manifest completely. There may be great differences in severity in different generations making predictions difficult. New cases may arise in a previously unaffected family. Achondroplasia is such an example.

Genetic counselling is available for those inherited conditions that are predictable in their pattern of inheritance. The main aims of such counselling are to determine the diagnosis of the disease, its genetic basis, analyse the family history and to provide information about the disorder and its probability of appearing in any offspring. Relatives may also be screened genetically.

SUMMARY

Pathological processes in conventional medicine are physical in nature and origin.

The primary process is inflammation that gives rise to characteristic symptoms of redness, pain, swelling, heat and loss of function.

Most disease labels in conventional medicine are merely descriptions of an inflammatory process.

There are many prescribed drugs available that have an anti-inflammatory effect.

Suppression of inflammation may cause worsening of the condition.

In general, inflammation may be divided into that which is associated with infection and that which is not.

Conventional medicine considers raised cholesterol levels and atheroma to be the main cause of ischaemic heart disease.

Haemorrhage, thrombosis and embolism are the three major disorders of blood leading to disease.

Oedema has many causes attributable to different organs. The precise cause can generally be determined from accompanying symptoms.

Genetics is arapidly developing area of medicine. Its application to health and disease is imprecise and would benefit from an open debate about its use.

---

[1] *Lancet* 1989; Jun 24th.

[2] *The Saccharine Disease* by Cleave (Wright, 1974).

[3] A study researching cholesterol levels showed that these were increased in people threatened with unemployment. These were much higher if there were sleep disturbances. *BMJ* 1990;Sept 8:461.

[4] It has been known for many years that the use of cholesterol-lowering drugs leads to serious problems. A trial of clofibrate in 1978 revealed an increase in suicide, aggressive behaviour and accidental death. A US trial in 1980 showed that low cholesterol levels are linked to an increased risk of cancer. *Journal of Chronic Disease* 1980;33:311-312.

It would seem the only conventional reason to prescribe such drugs is if the cholesterol level is very high, that is, at least in excess of 12 mmol/l (Normal 3.5 - 6.5 mmol/1).

5 Overt scurvy, Vitamin C deficiency, may be unusual in the UK but there are many people who eat inadequate diets either in terms of quantity or quality. This is particularly true in the elderly and those who live alone. It is always worth checking what people eat on a daily basis. You only have to see the average trolley of goods in your local supermarket to know that many people's diets leave much to be desired.

6 Other items that may form an embolus are atheroma, injected air, tumour cells and fat (from a broken bone).

7 Osmosis is a process where water passes from a less concentrated area to a more concentrated one through a semi-permeable membrane. Osmotic pressure, therefore, is the pressure exerted (in this case by blood) that draws water into the more concentrated area.

8 The Spleen, as understood by Chinese medicine, is responsible for many digestive processes. Such action is described as transformation and transportation and is described more fully in Chapter 13 – Gastrointestinal system.

4 INVESTIGATIONS

INTRODUCTION

Investigations are the tests that are carried out after a physical examination has been made and a case history taken. There are many different types used in many different situations. It is possible to categorise them according to their effect on the person. It is useful to think of them in terms of their degree of invasiveness. This information can be used as the basis of making an informed choice. A person may, for example, decide to request a less invasive test to minimise the potential harm.

Category of investigation	Meaning
1	Relatively non-invasive with little or no risk of illness
2	Invasive and carries a significant risk of morbidity
3	Invasive and may, in some circumstances, cause death

Table 4.1: Invasiveness of investigations – general categories

REASONS FOR INVESTIGATIONS

Doctors perform investigations for several reasons and these may be different to the reasons that patients consider important. Such tests aim to detect pathological changes within the body not discernible to the ordinary senses. No method of perception is infallible and all investigations must be considered in the light of other evidence. I would never recommend a course of action solely on the basis of an investigation. This is particularly true if the person feels healthy.

An investigation may enable the doctor to make or confirm a diagnosis. In some situations, an investigation helps to decide on the degree of pathological change. The disease may be staged as to its severity. This is invariably done in the case of cancer. Do not confuse this with prognosis. It is notoriously difficult to assess prognosis on the basis of the nature of physical disease and there are many people alive today who were told years ago that they only had several months to live.

In general, the degree of structural change has a poor relationship with symptoms. For example, some people with severe symptoms of pain and stiffness in the cervical spine may have minimal change on X-ray whereas some people with gross radiological evidence of degeneration may have little or no symptoms. The person must be treated, not the X-ray. Symptoms are the result of an *energetic* imbalance and are related to function more than structure. What something looks like is not so important as how it works.

Fear of a particular disease or process may lead to investigations. This is particularly true for infectious diseases, even where there is no conventional treatment. HIV infection is a case in point where the conventional treatment available makes little or no difference to the state of HIV infection and yet people may be advised to discover their HIV antibody status.

There are several reasons why someone may choose to have an investigation. I would suggest it is primarily for reassurance as there is a great sense of relief when they are done. This is before any result is obtained. It may be why such great disappointment is felt when the test comes back revealing abnormality. Investigations are seen as 'something being done' and are regarded as positive in themselves. They are seen as treatment or at least the initiation of treatment. This is potentially dangerous in the sense that investigations lead only to the gathering of information and, usually, have nothing to do with treatment. In addition, the almost blind faith in the power of investigations to reassure can lead to despair and depression if they do not live up to this expectation. So, many people seek to be reassured that they are well. The medical profession undertakes investigations for the exact opposite reason – to detect abnormality! This scenario certainly has the potential for disappointment at the very least. It is not possible to diagnose normality by investigation, only abnormality and even then not all abnormality. Therefore, it must only be regarded as an aid and not, as is so often the case, an end in itself.

There may be a risk of illness associated with an investigation that can be significant. The degree of risk is directly related to their invasiveness. There may be mortality – some investigations may actually kill the person.

The more routine an investigation, i.e. the more automatically it is done, then the less revealing it is. Routine X-rays of the lumbar spine, for example, which are used in cases of low back pain, reveal an abnormality in only 1 in 4000 cases. A survey of 595 people who attended a clinic in Switzerland showed that they had a total of 2,378 tests performed of which 65 per cent were considered to be routine. In only 0.3 per cent of cases did the results of such tests lead to a change in management. Over the next 15 months it was noticed that 60 per cent of the blood change abnormalities returned to normal. The conclusion of the report was that 30 per cent of these blood tests were unnecessary.[1] Not only is this a large expenditure in terms of money and time for the health services, it is unnecessary for health, may damage the person and leads to increased levels of anxiety.

Screening procedures are the use of investigations in people with no symptoms or known health problems. They serve to provide employment for a large number of medical and paramedical staff. There has never been a recorded instance of mass screening campaigns changing the course of a disease. Why is this? The degree of invasion and the anxiety produced as a result seems to be counterproductive.[2] Although some problems will be revealed others will be caused. In addition, conventional medical treatment may make no difference to the course of a detectable abnormality and may lead to other problems.

This does not mean that an individual investigation done in an individual case for an individual problem is without benefit. A person may decide that they would benefit from the knowledge such an investigation may give them. The widespread, indiscriminate use of investigations, however, is of no benefit.

The golden rule of all investigations is: *only perform an investigation if the result will change the management of the case.* For example, if a woman is not going to take female sex hormones for a gynaecological condition there is no point in ascertaining levels of oestrogen and progesterone. If a person is not going to have a coronary bypass operation, there is no point in an angiogram to determine the state of the coronary arteries. If the person is not going to have chemotherapy or radiotherapy for cancer treatment, there is no point in removing lymph glands or other structures to make a conventional decision about staging.[3]

TYPES OF INVESTIGATIONS

BLOOD TESTS

Full blood count

This is a general investigation of the blood and has an invasiveness of Category 1. The tests available, their results and meaning are shown in Table 4.2. Where only one figure is shown, this is the upper limit of normal. There is always a degree of error and so minor deviations from the normal can usually be safely ignored. If a result is abnormal then repetition may reveal 'return to normal'. This could indicate an initial error or a minor problem that has now subsided.

Test	Normal range[4]	Meaning
Haemoglobin (Hb)	Male – 13.5-18 g dL^{-1} Female – 11.5-16.5 g dL^{-1} Pregnancy – 6.8-9.3 g dL^{-1} New–born – 17-22 g dL^{-1} Infant – 6.8-7.8 g dL^{-1} Child – 12-14 g dL^{-1}	Low in all types of anaemia
Mean corpuscular volume (MCV) – size of red blood cells	80-96 fL	Low in anaemia of iron deficiency and chronic disease, chronic blood loss and pregnancy. High in Vitamin B_{12} and folate deficiency anaemias, malabsorption, malnutrition and aplastic anaemia.
Mean corpuscular haemoglobin (MCH) – amount of haemoglobin in red blood cells	27-31 pg	Reduced in all types of anaemia.
Mean corpuscular haemoglobin concentration (MCHC)	32-35 g dL-1	Low in iron deficiency anaemia, pregnancy and chronic disease.
Haematocrit or packed cell volume (PCV) – volume when red blood cells are packed together	Male – 40-54 per cent (0.40-0.54 L L^{-1}) Female – 32-42 per cent (0.32-0.42 L L^{-1}) Child – 32-42 per cent	Low in anaemia. High in polycythaemia and dehydration.
Red blood cell count	Male – 4.5-6.5 x 10^{12}/l Female – 3.9-5.6 x 10^{12}/l	Low in haemolytic and aplastic anaemia. High in polycythaemia.

White cell count (WCC)	Adult – 4000-10000 x 10^9/L Child – 10000-20000 x 10^9/L	Low in some leukaemias, viraemia and the elderly. High in bacterial infection and some leukaemias.
Neutrophils	2.5-6.5 x 10^9/L (40-60 per cent)	Low in viral infection, overwhelming bacterial infection Vitamin B_{12} deficiency, folate deficiency, leukaemia, aplastic anaemia and SLE. High in bacterial infection and herpes zoster. Very high in pneumococcal pneumonia.
Basophils	0.01-0.1 x 10^9/L (0-1 per cent)	High in chronic inflammation and hypothyroidism. Very high in chronic myelocytic leukaemia and polycythaemia.
Eosinophils	0.05-0.4 x 10^9/L (1-3 per cent)	Low in acute bacterial infection and corticosteroid treatment. High in allergy, hay fever, polyarteritis nodosa, Hodgkin's disease and parasitic infestation. Very high in malignancy and eosinophilic leukaemia.
Monocytes	0.2-0.8 x 10^9/L (4-8 per cent)	Low in chronic infection and Hodgkin's disease.
Lymphocytes	1.5-3.5 x 10^9/L (20-40 per cent)	Low in stress, injury, haemorrhage, overwhelming infection, Hodgkin's disease and the elderly. High in chronic infection, acute viral infection and acute lymphatic leukaemia.
Platelet count	150-350 x 10^9/L	Low in thrombocytopenia. High in chronic leukaemia and polycythaemia.
Erythrocyte sedimentation rate (ESR)	Male – 0-10 mm/hour Female – 0-20 mm/hour Child – 0-20 mm/hour	Non-specific test of inflammation. High in pregnancy, infections and some malignancies. Very high (50 mm or more) in autoimmune disease.

Table 4.2: Full blood count - components, results and interpretation

Serum tests

These have an invasiveness of Category 1. They are investigations carried out on the blood but relating to the presence of substances such as nutrients, waste materials and the like.

Test	Normal range	Meaning
Acid phosphatase	1-5 U L^{-1}	High in malignant disease of the prostate and acute myelocytic leukaemia.
Alanine aminotransferase (ALT) formerly glutamic pyruvic transaminase (SGPT)	5-40 U L^{-1}	High in obstructive jaundice, chronic hepatitis, malignant disease of the liver, heart attack and glandular fever. Very high in acute hepatitis.
Albumin	35-55 g L^{-1}	Low in liver cell death, cirrhosis, malnutrition, malabsorption, some types of glomerulonephritis and leukaemia. High in shock and dehydration.
Alkaline phosphatase	25-115 U L^{-1}	Low in hypothyroidism. High in malignant disease of bone, rickets, Paget's disease of bone and secondary malignancy of liver.
Amylase	<220 U L^{-1}	Low in hepatitis, toxaemia of pregnancy. High in acute pancreatitis, malignant disease of the pancreas, mumps, salpingitis, perforated duodenal ulcer, liver disease and ruptured ectopic pregnancy.
Aspartate aminotransferase (AST) formerly known as glutamic oxaloacetic transaminase (SGOT)	8-40 U L^{-1}	High in obstructive jaundice, acute hepatitis, cirrhosis, heart attack, malignant disease of the liver, haemolytic jaundice and injury.
Bicarbonate	22-31 mmol L^{-1}	Low in hyperventilation, diabetes mellitus and severe kidney disease. High in potassium depletion, vomiting and Cushing's syndrome.
Bilirubin	Total 20 mcmol L^{-1} Direct 1.6 mcmol L^{-1} Indirect 2-13 mcmol L^{-1}	Indirect is high in haemolysis. Both are high in hepatitis, biliary obstruction and toxaemia.
B$_{12}$	200-900 ng L^{-1}	Low in pernicious anaemia. Calcium 2.2-2.7 mmol L^{-1}. Low in Vitamin D deficiency, renal failure and nephrotic syndrome. High in osteoporosis, malignancy, sarcoidosis, excess calcium intake, Hodgkin's disease, Paget's disease of bone and with thiazide diuretic use.
Carbon dioxide	4.8-6.1 kPa (36-46 mmHg)	Repeated measurements are taken in severe respiratory disease and give a reliable guide to lung function.
Chloride	97-108 mmol L^{-1}	Low in dehydration and with diuretic use. High in excess fluid intake and dehydration.
Cholesterol – HDL cholesterol LDL cholesterol	3.5 – 6.5 mmol L^{-1} Male – 0.95 - 2.15 mmol L^{-1} Female – 0.7 – 2.0 mmol L^{-1} 1.55 – 4.4 mmol L^{-1}	Low in acute hepatitis, hyperthyroidism, acute infections, uraemia and malnutrition. High in hypothyroidism, diabetes mellitus, nephrotic syndrome, chronic hepatitis, cirrhosis, elderly and familial hypercholesterolaemia
Creatine kinase (CPK)	Female – 24-170 U L^{-1} Male – 24-195 U L^{-1}	High in heart attack, muscle injury, dystrophy and polymyositis.
Creatinine	0.06-0.11 mmol L^{-1}	Low in pregnancy. High in renal failure and urinary tract obstruction.

Follicle-stimulating hormone	Female – 2.5-10 U L^{-1} (early cycle), >30 U L^{-1} (post-menopausal)	High at peri-menopausal and post-menopausal times. High in ovarian failure.
Globulin	Total – 20-35 g L^{-1} Alpha1 – 2-4 g L^{-1} Alpha2 – 4-8 g L^{-1} Beta – 6-10 g L^{-1} Gamma – 6-15 g L^{-1}	Total is in malnutrition and lymphatic leukaemia. Alpha1 is low in nephrotic syndrome. Gamma is low in nephrotic syndrome, leukaemia and with corticosteroid treatment. Total is high in cirrhosis, chronic hepatitis and SLE. Alpha1 is high with oestrogen treatment. Alpha2 is high in acute infections, heart attack, injury and nephrotic syndrome. Beta is high in cirrhosis, hypercholesterolaemia, nephrotic syndrome, pregnancy and hypothyroidism. Gamma is high in infection, autoimmune disease and cirrhosis.
Glucose (fasting)	4.5-5.6 mmol L^{-1}	High in diabetes mellitus, hyperthyroidism, overactivity of adrenal cortex (includes treatment with corticosteroids) and liver disease.
Iron	Male – 15-30 mcmol L^{-1} Female – 14-28 mcmol L^{-1}	Low in iron deficiency anaemia, dietary lack, malabsorption, chronic blood loss, Hodgkin's disease and the elderly. High in other anaemias.
Lactate dehydrogenase	120-280 U L^{-1}	High in heart attack, kidney damage, acute hepatitis, polycythaemia and pernicious anaemia.
Lipids (total) Luteinising hormone (LH)	4.0-10.0 g L^{-1} Female – 25-70 U L^{-1} (whilst ovulating), >30 (post-menopausal)	High in diabetes mellitus and hypothyroidism. Low in infertility. High at ovulation.
Magnesium	0.7-0.9 mmol L^{-1}	Low in alcohol abuse, cirrhosis, malabsorption, chemotherapy for malignant disease and with diuretic use.
Oestradiol (oestrogen)	Female – 500-1100 U L^{-1} (whilst ovulating)	Low in post-menopausal women (< 150 pmol/L) – this is normal since the menopause is not a disease state.
Oxygen	10-13.3 kPa (75-100 mmHg)	Repeated measurements are taken in severe respiratory disease and give a reliable guide to lung function.
Paul-Bunnell test	up to 1:128	High in glandular fever.
Phosphate	0.9-1.5 mmol L^{-1}	Low in rickets, osteomalacia, insulin treatment and after meals. High in kidney disease.
Potassium	3.5-5.2 mmol L^{-1}	Low in fluid loss, diuretic use, malabsorption, purgative use, diabetes mellitus and with corticosteroid use. High in acute renal failure and uraemia.
Progesterone	>30 nmol L^{-1} – second half of cycle	Reduced in progesterone deficiency that may be found in irregular periods, infertility, habitual miscarriage and heavy menses (in the majority of cases there is no abnormality).
Prolactin	<400 mU L^{-1}	Female infertility. High in pituitary tumours and overactivity, brain injury and unknown causes.
Prostate-specific antigen	up to 4.0 mcg L^{-1}	Markedly raised in prostatic cancer.
Protein (total)	60-80 g L^{-1}	Low in nephrotic syndrome, chronic renal failure and malnutrition.
Rheumatoid factor	Absent	Positive in 75 per cent of people with rheumatoid arthritis and in many normal people.
Sodium	137-150 mmol L^{-1}	Low in dehydration, oedema, Addison's disease and acute renal failure. High in dehydration.

Thyroxine (total) Thyroxine (free) Tri-iodothyronine	58 – 174 mmol L^{-1} 10 – 22 pmol L^{-1} 1.07 – 3.18 nmol L^{-1}	Low in hypothyroidism, nephrotic syndrome and phenytoin use. High in hyperthyroidism, pregnancy and with female sex hormone use
Thyroid-stimulating hormone	0.3 – 4.0 mU L^{-1}	Low in hyperthyroidism, high in hypothyroidism
Triglycerides	Male - 0.7-2.1 mmol L^{-1} Female - 0.5-1.7 mmol L^{-1}	High in nephrotic syndrome and chronic renal failure.
Urea	3.2-6.6 mmol L^{-1}	Low in liver failure, severe weight loss, diabetes insipidus and pregnancy. High in nephritis, urinary tract obstruction, dehydration, bleeding in the gastrointestinal tract, shock, underactivity of adrenal cortex and the elderly.

Table 4.3: Serum investigations – substances tested, results and meaning

ELECTROCARDIOGRAPHY (ECG)

This is non-invasive and is Category 1 unless done whilst exercising. It merely records electrical activity of the heart during the cardiac cycle. From this information, it is possible to infer certain structural changes. Abnormalities detected include cardiac arrhythmias, enlargement of certain areas of the heart, heart attack, angina pectoris (usually only if an exercise ECG is abnormal), pulmonary embolism. In the case of heart attack, it may take 24 hours for the ECG to become abnormal. A 24-hour recording is done in cases of arrhythmia.

An exercise ECG is used to diagnose the angina pectoris and is of Category 3 invasiveness. The resting ECG is usually normal in this condition, and so measurement whilst exercising may provide evidence of ischaemia. An exercise ECG leads to heart attacks in 0.05 per cent of cases and has a death rate of 0.01 per cent.

ELECTROENCEPHALOGRAPHY (EEG)

This is the cerebral equivalent of the ECG and is non-invasive of Category 1. It measures the electrical activity of the brain. The main use is to diagnose epilepsy but abnormalities are also seen in encephalitis, dementia and hypoglycaemia. It may be normal between epileptic attacks. Some people with epilepsy have normal EEGs and some 'normal' people have abnormal EEGs.

ELECTROMYOGRAPHY (EMG)

This has an invasiveness of Category 2. It is a measurement of the electrical activity of muscle made by inserting a needle electrode into the muscle. Abnormalities detected include myopathy, myasthenia gravis, nerve entrapment syndromes and neuropathy. It is a particularly painful investigation.

PULMONARY FUNCTION TESTS

These have an invasiveness of Category 1 unless drugs are given to monitor their effect in which case it is Category 2. They are performed as an outpatient and involve breathing into various instruments to measure force of expiration and lung volume. They give a quantitative measure of lung function and can be repeated to check on changes in response to treatment. They may have a role to play for the holistic practitioner who would like objective evidence of improvement. Abnormalities detected include obstructive airways disease such as asthma, chronic bronchitis and emphysema.

SKIN TESTS

These have an invasiveness of Category 2. They are used to test for allergic responses to a variety of substances. A scratch is made on the skin and the test substance placed on the wound. Some days later the area is tested for evidence of an allergic response. In my experience they are of minimal help since there is little relationship between the results of the tests and the symptom picture. They also serve to reinforce the mistaken belief that manipulation of the external environment can lead to health. In some cases the removal of an offending allergen may markedly reduce symptoms but what may happen is that the pathology moves somewhere else or the person then develops an allergy to something else.

X-RAYS

These have an invasiveness of Category 2. Medical sources of radiation are the commonest cause of exposure to radiation other than natural sources. The risk increases proportionally to the degree of exposure to radiation. Such radiation leads to increases in the rate of malignant disease such as cancer and leukaemia. Radiologists and radiographers have a higher incidence of these than the general population. Although there is minimal risk with one X-ray investigation, care needs to exercised in the case of repeated usage. It has been estimated that the effects on health of one barium examination of the intestines is the equivalent of smoking 20 cigarettes for a year. The effects are much greater on children and babies.

PLAIN X-RAYS

These are the simplest X-rays since they use a relatively low dose and are taken without the aid of radio-opaque substances. Their use in summarised in Table 4.4.

Organ/structure studied	Abnormality detected
Chest	Structural defects
Lungs (via chest X-ray)	Collapse, pleural effusion, pneumonia, fibrosis, infections such as tuberculosis, sarcoidosis, cancer, lymphatic gland enlargement, increased or decreased pulmonary blood flow
Heart (via chest X-ray)	Enlarged heart, abnormal heart shape, pericardial effusion (large), calcification
Abdomen (gall bladder)	Gall stones (10 per cent are seen)
Abdomen (pancreas)	Calcification
Abdomen (kidney)	Kidney stones (90 per cent are seen), bladder stones, calcification
Abdomen (peritoneal cavity)	Air in the peritoneal cavity due to perforated ulcer
Skull	Fractures, erosion of bony structures by tumour, calcification
Spine	Fractures, degenerative changes, vertebral collapse, tumours
Bones	Fractures, osteoporosis, rickets, osteomalacia, tumours
Joints	Arthritis

Table 4.4: Plain X-rays

Computerised axial tomography

This is an X-ray examination that uses increased doses of radiation in order to give more detailed information about the tissue examined. This investigation can also be known as a CAT scan or an EMI scan (after the company which makes the equipment). The use of this type of scan is summarised in Table 4.5.

Organ/structure studied	Abnormality detected
Lung	Cancer, sarcoidosis, lymphoma, dust diseases (in each case provides more detail than can be detected by plain X-rays)
Abdomen	Lymphatic gland enlargement
Liver	Tumours
Gall bladder	Gall stones
Pancreas	Tumours
Brain	Tumours, haemorrhage, haematoma, atrophy, pituitary disease (misses abnormalities <1 cm diameter or close to the skull)
Spine	Tumours, disc prolapse
Kidney and urinary tract	Tumours of kidney, bladder and prostate
Adrenal	Tumours

Table 4.5: Computerised axial tomography

Barium studies

Barium is radio-opaque and such studies can reveal information about organs of the gastrointestinal tract that is not easily displayed on plain films. They can diagnose a wide range of disorders such as carcinoma, ulcers, polyps, strictures, diverticulitis and the inflammatory bowel diseases. They can be done on an outpatient basis. Screening is carried out at the same time. This involves observation of the movement of the intestine during the investigation. This necessitates exposure to more radiation than would be the case if only static pictures were taken.

Barium meal

This is used to examine the upper gastrointestinal tract of oesophagus, stomach, duodenum and jejunum. If the passage of the barium into the small intestine is observed then abnormalities of the ileum can be diagnosed. People are X-rayed with their head down to try to demonstrate reflux from the stomach to the oesophagus or the existence of a hiatus hernia. Prior to a barium meal nothing is eaten or drunk from the previous night. Abnormalities detected include reflux into the oesophagus, hiatus hernia, oesophageal cancer, gastric ulcer, gastric cancer, duodenal ulcer and Crohn's disease.

Barium enema

This is used to examine the large intestine and terminal ileum. The lowest part of the rectum must be examined by other means such as rectal examination or sigmoidoscopy. Prior to the investigation, people are put on a low fibre diet for 3 days and laxatives for 1 day before the investigation. A colon washout is performed immediately prior to the X-ray. This is why people who have this test can feel so tired. The use of laxatives and a colonic washout lead to the loss of energy and fluid from the body thus causing fatigue. Abnormalities detected include cancer of the large intestine, ulcerative colitis and diverticulitis.

Cholecystogram

Gallstones can be detected merely by a plain X-ray of the abdomen in only 10 per cent of cases. Because of this, dye studies are the norm. It is not used in jaundiced people as the secretion of bile is disturbed and so the dye does not enter the gall bladder. This investigation has been replaced by ultrasound examination in many situations. Oral cholecystograms involve taking a dye in tablet form which is later found concentrated in the gall bladder. Some hours later, X-rays of the gall bladder are taken before and after the ingestion of fat. Abnormalities detected include gallstones.

Percutaneous transhepatic cholangiography

This has an invasiveness of Category 3. It is used to obtain information about the biliary system. A needle is passed through the skin and superficial tissues into the liver, after injection of a local anaesthetic, to allow the injection of dye into the biliary system. X-rays are taken subsequently. Abnormalities detected include obstruction of the biliary system. Complications include bleeding, infection of the biliary system and septicaemia.

Intravenous pyelography (urography)

This is the injection of dye that is excreted by the kidney and allows X-ray examination of the kidney and urinary tract. This has an invasiveness of Category 2 since some people are severely allergic to the dye leading to anaphylactic shock and occasionally convulsions.

It is used to define the size and shape of the kidneys as well as urine flow out of the urinary tract. Abnormalities detected include stones, obstruction to urine flow, long-term kidney disease such as pyelonephritis or glomerulonephritis and tumours of the kidney and bladder. Studies of bladder function and emptying can be made by taking films whilst the person is urinating.

Myelography

This has an invasiveness of Category 2. It is the injection of dye into the subarachnoid space, usually in the lumbar (occasionally cervical) area, to allow X-ray or computerised axial tomography of the structures around the spinal cord. Lumbar puncture – see Page 41 is performed first and then dye injected.
Recently a newer type of dye has been used which is water-soluble. In the past, a heavy oily dye was used which remained in the area for a long time and has been implicated in leading to arachnoiditis. This is an unusual inflammation that causes headaches and nerve problems including tingling and weakness. It may be severe in its manifestations. Abnormalities detected by myelography include spinal tumours and prolapsed disc.

CARDIAC CATHETERISATION

This has an invasiveness of Category 3. It is the passage of a tube (catheter) into the heart. The right side of the heart is accessed via a vein, usually in the neck. The left side of the heart is accessed via an artery, usually the femoral artery in the groin. There are several uses of this procedure enabling blood samples to be taken, pressures measured or dye injected (angiography) depending upon the actual clinical situation. Abnormalities detected are included in Table 4.6 with regard to angiography.

Angiography

This is the injection of dye into the vascular system and can give information about the blood supply. It is used to investigate structures such as the heart or the circulation of any organ or area of the body. Its use is summarised in Table 4.6.

Organ/structure studied	Abnormality detected
Heart	Aneurysm, cardiomyopathy
Coronary arteries	Atherosclerosis
Liver	Tumours
Brain	Vascular abnormalities such as thrombosis or aneurysms
Carotid artery	Narrowing, atherosclerosis
Vertebral artery	Narrowing, atherosclerosis
Kidney	Tumours, renal artery disease in, e.g. hypertension

Table 4.6: Angiography

SCANS

This is a general term used to describe methods of obtaining an idea of internal structures without needing to resort to surgery. They utilise various means including radiation, magnetic fields and ultrasound. Invasiveness depends upon the particular type. Each is indicated separately. Computerised axial tomography (CAT) described above may be designated as a scan.

Ultrasound scans

These are described in conventional textbooks as being non-invasive which is not true. Their invasiveness is Category 1 unless applied to pregnant women where the effect on the baby will be in Category 2.

Such scans involve the use of sound waves to bounce off tissue of differing depths and types. A cross sectional image of the organ or area, e.g. the abdomen, is obtained. They are commonly used in obstetric practice and increasingly so.[5, 6] I trained in medicine in the mid-1970s and it was then performed for specific indications in early pregnancy. Now, it is almost universal with, in some centres, two or more ultrasounds during pregnancy. It is used in 85 per cent of pregnancies in England, between 15 and 40 per cent in US and 100 per cent in Germany.

Organ/structure studied	Abnormality detected
Heart (echocardiography)	Valve disease, infective endocarditis, cardiomyopathy, pericardial effusion, congenital heart disease
Liver	Tumours (over 1 cm in diameter), cirrhosis
Gall bladder	Gall stones (98 per cent accuracy)
Pancreas	Tumours
Abdomen	Tumours
Kidney and urinary tract	Tumours, cystic kidney disease, kidney size and urine obstruction in kidney failure, prostate tumours
Pelvic organs	Uterine fibroids, ectopic pregnancy, foetal abnormality, tumours, abnormal placental site

Table 4.7: Ultrasound examination

Ultrasound provides information about the foetus such as gestational age, stage of development and the normality of internal organs as well as the site of the placenta. They are usually performed at around 10-12 weeks and later in pregnancy at around 36 weeks. The other uses of ultrasound scans are summarised in Table 4.7.

There are several causes for concern to consider. It may not be of any value in changing outcome. Routine ultrasound scanning during pregnancy does not result in an increase in the number of live births or reduce the chances of infant illness in the 28 days following birth. Scanning can detect foetal growth retardation and multiple pregnancies but early detection does not affect the management of either of these conditions.[7] There is much evidence to suggest that such procedures are harmful to the foetus.[8] This is another example of the medical profession using techniques with no long-term follow-up of possible effects and with no *informed* consent obtained from pregnant mothers. If you observe a foetus who is undergoing ultrasound examination, he/she will hold their hands up to their ears and move away from the source of the sound. Whilst it may be reasonable in some circumstances to perform ultrasound in pregnancy, it is unreasonable to subject every mother regardless of her personal situation.[9] In addition, there have been many articles in the professional journals about the uselessness of mass ultrasound screening and yet it is continued.

It is easy to misinterpret results and there are cases of women told of abnormalities detected only to find later that the aborted foetus or newborn baby is normal. Conversely, some women are told that their baby is normal only to find later that it is not. This fallibility, of course, is true of all investigations.

Experiments into the safety of ultrasound are usually done with continuous wave or high intensity pulse lengths. The ultrasound used in clinical practice is not of these types. Finally, it is difficult to relate tests in animals to those in humans. The tragedy of thalidomide and other drug effects confirm this fact.[10]

The adverse effects of ultrasound are thought to be caused by the generation of heat or by mechanical effects. It is stated conventionally that ultrasound does not cause damage to the foetus but the truth is that this is not known. The possibility exists, however, and there is some disturbing evidence.[11-26] It would seem that the potential for harm is greater at the earlier stages of development.

There are several stated aims for performing ultrasound scans in early pregnancy. These are –

- to determine the age of foetus
- to diagnose multiple pregnancy
- to diagnose foetal abnormalities
- to locate the placenta – thus determining the likelihood of placenta praevia.

The age of the foetus and the possibility of multiple pregnancy can be determined by clinical examination. If the foetus is 'large-for-dates', that is, the size of the uterus is larger than expected, it may indicate that the foetal age is not as expected or that more than one foetus is present.

The detection of foetal abnormalities is only necessary if the mother is contemplating termination of the pregnancy. If this is not the case, and there are moral and religious beliefs to be considered here, there seems little point in performing potentially hazardous investigations just for information. It also important to consider the possibility of error as investigations are not infallible. There are several court cases currently pending where terminations were performed only to discover that the foetus was normal.

It may be important in later pregnancy to determine the site of the placenta where there may be a possibility of placenta praevia. This is the presence of the placenta near the cervix and is discussed on Page 331. It is impossible for the baby to be born vaginally and a Caesarian section is necessary. This condition can be suspected if the head of the baby does not go down into the pelvis in late pregnancy. It would seem sensible to reserve ultrasound for those cases and at that stage. In this way, the foetus is not exposed at early stages of its development. In any event, diagnosis by ultrasound of placenta praevia in early pregnancy is unreliable and, conventionally, is always followed by a repeat examination in the final months.

I would consider the following to be reasonable considerations for the use of ultrasound in pregnancy –

- confirmation of life or death of the foetus after threatened miscarriage (to detect missed or incomplete miscarriage)
- localisation of placenta in those cases where the foetal head does not engage.

Radionuclide scans

These have an invasiveness of Category 2. I have read medical textbooks where these procedures are described as being 'safe and non-invasive'. This reveals, at the least, an interesting use of the English language.

The scans are performed by injecting radioactive materials (isotopes) and a radiation monitor is used to determine the uptake into the relevant organ. They are performed in many conditions. People may feel unwell for several weeks after this procedure as would be expected from the injection of radiation into the body. Their uses are summarised in Table 4.8.

Organ studied	Isotope	Abnormality detected
Heart	Thallium^{201} or technetium^{99}	Myocardial infarction, angina pectoris
Lung	Technetium^{99} or xenon^{133}	Pulmonary embolus (may not give definitive result)
Liver	Technetium^{99}	Cirrhosis, alcoholic hepatitis
Gall bladder	Technetium^{99}	Acute cholecystitis
Oesophagus	Technetium^{99}	Oesophageal reflux
Stomach	Technetium^{99}	Slow gastric emptying
Small and large intestine	Radioactive white blood cells	Inflammatory bowel disease
Brain	Technetium^{99}	Tumours, haematoma, infarction
Kidney	Technetium^{99}, iodine^{123} or gallium^{67}	Renal artery disease, obstruction to urine flow, bladder emptying, kidney size and shape, inflammation

Table 4.8: Radionuclide scans

Magnetic resonance imaging

This is relatively speaking a recently developed investigation and uses magnetic fields to give more detailed information of internal organs than some other tests. It has an invasiveness of Category 2. The use of magnetic fields in this way may lead to health problems but they are too new for any firm conclusions to be drawn. However, magnetic fields in other situations such as those formed by overhead electricity pylons have been implicated in several disorders including suicide, psychological disturbances, leukaemia and cancer.[27]

Organ/structure studied	Abnormality detected
Heart	Structural defects
Lungs	Tumours, lymphatic gland enlargement
Liver	Tumours
Brain	Tumours, multiple sclerosis (not definitive)
Spine	Tumours, spinal cord compression

Table 4.9: Magnetic resonance imaging

ENDOSCOPY

In general these have an invasiveness of Category 3 since perforation of the organ is a risk. If a general anaesthetic is required this would entail increased risk. In the latter case especially, careful thought has to be given to whether similar information may be obtained by other means. Some endoscopy procedures also allow treatment to be performed and are not just investigative.

Endoscopes are instruments that allow the operator to directly see the internal structure of the body. They provide access to internal organs for biopsy, sampling of secretions or cells, injection of investigative media such as dyes and may allow the application of treatment for some conditions. They are usually performed in the outpatient department but some require a general anaesthetic.

Bronchoscopy

This is performed under local anaesthesia to the throat and intravenous sedation with diazepam. Amnesia of the events during the investigation is a result of such sedation. It allows the direct examination of the larger airways. Sputum and biopsies may be obtained at the same time. It is a useful method to remove aspirated objects. Abnormalities detected include cancer, tuberculosis and a variety of other lung infections.

Upper gastrointestinal tract endoscopy

An oesophagoscope, gastroscope or duodenoscope is used to examine the upper gastrointestinal tract. The same instrument may be used to examine all organs. The person has nothing by mouth overnight and is examined as an outpatient. Intravenous sedation, usually with diazepam, is given as well as local anaesthetic spray on the throat. Intravenous diazepam is used partly since it induces sedation but also because amnesia is a common effect. Abnormalities detected include reflux oesophagitis, oesophageal cancer, gastritis, gastric ulcer, gastric cancer, duodenitis and duodenal ulcer.

An additional procedure is endoscopic retrograde cholangiopancreatography (ERCP) where a tube is passed in to the common bile duct or pancreatic duct. Secretions can be obtained for analysis as well as dye injected for X-ray studies. Risks of this procedure include infection of the biliary system and pancreatitis.

Colonoscopy

A colonoscope can allow examination of the large intestine and terminal ileum. There is some preparation involved as with a barium enema. People have only fluids the day prior to the test and are given a stimulant laxative. On the day of the investigation they are given sedation, usually diazepam, and an opiate analgesic, e.g. pethidine. The terminal ileum is reached in 80 per cent of cases. There is a mortality rate of 1 in 100,000. Abnormalities detected include cancer of the large intestine, Crohn's disease, ulcerative colitis, diverticulitis and polyps.

Cystoscopy

This is a specialist investigation of the urinary tract. It is a form of endoscopy (see above). Cystoscopy allows examination of the bladder wall and urethra. It is done under either local or general anaesthetic. The indications for its use are haematuria and urinary tract infection. Diagnosis can be made of stones, tumours and prostatic enlargement. The instrument may remove stones and biopsy can be simultaneously performed. The complications include haemorrhage, perforation of the bladder, urinary retention and infection.

Large intestine endoscopy

A proctoscope and sigmoidoscope are short instruments used for direct viewing of the rectum and lower sigmoid colon in an outpatient setting. Both are relatively painless and require no preparation or sedation. Abnormalities detected include haemorrhoids, polyps, ulcerative colitis, fissures, cancer of the rectum and anal margin. A longer sigmoidoscope is available which is used after an enema. This allows more of the colon to be examined and 70 per cent of colonic tumours can be reached.

Laparoscopy

A laparoscope is an instrument that is used to examine the abdominal cavity. It is necessary to pump air into the abdomen to separate the organs and allow clear access. The presence of air forces the diaphragm up and so respiration is impaired. A general anaesthetic is administered to prevent respiratory difficulties.

It is mainly used in gynaecological conditions to allow examination of the pelvic organs. Treatment can be administered at the same time. Abnormalities detected include ovarian disease, endometriosis, pelvic inflammatory disease, uterine fibroids and tumours.

Risks of general anaesthesia

No one knows the true incidence of problems due to anaesthesia since complications may be described as being due to the original disease. Death due to anaesthesia may be misrepresented as being caused by the original condition requiring treatment. During my medical education an anaesthetist told me that there are three stages of anaesthesia – awake, asleep and dead. Although this was an attempt at a medical joke, the reality may not be far away. Severe problems with anaesthesia are clearly uncommon but minor degrees of illness may be more frequently encountered.

The risks of anaesthesia include:

- death rate of 1 in 5000 but this risk is increased for the young and the elderly
- heart attack especially in those who have had a previous attack (particularly in the preceding 6 months).
- injury whilst unconscious during transfer off and on the operating table
- psychological reactions – lack of concentration, poor memory, disordered mental function. These can last for at least 6-8 weeks after an anaesthetic
- babies – if delivered by Caesarian section – breathing difficulties, slowness and dullness.

Epidural anaesthesia is less dangerous than general anaesthesia. Headaches and back pain are common. These may last many months. Babies delivered by Caesarian section suffer from slowness and dullness for at least 6 weeks. They are twice as likely to develop jaundice.

Risks of surgery

The risks of surgery include:

- infection – 3000 people die from post-operative infections in the UK each year. Over 30 per cent of women who have a hysterectomy develop post-operative infections
- blood transfusion – may result in HIV infection, hepatitis, mismatching, reactions to the transfused blood – one death in 9000
- haemorrhage
- embolism
- shock
- injury from error during the operation
- scars and cosmetic considerations
- pain
- psychological reactions
- wrong operation.

BIOPSY

This is the examination of pieces of tissue obtained by various means. It is the only way in which many diseases such as cancer can be definitively diagnosed and treated by conventional medicine. This is because the exact cell type and structure needs to be known. I have included in this section all types of tissue and body fluid sampling.

Sputum analysis

This has an invasiveness of Category 1. Naked eye inspection may reveal the presence of blood (if red) or of inflammation (if yellow or green). Further studies of culture are performed to detect bacterial infection. The antibiotics that are most effective can then be determined. The presence of cells can be checked and whether or not they are abnormal. This may be used to diagnose cancer of the lung. It is of variable reliability.

Urine analysis

This has an invasiveness of Category 1. There are several tests that can be performed on a fresh urine sample. They are cheap, non-invasive and easy to perform.

Dipstick testing

The urine can be examined by the naked eye and more detailed information obtained by testing by various dipsticks easily available from the chemist. This may be of help to the holistic practitioner in monitoring people with diabetes mellitus or checking for abnormalities in people with symptoms of kidney disease. Substances that can be detected include blood, protein, ketones and sugar.

Blood in the urine (haematuria) can be seen with the naked eye. In less severe cases it may impart a smoky appearance, though it is invisible in many cases. It may be in urine as a contaminant in women who are menstruating. In other cases it may be further studied by urine microscopy (see below). Diseases that may cause haematuria include cystitis, pyelonephritis, bladder tumours, kidney tumours, kidney and bladder stones. Trauma can also result in haematuria.

Protein in the urine (proteinuria) is often mistakenly viewed as being synonymous with infection and people are given antibiotics. Further study by culture is necessary to confirm or exclude infection. There are several causes of proteinuria and they include infection of the urinary tract, contamination by skin/hair and so on, inflammatory diseases of the kidney of which there are many. Blood in the urine will test positive for protein. It is reasonable to check two or three times if protein is detected before thinking about further investigation especially if there are no symptoms.

Sugar in the urine (glycosuria) is almost always indicative of diabetes mellitus. It is more likely to be present in urine passed some time after a large carbohydrate intake.

Ketones in the urine (ketonuria) indicate that the body is obtaining energy from supplies of fat rather than sugar. Ketones are a breakdown product of fat metabolism. They are seen in diabetes mellitus when hyperglycaemia is present and in fasting.

Bacteria may be tested using special dipsticks. They rely upon detecting nitrites but are unreliable indicators of infection.

Microscopy

This aims to detect several abnormal constituents. White cells in the urine indicate inflammatory disease which may or may not be infective in origin. Red cells will be seen in those people with haematuria.
Casts are collections of cells that have the shape of the tubules of the kidney. The types and their meaning are summarised in Table 4.10.

Cast	Meaning
Hyaline	Normal especially after exercise
Fine	Normal especially after exercise
Granular	Kidney disease
Red cell	Kidney disease
White cell	Pyelonephritis
Tubular cell	Acute tubular necrosis

Table 4.10: Urinary casts and their meaning

Bacteria may occasionally be seen and would suggest infection but it is important to be guided by the symptom picture. This is true, of course, of all investigations.

Urine culture

This has an invasiveness of Category 1. Urine is cultured to see if bacteria can be grown. This would suggest that infection is present but see Chapter 5 on infectious disease for a discussion of the relevance of such a finding especially in the asymptomatic. Subsequently, tests are performed on the bacteria to discover which antibiotic(s) are effective. This investigation is the preferred way to manage all urinary tract infections to prevent overuse of antibiotics or their inappropriate use. It takes 2-3 days for results to return from the laboratory.

Semen examination

This is a non-invasive examination. Some religious groups do not permit masturbation and in such a situation semen is obtained for investigation by a post-coital examination of the woman.

Normal values are:

- Volume 3.5ml
- pH 7.4
- Sperm count 60,000,000 to 200,000,000
- Motility – 90 per cent at 45 minutes and 65 per cent at 3 hours
- Abnormal forms 10-20 per cent.

Lumbar puncture

This has an invasiveness of Category 3. Cerebrospinal fluid is obtained by inserting a needle through an intervertebral space in the lower lumbar spine. Common problems after this procedure are severe throbbing headache and lower back ache. Milder headaches and low back pain may last for several months after the procedure. It must be used with great care if there is evidence of a cerebral tumour. In such cases the increased pressure in the skull can force the brain stem down into the cervical spine with possibly fatal results. Abnormalities detected include meningitis, encephalitis, multiple sclerosis (not definitive), subarachnoid haemorrhage and tumours.

Cervical smear

This has an invasiveness of Category 2. It is a sample of cells taken from the uterine cervix. A wooden spatula is used to scrape cells from around the cervix and they are smeared onto a slide for examination under a microscope. There are various grades of abnormality – see Chapter 18 – Women's Health.

Smears frequently lead to a small amount of vaginal bleeding and some women develop irregular periods or heavy periods for a short time. In Chinese medical terms they stagnate the energy of the Liver and so drinking lemon juice just before and after may prevent any adverse reactions.

Foetal biopsy

All current methods of determining the appearances of foetal cells are invasive and carry a definite risk to the foetus. There are currently three routine ways of obtaining foetal tissue. These are amniocentesis at 15 to 20 weeks' gestation, chorionic villus sampling at 10 to 12 weeks and umbilical blood sampling after 18 weeks. In addition, experimental invasive foetal sampling methods such as early amniocentesis, late transabdominal chorionic villus sampling, skin biopsy, liver biopsy, and muscle biopsy are being used. Research is currently being carried out to develop possible tests for non-invasive diagnosis by identifying foetal cells in the mother's blood[28] but this method is not yet at the clinical stage.

There are blood tests available, which measure levels of substances that may indicate foetal abnormality.[29] They are performed in the second-trimester and may detect conditions such as open spina bifida,[30] Down's syndrome, trisomy 18, multiple pregnancy and adverse pregnancy outcome. The investigations measure levels of alpha-foetoprotein, human chorionic gonadotrophin and unconjugated oestriol.[31] Such blood tests may be used as a screening for those who can be offered ultrasound examinations, amniocentesis or other intervention.

The blood testing of alpha-foetoprotein is most accurate when done between 16 and 18 weeks. When time is allowed for the return of the results it can be seen that any subsequent termination of pregnancy is late. In some cases it may be approaching the stage where survival would be possible if the foetus were delivered prematurely.

The administration of vitamin supplements and especially folic acid[32] can prevent neural tube defects.

Foetal blood sampling involves the removal of blood from the umbilical cord under ultrasound guidance. Complications that can occur include bleeding, local collection of blood, transient decrease in foetal heart rate, premature labour, abruptio placentae, or premature detachment of the placenta.[33]

I know of a woman of 25 years who had these blood tests at an early stage of pregnancy. She was unsure whether they were necessary but the expectation was she should have them. She would clearly have been considered unusual if she had declined and gave into the pressure from the hospital. The tests were abnormal and she was told that an amniocentesis was necessary. She was unsure whether to proceed because of the risk of death to the baby but decided she had to know. She spent several weeks of worry and anxiety before the amniocentesis result came back showing no abnormality. It was only at the stage of the amniocentesis that the hospital discussed the possibility of termination with her.

Amniocentesis [30]

This has an invasiveness of Category 3 due to the risk to the baby. This is a way of obtaining samples of amniotic fluid – the fluid surrounding the foetus in the uterus. It is performed at about 15-20 weeks. The sample is examined to detect foetal cells for determination of sex, chromosomal abnormalities and serious abnormalities such as spina bifida. It is offered mainly to women in their thirties and older, when foetal abnormalities do tend to be more common. It is only of use to those who would consider termination of pregnancy if the results were positive, since the risks to the baby subjected to testing would serve no purpose otherwise.

It is performed under ultrasound control so that the risk of damage by the needle to the foetus, placenta or maternal organs is minimised.

The procedure can involve discomfort as the needle is inserted into the uterus. Complications include miscarriage (1 per cent), neonatal respiratory difficulties, postural deformities and Rhesus sensitisation. After amniocentesis, a total of 5.7 per cent of pregnancies end in miscarriage, termination of pregnancy, stillbirth or neonatal death.

Chorionic villus sampling [35]

This has an invasiveness of Category 3 due to the risk to the baby. This is performed for the same reasons as amniocentesis. Samples of the chorion are obtained for examination. It is done by either a transabdominal approach similar to the method of amniocentesis or by a transcervical approach.

The risks of transcervical sampling are greater than those of the transabdominal approach. Whichever is performed, it is essential to determine that the operator is skilled in its use. Some experience is obtained by training on women undergoing termination of pregnancy.

Complications of this procedure include miscarriage (1-5 per cent for the transabdominal approach and 2.5-10 per cent for the transcervical approach), intrauterine infection, septic shock, Rhesus sensitisation and foetal abnormalities. Vaginal bleeding as evidenced by spotting is common and is seen in up to 60 per cent of women. There may be associated lower abdominal discomfort. If the bleeding is heavy then miscarriage occurs in 25-50 per cent of these cases. If mild vaginal bleeding occurs then there should be abstinence from sexual intercourse. Even if no bleeding occurs, abstinence for one week after the sampling is advisable. After chorionic villus sampling, a total of 7.2 per cent of pregnancies end in miscarriage, termination of pregnancy, stillbirth or neonatal death.

Chorionic villus sampling during the first nine weeks of pregnancy has a risk of causing limb deformities.[36] This is because the crucial time of limb development is nine weeks. No-one knows what damage is done to the placenta by this procedure. It has been recommended that it is not done until after 9 weeks.[37] As a consequence there is a move to bring amniocentesis forward from 16 weeks' gestation to 14 weeks or before. The result will be that a significant proportion of amniotic fluid will be removed at a critical stage of foetal lung development.

Joint aspiration

This has an invasiveness of Category 2. Fluid is removed from joints in cases of joint swelling. This may diagnose infective arthritis and gout. Treatment may also be given at the same by allowing drugs, e.g. corticosteroids to be injected into the joint. Removal of the fluid may also constitute treatment to relieve swelling or discomfort. Complications include infection (1 in 10,000), inflammation and increased risk of joint deterioration.

Pleural aspiration

This has an invasiveness of Category 3. Fluid is removed from the pleural cavity in cases of pleural effusion for examination and culture. Causes of pleural effusion include cancer, tuberculosis and mesothelioma.

Pleural biopsy

This has an invasiveness of Category 3. It is performed through the chest wall under local anaesthesia. It is positive in 60 per cent of cases of mesothelioma and 80 per cent of cases of tuberculosis.

Brain biopsy

This has an invasiveness of Category 3. Brain tissue from a frontal lobe is taken in cases of suspected inflammation and degeneration of the brain. Biopsy of brain tumours under CT scan is now commonly performed.

Liver biopsy

This has an invasiveness of Category 3. Liver tissue is obtained by needle biopsy through the abdominal wall. Local anaesthesia is used. Abnormalities detected include hepatitis, cirrhosis, tumours, and metabolic disease. Complications include bleeding into the peritoneal cavity (common) or biliary system, infection including septicaemia, pleurisy, and peritonitis. Death occurs in 2 per 100,000.

Renal biopsy

This has an invasiveness of Category 3. It is performed by needle through the loin whilst viewing with ultrasound. Abnormalities detected include glomerulonephritis and the causes of kidney failure. Complications include pain in the loin and shoulder tip, infection, haematuria (20 per cent), haematuria requiring blood transfusion (3 per cent), haematuria requiring surgical intervention or removal of kidney (0.5 per cent), death (0.1 per cent).

SUMMARY

Investigations are commonly used in many situations.

In some cases, investigations and treatment may be combined.

There are different levels of invasiveness and some investigations may lead to illness or death.

Everyone has the right to request a different investigation to obtain the same or similar information.

No investigation must be performed if it does not change the management of the case. The only exception to this may be the use of completely non-invasive tests that carry no risk of damage to the person.

---

[1] *Annals of Internal Medicine* 1991;114(5):432.

[2] There have been several studies that cast doubt on the oft-stated belief that screening leads to reduction in disease. Breast cancer investigations using mammography are a case in point where the incidence may be increased in the study group. This may be due to several factors such as trauma to the breast by mammography where the breast is squeezed between X-ray plates and the anxiety generated by the test, waiting for the result, recall for further investigation, false positive results. *Journal of Clinical Epidemiology* 1990;43(3):215-25 states that '.... for each woman who can derive a direct benefit in terms of a prevented breast cancer death, hundreds of women have to suffer the anxiety of a positive screening mammography. Moreover, it is possible that adverse effects of breast cancer screening may contribute to mortality from other causes.'

[3] The staging of malignant disease is discussed in Chapter 6.

[4] Normal here refers to the usual result. This explains why some people may have results slightly outside of the quoted range with no problems. Different laboratories may work to slightly differing ranges of normal.

[5] Doubts are occasionally expressed about the wisdom of routine ultrasound testing. The degree of anxiety generated is an important factor to consider particularly if the investigation reveals an abnormality of little significance, an abnormality for which there is no treatment, an abnormality which cannot be addressed until after delivery or an image which is difficult to interpret (this is becoming increasingly common as equipment is more sensitive). See *Journal of Family Practice* 1989;9(6):660-4 for a discussion on the routine use of ultrasound scans in pregnancy.

[6] *Report of the Royal College of Obstetricians and Gynaecology Working Party on Routine Ultrasound Examination in Pregnancy 1984* discusses the indications and risks of ultrasound.

[7] Bucher, Heiner C. *et al. British Medical Journal,* 1993;307(6895):13(5).

[8] Diagnostic Ultrasound Equipment Federal Register, Part III, 2 Feb. 1979. Animal studies of ultrasound examination reveal that there may be altered emotional behaviour, delayed muscle and nerve development, increased death rates and changes to the electroencephalogram.

[9] *The American Way of Birth* by Jessica Mitford (Gollancz, 1992). This is a thorough description of the medicalisation of the birth process as has occurred over the past 30-40 years. Ultrasound is discussed in clear detail on pages 103-106. This book is recommended reading for every pregnant couple and every practitioner dealing with pregnancy.

[10] Animal tests may show no effect but this does not mean that the same will be true in humans.

[11] Flynn 1982, Edmonds and Sancier 1983

[12] Suppression of immune response in mice after spleen exposed to diagnostic ultrasound (Anderson and Barrett, 1970).

[13] Disruption of platelets by use of continuous wave ultrasound. No effect on human platelets has been identified (Zarod and Williams, 1977).

[14] Increase in foetal abnormalities (exencephaly and skeletal abnormalities) in mice when exposed to continuous ultrasound at day 9 of gestation (Shoji *et al*, 1971 and Shimizu and Shoji, 1973).

[15] Weight reduction of foetus following exposure to ultrasound in utero (O'Brien, 1976, 1983, Fry *et al*, 1977, 1978, Stolzenberg *et al*, 1980).

[16] Affect on cell division of rat's liver (Kremkau and Witcowski, 1974).

[17] Increased chromosome fracturing after exposing human lymphocytes to diagnostic levels of ultrasound (MacIntosh and Davey, 1970).

[18] DNA changes in human lymphocytes exposed to diagnostic ultrasound (Liebeskind *et al*, 1979, Haupt, 1981)

[19] Alterations in reflexes and emotional and cognitive behaviour after continuous wave ultrasound (Murai *et al*, 1975).

[20] A survey of 10,000 babies in Canada showed some to be underweight (Bolsen, 1982).

[21] Comparison of 426 children who had prenatal ultrasound against control group of 381 from 1966 to 1972 revealed a higher rate of dyslexia in the ultrasound group. This was considered to be statistically 'insignificant' by the researchers.

[22] According to the Royal College of Obstetricians and Gynaecologists there are no studies to suggest an effect on the incidence of cancer. However, Dr Alice Stewart is currently conducting a study on 234,764 children who died of cancer between 1953 and 1981. She states 'an early examination of the data indicated that children above the age of 6 who were examined in utero by ultrasound have an increased risk of childhood cancer.'

Certainly the information above indicates effects on the immune system.

[23] An Australian study in 1993 showed that pregnant women who had frequent ultrasounds were more likely to give birth to underweight babies.

[24] A Norwegian trial showed that by the age of 8 or 9, children who had received prenatal ultrasound had a higher frequency of left-handedness.

[25] A study of 2600 women at Queen Charlotte's Hospital, Chelsea found that those who received routine ultrasound were more likely to have miscarriages – 17 deaths compared to 7 in the control group. *Lancet* 28th November, 1992.

[26] Ovarian ultrasound may precipitate premature ovulation. Testart *et al, British Journal of Obstetrics and Gynaecology,* 1982.

[27] *Subtle Energy* by John Davidson (C.W. Daniel, 1987). This is a clear account of energies as described by various medical systems as well as discussing planetary energy. The problems caused by pollution due to radiation of all types including electromagnetic are described in Chapter 4. Also see *Electromagnetic Man* by Cyril Smith and Simon Best (J.M. Dent, 1990)

[28] Chueh, Jane, *et al. The Western Journal of Medicine* 1993;159(3):308(4).

[29] Tests may give false-negative results. That is, they suggest normality when the foetus is abnormal. Effects in this direction include foetus older than expected, multiple pregnancy, low weight of the mother (less than 90 lb) and race. Women of African extraction have normally higher levels.

False-positive results may also be found in about 5 per cent of cases. That is, abnormality is suggested when the foetus is normal. Effects in this direction include foetus younger than expected, insulin-dependent diabetes mellitus in the mother and her being overweight.

[30] This is one of several conditions that are known as neural tube defects. The others are acrania (anencephaly) and encephalocele.

In the United States, the incidence of neural tube defects is 1 to 2 per 1,000 births.

[31] See Rose, Nancy C. *et al. The Western Journal of Medicine* 1993;159(3):312(6) for a discussion of their uses.

[32] Results of the Medical Research Council Vitamin Study. *Lancet* 1991;338:131-137.

[33] Ghidini, Alessandro, *et al. American Journal of Obstetrics and Gynecology,* 1993;168(5):1339(6).

[34] *Prenatal Diagnosis in Obstetric Practice*, Ed. by MJ Whittle and JM Connor (Blackwell, 1989)

[35] *Prenatal Diagnosis in Obstetric Practice*, Ed. by MJ Whittle and JM Connor (Blackwell, 1989). *A Practical Guide to Chorionic Villus Sampling* by David Liu (Oxford University Press, 1991)

[36] Saul, Helen. *New Scientist* 1993;138(1868):12(2).

[37] *Lancet;* 341:468.

5 INFECTIOUS DISEASE

INTRODUCTION

I have included some infectious diseases in this Chapter. Most can be found in their corresponding chapter according to their main symptoms. For example, acute bronchitis is in Chapter 8 – Respiratory system, skin infections are in Chapter 11 – Dermatology and so on.

Infections are considered by conventional medicine to be of great importance in causing disease. The idea of a transmissible agent, which people 'catch', has existed since the beginning of time and such ideas have attained almost supernormal significance. Large amounts of energy and time are spent studying tiny organisms and inventing new ways to kill them. Infection and its control hold the Western world in a mystical spell.

Lucretius who lived 99-55 BC said: 'Invisible animals enter via the nose and mouth and cause difficult diseases.' Before the discovery of bacteria, it was known that removing pump handles from contaminated wells during a cholera epidemic could stop the spread of the disease.

With the discovery of organisms in the latter half of the 19th century, there seemed to be incontrovertible evidence that these cause disease. Pasteur's theories of disease causation by infectious agents known as bacteria (viruses and other organisms were added later as they were discovered) were generally accepted and conventional medicine holds the views that destruction of these will lead to recovery. This has led to the development of pasteurisation, vaccination, antibiotics and a whole system of medicine that is geared to the detection of external agents.

Antoine Bechamp,[1] a contemporary of Pasteur, suggested that organisms already exist in tissues and are not a problem until there is a change in the immune system[2] that would allow such organisms to cause disease. This viewpoint has been suppressed. For the practitioner of holistic medicine, such ideas are of great interest since they support the view that it is the immune system, the energy of the person, which is the important factor.

Koch, who discovered the TB bacterium, postulated four things that should always be true in an infectious disease:

- the organism must always be present in all cases of the disease
- the organism should be obtainable and it should be possible to grow it in a culture
- organisms from such cultures must produce the disease when injected into a healthy person
- the organism must be recoverable from that person.

Even if these four statements were always true,[3] there is one vital component that is not given any importance and that is the person themselves. Why is it that in any epidemic there are certain people who are exposed but who do not contract the disease? Why is it that if people do contract the disease, it takes different forms with each of them? The answer of course is that each person's condition is different and it is this that is of overriding importance in the discussion of infectious diseases. It was this very thought that led Pasteur to say later in life: 'The condition is everything, the germ is nothing.'

It is a common observation that organisms, of the exact type associated with disease, are found in normal, healthy individuals. People only become ill when some other factor occurs. Susceptibility, therefore, is the preceding state that leads to the appearance of disease that is called infectious. The organism is very much the secondary phenomenon.

The original work of Bechamp included the observation that there are tiny organisms present in all tissues as well as supposedly inanimate matter such as chalk. He called them microzymas or small bodies. Subsequently, other workers have described such bodies including Rife[4] who invented a microscope capable of observing living tissue at many times the usual magnification and Gaston Naessens.[5]

Naessens, a French biologist, has found that there are tiny particles in living tissue that have a life cycle. These are almost certainly the microzymas of Bechamp. By careful observation, they can be discovered in tissues of healthy people but in people with disease states they can be observed to undergo an abnormal life cycle. In this case, they can take on the appearances of bacteria, viruses or fungi depending upon the stage of their development. The prerequisite for this is a disordered immune system. Recovery is associated with the disappearance of the abnormal forms.

This flies in the face of the conventional view, which states that bacteria, viruses, and fungi cannot change from one form into the other. They are considered to be fixed. The discoveries of Bechamp, Rife and Naessens reveal that this is not true. Organisms arise from material in the body, as well as existing in many other places, and are capable of dynamic change.

The consequence of this misunderstanding of the origin of 'infection' is that chemicals are given to kill organisms and vaccination is given in an attempt to prevent their existence. In reality, it is not the organism that is the problem. It is only the result of a prior imbalance. The true cause is a disturbance in the energetic state of the person, this is then followed by the appearance of symptoms. If a doctor discovers an organism in someone, this is regarded as the cause to be attacked. If not, then some other reason is suggested for the cause of the inflammation. Other drugs may be given, e.g. corticosteroids, anti-inflammatory agents or antihistamines. Conventional medicine has been diverted down a blind alley.

In energetic medicine, for example, traditional Chinese medicine, it *is* possible to talk about external pathogenic factors such as WindHeat or WindCold or DampHeat invading the body and causing disease. These are not the same as bacteria or viruses and they more importantly describe the internal condition of the person. The symptoms of such external pathogenic factors are manifest on the surface of the body and it does not necessarily mean that the problem has come from the outside. It is the balance of the relative strengths of pathogenic factor and the Qi or vital energy of the body that is the important question.

These ideas are clearly illustrated by the following quotation:

'Shao Yu replied: The wind generated by the heaven is fair and square to all the people without discrimination, but those who offend it will be under attack and those who avoid it will be free from attack. Therefore, people become sick, not because of the vicious energy of the wind which comes to attack, but rather because they themselves offend the wind.' [6]

This is why antibiotics which lead to continuance of the pathogenic factor in the body and vaccination which is the deliberate introduction of the pathogenic factor into the body and at deep levels result in ill health.

A further example of Chinese thought may help to illustrate these ideas.

'Chi Po replied: Wind, rain, cold, and heat cannot harm the human body unless the latter is already in deficiency. Some people do not become sick in the face of sudden gale and rainstorm, because they are not in deficiency so that the vicious energies cannot do them any harm. When people become sick due to external energies, it is because their bodies are already in deficiency so that they are susceptible to the attack of deficiency energies which come to reside in their bodies as guests.' [7]

There may be several sequelae of 'exposure to infecting organisms' and the same is true for the consequences of vaccination – Table 5.1.

Not susceptible	Susceptible
No disease – so no symptoms	Strong symptoms – defence system strong and likely to have successfully thrown off the invasion.
	Mild illness – weak reaction by defence system so organism is not thrown off. Likelihood of chronic disease. Mild symptoms can also indicate mild problem. Differentiation is by careful questioning and determining the general state of health.[8]
	Complications such as meningitis, otitis media weak – defence system that is somewhat overwhelmed. If death does not intervene then health may be affected chronically.

Table 5.1: Energetic view of consequences of contact with 'infecting organism'

In energetic medicine, because the person is seen to be an interconnected whole, there are different levels at which disease may manifest and to which it may descend. It would seem to be more important to emphasise climatic factors, their influence on health and the person's underlying energetic condition, than the nature of infecting organisms. I shall return to these ideas later when dealing with specific diseases such as the common cold. The six climatic factors are heat, cold, damp, wind, dryness and summer heat.

ACUTE AND CHRONIC DISEASE

Acute disease may be defined as a disease of rapid onset and short duration (usually with strong symptoms) that either ends in recovery or death. People who have an acute disease know that they are ill. It is clear cut and indicates that the person is of relatively strong energy. For an acute manifestation to take place there must be strong energy in the system. This is why children tend to have acute illnesses since their energy is strong.

Chronic disease can be defined as a disease of slow onset and long duration that ends in gradual deterioration of health. The symptoms are more vague than those of an acute problem. This picture indicates that the person's energy is weaker. There are some instances of very few symptoms despite serious chronic disease, e.g. elderly people with bronchopneumonia may have little in the way of cough or fever. They may only present with breathlessness or perhaps confusion.

There are diseases that do not fit easily into either category and these are usually the acute manifestations of a chronic illness. I would argue that in fact virtually all acute disease is a manifestation of a chronic imbalance and to only treat the acute manifestation will not lead to removal of the chronic problem. However there are some diseases which are clearly acute in nature and I would put the childhood infectious diseases in that category.

Conventional views of infection

Conventional medical textbooks classify infectious disease according to the causative organism. This is in accordance with the belief that such organisms are fixed, unchanging entities. For the holistic practitioner this is not a helpful method since you are not going to treat the organism.

Organisms
There are several which are considered capable of causing infection.

- bacteria – cocci, e.g. staphylococci, streptococci, pneumococci (pneumonia), gonococci (gonorrhoea), meningococci (meningitis); bacilli, e.g. tetanus; spirochaetes, e.g. syphilis; vibrio, e.g. cholera
- viruses, e.g. measles, mumps, rubella, chickenpox, influenza, polio
- fungus, e.g. Candida ('thrush'), tinea (ringworm)
- protozoa, e.g. trichomonas, giardia, amoeba, malaria
- parasites, e.g. worms. This is technically an infestation but it is useful for our purposes to consider with the above.

Mode of transmission
Certain diseases are thought to be spread in particular ways. These depend primarily upon the site of the disease. For example, respiratory disease will be mainly spread through sneezing or coughing, bowel disease through contact with faeces.

- droplet spread, e.g. sneezing, coughing, dust. Diseases include influenza, whooping cough, pulmonary tuberculosis, common cold
- contamination of food/water. Diseases include gastroenteritis, dysentery, cholera, typhoid, polio
- implantation including wound contamination. Diseases include skin conditions caused by streptococci and staphylococci, tetanus
- direct contact. Diseases include scabies and the sexually transmitted diseases of syphilis and gonorrhoea
- injection into the body, e.g. injections, insects. Diseases include HIV infection, hepatitis, malaria, yellow fever. I would include transplacental spread here since the mode of transmission is similar, i.e. via the blood. Diseases include rubella, syphilis, HIV infection.

Incubation period
The incubation period is the time between invasion of the organism and the development of symptoms. It may be of importance in informing people of the natural history of an infectious disease. They are often variable and you will see times such as 7-10 days. This would seem to confirm that it is the person rather than the organism that is the important factor.

Notification of infectious disease
There are certain infectious diseases that are notified to the Department of Health in the UK. This only applies to registered medical practitioners and does not affect holistic practitioners. The reason for notification is to compile the incidence of infectious disease as well as instituting specific public health measures, if necessary.

Public health legislation and its observance is an important factor in the prevention of disease as it stops the contamination of water and food as well as laying down standards for living and working conditions.

HOLISTIC CLASSIFICATION OF INFECTIOUS DISEASE

The important factors in deciding upon a classification are the underlying state of health of the person and the site of manifestation of the symptoms. These are interconnected and lead to disease appearing at a particular level in the individual.

There are several diseases of childhood that are universal and they are necessary for normal development. The immune system requires exposure to experiences to aid maturation just as we need other kinds of experience to help our mental and emotional development. The diseases of measles, mumps, rubella and chickenpox are essential for the healthy development of our immunity. The practice of mass vaccination naturally has consequences for the immune system since it will be weakened if these illnesses are suppressed. Such a practice leads to the development of other disease, perhaps more serious, at a later date.

Other diseases are the result of disordered immunity and occur in susceptible people. These include streptococcal infections, glandular fever, herpes zoster, myalgic encephalomyelitis (ME) and AIDS. The depth at which they occur reflects the energy of the person, i.e. the state of the immune system. Table 5.2 illustrates the application of these ideas to a list of infectious diseases with superficial, acute disease at the top and deep, internal, chronic disease at the bottom. Consider this merely as a guide to deciding on the severity of the problem and not as a rigid plan to be applied at all costs. People with strong energy manifest disease that is associated with clear bacterial illnesses such as scarlet fever (streptococci) or boils (staphylococci) that are relatively 'old-fashioned' now. The newer diseases such as AIDS, legionnaire's disease, non-specific urethritis are associated with strange, unusual organisms.

Acute disease, strong energy

Childhood illnesses – rubella, measles, chickenpox, mumps: normal
Common cold
Staphylococcal infections, e.g. boils – localised superficial problems
Streptococcal infections, e.g. impetigo, cellulitis – spreading superficial problems
Influenza
Glandular fever – acute attack mainly causing sore throat and enlarged neck glands
Acute bronchitis
Pneumonia
Glandular fever – chronic attack with chronic debility and weakness
Myalgic encephalomyelitis
Tuberculosis
Syphilis
Acquired Immune Deficiency Syndrome

Chronic disease, weak energy

Table 5.2: Classification of infectious disease according to energetic principles

NORMAL CHILDHOOD ILLNESSES [9]

Measles

This is an almost universal disease of childhood with epidemics every second year. Passive immunity is obtained from the mother (provided she herself has natural immunity) particularly if the child is breast-fed. Most cases occur in childhood. The incubation period is 10-14 days. It is the strongest of the childhood illnesses of this type and is responsible for a high mortality in countries where malnourishment is common.

Symptoms
Firstly there is a catarrhal stage that is common to all the infectious fevers of childhood. There is fever, runny nose, sneezing and a harsh irritant cough. The eyes are invariably affected with swollen eyelids, red and sore eyes (conjunctivitis). There may be photophobia. At this stage it is very difficult to distinguish from the common cold. There are, however, the presence of Koplik's spots which are tiny areas the size and appearance of a grain of salt with surrounding inflammation. They are present in the mouth on the mucosa opposite the upper molars. They appear around 3-5 days before the rash.

The rash arrives around day 3-5, begins behind the ears and rapidly spreads to the sides of the neck, forehead, face and then the trunk and limbs. As the rash appears the fever subsides and the child becomes subjectively improved. The eruption is pink at first and deepens to a dull or purplish red. As it does so the appearance becomes more papular and areas coalesce into larger patches. There is generalised lymph node enlargement. The process from appearance of the rash takes place over about 24-48 hours and then fades to a brownish colour. By the end of 7-10 days the rash has gone.

Complications

Complication	Symptoms to look for
Febrile convulsions	Increasing fever, irritability, stiff neck, photophobia, twitching
Pneumonia	Cough, breathlessness, increasing fever
Otitis media	Earache, fever remains high
Corneal ulceration	Continuing eye symptoms which worsen, pain in the eye

Table 5.3: Complications of measles

Treatment

There is no specific conventional treatment. Antibiotics will be used in cases of complications. Some practitioners use antibiotics in uncomplicated cases of measles to 'prevent' further infection such as otitis media or pneumonia. This practice is dangerous as any infection which does then occur will be by organisms resistant to that antibiotic. This is in addition to the usual side-effects of antibiotics. Vaccination is administered as part of the MMR (measles, mumps and rubella) vaccine – see Page 66.

Holistic management

Measles is an almost invariable event of childhood or at least used to be until vaccination altered the pattern of its development. It is necessary for the normal development of the immune system. If it does not appear, is only mild (perhaps the rash does not fully appear) or treated with conventional medication, there may be problems later with other, more chronic disease. A healthy immune system will experience this condition at the appropriate time, i.e. during childhood. A common observation is that childhood diseases in adult life commonly lead to complications.

Treatment is not often needed since it is a normal disease of childhood and there is no need to interfere if progress is normal. I would treat if the eruption of the rash was not full or stopped emerging. A continuing fever and feelings of ill health will accompany this. In these cases there is a risk that either a complication will appear or future health problems. If children have a simple, naturopathic approach or are treated with homoeopathy or acupuncture they seem to be better after the illness than before. It is as if they have been exposed to an experience that they have passed with success.

Children who have had antibiotics during the course of measles undoubtedly take longer to recover to full health, regain energy and appetite. Some may go on to develop syndromes of 'never well since' with a variety of manifestations. These complications, as well as problems in the ears, eyes and lungs, are prevented by prompt treatment by holistic medicine. Similar difficulties occur in children who are debilitated prior to the illness.

In terms of Chinese medicine, this illness is due to Wind-heat invasion. This does not mean that the problem comes from the outside but that the manifestation is on the exterior of the body. It is due to the release of heat toxins that gathered during the time in the uterus.

Measles vaccination as with all vaccines, weakens the immune system because this avenue of expression has been removed. Some cases of encephalitis, multiple sclerosis and other neurological disorders are linked to previous infection with the measles virus.[10]

Mumps

This is a viral illness that may go unrecognised because it can be mild in its manifestations. The incubation period is 18-24 days. It affects young children and adults and is very unusual before the age of 2 years. The main areas affected are the salivary glands, central nervous system and endocrine glands such as the pancreas, ovaries and testes.

Symptoms

The beginning of the illness is non-specific with fever, headache and poor appetite. Pain at the angle of the jaw heralds the development of parotid salivary gland swelling. This is usually bilateral but is occasionally one-sided. There is swelling of the three groups of salivary glands – parotid, sub-mandibular and sublingual although the parotid is the classical site and usually the most noticeable. Dry mouth with a coated tongue is a key feature.

The illness is more severe in adults and there may be a few days of fever, shivering and stiffness in the jaw before the glandular enlargement. In this post-pubertal group the gonads are affected with the male affected much more than the female. One in four such males will develop orchitis and if this is bilateral then infertility is a risk. This is extremely rare.

There is pain and swelling of the testis with or without a high fever and there may be mental symptoms of a mild delirium or depression.

The central nervous system may be affected with the development of meningitis or encephalitis. It is the commonest viral cause of encephalitis. It is easy to see how mumps vaccination may be implicated in nervous system disease including autism. The symptoms include headache, delirium and hallucinations. The nervous system manifestations may be the only evidence of mumps – 30 per cent with these symptoms have no salivary gland symptoms. There can be paralysis due to affection of the cranial or peripheral nerves and this can be permanent.

Pancreatic involvement is evidenced by pain in the epigastrium, vomiting and anorexia. There may also be endocrine involvement in some with glycosuria, which may persist into the convalescent phase. Rarely the heart, liver, joints and breasts may be involved.

Complications

Complication	Symptoms to look for
Orchitis	Pain and swelling in testes – affects 25 per cent of those affected who are post-pubertal. Sterility may occur if both testes are involved. This is very unusual and in any case is virtually always transient
Pancreatitis	Epigastric pain radiating through to the back. Vomiting
Oophoritis	Iliac fossa pain in females. Only if post-pubertal
Meningitis, encephalitis	Occipital headache, neck stiffness, photophobia

Table 5.4: Complications of mumps

Treatment
There is no specific conventional treatment although corticosteroids may be given for the complications that are usually seen in adults. Care of the mouth is important. Mumps vaccination is given part of the MMR (measles, mumps, rubella) vaccine – see Page 66.

Holistic management
The general comments I made with regard to measles are relevant here. Care of the mouth is particularly important in cases of mumps because the salivary glands are affected causing dry mouth. It is interesting to note that it is glandular tissue of varying types that is particularly affected in this illness.

In terms of Chinese medicine, this is a case of Invasion of Wind-heat of Shaoyang type leading to Stagnation of Qi (swelling behind the ears). In most cases it is mild with little constitutional upset.

Rubella

This is also a viral disease that can be mild with about 50 per cent of cases going unrecognised particularly in the under fives. The peak incidence is at 15 years of age. Prior to vaccination, most cases occured in childhood so that by the age of 18-20 years around 80 per cent of people had had it. The incubation period is 2-3 weeks. The person is infective from 1 week before the rash appears until 4 days after it appears.

Symptoms
Usually the rash is the first indication of the disease although adults may suffer more systemic symptoms with an initial illness of painful stiff neck, headache and general malaise for 24 hours. Some people may have a mild conjunctivitis or sore throat with slight redness of the soft palate and inside of the mouth. There is generalised enlargement of the lymph glands but especially the sub-occipital and post-cervical groups. If there is marked lymph gland enlargement the spleen may be palpable.

The rash is small, discrete, pink and macular. The spots are around 1-3 mm in diameter. They are seen first on the face and neck rapidly spreading to the trunk. It rarely lasts more than 24-48 hours.

Complications

Complication	Symptoms to look for
Arthritis	Pain and swelling of small joints in the hands and feet. Appears in adults by around 7 days, may be severe for a few days but subsides by 3-4 weeks
Meningo-encephalitis	Headache, neck stiffness, photophobia
Foetal abnormalities	There is a risk of foetal abnormality if a pregnant woman contracts the disease due to congenital rubella syndrome – 20 cases per year in the UK with 362 confirmed infections in 1987.[11] The risk varies from 70 per cent during the first 4 weeks to virtually zero at 4 months. It causes low birth weight, delayed teething, microcephaly, cataract, deafness and congenital heart defects. A termination of pregnancy is offered in these cases

Table 5.5: Complications of rubella

Treatment
There is no specific conventional treatment. Rubella vaccination is given as part of the MMR (measles, mumps, rubella) vaccine – see Page 66.

Holistic management
The general comments made under measles are also relevant here. Rubella is mild in virtually all cases. The issue is around mass vaccination aimed at preventing rubella in females of childbearing age. It seems expensive to routinely vaccinate every female when most of them will contract rubella naturally.

There is no attempt made to assess immune status prior to vaccination so most will be unnecessary both from a financial and a medical viewpoint. There is no hard evidence that artificial rubella immunity lasts for a significant period of time. It may only last for a few years in which case it increases the risk of women contracting the disease during their childbearing years – the very situation to be avoided. A much better idea is to have rubella 'parties' where any cases of rubella in the area invite other children to meet them and pass it on naturally. Rubella is one of the normal childhood diseases necessary for healthy development and seems to protect against arthritis in later life. Women planning to conceive should be encouraged to verify that they are rubella immune.

In terms of Chinese medicine, this is similar to measles in that it an attack of Wind-heat Invasion.

Chickenpox

This is a viral illness also known as varicella and is associated with the same organism as herpes zoster (shingles). It is possible to contract chickenpox from a case of herpes zoster and vice versa. It usually appears in the 5-15 years age group. The incubation period is 14-21 days.

Symptoms
In children the first sign is usually the appearance of an itchy rash but in adults there may be a short constitutional upset. Adults tend to have a more severe version of the illness. People who receive corticosteroids or immunosuppressants are in particular badly affected. Chickenpox is the feared infectious disease in units treating childhood leukaemia where an infection may prove fatal due to the suppression of the immune system implicit in the conventional treatment of the disease.

All herpes infections have similar rashes. The first appearance is that of a macule which, over a period of 18-24 hours goes through the stages of papule, vesicle and pustule. The rash is more marked on the trunk and in areas such as the axilla. The mucous membrane of the mouth is also affected. New spots continue to appear throughout the illness so cropping is seen – spots at different stages.

Complications

Complication	Symptoms to look for
Skin infections	Redness around the pustules and more discharge. In very severe cases there is bleeding into the vesicles
Encephalitis	Occipital headache, neck stiffness, photophobia
Pneumonia	High fever, cough, breathlessness, the child is ill. Rare in children but 20 per cent of adults may develop respiratory symptoms

Table 5.6: Complications of chickenpox

Treatment

There is no specific conventional treatment. Symptomatic treatment by bathing and keeping the skin clean is important for prevention of skin infection. Antibiotics will be given if there is such infection. Chickenpox vaccination – see Page 70 – has been available since 1995 and is available in the USA. It is currently only available in frozen form and as most GP surgeries in the UK do not have freezers it is not yet used there.

Holistic management

The general comments made about measles are also relevant here. This is a useful illness from an holistic point of view since it usually mild, there is no vaccination currently available and there is no conventional treatment. It is innocuous in most people.

In terms of Chinese medicine, this is caused by an Invasion of Damp-Heat.

Whooping cough

This disease is different from the 'normal' childhood illnesses discussed above because it involves a degree of disordered immunity in order to develop in the first place. It is frequently mild in the West although may be debilitating. Excellent treatments exist by methods of holistic medicine.

Whooping cough is associated with the bacteria, *Bordetella pertussis*. There is an epidemic every 3-4 years with any age affected but especially children. The greatest risk to children is during the first year of life when it may be life-threatening. The incubation period is 8-14 days.

Symptoms

The initial symptoms are those of a catarrhal nature with runny nose, red, sore and watery eyes and a harsh cough. This is a common picture of many childhood illnesses and is relatively non-specific. The child becomes progressively more 'mucoussy' and the cough worsens.

After 7-10 days the typical paroxysms of coughing appear. They last for several minutes and the child becomes red in the face (blue in severe attacks). There may be subconjunctival haemorrhages at this time with ruptured blood vessels in the conjunctivae leading to the appearance of bright red areas there. Nosebleeds may also occur.

An attack usually ends in retching or vomiting. It is here that the characteristic whoop is heard which is a sharp inhalation of breath after a prolonged bout of coughing. The whoop is not common and is more likely to be heard in severe cases or in very young children (less than 1 year).

At this time the child is actually less infective although thoroughly miserable with swollen eyelids and a constant sticky nasal discharge. The paroxysms are precipitated by factors such as cold air, smoky atmosphere, stress, sudden noises and posture. They are classically worse at night at around 2-3 am. The attacks are maximal around the third week and subside by 6-7 weeks. The cough may return with any subsequent upper respiratory tract infection for up to a year later.

Complications

Complication	Symptoms to look for
Otitis media	Pain in the ear, fever remains high or returns, redness of eardrum
Pneumonia	High fever, cough, breathlessness, the child is ill
Cerebral haemorrhage	Headache, central nervous system symptoms such as paralysis, numbness
Convulsions	Unconsciousness, jerking of limbs

Table 5.7: Complications of whooping cough

Treatment

There is no specific conventional treatment available. Antibiotics are usually given to eradicate the bacterium responsible. Such conventional treatment does not affect the symptoms and the only help offered is cough remedies which are of limited benefit or the treatment of complications. Whooping cough vaccination is administered as part of the DPT (diphtheria, pertussis, tetanus) vaccination – see Page 66.

Holistic management

I would always treat whooping cough since it is due to a pre-existing lung weakness. It is very amenable to treatment by holistic medicine. I have seen children who have had problems for weeks and yet find that a single homoeopathic remedy can cure the cough almost overnight. Holistic treatment is more difficult if the child has received antibiotics. If the illness has been long-term then treatment of any underlying lung condition may have to be undertaken after the acute episode has subsided.

In terms of Chinese medicine, this is known as 'hundred day cough' and reflects the duration of many cases. It is considered to be due to Wind-heat invading the Lung leading to Phlegm-fire in the Lung.

CHRONIC INFECTIOUS DISEASE

In this section, I have listed four diseases. They are good examples of chronic disease associated with organisms. They illustrate the point that what is important is the depth of the pathology not the supposed organism which may or may not be present. Other infectious diseases are described in their relevant chapter.

Glandular fever

This is a viral illness associated with a herpes-like organism called the Epstein–Barr virus. It affects people mainly in the 15-25 year age group. The incubation period is variable; 1-4 months but often 4-20 days. Although many people are exposed to the virus only a few develop symptoms.

Symptoms

The onset may be gradual or sudden. There is a fever of around 104°F (40°C) and a sore throat sometimes with a membrane over the tonsils. The degree of discomfort is more than with the usual tonsillitis and swallowing may be difficult and painful. Lymph gland enlargement is generalised but more marked in the neck. The glands are usually tender. The spleen is palpable in one third to one half of cases. For this reason anyone with glandular fever must avoid all sports. Ruptured spleen is an unusual complication but may be fatal.

Rashes are seen in around 5 per cent of cases and can take several forms. Macules may appear at the end of week one and resemble rubella whilst some develop petechiae on the hard and soft palates. The fever is of variable duration. Jaundice occurs in around 5 per cent although liver involvement is present in virtually all cases as evidenced by liver function tests becoming abnormal. Chronic tiredness is said to occur in about 15 per cent of cases (according to the textbooks) but in my experience it is much more common.

Complications

Complication	Symptoms to look for
Meningitis, encephalitis	Occipital headache, photophobia, neck stiffness
Peripheral neuritis (rare)	Tingling and numbness in the hands and feet
Mesenteric adenitis	Abdominal pain resembling appendicitis
Haemolytic anaemia	Jaundice, pallor, tiredness and other symptoms of anaemia
Rupture of spleen (very rare)	Severe abdominal pain, shock with low blood pressure, rapid and thready pulse

Table 5.8: Complications of glandular fever

Investigation

The white cell count shows atypical monocytes in most cases. Eighty per cent of cases show a positive reaction to the Paul-Bunnell test. One fifth of people never become positive.

Treatment

There is no specific conventional treatment. It is supportive only although antibiotics are usually given. Penicillin causes the appearance of a rash in over 90 per cent of cases with an associated marked debility. In the US this can lead to charges of negligence for which there is no legal defence.

Holistic management

In terms of Chinese medicine, this is an Invasion of Damp-heat. Most cases occur in students either at school or university. It seems to be a result of excessive work and study as well as emotional stress particularly about examinations and career choices. This combination of factors typically depletes Spleen (digestive) energy and so makes the body susceptible to such an invasion.

Treatment needs to be aimed at these underlying factors as well as the acute manifestations. Typically the acute illness subsides into a chronic period of ill health lasting anything from a few weeks to many months. The distinction between this and conditions such as ME and post-viral fatigue syndromes in general is rather blurred.

Consideration of many aspects of life such as diet, relaxation and rest, attitudes to work and study as well as relationship issues can all be helpful.

The diagnosis may not be clear because the 'tests' are normal and it may be difficult to distinguish between this and ME. In fact the label is unimportant since the causes are similar and diagnosis and treatment is taking place on an energetic basis (by homoeopathy, acupuncture and so on).

I have treated people who have tested positive for glandular fever. As their condition fluctuated with relapses due to stressful situations the tests have also fluctuated. Tests tend to be negative at times of good health and positive at times of poor health. This is difficult to understand conventionally as in conventional thought you either have something or you do not.

Herpes infections

Herpes viruses are related and lead to a group of diseases that are recognised by the nature of the rash. This goes through the stages of macule, papule, vesicle, pustule and scab. Herpes diseases tend to become chronic so chickenpox may lead to *herpes zoster* in later life and *herpes simplex* is recurrent.

Herpes simplex

There are two types of *herpes simplex* depending upon the area affected. Type I affects the lips and around the mouth and is the typical 'cold sore' with which most of us are familiar. It recurs with tiredness and upper respiratory tract infections.

Type II affects the genital area and buttocks and has been more frequent since the 1970s. It is transmitted via sexual contact. It typically recurs when there is tiredness, overwork or as a result of sexual activity.

Treatment
Mild cases are untreated. High protection factor sunscreens are recommended to those who suffer a flare-up with the sun. Anti-viral agents such as acyclovir, valacyclovir and famciclovir are now available for this condition and they seem to prevent appearance of the rash in some people. They are taken orally. Acyclovir is also available as a cream to be used locally. The rash may then 'leak' out to appear at the edges of where the drug is applied topically. Some people would probably have to apply it all over their bodies to prevent it! Others may find that the rash does not appear but they develop internal problems in the bowel, lungs or brain. No conventional treatment prevents future attacks.

Holistic management
In terms of Chinese medicine, all the herpes viruses cause conditions considered to be Damp-heat in nature. Type I is an affection of the Stomach where the Damp-heat flares up into the Stomach channel and Type II is Damp-heat invading the Liver channel. Suppression by acyclovir may lead to conditions of internal Damp-heat. Some cases of herpes simplex correspond to invasion of the Lung and Stomach Channels by Wind.

Treatment needs to be constitutional in nature and results are usually very impressive for such conditions. You would expect this to be so since they manifest on the skin and are therefore relatively superficial.

Herpes zoster

This is a disease of the skin that is related to chickenpox as the same virus is involved. In this case the virus irritates the posterior root (sensory) ganglion of the spinal cord and so produces symptoms in the distribution of that nerve. The thoracic or lumbar area is usually involved but any area from the head to the lower limb may be affected.

The disease is also known as shingles and is typified by the appearance of a vesicular rash (classical herpes appearance) in the distribution of the posterior nerve root of one or more segments of the spinal cord. It may also be seen in the area of distribution of the fifth cranial (trigeminal) nerve.

It occurs mainly in the middle-aged and elderly and is triggered by stress or other episodes that lead to lowered immunity.

Some cases occur after a shock (such as a fall or bereavement), others occur in people with an underlying malignancy or pneumonia.

Symptoms

There is an initial illness of mild constitutional disturbance and fever. Pain develops in the affected areas and at this stage the symptoms may be mistaken for any number of conditions ranging from musculo-skeletal problems to heart attack. After 4 days the rash appears which passes through the typical stages of a herpes infection – macules, papules, vesicles and pustules. These rupture leaving dry, crusting areas. These may separate and leave white anaesthetic areas. The disease is usually one-sided.

As the rash appears the pain worsens and becomes neuralgic in nature. There is a continual burning soreness that is worse for contact or there may be an intermittent stabbing. Itching is seen in some people. Some cases persist and lead to post-herpetic neuralgia. This is a particularly debilitating condition since the pain is virtually continual.

The ophthalmic division of the fifth cranial nerve may be affected especially in the elderly, which in turn affects the conjunctiva and cornea. This may lead to keratitis and severe damage to sight.

Post-herpetic scars are usually permanently analgesic and in some cases the muscles of the affected area may be involved leading to paralysis which is also usually permanent.

Treatment

In recent years acyclovir, valaciclovir and famciclovir have been used to treat herpes infections such as simplex and zoster (see above). They are recommended orally in cases of facial shingles, those with immune suppression or in severe attacks where the sufferer is over the age of 50. Analgesics may also be given. In some cases, corticosteroids and antibiotics may also be given. People with herpes zoster require two weeks or so off work, partly due to the systemic nature of the illness and because they are infective.

Holistic management

Early treatment with acupuncture is well recognised as a means of preventing the complications of post-herpetic neuralgia. Holistic treatment will help the symptoms, which sometimes are severe.

Attention may have to be paid to the underlying condition since shingles occurs in people who already have some imbalance due to shock, an injury, emotional stress and so on.

Myalgic encephalomyelitis (ME)

This is also known as post-viral fatigue syndrome, post-viral syndrome and Royal Free disease. It is a relatively new disease although it was first described in 1934. It seems to be more common as the years pass and affecting younger people. Some conventional practitioners deny its existence but with increasing awareness and the presence of support groups, it is being taken more seriously. Many conventional textbooks still do not even mention it. It may occur in epidemics. It is a vague, ill-defined disease in many people.

Women seem to be three times more prone to its development than men. It chiefly affects the 30-40 years age group. It typically begins after an upper respiratory or gastrointestinal tract infection from which the person does not make a full recovery.

Symptoms

These can be vague and ill defined which reflects the underlying weakness of the person's energy. Muscle fatigue and pain are common with general malaise. The tiredness may, on occasions, be severe. Some people remain in bed all day and literally can do nothing. Others have to use wheel chairs because they are too weak to walk.

Headache, dizziness and fainting attacks may occur. The extremities are cold. Gastrointestinal symptoms include nausea, flatulence and diarrhoea. Mentally, there are problems with memory and concentration. The emotions are unstable with outbursts of anger or weeping. Sleep disturbance is common – either difficulty getting off to sleep or continual waking during the night. A rather unusual symptom is hyperacusis (sensitivity to sound), which is commonly seen with withdrawal syndromes from tranquillisers. The key, as always, is the individual and the symptom picture will vary from person to person.

In common with most chronic diseases, people with ME can be broadly divided into three groups depending upon their progress:

1. Recovery after a variable length of time.
2. Remissions for years with relapses at times of undue physical or mental stress.
3. Chronic progressive disability.

These groups reveal the state of energy of each person with those in the first group being the strongest and those in the last being the weakest.

Diagnosis

Conventional physical examination is normal as are laboratory tests and so the diagnosis is one of exclusion. In some people there may be evidence of a recent infection, usually viral. The commonest ones seen are Coxsackie A and B, echo and Epstein–Barr viruses. The latter is associated with glandular fever.

Treatment

There may be several approaches depending upon who is treating the person. People may be given antibiotics if there is evidence of any continuing infection (although this is more likely to be the precursor to the illness). Antidepressants are probably the most common medication offered, with or without tranquillisers. Counselling and psychological approaches may be used.

Holistic management

This illness is a collection of conditions in which each individual will have factors of varying importance. It is clearly an attempt by the body to switch off and gain some rest. Its initials, 'ME' say it all. It is about 'me' and how the person can recognise and meet their own needs. It often affects people who work hard and find it difficult to let go and relax. This may be why it is more common in women who are taught by society to look after the needs of others even to the point of ill health. Men on the other hand may find it easier to stop and rest. In addition, diseases that have a psychological component are usually under diagnosed in men.

In terms of Chinese medicine, the condition may be, at least at its outset, one of External Pathogenic Factor Invading as a consequence of underlying depletion of Qi or Blood. The origin may lie in such factors as overwork, emotional stress, not wanting to say 'no'. There is invariably use of antibiotic prescriptions. These can only make the problem worse since they further deplete the Qi and lead to Damp Accumulation. Frequently seen syndromes include Damp-heat in the Muscles, Shaoyang Level Patterns (Half Interior Half Exterior), Heat Lingering in the Interior as well as Qi, Blood and Yin deficiency.

A woman I treated with this condition had 2 years of upheaval due to her husband changing jobs and working away from home. She had to sell the house on her own and look after the children. After that period of time the family moved house (some 400 miles) to be with the husband. She moved to a new job, the children started a new school and then she developed toxoplasmosis, which is an unusual infection caught from cats. After 4 months of treatment with antibiotics she was so weak that she could only get out of bed for 4 hours each day. At that point her life was merely sleeping, eating and resting. The issue here is that the infection comes after – *it is the result not the cause.*

Treatment should be aimed at removing any Pathogenic Influence Remaining together with attempting to remedy the underlying condition. The use of drugs will only serve to worsen the already weakened state. Since Qi deficiency and Damp Accumulation are common, it is clear why antidepressants are often prescribed and produce short-term relief in some. Antidepressants are hot energetically and so stimulate the Qi and dry up the dampness. They primarily affect the Heart and Liver. In the short-term, there may be less aching and depression as the Damp is dried and the Heart and Liver Qi are heated and moved. Long-term of course, they can only disperse and weaken the Qi and further deplete the Yin and Blood.

Case one

A woman of 55 years came for treatment of tiredness for many years. She had a very pale complexion and frequently felt exhausted. She would often develop heaviness in the limbs. She had no other specific symptoms. I made a diagnosis of Spleen, Lung and Heart Deficiency with Damp Accumulation in the Muscles. I treated her with acupuncture and Chinese herbs for many months. At first she showed little sign of improvement other than minimal improvements in energy levels. After three months of treatment she felt markedly better and now, some 3 years later she has no symptoms. In my experience, Chinese medicine is a very effective form of treatment for ME and people with such symptoms can be encouraged that there is the very real possibility of improvement.

Acquired immune deficiency syndrome (AIDS)

AIDS was recognised as having been a cause of death in the UK in a seaman in 1959[12] but it was first described clinically in 1981. In conventional medicine it is seen as being due to the effects of HIV (Human Immuno deficiency Virus) infection, of which there are two types, HIV-1 and HIV-2. The person becomes vulnerable to certain infections and various rare malignant tumours develop.

T lymphocytes, which are involved particularly with resistance to viral and fungal infections, are affected. B cells, which are involved primarily with resistance to bacterial infection, are left intact. The reduction in lymphocytes is associated with the development of viral and fungal infections, parasitic infestations and certain tumours. This collapse of the immune system indicates the severity of the condition.

It was recognised fairly early that there are similarities between this disease and Hepatitis B in that a virus is involved, antibodies are present (which are an indicator of infection) and transmission may take place some time after initial infection. Transmission is similar in terms of contact with blood and body fluids. Although, HIV infection is conventionally thought to be the cause of AIDS, as with most chronic disease the causes are multifactorial.

A diagnosis of being HIV-positive leads to profound psychological effects on the person because of this assumed link with AIDS. In reality, it is not that clear-cut. AIDS is not necessarily associated with HIV infection, HIV infection does not lead inevitably to AIDS. Peter Duisberg, professor of molecular biology at Berkeley, a well-known proponent of the theory that HIV has a minor role to play in AIDS, states that it is the immune system that is the main problem. The body does a good job, in most cases, of dealing with the virus. It is when other factors come into operation that the syndrome of AIDS develops. These include drug use, poor diet, excessive sexual activity, stressful lifestyle and the other factors that can deplete the immune system.

There is much discussion about the origins of AIDS. There are several theories but the ones that seem most reliable are those that relate the disease to susceptibility. How can someone's immune system be so weakened that it lets in such a virus and, subsequently, opportunistic viral, fungal and parasitic infections? In Africa, the disease is most prevalent in the very countries where smallpox vaccination was pursued the most vigorously in the push to eradicate smallpox.

In the 1920s, trials of a polio vaccine were held which involved the injection of monkey serum into humans. There were already simian immune deficiency syndromes and one could argue that transmissible agents crossed from one species to another.

AIDS is seen in those with severely weakened immune systems. For example, in babies (where the immune system is immature) or in adults, where immunity has been weakened by drug use, suppressed disease, poor diet, irregular life-style and so forth. In Edinburgh in 1989 it was stated that 60 per cent of HIV-positive people had used intravenous drugs. This illustrates that HIV is a weak pathogen and only affects those with severely depleted immune systems.

The most dangerous situation for any immune system, healthy or not, is a bypassing of the normal layers of protection by the injection of contaminated blood or body fluids. The first groups to be affected were drug addicts who injected (13 per cent) and male homosexuals (71 per cent). This situation mirrors Hepatitis B and C, which have the same methods of transmission. The other similarity is that whilst most people with HIV disease suffer little or no illness as a result, they may still be infectious to others. Only a minority will go on to develop AIDS.

No one knows how many people who are HIV-positive go on to develop full-blown AIDS. It depends upon many factors such as constitution, life-style, drug use/abuse,[13] work practices, sexual practices.[14] Conventionally, the incubation period for the disease is seen as being very variable. On average it is 28 months with a range extending from 9 months to 11 years. This latter figure is increasing as time passes and we move further and further away from the date of original discovery.

The first stage in this process is that contact is made with the virus. This is by means of sexual intercourse or passage of blood or body fluids into the body. If the person is susceptible then 'infection' occurs.

After a latent period which is not accurately known, antibodies are produced against the virus. This is the state of being HIV-positive. It is important to realise here that HIV-positive only indicates that antibodies are present. No antibodies, i.e. HIV-negative may still mean that the virus is present – Figure 5.1.

It is not clear how long it takes for a person to become HIV-positive after contact but it can certainly take three months and occasionally longer. Some people never develop antibodies. During this period, a person would be HIV-negative but infectious. In a study of HIV-negative homosexual men engaged in high-risk sexual behaviour, almost one quarter (23 per cent) were found to have the virus. Most of these remained HIV-negative for up to 36 months.[15]

Prevention of HIV infection is pursued by health authorities with recommendations to use condoms and avoid so-called high-risk sexual behaviour – anal intercourse and vaginal intercourse without condoms, any act which draws blood, any sexual practice which involves contact with urine or faeces, sharing sex toys, and sex during the menstrual period if the partner has open cuts or grazes or sores on their hands or body.

Added to the uncertainties about the testing for antibodies, is the certainty that if a person's HIV status becomes generally known there is a social stigma. People lose their jobs, children are banned from school, there may be general social ostracism. Getting insurance or a mortgage becomes almost impossible. It may be difficult even if it is discovered that the test is negative since some may take the view that if there had been no risk why would the person have chosen to take the test in the first place? If the test is positive then there is pressure to take conventional medication.

If someone were thinking of checking their HIV status then I would consider the following to be useful advice:

- have counselling before the test to discuss the issues that are important to you. It may be preferable to use a counsellor who is not involved in the unit doing the testing since vested interests are better avoided.
- a normal test does not prove there is no problem.
- a positive test only tells you if you have antibodies. It gives you no information about your general level of health.
- medical confidentiality is not absolute so have the test under an assumed name and certainly never through medical practitioners you know unless you can be absolutely certain of their reaction. Specialist clinics for sexually transmitted disease tend to be more helpful.
- be very careful about whom you tell, since the consequences of this becoming generally known can be severe.
- the main issues are around health and general life-style and these can be addressed whether you know your HIV status or not.

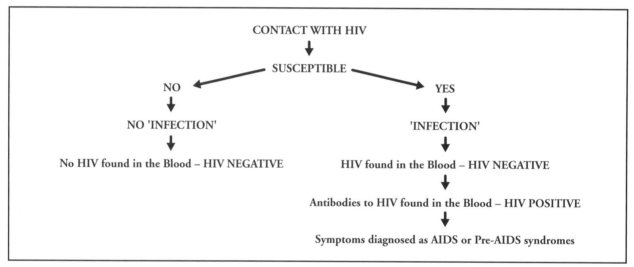

Figure 5.1: Flowchart of sequelae of contact with HIV

Symptoms

The initial symptoms of HIV infection can be acute fever with lymphatic gland enlargement, muscle pains, tiredness, sore throat and on rare occasions a mild pink rash some 6 – 8 weeks after initial contact. It lasts for a few days and is followed by a symptom-free period. Blood tests reveal a reduced lymphocyte and platelet count and raised liver enzymes.

Whether there is progression to further clinical conditions clearly depends upon the general state of health of the person. If the lifestyle is one of depletion then this tends to lead to deterioration in the immune system. If the lifestyle is more moderate and strengthening then there is every reason to suppose that a long and healthy life will follow.

Symptoms that may indicate the development of AIDS or a pre-AIDS syndrome are:

- generalised lymphatic gland enlargement.
- profound fatigue, persisting for weeks with no obvious cause.
- unexplained weight loss (more than 10 lb in 2 months).
- severe night sweats that may occur on and off for several weeks.
- fever lasting more than 10 days.
- diarrhoea lasting more than 1 month.
- cough lasting more than two weeks and not due to smoking. This may be associated with shortness of breath, persistent sore throat and difficulty in swallowing. The white spots of 'thrush' may be visible in the mouth.
- signs of individual cancers such as purplish or pink blotches in the skin (Kaposi's sarcoma).

The three main problems for people with AIDS are infections, cancers and other immune disorders.

Infections are due to viruses, fungi or parasites. Pneumonia due to the unusual parasite *Pneumocystis carinii* is the most common disorder. The most common fungal infection is *Candida albicans* ('thrush'). The most common viral infection is herpes simplex ('cold sores'). Other infections found with AIDS are unusually severe attacks of herpes zoster ('shingles'), toxoplasmosis and tuberculosis.

Two types of cancer are seen with AIDS. These are Kaposi's sarcoma (KS) which is a rare cancer of skin presenting as purplish blotches and lymphoma.

Other immune disorders include haemolytic anaemia and idiopathic thrombocytopenic purpura.

Investigations

When AIDS has begun to develop, lymphocyte (CD4) counts fall. If the level falls below 200, the patient is at serious risk of other infections. HIV RNA levels are also assessed as high levels are associated with progressive disease.

Treatment

The main aims of conventional treatment are to maximise the health of the patient, prevent further transmission of HIV and to provide support to the patient and their family. Advice is given about reducing the possibility of HIV transmission and recommendations made about sexual practices and the use of condoms. Breast-feeding is generally advised against as transmission of HIV to the baby occurs in up to 20 per cent of cases.

There are now several antiretroviral drugs available. There is no claim that these cure the disease but they are used conventionally in an attempt to control the HIV infection. The belief is that if the virus levels can be reduced as much as possible, further damage to the immune system can be minimised. The drugs currently available are shown in Table 5.9. Several drugs may be used together

Drug group	Drug name	Comments
Nucleoside-analogue reverse-transriptase inhibitors (NRTIs)	Zidovudine (AZT)	Originally developed as a chemotherapy treatment for cancer. Side-effects include nausea, insomnia, myalgia, severe headache, rashes, vomiting and fever. A severe polymyositis syndrome of muscle aches and pains can occur with prolonged therapy. Red blood cells swell up commonly (megaloblastic changes). Bone marrow suppression leads to neutropenia and thrombocytopenia.
	Didanosine (DDI)	Side-effects include nausea, diarrhoea, pancreatitis and polyneuropathy.
	Zalcitabine (DDC)	Side-effects include polyneuropathy and mouth ulcers.
	Lamivudine	Similar side-effects to zidovudine (AZT) occur with bone marrow suppression also being a problem.
	Stavudine (D4T)	Side-effects include polyneuropathy.
Non-nucleoside reverse-transcriptase inhibitors (NNRTIs)	Nefirapine Delavridine	These drugs cannot be used with saquinavir (see below) because of similarities in their actions. Side-effects include rash and raised liver enzymes.
Protease inhibitors	Ritonavir	There are several drugs that cannot be given with this due to serious adverse interactions. Side-effects include nausea, diarrhoea, vomiting and tingling with numbness.
	Saquinavir	Side-effects include nausea, diarrhoea and abdominal pain.
	Indinavir	Side-effects include kidney stones and raised bilirubin levels in the blood.
	Nelfinavir	A very newly developed drug.

Table 5.9: Drug treatments of HIV infection and AIDS

Holistic management

Many of the approaches described in Chapter 6 and the treatment of cancer are valid here. A multiple approach must be taken, and a complication is conventional treatment which is heavily suppressive and strongly advocated by conventional practitioners. Energetically, it may be helpful to consider the antiretroviral drugs as similar in action to chemotherapy agents used in cancer.

The key is the immune system, as in so many cases, and it is important to pay attention to diet, mental/emotional factors as well as perhaps a specific therapy. The people who do the best in terms of quality and length of life are those who pursue a holistic approach.

If you look at Figure 5.1, you can see that as a person improves their situation he/she will be nearer the top of the diagram. Some people become asymptomatic with treatment and then HIV-negative as the blood clears and the antibodies disappear.[16]

People with HIV infection and AIDS will require a lot of support. If we can offer support, practical help and measures which can increase the strength of the immune system then definitely beneficial results will be obtained.

HISTORICAL DISEASES

These diseases are unusual in the West but their importance lies in the widespread use of vaccination in the belief that such practices will prevent their re-emergence.

Tetanus

This is associated with a bacterium – *Clostridium tetani*. It is found in ground that is contaminated with the faeces of animals such as the horse and cow. Spores develop which resist heat and dryness and so can survive for long periods. There has never been a recorded instance of tetanus resulting from the bite of a domestic animal.

The bacterium grows in conditions where there is no oxygen and so thrives in deep penetrating wounds particularly where there is much tissue damage. Crushing injuries in agricultural workers are a special risk as are neglected wounds (e.g. battlefield injuries).

The bacterium produces toxins that affect the central nervous system. Symptoms develop after an asymptomatic period of variable time depending upon the site of the wound and its proximity to the central nervous system.

The first signs are those of restlessness with muscle twitching then stiffness of the neck. Soon the jaw muscles are affected (hence its popular name – 'lockjaw'). Later there is more generalised stiffness and convulsions. These are precipitated by stimuli such as noise or light. Death, if it occurs, is due to exhaustion, cardiac insufficiency or pulmonary collapse. Some cases are very mild and certainly not all lead to such severe problems.

Treatment
Injections of antitoxin are given as soon as there are suspected problems and antibiotics to remove any remaining organisms. Convulsions are treated with anticonvulsants. Treatment is mainly supportive to deal with any manifestations in a particular case.

The key is wound hygiene and so tetanus is rare now in the developed world where wounds tend not to be neglected. Vaccination is still routinely given to all children as part of the DPT (diphtheria, pertussis, tetanus) vaccine – see Page 68 – and in response to minor wounds and the bites of dogs and cats. I would estimate that many are given unnecessarily even from a conventional viewpoint.

Antibiotics are usually injected at the same time to 'prevent' wound infection. As mentioned later, the use of antibiotics for prophylaxis is usually counter-productive. It increases the likelihood of infection by more resistant strains of bacteria in a situation where infection probably would not have occurred anyway.

Diphtheria

This is a bacterial disease caused by *Corynebacterium diphtheriae*. The main feature of the disease is that the organism produces a toxin that affects the heart and the central nervous system. This is not true in every case and some people may only have a very mild attack.

Symptoms
The incubation period is very short, in the order of 2-4 days. The nose and tonsils are the usual sites of affliction. The person is clearly ill with malaise, pallor and mild fever. There is sore throat with a characteristic greyish-white membrane on one or both tonsils which is firmly attached. There will be enlargement of the associated lymph node groups. In severe cases toxins are released which affect the cardiovascular and/or central nervous systems.

This disease is rarely seen in the West now. It is a problem exacerbated by poor housing, poor nutrition and inadequate public health measures. Therefore, there has been a great reduction in the numbers seen in the last 50 years or so with the result that most people have never seen a case. In 1984 there were only two cases in the UK.

Treatment

Injections of antitoxin are given to neutralise the toxins released by the organism. Supportive treatment may be required if circulatory failure intervenes. Vaccination is routinely given to all children as part of the DPT (diphtheria, pertussis, tetanus) vaccine – see Page 69.

Complications

Complication	Symptoms to look for
Circulatory collapse	Low blood pressure, rapid and thready pulse, grey and pale complexion, reduced urine output, proteinuria
Nerve involvement	Altered speech, regurgitation of fluids into the nose when swallowing, blurred vision, double vision, difficulty swallowing, numbness and tingling in the limbs (legs more so than arms)

Table 5.10: Complications of diphtheria

Holistic management

The importance of this disease for holistic medicine lies merely in the public health application of its vaccination. No practitioner in the West is likely to see this condition.

Polio

This is a viral disease that is transmitted by the faecal-oral route. The large epidemics of the 1940s and 1950s were almost certainly associated with the fad of tonsillectomy. Removal of such an important lymphatic gland at the entrance to the lung and stomach has potentially serious consequences. Since that time, the number of cases has gradually declined and now the only cases are either caused by the vaccine or are due to ingesting contaminated food or drink. This does not happen in the West because sewage and drinking water are separated. Epidemics tended to occur in the late summer and early autumn.

Although polio vaccination is assumed to have led to reductions in the incidence of the disease, the diagnosis of polio was changed in the 1950s to specifically exclude anyone who had had polio vaccination. Therefore, although there are many cases of polio-like syndromes in the West they are not labelled as such. They are diagnosed as Guillain–Barré syndrome, aseptic meningitis and the like.

Symptoms

Many people in an epidemic will be infected with the virus but only a minority will develop symptoms and not all of these will be severe. The virus affects the motor nerve cells in the spinal cord, which may lead to paralysis.

The incubation period is 7-12 days. There is mild fever, generalised aches and pains which in some leads to weakness and paralysis. The site of the paralysis depends upon the part of the spinal cord and brain involved. In some instances the muscles of respiration are affected requiring mechanical assistance (e.g. an 'iron lung') to prevent death due to asphyxiation.

Treatment

There is no definitive treatment available. Prevention is important and public health measures to protect water and food supplies are essential. If a person develops symptoms then complete rest will minimise the severity of the attack. Massage plays an important part in aiding recovery. Vaccination – see Page 69 – is given to all babies.

Holistic management

The importance of this disease for holistic medicine lies in the public health application of its vaccination. Related diseases such as Guillain–Barré syndrome are more commonly seen. They frequently occur after polio vaccination. There are treatments available such as massage, Chinese herbal treatments, homoeopathic remedies and Ayurvedic treatment and such natural approaches are used where polio is still found.

Antibiotic use

Antibiotics, strictly speaking, are drugs that kill bacteria or prevent their growth. For the purposes of discussion, I include all the drugs that are used against infecting organisms. These are antifungal, antiviral, antiprotozoal and antiparasitic drugs.

Such chemicals can be used either when an infection occurs or as prophylaxis (to prevent the occurrence of infection).[17] Prophylactic use tends not to prevent infection, but to lead to the appearance of resistant organisms when infection does actually happen.

There is a general view that antibiotic use is harmless or at least only leads to minor problems. Antibiotics are powerful in their effect and are particularly harmful in the case of children who are more susceptible to their effects. There are the well-known problems of diarrhoea and vaginal thrush due to eradication of the usual resident bacteria as well as disturbance to Vitamin B absorption. Also the use of antibiotics leads to a general weakening of the immune system. This is well recognised amongst mothers of young children who may have received recurrent doses of antibiotics. The child then becomes susceptible to every passing infection.

Different antibiotics tend to be used for different infecting organisms but this is not particularly important for the practitioner of holistic medicine. It is more helpful to know how to ameliorate their harmful effects and withdraw them when appropriate.[18]

In terms of Chinese medicine, most antibiotics are Cold and Damp in nature leading to depletion of Spleen Qi deficiency, Damp Accumulation in the Middle and Upper Jiaos and Qi depletion of other organs as a consequence especially the Lung and Kidney. There is often Heat in the Lung after such treatment particularly in the case of children. If the original diagnosis is one of External Pathogenic Factor then the consequence may be External Pathogenic Factor Remaining.

The sulphonamide group of antibiotics seem to be different and lead to superficial heat reactions and are warm and dispersing in nature. They are especially a problem, therefore, in people with Blood or Yin deficiency conditions.

Antifungal and antiprotozoal agents are heating and drying and can be extremely strong in their action. Antifungal drugs particularly affect the Liver and Spleen leading to nausea, vomiting, hypochondriac pain and in some cases, jaundice.

The so-called antiretroviral drug, AZT, used in the treatment of HIV infection and AIDS, was originally developed as a cancer chemotherapy drug – see Page 59. Such agents are strongly heating and lead to Deficiency of Qi, Blood and Yin, Rebellious Stomach Qi, Stomach Heat and Heat in the Blood.

VACCINATION

Vaccination[19] is the introduction of 'foreign' material into the body in an attempt to prevent disease. The term originally derived from using cowpox to protect against smallpox. The intention is to make people immune to the specific disease by stimulating the production of antibodies that would be generated if the person were to develop the disease naturally. The belief is that the already present antibodies will either resist the disease in its entirety or lead to a milder disease. It is a common practice and mass vaccination campaigns are carried out, particularly on children.

This sounds very reasonable and is information we are all familiar with. However, the immune system is much more than the presence or absence of antibodies. These are found in the blood and so, hierarchically, are at a deep level of the person. The immune system as a whole is made up of many different layers from the superficial tissues such as skin, secretions such as sweat and tears, defence mechanisms within each organ such as mucus production in the lungs. In addition, there is an outer level of energy that resists the inward movement of disease. In Chinese medicine this is known as Wei Qi.

Once disease has descended into the deeper levels only then are antibodies produced. Antibodies are only produced when the disease is already a relatively severe problem for the body. Antibodies indicate disease not health. In cases of polio, for example, the virus first enters the body and symptoms appear after the generation of antibodies. If antibodies are not produced, as in the majority of cases of polio virus infection, there is no paralysis.

Vaccination bypasses these subtle levels of the immune system. It is clearly not the best way to minimise a person's susceptibility since other levels need to be addressed at the same time. We only develop an infectious disease, and indeed any disease, if we are susceptible. The question is does vaccination change that susceptibility and if so, is it in the direction of health or of disease?

Vaccination developed from a procedure carried out by a Dr Jenner in 1792 when he used cowpox to try and prevent the development of the more serious smallpox. Edward Jenner, a country doctor, noted that dairymaids who had contracted cowpox were protected against smallpox. He inoculated a healthy boy, James Phipps, with pus from the arm of Sarah Nelmes, a dairymaid who was suffering from cowpox. Some weeks later he inoculated Phipps' arm with material from a case of smallpox. The boy remained healthy. Jenner published these results and the medical profession immediately took on the idea.

As a result, vaccination has become accepted as an essential part of the armoury of conventional medicine to fight infections. Large-scale vaccinations of the population were used from the early part of the 20th century and were compulsory until the 1950s and remain so in the USA.

The idea that you actually eradicate disease is, at the least, philosophically contentious. If it were possible, where would the underlying imbalances go?[20] There is no such thing as perfect human health. If people are prevented from having relatively mild infectious diseases what will be the long-term consequences? There are three ways of looking at vaccination. Is it safe, is it effective and are there less harmful ways of resisting disease?

Is it safe?

There is increasing evidence that vaccination is a major cause of ill health, both in the immediate aftermath of its administration and in later years. There are several reasons for this not the least that the immune system is being challenged with a noxious stimulus at a deep level. There are theoretical and pragmatic reasons why this practice may lead to disease.

It is certainly true that vaccination has an effect on the body. However, the perceived result may not be the real result. By applying principles of energetic medicine we can see that there are two possibilities following vaccination. It can either have an effect or it cannot. The vaccination can only affect the person if they were already susceptible to that particular disease. If there is no susceptibility then neither the disease nor the vaccination can affect the person.

Three reactions are possible if the person is susceptible:

- Mild, with local irritation – this infers that there is a connection energetically with the vaccine but the person's energy is not strong enough to entirely throw off the injected material. It remains in the system manifesting later as a chronic condition. In terms of Chinese medicine this may be analogous to a case of Pathogenic Factor Remaining in the body.

- Stronger reaction such as fever where the body's energy is strong and may throw off the vaccine completely.

- Very strong reaction such as encephalitis, brain damage, meningitis, paralysis. There is susceptibility and the person's energy is so weak that the vaccine enters deep into the body and damages vital organs or in some cases causes death.

If a person has a vaccination and later does not develop the disease, there are several possibilities:

- no susceptibility – vaccination has no effect and the person would not have developed disease anyway.
- the disease develops but is unrecognised – this is common since medical practitioners are reluctant to diagnose, for example, whooping cough in those who have been vaccinated as this would lead to doubts being cast upon the effectiveness of the vaccine. Also, when a disease occurs for which the person was vaccinated, it is frequently different in its manifestation as the vaccine will have altered the person's health.
- immune system damaged – energy of the person has been impaired so that manifestations of acute disease are not possible. Some time in the future there may be the appearance of a chronic disease.

Specific examples of the difficulties arising from vaccination may also be found in the literature. In the case of smallpox vaccination its use caused far more deaths than the actual disease. Between 1953 and 1961 in a population of 47 million there were 11 deaths from smallpox. In the same time there were 37 deaths from the vaccination but in only 0.5 million people vaccinated. This gives an excess of deaths in the case of smallpox vaccination 316 times that of the disease itself.[21]

In the 25 years ended December 1962, nearly two thirds of the children born in England and Wales remained unvaccinated for smallpox yet only four children under 5 died from smallpox. In the one third who were vaccinated, no less than 86 children under 5 were killed by vaccination and many more were seriously injured by it.[22]

In a military hospital in 1944, 100 consecutive cases of smallpox were studied and 96 per cent of those were vaccinated. Seventy per cent had been vaccinated within the last two years. Fourteen cases died and of these only 1 had not been vaccinated. It can be concluded that vaccination failed to prevent smallpox and death from smallpox.

However smallpox is no longer a problem since there have been no recorded cases since the late 1970s. It has always been attributed to the practice of vaccination but I would suggest that contact tracing and isolation were at least as important if the effectiveness of the vaccine is as indicated by the figures above.

An added difficulty with vaccines is the methods employed in their production. In the case of live vaccines, they are cultured using animal cells. Rubella vaccine has been grown using the tissue of aborted foetuses, polio on monkey kidney cells, measles on chick embryos and so on.[23] Various additives are also used to boost antibody responses, for sterilisation and to stabilise them. Substances such as thimerosal (a mercury-based preservative[24]), aluminium sulphate and formalin are routinely added. Others include phenol (a disinfectant), ethylene glycol (main constituent of anti-freeze) and benzethonium chloride (antiseptic).

Is it effective?

The major difficulty in assessing the adverse effects of vaccination is a lack of information. There are no controlled clinical trials carried out on the effectiveness of vaccination and there is no attempt to gather information about short-term and long-term effects. During the introductory phase of a vaccine's development, attention is given to immediate effects. However, frequently this specifically ignores adverse reactions after an arbitrary period of time – usually 48 hours. Some researchers have gathered information from parents of vaccinated children by more proactive methods and this would seem to be an effective method.[25-26] Certainly, more reactions will show up than in the current system that relies almost solely on medical practitioners reporting what they consider to be adverse reactions.

Conventionally, the reduction in cases of infectious disease over the past 100 or so years is attributed to the use of vaccinations and antibiotics.[27-28] The incidence and mortality rate of many infectious diseases has indeed reduced over the years but is this as a result of vaccination? Almost 90 per cent of the total decline in childhood mortality between 1860 and 1965 occurred before the introduction of antibiotics and mass vaccination.

There are many reasons why diseases change. Some like scarlet fever, for which there is no vaccination, become milder whilst others become more severe. Complex sociological, economic and political factors operate. The only factor with which there is *no* correlation is medical practice.[29]

This is used as evidence of the need and efficacy of past, present and future vaccination schemes. However, if we consider the true cause of infectious disease, which is susceptibility, and accept that organisms are the effect not the cause, perhaps things are not as they may seem. If one looks at the available data it becomes clear that the death rates from infectious diseases began to decline long before mass vaccination came along.

Figure 5.2 shows that a great reduction in the death rate from tuberculosis took place well before the common use of antibiotics in the 1940s or mass vaccination in the 1950s. The first sanatorium was not opened in New York until 1910 so it is clear that improvements in living standards which began in the latter part of the 19th century are responsible for changes in death rates.

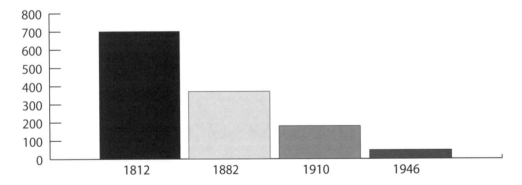

Figure 5.2: Death rate in New York from tuberculosis (/10,000) [30]

Frequently, parents and the public are exhorted to have vaccinations because the disease is dangerous or may be fatal. This is rarely true in the West now and those who are already ill are the ones who have difficulties with childhood diseases. Of 132 deaths from measles discussed in the *Lancet*, half were in children with serious chronic disease or disability, who had at best a short expectation of life. That is, they were due to die soon anyway.[31] Conventional medical sources are clearly at a loss to understand the effects of vaccination when the same article states: 'The effect of measles vaccination on mortality has proved difficult to assess. This is surprising...'.

Are there less harmful ways of resisting disease?

Health, as all holistic practitioners know, is the result of an internal energetic balance, Chinese medicine seeks to harmonise Yin and Yang. Homoeopathy aims to nurture a strong and vibrant vital force. There are many and varied ways in which health can be attained and maintained. There are non-toxic methods that gently balance and nourish us. People can be encouraged to pursue these and thereby gain confidence in their own natural healing ability. Many people resort to vaccination because they are frightened of disease and symptoms. They have lost contact with what is healthy and what is not. Education is a large part of our work as holistic practitioners so as to encourage and facilitate people to explore health and what is appropriate for people themselves. Sadly, it is possible to frighten people with information about the negative aspects of vaccination. This is never healthy or helpful. In my practice, I guide people towards different sources of information so that they are aware of the pros and the cons of vaccination. Then they can decide for themselves the most appropriate course of action to take.

Measles vaccination

Mass vaccination[32] began in 1968 with an uptake rate of 71 per cent in 1986 (in some areas 29 per cent, in others 89 per cent). In the case of measles the death rate showed a similar marked fall before the introduction of mass vaccination and before the introduction of antibiotics in any great quantity. The argument for the introduction of measles vaccination is that it kills some children. Whilst this is true we have to consider whether it protects *at all*. Figure 5.3 illustrates the changes in deaths from measles over the past century. It is clear from this the effect of mass vaccination on death rate.

An epidemic of measles in the US in 1990[33] has cast doubts on whether vaccination is as effective as has been thought.[34] There was the highest number of cases for the previous 10 years. It seemed from comments by scientists at the Centre for Disease Control in Atlanta that up to 40 per cent of cases had been vaccinated. Since only half of the children had been vaccinated the conclusion is self-evident – vaccination is of no use. As a result, the Centre of Disease Control has recommended that everyone have a *second* vaccination. Some states have introduced legislation to make this legally enforceable. Presumably we shall see pressure for a third vaccination ..... and a fourth .... and a fifth.

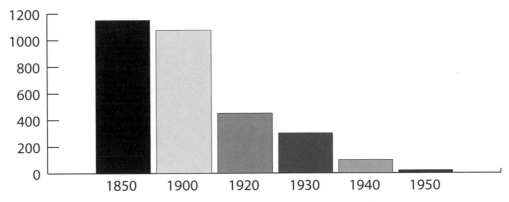

Figure 5.3: Deaths per million from measles[35]

Measles is generally given now as part of the measles, mumps and rubella vaccination. There are several possible known sequelae of measles vaccination. These include:

- fever in up to 15 per cent – begins 5-6 days after vaccination and lasts for 2 days
- febrile convulsion will occur in some with fever
- rash in 5 per cent – begins 7-10 days after vaccination and lasts for 2-4 days
- encephalitis
- encephalopathy
- syndrome of muscle weakness, wasting, tingling and numbness (Guillain–Barré syndrome)
- Reye's syndrome
- squint
- blurred vision and other visual disturbances
- hearing loss
- lack of coordination and balance
- arthralgia
- arthritis
- allergy
- bruising or other bleeding abnormalities
- weight fluctuations in the weeks or months after vaccination[36]
- decreased lymphocyte number and activity.[37]

Rubella vaccination

In the case of rubella, German measles, the problem is not the person with the disease but the foetus in cases of pregnancy. Therefore, vaccination of pre-pregnant females is advocated. It was introduced in 1970. However over 2 per cent of susceptible pregnant women still develop rubella and so rubella is now given to children of both sexes between the ages of 12 and 24 months. In spite of high vaccination rates there has been no detectable reduction in the numbers of babies born with congenital defects.[38] In fact, in Greece there were many more cases in 1993 (25 cases – 24.6/100,000 births). It seems that if there were any results of the rubella vaccination campaign in Greece, it was to push susceptibility into the childbearing years.

In the 1960s the average age of contracting rubella was 8 years, in 1993 it was 17 years.

As vaccination was offered only to females before 1988 it provided a good opportunity to study the differences in the occurrence of the disease in males and females. A Glasgow practice investigated people's immunity to rubella after a vaccination take-up level of 86-87 per cent. There was no significant difference in the incidence of German measles between males and females.

Certainly, any vaccination offered should only be done after the immune status of the child has been previously ascertained. Since many cases of rubella are sub-clinical, children may in fact have had the disease without knowing. Any immunity gained from the vaccination lasts for a variable length of time and there is little information concerning long-term immune states. Reinfection does occur in vaccinated individual individuals with figures quoted of around 50 per cent and if in pregnancy can lead to foetal abnormalities.[39] Complications after the vaccine are common especially joint pains, which with naturally contracted rubella is only seen with more severe cases in adults. Up to 40 per cent of those receiving vaccination in mass campaigns develop joint pains.[40] The most effective way of attaining immunity seems to be 'rubella parties' where children are actively put into contact with someone with rubella in order to develop the disease and gain natural immunity. Rubella is generally given now as part of the measles, mumps and rubella vaccination. There are several possible known sequelae of rubella vaccination. These include:

- 40 days after vaccination a typical reaction is pins and needles, pains in the arms or pain in knee with desire for crouching
- multiple nerve problems with weakness and tingling
- tingling and weakness of the hands (carpal tunnel syndrome)
- syndrome of muscle weakness, wasting, tingling and numbness (Guillain–Barré syndrome)
- reduced platelet count
- suppression of cellular immunity
- blurred vision (optic neuritis)
- pins and needles, numbness in the face

Mumps vaccination

This was introduced in 1988 in the UK. At the same time mumps was made a notifiable disease. This will make the subsequent analysis of the effects of mumps vaccine impossible since the figures before and after that date cannot be directly compared. It is given as part of the measles, mumps, rubella vaccine (MMR) at the age of 12-18 months.

There are several possible known sequelae of mumps vaccination. These include:

- low grade fever
- inflammation of the parotid gland
- pain and swelling of the testes (orchitis)
- weakness, numbness and tingling (neuritis)
- encephalopathy
- nerve deafness
- allergic reactions
- a post-vaccination syndrome of glandular swelling, tiredness and malaise

A current debate is whether MMR vaccination is implicated in the development of autism. Certainly, holistic practitioners commonly report that such vaccines can have marked effects on a child's development. I have seen all too frequently such changes after vaccination. There is some research evidence also to support this view.[41] A London-based firm of solicitors, Hodge, Jones and Allen, say that autism is by far the most common adverse reaction of vaccination they come across in their work with the parents of vaccine damaged children.[42]

Whooping cough vaccination

Mass campaigns for this vaccine began in 1956 with a 67 per cent uptake rate in 1986. The changes in the death rate from this disease are shown in Figure 5.4 – date of mass vaccination marked with an arrow. The case of whooping cough vaccination is of interest as the problems surrounding whooping cough vaccination have been known for years and several authorities warn of the dangers of neurological damage following such procedures. Several European countries have now stopped such vaccinations.

A difficulty with determining whether vaccination leads to specific conditions is that there is no gathering of data. An important issue with regard to mass vaccination is that it is a worldwide experiment with human immune systems and no-one is gathering information in an organised way. Harris Coulter, the well-known author and medical researcher, questioned many people about the health of their children following vaccination. His books 'The Pertussin Vaccine: A strong contra view' and 'DPT – A Shot in the Dark' detail the results of his work in the US. Side-effects from vaccines and especially whooping cough vaccination are far more common than previously known. In his first book he says 'Our estimate of the prevalence of these disorders is based upon a study done in 1979 at UCLA under FDA sponsorship. Its findings (confirmed by two other studies) suggest that at least 1000 babies die as a result of DPT vaccine every year, with these deaths being classified as SIDS (Sudden Infant Death Syndrome)...... The UCLA/FDA study also suggests that at least 11-12000 cases of permanent damage (mostly neurological) are caused by the vaccine every year.'

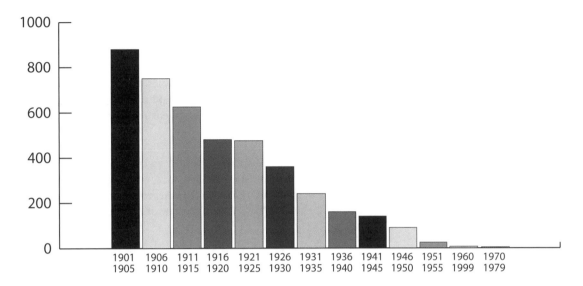

Figure 5.4: Deaths from whooping cough per million children aged under 15 years [43]

Trials in Sweden of an acellular whooping cough vaccine (the type usually used in the UK is whole cell vaccine) were stopped after a report of three deaths from the vaccine. The Swedes are very cautious about such trials and stated that they thought it 'unethical to test a dubiously needed vaccine on their population.' [44]

There are several possible known sequelae of whooping cough vaccination. These include:

- local swelling and pain
- fever
- anorexia
- irritability
- vomiting
- sleepiness
- crying – cannot be consoled
- episodes of decreased responsiveness and flaccidity
- convulsion
- acute encephalopathy leading to death or permanent brain damage.

Meningitis vaccination

There are currently two vaccines given against meningitis. The so-called Hib vaccine for *Haemophilus influenzae* type b is given at 2, 4 and 6 months with the DPT and polio vaccines. It was first used in the US in 1985 and the UK in 1992. Hib affects children under the age of 5 and causes meningitis and upper respiratory tract infections. The initial vaccine actually increased the risk of Hib meningitis and was abandoned in 1992.[45]

A new vaccine was developed in the late 1980s and licensed for use. The oft-quoted trial to support its use was on Navajo infants.[46] The trial was terminated because of an increased risk to the vaccinated children of infections. Although there were not due to *Haemophilus influenzae B*, these children were clearly suffering from a depleted immune system when compared with the control group. Vaccination, of course, is one of the most powerful factors in damaging the immune system.

A new vaccine released in October 1999 in the UK and September in Ireland is for meningitis C and septicaemia. It will be given at 2, 3 and 4 months of age, along with the DPT, polio and Hib vaccines, again at 12-15 months with the MMR, at 5 years old with the pre-school boosters and at 15-17 years of age, as well as older students entering university. The aim in Ireland is to vaccinate everyone up to the age of 22 years.

A similar scheme has been in operation in New Zealand for several years where babies under a week old are given vaccines. In 1987, in New Zealand, the Health Department began a trial of vaccinating children against meningitis. There was a high incidence of adverse effects leading to abandonment of the trial after public outcry. The campaign was eventually restarted with booster injections for everyone except those who had a reaction to the first thereby rendering useless any analysis of results.[47]

The efficacy of both the old meningitis C vaccine and the new one is not very good. In Australia in 1996 there was an outbreak of meningitis in which 426 people came down with the illness. They didn't use the vaccine during this outbreak because they said that *it is just not particularly good* and *it is expensive and it offers no long-lasting protection*.[48] According to the Public Health Laboratory Service, the old vaccine doesn't work and neither does the new one.[49]

A secondary school in Etwall, Derbyshire, took part in the vaccination campaign and subsequently 70 pupils were admitted to hospital suffering from collapse, extreme headaches and sickness. The authorities said they were suffering from vaccine-related anxiety and stress and there was no need for concern! Only 237 children had the jab to that point and more than half reported side-effects. The children and parents involved probably felt differently.[50]

The Food and Drug Administration in America have also refused to approve a similar vaccine because of fears it may cause an epidemic of insulin-dependant diabetes. The vaccine (based on the pneomococcal virus) is also very similar to Hib vaccine, except that it contains seven different organisms. A study was done over 10 years where one sample of children were given 4 doses of Hib vaccine and another sample of children weren't given any. The rate of diabetes increased by 26 per cent in the vaccinated children.[51]

North American Vaccine, pneomococcal vaccine manufacturers, have stated that as with any vaccine *there is a very small risk that serious problems, even death, could occur after getting a vaccine*.[52] Some medical practitioners are very circumspect in the use of this vaccine.[53]

Meningitis is clearly a serious disease but the best way to attempt to avoid these disorders or to minimise their effects is to strengthen the immune system. Holistic medicine is very good at this because it has the philosophical understanding of health and disease. There are several possible known sequelae of meningitis vaccination. These include:

- fever
- local pain and redness
- disturbed sleep
- extremely sore arm for a few days
- irritability
- headaches
- crying
- drowsiness
- anorexia
- diarrhoea
- vomiting
- myalgia.[54]

Tetanus vaccination

Routine vaccination for tetanus began in 1961. It is routinely given to everyone in the UK. The disease is a rare infection gained from infected deep tissue – injuries caused by a penetrating wound. Wound hygiene is of paramount importance in these situations and there is doubt as to the efficacy of the vaccine. Certainly, there are homoeopathic remedies available that can specifically prevent problems after perforating injuries. Immunoglobulin is given to those with a high likelihood of developing the disease such as neglected perforating wounds.

There are several possible known sequelae of tetanus vaccination. These include:

- local reaction in up to 95 per cent – the likelihood of this increases with each dose
- arthritis[55]
- oedema
- redness in 25-30 per cent
- enlarged lymphatic glands
- fever
- numbness, pins and needles (peripheral neuropathy)

- convulsions
- allergic reactions.

Diphtheria vaccination

Diptheria, the third component of the triple vaccine (DPT), is extremely rare in the West and yet the vast majority of the population is still vaccinated. The rationale behind this seems dubious to say the least. What is the point of vaccination against a non-existent disease?

The late Dr Robert Mendelsohn, a US paediatrician, was well known for his opposition to many conventional treatments of little or no use. He stated that there is as much likelihood of contracting diphtheria in the US as being bitten by a cobra.[56]

There are several possible known sequelae of diphtheria vaccination. These include:

- local reactions
- arthritis
- encephalopathy – this has been reported in one study and showed an increase in central nervous system damage.[57]

Polio vaccination

Polio rarely occurs in developed countries and then usually only in vaccinated cases. Vaccination, using a live vaccine, is the introduction of live polio virus into the environment. There are many instances of parents and carers developing the disease from their recently vaccinated children. In societies where sewage has been separated from drinking water it is extremely rare.

The immune status of the person is important as evidenced by the fact that the epidemics of polio in the 1940s and 1950s occurred mainly after tonsillectomy. Polio virus is found in those who do not contract the clinical disease with the ratio of infection with no symptoms to disease being 1000:1 in children and 75:1 in adults. Certainly, of all the vaccinations polio is the most 'natural' in terms of how it is administered. The most hazardous technique is to inject infective material directly into the blood stream as occurs with the rarely used Salk vaccine. The two polio vaccines – the live oral or the killed injection – present a dilemma – either introduce live polio virus into the community or risk damage to the immune system with injected morbid material.

However, neither may be particularly effective in terms of protection. Despite the introduction of vaccination into Africa, Asia and South America the disease has actually *increased* considerably.[58] The decline in polio cases in Europe occurred at exactly the same time as the decline in the USA although there was no mass vaccination in Europe at that time. A major difficulty with assessing the incidence of polio is that the criteria for diagnosing polio were changed in 1956 following the introduction of vaccination. Now it is no longer possible to diagnose polio in anyone who has been vaccinated. The incidence of other neurological diseases, such as aseptic meningitis and Guillain-Barré syndromes, has increased dramatically since then. When these diseases are included with cases of polio, it is clear that the incidence of such disease has remained the same.

A far greater tragedy in connection with polio vaccination is the contamination of supplies of vaccine with simian immunodeficiency virus (SIV – particularly SIV-40) in the 1950s. SIV was first described in rhesus monkeys in 1985, these being the main source of tissue for polio vaccination. There is hard evidence and very real fears that SIV infection in infants in Africa led to the development of HIV in humans in later years.[59] Manipulations to the immune system of young children and babies by researchers and pharmaceutical companies who have limited understanding of the intricate workings of the immune system can only have disastrous results for our health and the health of future generations.

Influenza vaccination

Influenza can be an unpleasant and occasionally fatal disease. It is the economic effects of time lost from work and the occasional deaths that encourage medical authorities to vaccinate against influenza. There have been many articles both in the press and the medical journals about the ill effects of influenza vaccination and also its lack of effectiveness. A *Lancet* article in 1974 quoted the results of vaccinating large numbers of staff in the Post Office: '...the annual offer of an injection of influenza vaccine in a large industry has not resulted in a significant reduction in sickness'.

Adverse reactions after influenza vaccination include:

- fever
- allergic reactions (can be fatal)
- rheumatic disease[60]
- encephalopathy
- Guillain-Barré syndrome[61]
- encephalitis.

Tuberculosis vaccination

This is by means of the BCG (Bacille Calmette-Guérin) vaccine. As stated above, the incidence and death rate of tuberculosis dropped sharply before the advent of vaccination and indeed antibiotics. It is a disease of the poor and malnourished. The USA for example has never used BCG in their vaccination schedules and yet they show the same rate of fall in the number of cases as the UK. There have been some trials of BCG vaccination and they reveal variable effectiveness from 0 to 75 per cent.[62] In France, an outbreak of TB affected 62 hospital workers, all of whom had been vaccinated.[63]

Hepatitis vaccination

Hepatitis B was generally a disease of intravenous drug users and homosexual men. Now that people are exposed to infection through medical procedures such as transfusion and the injection of substances derived from blood, infection is much more common.[64] Infants are recommended to receive Hepatitis B vaccination by the WHO. In Italy the vaccine is compulsory. As Hepatitis B only affects so-called high-risk groups (some healthcare workers, patients in haemodialysis, the sexually promiscuous and intravenous drug users) there seems little point in vaccinating infants.

Adverse reactions to the Hepatitis B vaccination include:

- rash
- itch
- pain in muscles and joints
- headache
- fever
- nausea and/or vomiting
- malaise
- redness at the injection site
- fatigue
- dizziness
- vertigo
- demyelination syndromes
- convulsions
- Bell's palsy
- Guillain-Barré syndrome[65]
- sciatica
- neuropathy
- spinal cord inflammation
- visual disturbances
- psychological symptoms.

Hepatitis A vaccination is most frequently given to travellers visiting countries where the risk of infection is increased due to contamination of water supplies. It is repeated after one year to boost antibody levels and then repeat every 10 years. Most adverse reactions are centred around the digestive system as would be expected as this is a disease of that area. Pancreatitis can occur after Hepatitis A vaccination.[66]

Chickenpox vaccination

It was always stated that the favourite infectious disease was chickenpox because it is generally mild with no severe effects and there is no vaccination. This is true no longer since a licence for a chickenpox vaccine was issued in 1995 in the US. The main danger of chickenpox is to those whose immune systems are depleted – people receiving chemotherapy for cancer or leukaemia and those taking corticosteroids.

Adverse reactions of chickenpox vaccination include:

- swelling and redness at the site of injection
- fever
- chickenpox rash
- upper respiratory tract symptoms
- cough
- pneumonia
- nephritis
- irritability
- anxiety
- fatigue
- insomnia
- diarrhoea
- constipation
- loss of appetite
- nausea and/or vomiting
- ear infection
- headache
- teething
- malaise
- abdominal pain
- enlarged lymph glands
- muscle and joint pains
- rashes.

Comments

The foregoing discussion of vaccination may present information that is new to you. Certainly, during my training at medical school and beyond, I was completely unaware that this information existed. I would only ask you to consider this information and decide for yourself. Many people have serious misgivings about vaccination and seek help from holistic practitioners. I would hope that the information I have quoted here and other sources will be more widely available in the future.[67]

Vaccination	Age
Diptheria, tetanus, whooping cough (pertussis) – DPT or triple vaccine	May vary according to the preferences of your region but when I qualified it was 5, 7 and 13 months. Now it is more likely to be 2, 3 and 4 months
Polio (oral)	With DPT vaccine
Meningitis (*haemophilus influenzae* – Hib)	With DPT vaccine
Measles, mumps and rubella (MMR)	12-18 months [68]
Diphtheria, tetanus and polio (oral) booster	3-5 years
Meningitis (*haemophilus influenzae* – Hib) booster	3-5 years
Measles, mumps and rubella (MMR) booster	3-5 years
Tetanus booster	Every 5 years
Bacille Calmette Guérin (tuberculosis) BCG	As a baby in inner city areas where tuberculosis is increasing. At about 12-14 years otherwise
Diphtheria, tetanus and polio (oral) booster	13-18 years

Table 5.11: Current vaccination schedule in UK

Vaccine	Presentation	Conventional contraindications
Cholera	Killed organisms injected	Acute illness, fever, hypersensitivity (may result from repeated vaccinations)
Diptheria	Toxin injected (alone or as part of DPT or as part of DT)	Acute illness, fever
Hepatitis B	Killed organisms injected – two types, one from human plasma and the other from yeast cells	Severe infection
Hepatitis B – for contacts	Human immunoglobulin	Lasts a few weeks only. Not to be given within 3 weeks of a live virus vaccination. Live virus vaccinations must be given over 3 weeks before or 3 months after
Hepatitis A	Human immunoglobulin	For contacts. Lasts a few weeks only. Live virus vaccinations must be given over 3 weeks before or 3 months after
Haemophilus influenzae b (Hib)	Killed organisms injected	Hypersensitivity to vaccine components or to previous Hib vaccine, fever
Influenza	Killed organisms injected	Hypersensitivity to egg, acute illness, fever, pregnancy. Children under four years
Measles	Live organisms injected – contains neomycin and polymyxin (alone or as part of MMR)	Acute illness, fever, lymphatic system malignancy, pregnancy, people receiving immunosuppressants, corticosteroids or radiotherapy, allergy [69] to neomycin or polymycin, hypersensitivity to egg
Measles, mumps, rubella (MMR)	Live organisms injected	See individual entries under measles and rubella
Meningitis C	Killed organisms injected	Hypersensitivity to vaccine components or to previous meningitis vaccine, fever
Polio	Live organisms (oral) – usual in UK – contains small amounts of penicillin, streptomycin, polymyxin, neomycin. Killed organisms (injection) – contains small amounts of penicillin, streptomycin, neomycin	Acute illness, fever, vomiting, diarrhoea, malignancy of the lymphatic system, in the first four months of pregnancy, hypersensitivity to the antibiotics contained in the vaccine
Rubella	Live organisms injected (alone or as part of MMR)	Acute illness, fever, malignancy of the lymphatic system, pregnancy, people receiving immuno-suppressants, corticosteroids or radiotherapy, hypersensitivity to neomycin or polymycin. Avoid pregnancy for one month after vaccination
Tetanus	Toxin injected (alone or as part of DPT or as part of DT)	Acute illness, fever
Tuberculosis (BCG)	Live organisms injected – unless newly born everyone must have skin test first to check for hypersensitivity to the vaccine	Acute illness, fever, positive sensitivity to the vaccine, generalised septic skin conditions (if eczema is present than may be vaccinated on normal skin area), people receiving immunosuppressants, corticosteroids, radiotherapy, malignancy of the lymphatic system
Typhoid	Killed organism injected	Under 1 year of age, acute illness, fever, typhoid outbreak, hypersensitivity (may result from repeated administration)
Whooping cough	Killed organism injected (alone or as part of DPT)	Acute illness, fever, history of severe reaction to a previous dose. Special care in those with cerebral damage, history of convulsions in child or immediate family

Table 5.12: Commonly administered vaccinations – methods and effects

The conventional contraindications are reasonable as far as they go but I would add some of my own. Avoid vaccination in the following situations:

- any chronic disease but particularly neurological conditions, allergic conditions or conditions where allergy is a factor
- acute illness
- allergic or hypersensitivity reaction to a previous vaccination (of any kind)
- current treatment with any drug which depletes the immune system including antibiotics
- pregnancy
- breast feeding
- anyone with an immature immune system – this is certainly everyone under the age of six months of age but strictly speaking means anyone under about 18 years of age.

Vaccination and foreign travel

Some people say to me that they accept the arguments about vaccination in this country but what about travel to other countries? If the statements about vaccination here are true, they must also hold true for diseases such as hepatitis, typhoid and cholera.

Compulsory vaccinations are restricted to yellow fever in some African and South American countries. In addition, specific vaccinations such as cholera or typhoid may be compulsory from time to time in areas where there is an outbreak. All other vaccinations and treatments are recommended only.

It would seem sensible to avoid contact, as much as possible, with contaminated food and water, biting insects and so forth. Travel does entail a certain degree of risk. It is clear that vaccination does not remove such risk. We all have to make decisions for ourselves based upon information and our personal preferences.

HOW TO RECOGNISE SERIOUS CONDITIONS IN ACUTE INFECTIOUS DISEASE

A common question that is asked by holistic practitioners is how to recognise when people may have disease that is life-threatening or dangerous. In such cases hospital treatment may be required or the help of a conventionally trained practitioner. The table below is a guide to what to look for. With children, be more circumspect because their symptoms change more quickly and more frequent monitoring will be necessary. In terms of acupuncture you would treat the person every day or so, and in the case of herbs perhaps give enough for two or three days. Also, you may need to be available by telephone.

Symptom	Comments
Fever very high	104°F (40°C) and above indicates potentially severe disease. Strong vital energy but the process may damage the person
Fever mild	Perhaps 99-100°F (37.2-37.8°C) may indicate mild disease but could be the beginning of severe disease in a weak person, i.e. vital energy too weak to generate fever
Fever prolonged	Most fevers last a day or so. If several days have elapsed then the concern is that the person is not strong enough to throw off the problem
Dehydration	This may result from loss of fluids, e.g. diarrhoea and vomiting or lack of intake. In babies look for dry skin/lips, decreased skin elasticity, strong urine, scanty urine or even dry nappy, sleepy, lack of responsiveness. In older people there will be reported thirst also
Symptom severity	The stronger the symptoms, e.g. lots of diarrhoea, lots of vomiting, then the more potentially serious they are. However be careful since weak people have weak symptoms, e.g. pneumonia in the elderly or people with AIDS may present only with breathlessness and no cough or fever. Assess each case carefully
Site of symptoms	Are these in the superficial levels of the body or involving internal organs? If symptoms occur indicating pathology in the lung, kidney, liver, heart or central nervous system then these are clearly more worrying. In terms of Chinese medicine, worry more if the symptoms are at deeper levels of the Taiyin, Shaoyin and Jueyin
Progression	Assess the direction of the pathology. Is it moving to internal organs or more superficially? Of concern is if symptoms start to appear indicating pathology at a deeper level, e.g. in the case of the respiratory system – sore throat with fever progressing to cough then breathlessness and finally confusion – an effect on the deepest level (mental)
Pulse diagnosis (Chinese medicine)	If you treat a person with an External Pathogenic Factor and the pulse is superficial, floating and even overflowing then after treatment you would expect the pulse to moderate. If this does not occur it indicates that the External Pathogenic Factor may be stronger than the upright Qi. Careful assessment of the case is then necessary as treatment is likely to be difficult. The next thing to happen may be collapse of the energy

Table 5.13: How to recognise serious conditions in acute 'infectious' disease

SUMMARY

The presence of organisms does not indicate disease as they are often found in 'normal' healthy people.

Any pathogenic influence of organisms must be the *result* of a pre-existing imbalance and not the cause.

Symptoms are the key to treating these diseases.

Ignore the organism and take the case.

Make a judgment as to the severity of the case based on the symptom picture.

Antibiotics are safe to stop *unless* the condition is severe or it is a case of long-term prescription.

Antibiotics are usually used inappropriately.

---

1 *Pasteur Exposed* by Ethel Douglas Hume (Bookreal, 1989). This book, originally published in 1923, clearly delineates the rival theories pursued by Bechamp and Pasteur and their attempts to find the truth by experimental methods. Pasteur was very much the seeker of fame and is the one who has been recognised by history. Bechamp, whose main work was blatantly plagiarised, worked away quietly and diligently to support the theory that it is the 'soil' – the immune system – which is the key, not the organism.

2 I would remind you of my comments in Chapter 2 about the immune system. I use this term throughout the book to refer to a wide, energetic view that includes superficial energetic levels, skin, mucous membranes, muscles and joints, bowels, internal organs and finally blood.

[3] The existence of organisms and their appearance are interesting to consider. Diseases of similar appearance may or may not have the same organisms associated with them. Many organisms associated with disease are present in the environment and ourselves all the time. Symptoms appear, i.e. disease is diagnosed, only when the conditions are right. There is no relationship with the organism itself as an external entity.

[4] Royal Raymond Rife, inventor of the Rife microscope in the 1920s, used this instrument to study tissue at magnifications far in excess of any equipment then available. However, his discoveries were so at variance with medical thought, then and now, that it has been difficult to even hear about them. See them *What Has Become of the Rife Microscope* by Christopher Bird, *New Age Journal,* March 1976.

[5] *The Persecution and Trial of Gaston Naessens* by Christopher Bird (Kramer, 1991).

[6] *The Yellow Emperor's Classic of Internal Medicine* (known as the *Neijing*). Translation by Henry Lu. Volume IV, 46.1.

[7] *The Yellow Emperor's Classic of Internal Medicine* (known as the *Neijing*). Translation by Henry Lu. Volume IV, 66.2.

[8] Do not confuse absence of disease (which has no symptoms) with mild disease (which has weak symptoms).

[9] The skin rashes of childhood appear as macule, papule, vesicle and pustule. These terms are explained in Chapter 11 – Dermatology.

[10] *Annals of Neurology* 1981;9:17-20.

[11] *Immunisation against Infectious Disease* DHSS leaflet, 1988.

[12] *Lancet,* July 7th 1990:51.

[13] I would include the use of prescribed drugs here as well as 'recreational' drugs.

[14] There is a recognition in Chinese medicine that excessive sexual activity particularly when emotionally disturbed, under the influence of drugs or when tired is more depleting to the body's energies.

[15] *New England Journal of Medicine* June 1st 1989:1458-62.

[16] There are many practitioners of holistic medicine who are working with HIV-positive people and people with AIDS. As with the holistic treatments of cancer, they are under supported although there are some well-organised support groups in the UK and particularly the US who are more involved in such treatment. Recently the work of Chinese medical practitioners in Africa has proved that Chinese medicine has much to offer for patients.
An unpublished trial by Professor BoPing Wu of the Academy of Traditional Chinese Medicine in Beijing working in Tanzania summarised the treatment of 158 HIV-positive patients between 1988 and 1991. The T4 cell count increased in 31% and 7% became HIV-negative.

[17] In good conventional practice, prophylaxis is restricted to specific situations where risk is known and not merely suspected. In routine clinical practice, a different pattern of behaviour is often evident. 'Failure to establish and adhere to such guidelines has made unnecessary chemoprophylaxis the commonest form of antibiotic misuse in hospitals' *Antimicrobial Chemotherapy,* Edited by D. Greenwood (Baillière and Tindall, 1983). Of course, 'antibiotic misuse' is not confined to hospitals.

[18] 'The Prescribed Drug Guide – A Holistic Perspective', Dr S Gascoigne (Jigme Press, 2001) is a comprehensive account of how to categorise the strength of drugs, how to manage patients who take them and how to reduce or withdraw them safely in selected cases.

[19] Although the terms vaccination, immunisation and inoculation have slightly different definitions, I shall use the word vaccination to embrace them all.

[20] There is a noted connection between the development of lymphomas (malignant disease of the lymphatic system) and vaccination particularly polio and BCG. *Eur J Cancer Prev* 2000;9(1):59-64.

[21] Reports of the Registrar General.

[22] Parliamentary reply, February 12th 1964.

[23] *The Vaccination Bible* edited by Lynne McTaggart (What Doctor's Don't Tell You, 2000).

[24] Hepatitis vaccination is a significant source of mercury found in babies, *J Paediatr* 2000;136(5):679-81.

[25] *A Shot In The Dark* by Harris Coulter and Barbara Loe Fisher (Avery, 1991).

[26] Viera Schreibner in her seminal work, *Vaccination - 100 years of Orthodox Research shows that Vaccines Represent a Medical Assault on the Immune System* (V Schreibner, 1997) details the work of herself and her late husband into developing a breathing monitor for babies. They rapidly realised that changes in respiration occurred frequently after vaccination. This led in some cases to Sudden Infant Death Syndrome. The changes in respiration were most marked in the first 2 weeks but also up to 25 days after vaccination. These are the cases specifically excluded from conventional assessments of adverse reactions to vaccination. Viera Schreibner in her book has detailed information obtained from respected medical journals of the adverse reactions of vaccination.

[27] It is often stated that modern medicine, including the use of vaccines and drugs such as antibiotics has been responsible for the improvement in life expectancy. In 1841 in Britain, a man of 50 years had a life expectancy of 20.0 years. In 1976 it was 22.7 years. This is a remarkably small improvement. The overall increase in life expectancy from birth has been due to decreases in infant mortality. This has declined due to changes in living conditions and not to medical treatments.

[28] More recent advances may be put into perspective by the following. 'There have been considerable advances in some rare conditions but with perhaps two exceptions, peptic ulcer and renal failure, there is no major common disease in which it is possible to demonstrate convincingly that those receiving the best treatment in 1985 are much better off than those who received the best treatment in 1960.' *Oxford Textbook of Medicine*, Volume 1: Page 2.1 (Oxford University Press, 1987).

[29] *Medical Nemesis* by Ivan Illich (Bantam, 1976).

[30] *Medical Nemesis* by Ivan Illich (Bantam, 1976).

[31] *Lancet,* August 1st 1981.

[32] In developing countries, there is the use of high strength vaccine in children under 1 year of age which causes increased mortality. *Lancet,* October 12th, 1991:903-906.

[33] *General Practitioner,* August 24th 1990.

[34] In 1978, an announcement was made in the USA of the goal of eliminating measles by 1982. History has revealed the worth of this rather grandiose scheme.

[35] *Epoch,* Volume 4, M. Nightingale 1982-3.

[36] *American Journal of Clinical Nutrition* 1977;30:592-98.

[37] *Clinical Immunopathology* 1981;21:341-50.

[38] Sir Henry Yellowlees, UK Chief Medical Officer, February 26th 1976.

[39] *Vaccines* by Plotkin and Mortimer (Saunders, 1988).

[40] *Science,* March 1977.

[41] Wakefield *et al. Lancet,* 28th February, 1998.

[42] *The Vaccination Bible* edited by Lynne McTaggart (What Doctor's Don't Tell You, 2000).

[43] *Epoch* Volume 4, M. Nightingale 1982-3.

[44] *New Scientist* 1989;1689:24.

[45] *Lancet* 1991;338:395-8.

[46] *New Eng J Med,* 1991;324:1767-72.

[47] Leaflet *Immunisation – Introduction to a New Perspective* by Marcus Williams.

[48] Australian Associated Press, 20/10/97.

[49] Public Health Laboratory Service – press statement, 1/10/99.

[50] BBC *News,* 19/11/99.

[51] BALTIMORE, *PRNewswire,* 8/11/99.

[52] North American Vaccine – vaccine information statement, 29/7/97.

[53] 'My general impression is that the incidence of meningococcal disease is still very low. It should be offered as an optional vaccine. If there are any outbreaks on college campuses, they should be taken care of locally. We are not really pursuing routine meningococcal vaccination or seeing it requested'. Joseph Horem, MD. *Paediatric News* 1999;33(9):51.

[54] Meningococcal C (meningitis C) vaccine fact sheet, Dept. of Health, UK, 1999.

[55] *Clin Exp Rheumatol* 2000 18(2):255 reported cases of arthritis following vaccinations against diphtheria, polio and tetanus.

[56] *Confessions of a Medical Heretic* by Robert Mendelsohn (1984).

[57] *British Medical Journal* 1981;282:1595-99

[58] World Health Organisation Bulletin, 1980.

[59] Melnick, J.L. *et al,* Excretion of SV-40 virus after ingestion of oral polio vaccines, *Proc Soc Exp Biol Med* 1962;109:965-968.
Shah K.V. et al., Serologic evidence for a simian-virus-40-like infection in man. *J Nat Cancer Inst* 1972 48:557-561.

[60] *Muscle Nerve* 2000;23(5):824-5.

[61] This syndrome was commonly found after the so-called 'swine flu' vaccination campaign in the US in 1976. Hundreds of cases of the syndrome were seen and dozens of people died within the four months of receiving the vaccination. Three billion dollars in compensation was paid out.

[62] Bailey et al., Tuberculosis prevention trial, *Madras Ind J Med Res* 1980;72 (suppl:1-74.

[63] Germanaud J. BCG vaccination and healthcare workers, *BMJ* 1993;306:651-2.

[64] Blood borne infections such as Hepatitis B and HIV are much less common now that blood and blood products are treated before they are used. Whether they are safe or not is a larger question!

[65] Shaw, F.E. *et al., Am J Epidemiol* 1988;127(2):337-352.

[66] *Eur J Med Res* 2000; 5(5):229-230.

[67] A clear and concise description of vaccination and its problems is contained in *Mass Immunisation – A Point in Question* by Trevor Gunn (Cutting Edge Publications, 1992). This is published in booklet form and is useful to have in the waiting room or to be given to patients.

[68] This vaccine (MMR) is given even with a history of these diseases or previous vaccination of measles.

[69] Allergy here indicates any allergic reaction to a substance of mild nature. Hypersensitivity refers to severe allergic phenomenona that would include wheezing, cyanosis, breathing difficulties, low blood pressure, fainting, shock and urticaria.

6 CANCER

INTRODUCTION

Cancer is a term that is applied to groups of cells that are malignant. Malignant cells are capable of rapid growth and do not respect normal tissue boundaries. Such cells, therefore, break out of their original site to spread either locally or through the blood or lymphatic systems. The name, cancer, is derived from the Latin for crab and this indicates its nature of grabbing or clawing at neighbouring tissue and invading.

Cancer is a powerful symbol in our society. A diagnosis of cancer leads to great consequences for the affected person and their family. It is very common with, on average, one person in three developing the disease and one in four dying of it. Very few families are untouched by it. Death is such a taboo in the West that the diagnosis of cancer frequently provokes shock, disbelief and huge psychological difficulties.

Cancer has always been with us and was described by the ancient Greeks. In this century, there have been increasing numbers of people with cancer – this has been described as an epidemic of cancer. This reflects the general increase in incidence of all chronic diseases. This is not due to more effective means of diagnosis (the majority of people are still diagnosed by the tried and trusted methods of old) or due to increased life expectancy. Changes in life expectancy have not occurred significantly over the past 50 years and yet more and more cancer has appeared in recent years.[1-2] There has been a genuinely measurable increase in the numbers of people who develop cancer. World Health Organisation figures show a 25 per cent increase in cancer in recent years that represents a real increase of 12 or 13 per cent.

It is often quoted that we are waging a war against cancer and terms such as these reveal much about conventional views of cancer.[3] Conventionally, it is believed that cancer comes from somewhere outside ourselves and that we are the passive victims of its invasion and assault. The cancer is seen as something that is alien and has to be attacked. Nowadays, there are theories that we are somehow genetically programmed, or not, to develop cancer. Whatever the current conventional medical fad, there is the continuing belief that there is little or nothing we can do to prevent it.

In reality, cancer does not come from elsewhere, our bodies manufacture it and it is a manifestation of an underlying energetic imbalance. This is no different, in principle, from the holistic view of other diseases – except that cancer may be life-threatening. Some of the emotion generated around cancer is also related to older ideas associated with diseases such as leprosy, syphilis, tuberculosis and plague. The person is often shunned and stigmatised by the diagnosis of cancer, they are seen as being a victim but also somehow tainted. People are treated in ghetto-like institutions and they are frequently subjected to treatments that seem, and indeed often are, worse than the original disease.

I am reminded here of the description of the death of Charles II and similarities with the treatment of some people with cancer. The King fell ill with a kidney complaint and a series of physicians proceeded to bleed him, use cupping glasses and scarification, administer purgatives, blister the skin of his shaven head ending with red-hot cautery. For four days and nights he was 'treated' by 14 physicians. At the end of this time he apologised for 'an unconscionable time a-dying'.[4]

I see many similarities with the treatment of cancer today. Some people are given treatment that is severely depleting, which may end in complete collapse of the immune system. Some people are given treatment when they are clearly in a terminal or pre-terminal state.[5] This causes difficulties for patients and their families since they may feel relief that 'something is being done' and believe there is no hope of recovery, whereas the conventional view is that death is inevitable. In such cases, having been weakened by the treatment, there can only be increased suffering at the time of death. There needs to be an acknowledgement that people worry not only about dying but also about *how* they may die.

It is this disquiet with the conventional treatment of cancer that has driven practitioners to seek out alternatives. When I trained in medicine and subsequently in practice, I had no idea that such alternatives even existed, let alone their success rates. Alec Forbes, who helped found the Bristol Cancer Help Centre, said that he chose cancer as the disease to treat by means of holistic medicine because it is the condition that is treated particularly badly by conventional medicine and particularly well by unorthodox means.[6]

TUMOURS

The technical word for a lump of any description is tumour (Latin, *tumor* – swelling). Confusingly, the word tumour is also used as a euphemism to indicate cancer. The idea of a lump, and the possibility that it may be cancerous, is frightening for most of us. However, not every lump is cancerous.

Tumours are classified by conventional medicine as either benign or malignant. This distinction can only be definitively determined by microscopic examination of the lump after removal from the body. The two words are very different in their associations. Benign conjures up feelings of friendliness, harmlessness, quiescence and reflects the connection with benevolent. The term malignant is quite different. Sharing a root with malevolent, you can see how a completely different feeling arises. Now thoughts appear of evil, invasion, despair, pain and death.

When people are asked to visualise lumps, two appearances are commonly seen – Figure 6.1. Visualisation can be a powerful method of treatment. The cancer is visualised and the image that comes to mind is transformed into healthy tissue or cleansed out of the body. As improvement occurs, the images will change to become less diseased and more positive. There are several excellent books on this subject that outline the methods used and the responses that are possible.[7]

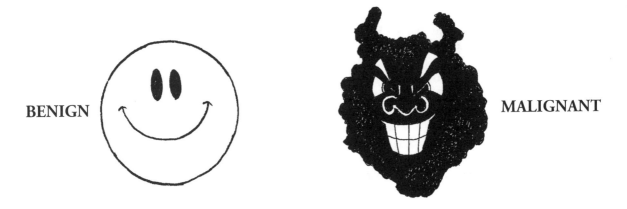

BENIGN   **MALIGNANT**

Figure 6.1: Common images of benign and malignant tumours

The duality of benign and malignant pervades the whole issue of tumours and cancer. There is a tremendous feeling of relief if people have a benign tumour. Great fear ensues leading to a desire to attack the cancer if people have a malignant tumour. There are many military metaphors in medical practice and none more so than in the field of cancer treatment. It is no accident that wars are fought against cancer as well as against foreign armies. Terms are used such as surgical strike, magic bullet, aiming and targeting. Always the emphasis is on aggressive treatment. Only the lump is considered as if the person to whom it belongs were merely an extraneous attachment.

CANCER

This is the second commonest cause of death in the Western World. The commonest cancers are in the lung, large bowel and breast. The conventional philosophical view is that all disease comes from outside the body. Thus, the causes of cancer are seen as external in origin. This is the basis of health education schemes to change behaviour, follow a more 'healthy' lifestyle and avoid known causes of cancer – see Table 6.1. Despite the work done in the 1950s by Sir Richard Doll in the UK outlining the connection between smoking and cancer, there is a deliberate lack of emphasis in conventional medicine regarding any connection between cancer and chemicals or radiation. The Imperial Cancer Research Fund in the UK states: 'One of the biggest myths in recent years is that there is a cancer epidemic caused by exposure to radiation, pollution, pesticides and food additives'.[8] What is not a myth of course is that the pharmaceutical companies producing chemicals to treat cancer often produce many other kinds of chemicals. There are powerful vested interests that seek to minimise the effects on our health of chemicals and radiation.

Event	Tissue affected
Ultraviolet light	Skin
Tar based substances	Skin
Aniline dyes	Bladder
Asbestos	Pleura
Benzene	Blood (leukaemia)
Vinyl chloride (PVC manufacture)	Liver
Radiation	Blood (leukaemia)[9]
Tobacco smoking[10]	Lung, lip, tongue
Drugs – female sex hormones	Breast, uterine cervix
Alcohol	Liver
Diet	Large intestine, oesophagus, stomach
Viruses	Uterine cervix – not proven

Table 6.1: Known or suspected causes of cancer

The holistic view is that there is a pre-existing susceptibility (see Chapter 5). Hence the 'causes of cancer' become merely triggers that lead to cancer in susceptible people. The real cause becomes a disordered vital force that manifests as a depleted immune system.

The immune system guards externally against invasion and internally detects and corrects imbalances. Cancer is arising all the time in our bodies.[11] When the immune system is healthy, these are dealt with before they become noticeable. If the immune system is depleted then the cancer can grow and become clinically identifiable. The holistic approach is to nourish and support the immune system so that it can deal with the cancer itself. The most appropriate treatment is generally to encourage the body to transform cancerous tissue – matter and energy – into healthy cells. In this way there is no waste. Surgery, where parts of the body are lost forever, means that this is not possible.

Therefore, prevention of cancer lies in maintaining a healthy immune system in all senses of the word. The tonsils, which are groups of lymphatic glands in the throat, serve to act as one of the first lines of defence. If they are removed our immune systems are weakened. It has been noted that children who have their tonsils removed are three times more likely to develop Hodgkin's disease, a malignant disease of the lymphatic system.[12]

Psychological traumas are the most powerful suppressors of the immune system. Cancer frequently follows a psychological shock such as bereavement, separation or other major life change.[13] Galen in the 2nd century AD stated: 'Melancholic women are more subject to tumours than sanguine women.' Burrows in 1723 said: 'Cancer is caused by the uneasy patterns and passions of the mind with which the person is strongly affected for a long time.' Sir James Paget in 1870 wrote: 'The cases are so frequent in which deep anxiety, deferred hope and disappointment are quickly followed by the growth and increase of cancer that we can hardly doubt that mental depression is a weighty addition to the other influences favouring the cancerous constitution.'

Here, we see two diametrically opposed systems – conventional medicine sees the cancerous lump as the problem which must be attacked and removed at all costs. Success is judged in terms of reducing or removing the lump with little mention of the person. Ironically, or not depending on your point of view, all the conventional treatments damage the immune system.

Holistic medicine sees the whole person and their immune system as the issue to be dealt with and so treatments are nourishing and strengthening. The so-called non-toxic cancer therapies, of which there are many, have been called the Gentle Method.[14] The person's energy is gently strengthened to the point where they, themselves, transform the cancer. The lump takes second place to the person and so may not change in size for a long time. It may even increase in size in the short term. A conventional doctor would see this as failure of the treatment. This can create difficulties when treating people with cancer.

The conventional definitions of response depend entirely on the behaviour of the cancer itself – Table 6.2. There is no mention of the person, quality of life or subjective changes in health. The condition of the person, conventionally, is not viewed in any depth. Any increase in general well being, appetite and so forth is of overwhelming importance in holistic medicine. Although welcomed by conventional practitioners, this is seen as being of less importance than the overriding issue of tumour size. The general condition of the person is mainly seen as important in relation to the ability to withstand conventional treatments such as radiotherapy or chemotherapy.

Complete response	Complete disappearance of all detectable disease
Partial response	More than 50 per cent reduction in the size of the tumour
No response	No change or less than 50 per cent reduction
Progressive disease	Increase in size of tumour at any site

Table 6.2: Conventional criteria for response of cancer to treatment[15]

Symptoms

Conventionally, symptoms are seen as a result of the presence of the cancerous lump itself. Any symptoms experienced before this is evident are not well understood by conventional practitioners. People with cancer may at first say that the lump was the first problem they noticed. On further questioning, however, they have had other symptoms – perhaps feeling tired, run-down or other more specific problems for some months or years before the diagnosis was made.

Some specific symptoms can be related to the lump itself. They may be understood as resulting from a progressive enlargement, which tends to invade surrounding tissue. The swelling itself is more or less obvious, depending upon its location. There may be enlargement of associated lymph glands. This is commonly due to inflammation and is a defence reaction. In some cases the cancer may have spread to these lymph glands. The lump is usually felt as being hard, irregular and immobile due to its invasion of surrounding tissue. This is in contradistinction to benign tumours, which are usually soft, smooth and mobile as they are surrounded by a capsule of tissue.

If the cancer is in an enclosed space such as the skull then symptoms of pressure will be more severe and become evident sooner and more severely. In this case, therefore, you see symptoms such as headache, vomiting, visual disturbances and eventually tiredness leading to confusion, sleepiness and coma.

A cancer in a hollow tube such as the gastrointestinal tract or adjacent to structures such as the common bile duct will lead to obstruction of that tube. In the case of the large intestine this leads to symptoms such as abdominal distension, constipation, colicky pain and eventually vomiting. In the case of the biliary system, there is the development of jaundice.

Since cancer may be an invasive process, bleeding will occur if the cancer breaks through onto a body surface such as the skin, mucous membrane, cervical canal and so on. This is why bleeding is always taken seriously. Symptoms such as haematemesis, haemoptysis, abnormal vaginal bleeding, bleeding in the stools may indicate cancer. This clearly depends on other factors such as age and lifestyle since there are many possible causes of each of these symptoms.

Pain and weight loss are usually thought of as common, early symptoms. In fact these occur late in the development of the disease and not in every case. Pain may be due to involvement of nerves, organ distension or general pressure. Typically, the pain is often dull and constant. Pain of this nature nearly always indicates a serious condition since energetically it reveals severe depletion of the person's energy. Pain that is sharp and changes from time to time is often indicative of a less severe condition. Weight loss occurs particularly with cancer of the lung and gastrointestinal tract. It is not seen in people with cancer of the breast or brain.

People will also have symptoms according to their own individual condition, which is of much more importance to practitioners of holistic medicine.

In rare situations, cancers produce hormones and syndromes of over production of hormones may present. They are usually antidiuretic hormone (ADH) or adrenocorticotrophic hormone (ACTH).

The key clinical picture that may indicate cancer includes:

- short history – weeks or months rather than months or years
- progressive – symptoms which develop over a short time with new ones developing indicating a progression, e.g. cough for 8 weeks with occasional haemoptysis over the past 3 weeks and the recent development of breathlessness
- lump
- bleeding.

If you see any of these, particularly the first two, you must always think of cancer as a possible diagnosis.

Conventional diagnosis of cancer

Conventional medicine always seeks to establish whether a lump is benign or malignant and the precise nature of the cells before any treatment or decisions about management can be made. This is because the tumour is considered to be the primary target for treatment. A biopsy[16] obtains samples of cells, which are examined microscopically to determine their appearance.

When cells are examined under the microscope, there is a remarkable resemblance to the diagrams on Page 78 of visualised lumps. A benign tumour is an accumulation of cells that reproduce in abnormal numbers but remain within the tissue of origin. They are relatively well behaved and do not stray outside a surrounding capsule. They are regular in size and shape, do not divide quickly and resemble their tissue of origin. A benign tumour may occasionally grow so large that it becomes a cosmetic problem. It may press on neighbouring structures. This is particularly true in the brain because the rigid skull does not allow expansion and so pressure symptoms are common.

Malignant tumours are capable of invading adjacent tissues and disseminating to form deposits in distant sites (metastasis). They are delinquent in nature and do not behave as normal cells. They do not seem to realise who they are or where they are. This loss of identity clearly reflects a serious problem and the deep pathology that must precede their appearance. The cells are irregular in shape and size, divide rapidly, do not resemble their tissue of origin so much and may outgrow their confining capsule. This is an imbalance of control rather than a problem with a few individual cells. The body has a control system to enable cells to know what they are, where they are and how much they should divide, develop and grow.

Although the distinction between benign and malignant is often clear-cut, this is by no means always the situation. Some cancers are designated latent (carcinoma-in-situ). That is, they have the microscopic appearance of cancer but do not break out of their capsule and remain in their tissue of origin. This serves to illustrate that there are different degrees of malignancy and carcinoma-in-situ will be present in someone whose immune system is relatively strong. In this case the cancer is being held in check, not receding and not advancing.

Conventional classification of malignant tumours

The classification of tumours is according to their cellular appearances. Names are given to indicate their tissue of origin. Some cases are difficult to determine their exact type and reflect a very malignant process. Of course, the more malignant the disease then the more imbalanced is the immune system.

1. Carcinoma: tissue of endodermal or ectodermal origin e.g. skin, bowel mucus membranes.
2. Sarcoma: tissue of mesodermal origin, e.g. muscle, bone.
3. Leukaemia/lymphoma: white blood cells/tissue from the lymphatic system.

Within each class there may be a subdivision depending on the precise cell type. For example, lung cancer may be squamous cell carcinoma, adenocarcinoma, small cell undifferentiated or large cell undifferentiated. The conventional significance is that some are affected more by radiotherapy or particular types of chemotherapy. In holistic medicine, the meaning is that those cancers that most resemble the organ of origin indicates a relatively strong immune system. The more undifferentiated are the cells, then the more disturbed is the immune system.

Staging

After a diagnosis of malignant disease has been made, investigations are performed to determine if the cancer has spread to distant sites. This is termed staging. Primary cancer is present only in its original site and the cells, although abnormal, are going to bear the closest relationship to those of the organ in which they are found. Secondary cancer is where cells develop in sites a distance away from the primary. Conventionally, these cells spread by means of the blood or lymphatic system or across body cavities. This process is known as metastasis.

The staging may be done in several ways. At the time of the original biopsy, lymph glands that drain the affected area may have also been removed. Scans are performed of bone and liver. A search is carried out in likely areas for evidence of further disease.

An assessment is made of the size of the primary tumour, the extent of local spread, lymph gland involvement and whether spread to distant parts has occurred. Staging is an indication of the degree of malignancy of the tumour and of the state of the tumour–person relationship. Many tumours are classified according to a TNM classification, T = tumour, N = nodes, M

= metastasis. T0 or T1 is an indication of the size of the tumour, M0 or M1 is an indication of whether there are metastases or not.

In some cases the cancer that has been diagnosed may be a secondary itself. For example, if a cancer becomes evident in the liver and is in several sites at once, it is likely that it has spread from somewhere in the gastrointestinal tract. In this case, a search will be made for the primary since treatment cannot begin until this is found and analysed. The fact that a primary is means that the imbalance must be severe.

In holistic medicine, what is important is the energy of the person. People who are relatively well localise a problem in one area of the body – whatever that problem may be. If their energy is depleted, the disease tends to spread and perhaps affect more internal levels or more important organs. Secondary cancer arises in those who are more depleted. Whether these cells travel round the body is, I think, irrelevant. The body is as capable of making 'secondary' cancer cells as it is of making 'primary' cancer cells.

Whether a cancer spreads or not is a function of the state of the person's energy. Conventional practitioners see it as a function of time and treat cancer as a surgical emergency. This haste and pressure can only serve to produce more anxiety and worry which in turns leads to further strain on the immune system. A large primary tumour indicates a healthier situation than a small primary tumour that may have spread early – Table 6.3.

Each position in Table 6.3 is a function of an individual's vital force, the strength of the immune system, of the upright Qi. It is *not* a question of time. If a person is very weak then they will move from the top to the bottom very quickly. This occurs when someone has a normal investigation one year and invasive cancer, perhaps with secondaries, the next. If someone has a relatively strong immune system then they will tend to remain at the top of the chart. Treatment here by *any* method will tend to be successful. Conventionally, surgery is used for primary tumours and this is relatively successful. This is to be expected. Treatment for people at the bottom of the chart by methods which serve to further deplete the immune system would be expected to lead to ill-health and possibly death.[17-18]

Health (strong immune system)
Malignant lump – primary
Secondary cancer
Widespread disease
Terminal condition
Death
Disease (weak immune system)

Table 6.3: Relationship between stage of cancer and strength of the immune system

Cancer spreads to different situations depending upon its original site – Table 6.4. The first spread is locally and to the relevant lymphatic glands. It is helpful to know the lymphatic drainage of the body as you will be able to know where to look for possible problems if you detect lymphatic gland enlargement – Table 6.5.

Primary site	Secondary cancer found in:
Lung	Liver, bone, brain, adrenal glands
Stomach	Liver, bone, brain, lung
Colon	Liver, lung
Breast	Liver, bone
Kidney	Liver, bone, lung
Prostate	Bone

Table 6.4: Site of secondary cancer

Lymphatic gland group	Area drained
Axillary	Front of chest, breast, upper back and shoulder, upper part of front and side of abdomen, upper limb
Supraclavicular	Skin of face and neck, external ear, lung, stomach (left side)
Inguinal	Penis, scrotum, vulva, perineum, abdominal wall below umbilicus, gluteal area, lower limb

Table 6.5: Main groups of lymphatic glands and the areas they drain[19]

Conventional treatment

The main aspect to consider in conventional medicine is whether the cancer is primary or secondary. In the case of only a primary tumour, the first sign of treatment is generally surgical. Depending upon the extent and type of the tumour, surgery may be followed by radiotherapy and/or chemotherapy. If secondary tumours are present, systemic treatment with chemotherapy and/or hormone therapy will be given. Response to treatment is evaluated according to the information in Table 6.2 on Page 80.

- In the case of primary tumours only, the treatment is usually local by either surgery or radiotherapy or a combination of both.
- If secondaries are present, systemic treatment with chemotherapy (and/or hormone) therapy will be given.
- There is an evaluation of the response to treatment as illustrated by Table 6.2 on Page 80.

These basic principles of treatment may change according to the preferences of the surgeon or physician in charge. Some people are given chemotherapy very early, others are given radiotherapy. There are many differences seen in clinical practice and from region to region and country to country.

Surgery

This is the conventional treatment of choice for most primary cancers. It may be used alone or with other treatments depending upon the cancer type and the preferences of the consultant in charge. After the development of anaesthesia and antisepsis in the latter part of the 19th century, surgery became very popular within the medical profession with ever more drastic operations being developed. There are risks involved with any surgery or anaesthesia – see Page 39.

Radiotherapy

The tumour is localised by the radiologist and multiple daily doses of radiation are given for a specified period of time. The practice in the UK and Ireland is to give the maximum permitted dose of radiation over one course and so people rarely have second courses. In the rest of Europe there seems to be lower doses given and so the courses can be repeated.

Radiation damages normal and malignant cells alike and so the radiation dose is aimed as accurately as possible. Despite this, many people experience marked symptoms. Treatment is usually continued for 3 to 6 weeks and causes a radiation-sickness syndrome of malaise, fatigue, nausea, anorexia and vomiting. This usually lasts for several months starting either during treatment or just after. It typically recurs with relatively normal periods in between.

The overlying skin becomes reddened and can break down. There are mouth and throat reactions. Thrush can be a problem. The bone marrow is affected if a large area is irradiated and so blood is checked regularly. Hair loss does not occur unless treatment is to the head when it is permanent. Radiotherapy to the gastrointestinal tract can cause difficulty swallowing, indigestion, diarrhoea, tenesmus and mucus per rectum.

Such treatment can be used in the case of secondary cancer to reduce the size of the cancer. In this case, it is only ever temporary in its effect and is merely aimed to give symptomatic relief only.

Chemotherapy

Chemotherapeutic agents cause toxic[20] side-effects that are worse the longer the treatment or the more agents are used. Frequently, several drugs are used in combination. They frighten people because they are concerned about their extreme effects. They are used routinely in about 50 per cent of people with cancer although it has been found that they are only of use in about 5 per cent of cases.[21-22]

The early agents were derived from nitrogen mustard, a chemical warfare agent. There are many different types now having effects in different parts of the cell metabolism. All cells have similar metabolism and so treatment affects all cells especially rapidly dividing cells as found in the gastrointestinal tract, bone marrow and skin (leading to hair loss). The maximum dose given is governed by the toxicity to the normal cells.

They are usually given repeatedly over periods of several months to several years. The toxic effect is monitored by noting symptoms and by regular blood checks. It is the state of the blood that is the controlling factor in the size of the dose given and the length of treatment. There may be intermittent administration to allow normal tissue to recover such as once every 3 or 4 weeks.

There are many side-effects because some damage to normal cells is inevitable. In the gastrointestinal tract there are mouth ulcers, nausea, vomiting and diarrhoea. There is hair loss which is usually reversible after the therapy ends. The blood is quickly affected and after 3-6 treatments most people have problems with tiredness, weakness, hair loss and signs of anaemia. Blood checks are done regularly and treatment may be stopped in those whose blood is affected severely.

There are often psychological problems involved in the illness and these may be magnified during treatment. Childhood growth may be stunted if treatment is given for a prolonged period of time. Intellectual impairment can occur, particularly in the treatment of children. Fertility is reduced in the case of post pubertal people, males being more affected than women. Chemotherapy agents are also carcinogenic and so cancer may develop after their use.

Hormonal therapy

Some malignant tumours develop in organs subject to hormonal control. Such cancers may also be hormone dependent and so manipulation of their hormone environment may affect their growth. Examples of such organs are the ovary, testis, uterus and breast.

Several methods may be used to apply these principles of treatment. The source of the hormone can be removed surgically. Alternatively, the levels can be manipulated chemically, either by using a drug that blocks the hormone or by administering its opposite hormone – Table 6.6.

Site of primary cancer	Treatment method
Breast	Administration of tamoxifen (oestrogen blocker) Removal of ovaries Administration of aminoglutethimide (adrenal blocker) Removal of adrenals Administration of androgens
Testis	Administration of oestrogen Removal of testes
Prostate	Administration of oestrogen
Ovary	Administration of progesterone
Uterus	Administration of progesterone

Table 6.6: Summary of hormonal treatments[23]

Biological therapy

This term applies to a relatively recently developed range of treatments that are considered to directly affect the immune system. Interferons are naturally produced by the immune system in response to viral infections. In recent years it has also been utilised in certain cancers as well as chronic infective hepatitis. Alpha-interferon has many and severe side effects including influenza-like symptoms, tiredness, loss of appetite, nausea, changes in liver function tests, suicidal behaviour, stroke and lowered white cell counts.

In cases where white cell counts are depleted by chemotherapy, granulocyte (G-CSF) and granulocyte/macrophage colony stimulating factor (GM-CSF) may be used especially in the US.

Holistic treatments of cancer

The essence of treatment by holistic medicine is to support and strengthen the immune system. At the same time methods may be applied against the cancer itself but this is a secondary issue. The prime concern is the state of the immune system. All the non-toxic cancer therapies have these aims in common.

Since disease always manifests at all levels of the person it is helpful to consider treatment at all of these levels to attain the best results. It is important to take multiple approaches with people to achieve this. Visualisation, dietary treatment and a specific form of holistic therapy are the minimum treatments I recommend.

The Hoxsey treatment is now situated at a clinic in Mexico after the US Government drove it out of the USA in the 1970s. The three strands of their treatment are healing through a positive attitude, diet and a herbal tonic. It is successful in having an 80 per cent cure rate[24] and these are usually people who have been through conventional medicine and are now categorised as untreatable. In conventional terms, they have a life expectancy in months rather than years.

Relaxation techniques can be taught quite easily and are extremely helpful. There is no doubt that visualisation adds power to the practice. Visualisation is an integral part of Buddhism and Hinduism and is a powerful tool for changing states of mind. Work has been done by physicians around the world to show that such treatments have proven, quantifiable results.[25]

Dietary treatment can be applied in many ways and my own methods, which reflect the principles of Chinese medicine, can be at variance with some of those used by other holistic cancer treatments. Diets consisting of large quantities of raw, cold food perhaps with the use of juice fasts, enemas and such like *are* detoxifying in nature. They aim to rid the body of the harmful substances that accumulate with time and lead eventually to disease such as cancer. From the Chinese medical perspective, however, they also remove valuable substances from the body and may be inappropriate in cases of depleted energy.

The precise details of diet depend upon the energetic diagnosis but there are some basic principles. The digestion, energetically, can be likened to a cooking pot. If cold and raw food is put into it then more energy has to be applied to the pot. Similarly, if people eat such food then more energy is required to digest the food. If there is already a digestive weakness or generally depleted energy this will be made worse. This is the reason why some people with cancer who eat raw, cold food in large quantities can get rapidly worse. I have seen people die due to following such diets.

General comments that are valid for most people are for cooked, warm food, no salt, no chemicals, the use of unbleached grains, no alcohol, tea or coffee. The emphasis is to be on vegetables, fruit (cooked) and grains. The principles of such treatment can be studied in several books on the subject of Chinese dietary therapy.[26]

Death is in the minds of everyone who has any contact with cancer and it is important that this is acknowledged. People may, for a variety of reasons, not be told their diagnosis. This prevents the person having access to information with which they may choose to change their lives. Elizabeth Kübler-Ross said it is not a question of whether to tell but when. People may also be told a conventional prognosis about length or quality of life when such pronouncements are notoriously inaccurate and often unnecessarily distressing.

Everyone has a right to knowledge so they can choose a course of action appropriate to them. The management of people with cancer is difficult but issues can be faced and explored so that emotions may be worked with and ultimately released. Suppression, particularly around the time of death, can only lead to more suffering and pain. There are several excellent texts that explore this.[27] Certainly some people do not want to know and it is important to respect this, but I believe that we should expect to tell people and to discuss the issues with them. The sense of relief that many people experience when they are shown that honesty and trust goes a long way to removing some of their problems. The hospice movement has, in the past few years, become a major benefit to people who are seriously ill and dying. Although they all too frequently depend upon drugs particularly for pain-relief, they are certainly aware of the issues that face people at death and are a great source of help. If people cannot be at home for their final days or weeks, a hospice can offer an appropriate alternative to hospital.

There needs to be the application of a specific method of treatment in addition to visualisation and diet. People with cancer are suffering from severe, degenerative disease and require help to deal with this. The main treatments that I advocate are herbalism with or without acupuncture and homoeopathy. In this way, the immune system of the person may be strengthened and internal blockages or deficiencies can be remedied. In my experience, the people who do best are those who reject conventional treatment and follow the methods outlined here. In this way, every treatment is designed to strengthen them and nothing depletes them.

In terms of Chinese medicine, many different syndromes can be diagnosed as cancer. The common occurrences are of Stagnation of Blood or Phlegm with underlying Yin or Yang deficiency. Such Stagnation is evident by the lump of the cancer but there is always an underlying chronic condition which is the predisposing factor in its development. The person's condition must be individualised for the most appropriate treatment to be applied.

The conventional treatments of radiotherapy and chemotherapy are part of an ancient method of treating tumours by escharotics. An escharotic is something that burns and has been used for centuries by herbal healers. Of course, the modern methods are much stronger and there is no way of using balancing treatments as with a complete herbal formula. Tamoxifen is an oestrogen blocker that is used after the primary treatment of breast cancer and is designed to prevent a recurrence. In energetic terms it should be considered the same as radiotherapy and chemotherapy. All these treatments are hot in nature, they damage the Spleen Qi and heat and dry the Blood particularly of the Liver and Kidney. Yin deficiency may result if the person is already Blood deficient.

The aim of conventional treatment is to melt the Stagnant lump of Phlegm or Blood with heat and this may have some results if the person is Yang deficient to begin with. If the person is Yin or Blood deficient, then the hot nature of the treatment may cause further Phlegm production as the Yin becomes more deficient. This would be evidenced clinically by the appearance of secondaries. In some people of course, the only way to remove a Phlegm lump is to dry all the body fluids and these are the people who die whilst having conventional treatment.

Cases

Describing case histories is the best way to summarise the holistic approach and to discuss issues around the treatment of cancer. I have outlined two cases here of radically different outcomes.

Case one
A woman of 40 years presented for treatment after a lump was removed from her right breast some 2 years previously and diagnosed as cancer. There was no other treatment given and 6 months before attending the clinic, she developed lumps in the scar of the operation and in the skin in several sites. These were diagnosed as secondary cancer in the skin. Bone and liver scans were normal She was given a course of chemotherapy for 6 months. There was no change in her condition except now she had developed breathlessness to the extent she could not walk upstairs without stopping.

She was told at this stage there was nothing more that could be done for her. She began a course of herbal treatment together with acupuncture, visualisation practice and sessions with a healer. The first reaction to treatment was that she felt better in herself with increased energy. Later the breathlessness began to subside. Within 3 months her skin lumps had disappeared. She was no longer breathless and could now walk with no problems.

After another 4 weeks she then noticed a lump begin to appear in her left breast. This gradually enlarged over a period of a week to become as large as a goose egg. This can now be classified as a primary cancer and if you study the Table 6.3 on Page 82 you will see that she has actually become healthier. She came originally with a secondary cancer and now had a primary. You would then expect this to reduce with treatment and eventually disappear. The conventional view, of course, sees this as another cancer that has to be treated in the same way as the first lump.

I informed her of my view of her progress but she decided to opt for a course of radiotherapy – five doses each week for 4 weeks. The breast lump quickly disappeared but within 1 week of the treatment she developed pain in the vertebrae and ribs. This was due to secondaries in the bone – worse than a secondary in the skin. Over the course of the next few weeks, many secondaries in bone appeared and were treated each time by radiotherapy locally. All the time her health was deteriorating and unfortunately she died some 4 weeks later.

There are several things to bring out here for discussion. People can improve even when apparently at an advanced stage of disease despite treatment by powerful suppressors of the immune system. Internal levels such as increased energy and well-being are the first changes seen. Treatment, if curative, may lead to the reappearance of old symptoms which in this case was primary cancer. People have strong faith in conventional medicine even if it is ineffective or leads to worse disease.

My personal view is that, in the end, people choose their own treatment plan and management. I do offer a holistic path for people and am, increasingly, keen that they have full knowledge of options. I have no problem offering people hope with my method of treatment since I know that this, in itself, can be therapeutic. I discuss conventional treatments and their effects with people so that they can decide which course of action is most appropriate for them.

Case two
A woman aged 44 years came for treatment. She was diagnosed as suffering from bone cancer some 10 years previously. The original site was the left mastoid area, which was treated with radiotherapy. Over the years, different areas of bone would be affected by cancer and each time radiotherapy was given. Each time the problem would disappear from that area only to reappear somewhere else.
Some 4 weeks before she sought holistic treatment, she developed generalised lymphatic gland enlargement, cough and breathlessness with multiple bony secondaries. Her other symptoms at that time were marked tiredness with very chilly feelings at 4am causing her to wake up. These are an indication that the energy is severely depleted.

The conventional treatment recommended was chemotherapy despite a poor prognosis and the likelihood of severe side-effects. She chose to decline this and decided to have treatment by means of Chinese herbs and acupuncture. She was also given dietary advice and recommended visualisation.

Again, the first changes were in general energy with increased well being, disappearance of the cold feelings in the morning and easing of cough and breathlessness. After 3 months of treatment virtually all the lymphatic glands had reduced in size and disappeared. She then began to develop pain behind the left ear with a feeling of 'drawing down' in the external auditory canal. On examination with an auriscope, there was a large, greyish cystic swelling obstructing the whole canal. This was the cancer affecting the mastoid area and surrounding tissues. Her hospital consultant wished to treat it with radiotherapy. As in Case 1, this is reappearance of the original primary cancer and is a curative event. Interference at this stage is dangerous and may lead to irrecoverable suppression. In this case, the decision was made to stay with holistic medicine only. Her view was that this was the only treatment that had ever really helped.

Over the next 6 months, the cystic swelling reduced in size and then disappeared. She still has some pain in the left mastoid 2 years later but remains well, is back at work and has few problems. I have no doubt that if she had received chemotherapy when recommended that she would not be alive.

The major difference between the two cases is that the second person had more faith in holistic treatment and managed to stay with the process. People are very fearful during their treatment, particularly if there is the appearance of unpleasant or worrying symptoms. They need a lot of support from us as practitioners, from their family, as well as information so that they can make informed decisions about treatment.

Cancer, and its treatment, draws a clear distinction between the opposing views of holistic medicine and conventional medicine. I believe that the more we can provide of a holistic path the greater will be the benefit to people's health. Ultimately, we can only offer what we believe to be true and so the priority is to have competence and confidence in our practice. This, together with diet, visualisation, healing and specific treatments, will definitely provide a vital service to people with serious health problems.

SUMMARY

The conventional view of cancer is that it is caused by external events.

The holistic view is that cancer is the result of a depleted immune system – susceptibility.

Conventional treatment focuses on the lump using surgery, radiotherapy, chemotherapy and hormones.

The holistic approach focuses on the state of the immune system by means of diet, visualisation and specific methods such as herbs or homoeopathy.

Cancer tends to spread to surrounding lymph glands and then distant sites.

The most effective results are obtained through multiple approaches. Mental and emotional issues are important factors that need to be dealt with using visualisation and counselling.

There are many sources of help and support for people whose illness is progressing towards death. Ultimately, the more comfortable we are with our own death, the more available we can be for people who are dying.

The conventional diagnosis may be cancer if you see any symptoms that have a short history and are of a progressive nature.

---

[1] *Chronic Disease and Public Health*, Edited by Lilienfeld and Gifford (John Hopkins Press, 1966). This reveals that there has been a real increase in the incidence of chronic disease including cancer. This is when other changes such as the age of the population has been taken into account.

[2] There has been an increase in cancer of 11 per cent in the last 40 years in real terms, i.e. taking account of population changes. National Cancer Institute (USA). See *Politics of Cancer* by Epstein (Sierra, 1978).

[3] There are moves within the conventional cancer establishment to present investigations and treatment in a more positive light. For example, there is a National Breast Awareness Month (NBAM) in the US each year. The aim of this, however, is to encourage women to seek mammograms and they are told that 'there are no practical ways to prevent breast cancer......the best opportunity for reducing mortality is through early detection' by mammography. The pros and cons of mammograms are argued elsewhere - see Page 366. The NBAM was conceived and funded by ICI in 1984. Its subsidiary is Zeneca Pharmaceuticals, the sole manufacturer of tamoxifen, the world's top-selling cancer drug. *Chicago Tribune,* October 26th, 1997, article by Dr Samuel Epstein.

4 *The Last Days of Charles II* by Raymond Crawford.

5 I have seen many occasions where a diagnosis of cancer has been made with a prognosis of surviving for a matter of months and yet people are still treated with chemotherapy. It is difficult, if not impossible, to see the therapeutic rationale for this. If people are not going to recover then why give them treatments that make them feel so ill? The answer lies partly in the doctor's desire to 'do something'.

6 Lecture given by Dr A Forbes at Bristol Cancer Help Centre, 1984.

7 *Getting Well Again* by Carl Simonton, Stephanie Simonton, James Creighton (Bantam, 1981).
Mind As Healer, Mind As Slayer by Kenneth Pelletier (Allen and Unwin, 1977), Pages 251-262 refer specifically to the management of cancer by visualisation methods. *Love, Medicine and Miracles* by Bernie Siegel (Rider, 1999).

8 *The Ecologist* 1998;28(2). This edition entitled, 'Cancer: Are the experts lying' is an in-depth analysis of current conventional ideas on cancer, its genesis and its treatment. It lucidly, and in detail, argues for a radical rethinking to a more holistic perspective.

9 There is a paradox here as conventional medicine acknowledges that radiation is the only known cause of leukaemia yet is slow to recognise that low levels of radioactive pollution can possibly cause leukaemia.

10 There is much emphasis on the avoidance of tobacco smoke, however, in rural China there is little difference in the rates of lung cancer between those who smoke and those who do not. Perhaps there are other factors at play here – the concept of susceptibility helps in explaining differences in cancer rates.

11 *Treatment of Inoperable Cancer* by W. Herberger (John Wright and Son, 1965).

12 *Lancet* 1971;1:431, *Lancet* August 16th, 1980: 338-9, *Journal of Paediatrics* 1958;52:339-61.

13 In *Mind As Healer, Mind As Slayer* by Kenneth Pelletier (Allen and Unwin, 1977) there is an excellent account of the commonly found personality traits found in people with cancer. See Pages 134-149.

14 *The Gentle Method* by Brenda Kidman

15 *Clinical Medicine* - Fourth Edition - Edited by Kumar and Clark (W B Saunders, 1998), Page 420.

16 This can be performed by surgery with local or general anaesthesia or by means such as cervical smear, sputum sample and aspiration by syringe and needle as in breast lumps.

17 *Cancer, The Alternative Method of Treatment of Cancer* by Isaac Bryant (Roberts Publications). There are several references here to increased death rates in people subjected to radiotherapy or chemotherapy.
Lancet March 15th, 1980; 580-2. This is an account of the decreased survival time of those with breast cancer treated with surgery and chemotherapy compared with those who only have surgery.
Although, the National Cancer Institute in the US, for example, regularly issue reports claiming improvements in survival rates in people with cancer, these are not supported by the facts. There has been little or no change in survival from the majority of cancers in the last 40 or 50 years.

18 It is one of the paradoxes of conventional medicine that the treatments with powerful effects on the immune system are reserved for those people who are weakest.

19 *Gray's Anatomy* Edited by Williams, Warwick, Dyson, Bannister (Churchill Livingstone, 1987 - 37th Edition).

20 The word 'toxic' is derived from *Taxus* – the yew. In recent years, Taxol, an extract from yew has been used to treat some cancers.

21 *Scientific American* November 1983, Volume 253. Article by John Cairns of Harvard University.

22 It is useful to think about the following observation. Chemotherapy cannot possibly kill all cancer cells since it kills normal cells at the same time. To kill all cancer cells by such a method would require the death of all cells. Hence it is left to the immune system to remove any remaining cancerous cells. Unfortunately, the immune system is particularly damaged by chemotherapy and so less likely to be able to help. This is a paradox which conventional medicine does not attempt to address.

23 These hormones are synthetic versions are carcinogenic themselves.

24 Mildred Nelson, *Hoxsey – A treatment for cancer,* US Film 1982. 'Cure rate' or survival rate are the terms used to mean that the person has survived for a certain period of time – usually 5 years. Conventionally, these are used to indicate whether a treatment is successful or not. I quote survival times as used by conventional medicine for each cancer in their relevant Chapters.

25 *Getting Well Again* by Carl Simonton, Stephanie Simonton and James Creighton (Bantam, 1981). This book was a great revelation to me. I read it when I was in general practice and prior to this I had great doubts about whether people could recover from serious chronic disease. An invaluable account of the power of visualisation.

26 *Chinese System of Food Cures* by Henry Lu (Sterling, 1986) and *Prince Wen Hui's Cook* by Bob Flaws and Honora Wolfe (Paradigm 1983). These are particularly useful for descriptions of the underlying principles of Chinese medicine and their application to diet.

27 *On Death and Dying* by Elisabeth Kübler-Ross (Tavistock Publications, 1986). An excellent account of the states of mind encountered during terminal illness and methods to ease the progression to acceptance.
The Tibetan Book of Living and Dying by Sogyal Rinpoche (Rider, 1992). This uses the insights of Tibetan Buddhism to help all of us gain an increased awareness of life and death. I cannot speak too highly of this book, which is written by one of the foremost spiritual teachers in the West.

7 CARDIOVASCULAR SYSTEM

INTRODUCTION

The cardiovascular system consists of the heart and blood vessels. Conventional medicine takes a physical view of the heart pumping blood through the vessels to complete a circuit. This can be likened to a domestic central heating system with a pump and tubes carrying fluid. This mechanistic view ignores any non-physical aspect.

Association	Comments
Propels Blood[1]	This is the familiar view of the heart as a pump
Governs Blood vessels	This association is familiar to the Western view
Houses the Mind	The word spirit may be used. It is the seat of consciousness and many disorders that are psychological in manifestation are classified energetically as Heart disorders
Paired organ is Small Intestine	This is how anxiety due to a Heart disturbance may lead to problems in the lower part of the body. The heat of the anxiety may be conducted through to the Small Intestine or Urinary Bladder leading to colitis, cystitis and so on
Opens into the Tongue	Heart disturbances can be manifest by speech problems such as stuttering. Blueness of the tongue is seen in conventional medicine as being caused by heart disease in some cases
Complexion	This is very much affected by the function of the heart
Arteries and arterioles	This is also understood from a conventional viewpoint
Colour – red	The Heart is said to 'stamp the Blood red'. It is interesting to note that many prescribed drugs for the heart are red in colour
Taste – bitter	Each major organ has an associated taste. In this case excess bitter food can damage the Fire element.
Season – summer	The energy of summer is of luxurious growth and blossoming. This can be compared to the energy of the Heart that is the major organ circulating blood around the body as well as housing the mind – our innermost spirit
Element – Fire	The Element correspondence reveals the connection of Chinese medical theory to nature. Each Element is connected to the others to provide, in health, a harmonious balance
Time – 11am to 1pm	The 'time' of an organ is when its energy it at its maximum. This explains why heart attack is commonly seen at around midday, as it is an excess of energy in the heart. Cardiac insufficiency, a deficiency of heart energy, is commonly seen around midnight
Emotions – joy and happiness	This association explains why loneliness and separation affects the heart
Mental aspect	Responsibility, gratitude, appreciation, politeness, humility

Table 7.1: Holistic view of the Heart[2]

Vitalistic principles (Table 7.1) reveal that the heart houses the mind and has an important role in mental and emotional aspects. The comments on the right of the Table explain the associations that are made by energetic medicine. The information here is derived from Chinese medicine. The underlying energetic principles are common to all methods of holistic medicine and there will be glimpses of recognition for other practitioners.[3]

The emotion that Chinese medicine associates with the heart is joy, although it may be more helpful to think of emotions such as love and compassion. In the West, this is seen on days such as February 14th – St Valentine's Day – when a heart is pictured in conjunction with ideas about love. This reveals again the basic split in Western life where the doctor is a 'fixer' of the machine and other aspects are reserved for special occasions.

The major factor to affect the heart is separation – separation from the love of others and separation from our own love. Heart disease is more common in social groups such as immigrant communities[4] and people who are socially more isolated or deprived.[5] The heart is the core – *coeur* – the innermost part and terms exist in common language such as heartache, broken heart, heartfelt and openhearted.

In conventional medicine, disturbances of the heart on an energetic level associated with anxiety, depression and so on are categorised as psychological disorders. In clinical practice, it is common to see groups of symptoms such as palpitations, breathlessness and anxiety indicating that the heart as a whole is involved.

ANATOMY AND PHYSIOLOGY

The conventional view of the cardiovascular system as a kind of domestic central heating system. Although this may seem simplistic, yet this is the underlying idea behind many conventional treatments. The anatomy of the cardiovascular system can thus be diagrammatically represented – Figure 7.1.

There are several facts of anatomy and physiology that are useful to know. I consider that most courses in these subjects are over detailed and reflect orthodox thinking rather than the particular needs of the holistic practitioner. To study cardiovascular system disease it would be helpful to be able to:

- Identify the surface anatomy of the heart and great vessels
- State the location and names of the peripheral pulses
- Describe the main structure of the heart, arteries, and veins and describe how the whole is divided into the systemic and pulmonary circulation
- Describe the events, including electrical activity, during the cardiac cycle
- Discuss the movement of fluids between the capillaries and the intercellular spaces.

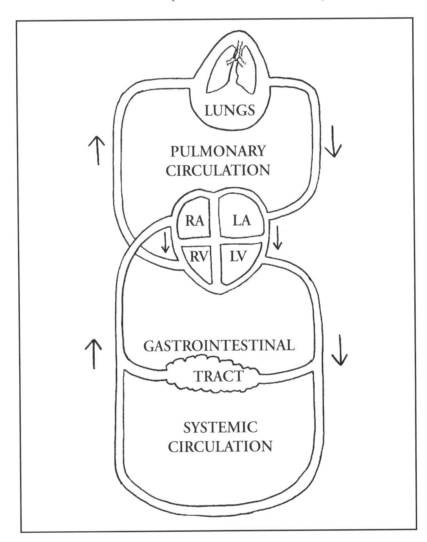

Figure 7.1: Diagrammatic representation of the cardiovascular system

CLASSIFICATION OF CARDIOVASCULAR DISEASE

Disease of the cardiovascular system is very common in the West causing 50 per cent of all deaths. The conventional classification of disease is according to its perceived cause – infection, degenerative processes such as atherosclerosis, thrombosis and so on. It is of more importance to an holistic practitioner to relate the disease labels to symptom pictures and underlying energetic states – Table 7.2.

Hypertension is missing from this list although it is invariably found in conventional textbooks in the section on cardiovascular disease. I describe hypertension in Chapter 9 – Urinary system, since I feel it is primarily a disorder of the kidney. It may well have effects in other areas but it is a misapprehension to state it is a cardiovascular disease.

Superficial, acute disease

Pericarditis
Peripheral vascular disease
  • Veins
  • Arteries
Angina pectoris
Myocardial infarction (heart attack)
Cardiac insufficiency (cardiac failure)

Internal, chronic disease

Table 7.2: Classification of cardiovascular disease

PERICARDITIS

This is an unusual condition, which, as its name implies, is an inflammation of the pericardium. The pericardium is the protective lining around the heart and so disease here is less severe than disease of the heart itself.

The pericardium may be involved with other disease such as heart attack, autoimmune conditions, tuberculosis and malignancy. In these cases there will be the symptoms of the original condition as well as the clinical appearance of pericarditis. However, viral pericarditis as described below is the commonest type.

Symptoms
Viral pericarditis is most common in young adults. There may be a preceding fever but the main feature is a sharp pain in the centre of the chest, which may radiate to the neck and shoulders associated with palpitations. It is better for sitting forward and worse for lying down, movement and breathing. The pain is similar to pleurisy but the presence of palpitations confirms that the pericardium is affected. It lasts for several weeks.

This illness occurs in people who are overworked and have a pre-existing heart imbalance. It is essentially energetic rather than structural. There are often relapses at times of stress or overwork.

Investigations
Diagnosis is made clinically with the help of ECG changes seen in the first week of ST segment elevation, which changes to T wave inversion. After recovery the ECG returns to normal.

Treatment
This is by means of aspirin or non-steroidal anti-inflammatory agents. Corticosteroids are given in severe cases.

Holistic management
The main issue here is to treat the underlying Heart imbalance after the acute attack has subsided. People with this complaint are often sensitive to external events in many senses and a combination of stress, worry and overwork has usually precipitated the attack. Some cases of pericarditis are secondary to more severe disease such as heart attack. These will be clear from the associated symptoms.

PALPITATIONS

These are a common symptom of heart disease. Palpitations are denoted in conventional medicine as 'disorders of rhythm and rate'. In conventional medicine, they are classified according to the particular appearance of the ECG. In this way, a precise pattern of disorder can be observed related to the passage of the electrical impulse across the heart muscle. It may originate from the sino-atrial node, atrium, atrio-ventricular node or ventricle.

For a holistic practitioner, precise diagnosis of this kind is not practicable. There is no access to an ECG, interpretation is difficult and such findings are, in any case, more relevant to conventional drug use. It is more helpful to relate to the symptom of palpitations. This is an awareness of the heart beating and occurs normally after exercise and in association with certain emotions. Even then if they were excessive or prolonged it would be considered as a symptom.

The important thing to determine with palpitations is whether there is underlying structural heart disease. Palpitations may result from emotional/energetic causes or be associated with more structural heart disease disrupting the flow of electrical conduction through the heart. The latter is clearly potentially serious and this is particularly true of those associated with ventricular disease.

Simply stated, a rapid pulse is more than 90 beats per minute and a slow pulse is less than 60 beats per minute. The more severe conditions are related to these extremes. A serious condition may be present if the pulse is very slow (<50/minute) or very rapid (>120/minute). Pulse rates such as these and symptoms arising from the ventricle of the heart would lead to severe disruption of cardiac function. Chest pain, oedema or loss of consciousness would point to this.

Treatment

Palpitations with no associated structural heart disease are treated by reassurance or with drugs such as tranquillisers or betablockers (see Table 7.3). Increasingly, betablockers are used early in the treatment of such symptoms and even in children.

Treatment (mildest to strongest)	Comments
Stimulate vagus nerve (vagotonic measures) • Valsalva manoeuvre[6] • Immerse face in water • Carotid sinus massage • Eyeball pressure	This increases the activity of the parasympathetic aspect of the autonomic nervous system, i.e. relaxatory mechanisms. This balances the sympathetic aspect, i.e. stimulatory or adrenaline effect
Oral drugs to prevent recurrence	Digoxin, betablockers, calcium antagonists or verapamil are given. Occasionally betablockers may be used to treat serious ventricular arrhythmias. This is usually sotalol
Intravenous drugs to control an acute attack	This is by means of adenosine or verapamil
Oral drugs for severe ventricular arrhythmia	Amiodarone, bretylium, disopyramide, dofetilide, flecainide,[7] ibutilide, lidocaine, mexiletine, procainamide, propafenone, quinidine, tocainamide. Patients who take these drugs need to be carefully monitored if they wish to reduce or withdraw them. Sudden withdrawal can be fatal
Electric shock – DC cardioversion	Used in relatively severe cases unresponsive to drugs
Pacemaker	Used in relatively severe cases unresponsive to drugs
Surgery – destruction of conductive pathway in the heart	An uncommon treatment

Table 7.3: Conventional treatment of palpitations

Holistic management

The conventional separation of emotional and structural aspects is very artificial. You cannot separate the function/structure of the heart as a pump of blood from its function/structure in housing the mind. It is vital to treat the person as a whole and particularly to consider emotional factors, long-term emotional suppression, separation, shock and bereavement, which may have a bearing. If a serious condition is suspected then can you deal with it? As a guide, any situation requiring drugs such as amiodarone or more severe cases as in Table 7.4 would be a potentially serious situation.

In terms of Chinese medicine, palpitations indicate a Heart-specific symptom. Therefore, any of the Heart syndromes may manifest palpitations amongst their symptoms.

If the case is complicated by drugs think about whether reduction is possible when you treat. Never reduce rapidly. In the case of ventricular arrhythmias you may need ECG monitoring as slow gradual withdrawal is performed. Remember that most cases of palpitations are not due to structural heart disease and so can be managed safely.

Case one
A woman of 45 years came for treatment with symptoms of hot flushes, sweating, anxiety, aggressive feelings and tiredness. She had suffered with palpitations some 8 years before and had a surgical ablation of an area of the heart transmitting electrical impulses. She also suffered with symptoms of abdominal bloating, pains in the abdomen and alternating constipation and diarrhoea particularly in stressful situations. She had symptoms of pre-menstrual tension each month with a lot of breast tenderness.

In terms of Chinese medicine, her diagnosis was Heart and Liver Blood deficiency with Liver Qi stagnation. She would also have presented with palpitations, but the operation some years before had prevented these appearing. After treatment involving tonifying Blood and relieving Liver Qi stagnation, she felt much calmer with reduced emotional flare-ups. During the course of treatment it became clear that problems in her childhood, particularly a violent father, had led to this situation. As she became stronger, she was able to remember more and become more aware of her feelings. Interestingly, her palpitations returned some months after beginning treatment, which I viewed positively as a return of old symptoms. Her consultant considered this to be impossible. These types of cases are difficult to treat as they involve deep emotional states, worrying current symptoms and long-term imbalances. There is much that can be done to help with care and the correct treatment. It is useful to consider additional help with perhaps relaxation, counselling or psychotherapy.

Case two
A woman of 58 years came for treatment complaining of palpitations, which were worse for exercise. She had had them for over 2 years since an attack of pneumonia. She had a history a several episodes of pneumonia especially as a child. Her appetite was poor and she was lacking in energy. Her medication was Sestril (once daily) and flecainide (twice daily). I made a diagnosis of Blood and Yin Deficiency and treated her with acupuncture and Chinese herbs. This was at a time when she was experiencing great personal and financial stress.

Some 2 months after beginning treatment, she came to the clinic unannounced one day with a left sided facial weakness, numbness in her left cheek and left hand. Her left arm and hand had been weak that morning but this had settled by the time I saw her. She was very worried by her symptoms. Her blood pressure was normal. This is the typical picture of a transient ischaemic attack (see Page 267).

I treated her daily for several weeks and these symptoms subsided. She was attending the hospital at the same time and they were keen for her to have anticoagulant treatment. They stopped her flecainide whilst awaiting her decision about taking this medication. For the next 3 to 4 months she would have frequent attacks of headaches, palpitations, tight feelings in her left jaw and tiredness. I continued to treat her during this time several times each week. Her general health improved with increases in energy although times of stress and overwork would cause her setbacks. When her energy was stronger, she had fewer headaches. Her blood pressure continued to be normal and over the course of the next few months she slowly reduced the Sestril until she stopped it completely some 8 months later.

I continued to treat her for 2 years in all and at the end of that time she was well with only occasional palpitations, She had no other symptoms and was on no medication. Whilst it was challenging at times to treat her, as it often is when people reject conventional investigations and treatment, in the end she did very well. She also had regular massage and aromatherapy, which was an additional invaluable support for her. She went through a difficult time with many personal and professional challenges and emerged much healthier both physically and mentally. It is important to know the limitations of what we can (and cannot) do but I am strongly of the opinion that it is important to support people in whatever they decide for themselves. Certainly, in some ways it is easier to treat such people since they generally have a strong spirit, their symptoms are not confused by the presence of drugs and our treatment is not undermined by conventional prescribing.

FAINTING

This is a temporary loss of consciousness (a few minutes) due to a fall in blood pressure. Less blood reaches the brain and as a protective mechanism, fainting ensues, producing a horizontal position that increases blood supply to the brain. There may be several causes of this common condition. Fainting during exercise almost always indicates a serious underlying condition. This suggests an obstruction to blood flow leaving the heart and must always be taken seriously.

Clearly, any loss of consciousness has to be carefully considered. It is important to determine the associated symptoms, any precipitating factors and sequelae. The common types are listed in Table 7.4.

Description	Comments
Classical faint – characterised by sweating, light-headedness, pallor, rapid pulse and then loss of consciousness – blood collects in the lower extremities. More likely in hot conditions and if hungry	Prolonged standing After illness, loss of fluid as with diarrhoea or vomiting On the sight of blood, unpleasant events Low blood pressure due to loss of fluids or blood Hypotensive drugs and vasodilators
Raised intra-thoracic pressure prevents venous return to the heart and so less blood for supply to brain	Excessive coughing, straining to urinate or defaecate
Poisoning	Toxic fumes, drugs
Epilepsy	This can superficially have the appearance of a faint but it lasts for longer, there is jerking of the limbs, there may be biting of the tongue and urinary incontinence
Central nervous system disorders	Head injury, 'stroke', and brain tumour. The latter two are discussed in Chapter 14 - Central Nervous System
Severe internal disease	These include failure of major organs such as heart, liver or lungs, diabetes mellitus,[8] obstruction to blood flow within the heart

Table 7.4: Loss of consciousness and its causes

PERIPHERAL VASCULAR DISEASE

Diseases of veins

Varicose veins

Veins contain valves, which aid the return of blood to the heart. When their function becomes defective, blood circulation is impaired and blood collects in the veins. In this condition, it is the legs that are affected. Any vein can be affected by varicosities, e.g. the anal veins (leading to haemorrhoids), and the veins at the lower end of the oesophagus (in cases of liver disease).

Varicose veins are common in people who have jobs involving a lot of standing such as shop workers although there is a large familial component. It is more frequently seen in women than men. Some cases of varicose veins occur following damage to the veins, for example after deep venous thrombosis.

Symptoms
There may be no symptoms other than the appearance of large, dilated veins. It is often the appearance that leads to requests for surgical treatment. Feelings of heaviness or tiredness in the legs are common. These are relieved by rest or by elevation of the limbs. Oedema and pigmentation occur in severe cases due to fluid leaving the venous circulation and entering the extra-cellular spaces. Pigmentation is due to the deposition of blood pigments in the tissues. Eczematous changes with itching (and even ulceration) can occur. There is often associated with infection.

Treatment
This is aimed at aiding return of venous blood upwards. Non-invasive approaches such as losing excess weight, doing gentle exercises, wearing support tights and taking adequate rest, especially with the legs raised, are all helpful. Surgery is a common procedure, which consists of stripping (i.e. removal) of the veins or by injecting phenol compounds into the vein to cause it to close down permanently. These are performed either for cosmetic reasons or because of severe symptoms. The varicose veins frequently return after a variable period of time and it is unusual to see complete removal of all affected veins.

Complications

Complication	Symptoms to look for
Varicose eczema	Itching, dryness and discolouration of the legs
Varicose ulcers	Ulceration of the leg above the ankle
Thrombophlebitis	Pain, redness, swelling of the superficial veins

Table 7.5: Complications of varicose veins

Holistic management

The treatment of varicose veins can be difficult particularly due to cosmetic considerations. It is certainly possible to relieve the symptoms of aching, heaviness and swelling but it is more difficult to deal with the appearance of the veins. Conventional treatment may miss some veins and they commonly return after some years. The removal of superficial veins can lead to reduced venous return in the legs and so causes symptoms of swelling and heaviness. There may be a consequent danger of deep venous thrombosis, as the symptom is driven to a deeper level.

In terms of Chinese medicine, the syndrome that usually corresponds to varicose veins is Sinking of Spleen Qi due to Deficiency.

Case one

A woman of 55 years came for treatment of her varicose veins. She would have heavy, aching feelings in her legs particularly when standing or at the end of the day which caused her a lot of difficulty as she worked in a shop. She had had varicose veins for some 30 years. She had difficulty losing weight and had gained around 20 lb in the previous 2 years. She would occasionally develop small itchy lumps on her legs which would bleed. They would begin as small areas under the skin. There were many cracked veins under the skin surface on her legs. She would experience numbness and tingling in her toes and lower limbs. Her back would ache at times and she could experience fairly severe bouts of low back pain. Her lower back would generally feel stiff. I made a diagnosis of Blood Deficiency, Spleen Qi Deficiency and Kidney Yang Deficiency. I treated her with acupuncture and Chinese herbs.

After one treatment of acupuncture, she felt slightly better with noticeably less numbness in her toes. Her pulses were generally stronger. After each treatment she felt slightly better and after 5 months she said that her energy was good and she felt happy. Her legs now felt much improved, the lumps had disappeared, there was no aching and her lower back felt much stronger and less stiff. After 8 months of treatment she is now fine with few symptoms. Her energy is good and she can now stand for long periods with little difficulty.

Superficial thrombophlebitis

This is an inflammatory disorder of the superficial veins, which is self-limiting in nature and never hazardous to life. It is usually associated with varicose veins, but may also occur after trauma or injection of irritant chemicals.

Symptoms

This condition is characterised by pain, swelling, redness and heat of the affected veins. The veins are tender and hardened.

Treatment

This is symptomatic by means of aspirin or non-steroidal anti-inflammatory agents. It is important to be able to distinguish this from the more serious deep venous thrombosis.

Deep venous thrombosis (DVT)

This is a potentially serious condition and is occasionally encountered in holistic clinical practice particularly with regard to its treatment by anticoagulant drugs. It is a much more serious condition than the previous one and you should know how to distinguish them, as the possible outcomes are so different. In this condition it is the deep veins of the calf that are affected. It is particularly important to be aware of the implications of treatment by anticoagulant drugs.

In health, blood is maintained in a fluid state. Clotting only occurs as a reaction to a specific event. There are some predisposing factors that may lead to clotting. These include:

- reduced blood flow
- post-operative states

- being elderly
- bed rest
- direct injury to the calf
- increased clotting tendency, e.g. post-operative, oral contraception/HRT, cancer, pregnancy.

Smoking increases any risk.

Symptoms

There is pain, tenderness and swelling of the affected leg. It is usually in the calf but may extend up into the thigh. There is marked pain on dorsiflexion of the ankle on the affected side. You should enquire about the previous history, which may indicate one of the factors mentioned above.

Complications

The main complication to be aware of is pulmonary embolism where a small area of clot breaks off and becomes lodged in the lung. It causes pleuritic chest pain, haemoptysis and breathlessness.

Diagnosis

Ultrasound may be used although the definitive test is by venograms. Dye is injected into the veins of the foot and X-rays taken to look at the deep venous system of the calf and thigh. A thrombosis will be seen as a shadow although the test is not infallible. Radioactive dyes may also sometimes be used.

Treatment

Anti-coagulant agents are given to prevent any extension of the thrombosis. These do nothing to get rid of clots that have already formed. The danger is considered to be from fresh clots as these break off fairly easily and may lead to the pulmonary complications. Anti-coagulation is continued for at least 6 months with regular check-ups at the hospital to ensure that the correct level of anti-coagulation is maintained. Warfarin is the most commonly used drug. Some people may be given such treatment on the assumption of a DVT with no radiological evidence.

Holistic management

In every case you should assess the severity of the condition and the underlying health of the person. It is always difficult to assess if it is wise to come off anticoagulants before the 'allotted time' is up – usually 6 months. I would suggest it mainly depends on the person's motivation as well as your assessment of the condition. Any withdrawal should be gradual to prevent the rebound effect of increased clotting. I would be less worried if the original situation were due to a specific event such as a surgical operation or in response to the oral contraceptive. If there were a long-standing blood disorder it would be wise to be more circumspect.

DISEASES OF ARTERIES

Raynaud's disease

This is an intermittent, symmetrical attack of pallor affecting the fingers (and occasionally toes) with no evidence of obstructive arterial disease. It is precipitated by cold and is more common in women. It is due to spasm in the arteries supplying the ends of the limbs.

In some cases it may be associated with an underlying autoimmune disorder such as systemic lupus erythematosus and scleroderma (when it is termed Raynaud's phenomenon). Some cases are due to pressure on the subclavian artery by a rib arising from the 7th cervical vertebra. In other cases it is associated with the use of vibrating tools such as pneumatic drills or chain saws where it is known colloquially as 'white finger'.

Symptoms

There is a classic sequence of whiteness, blueness and finally redness, which reflect changes in the arterial blood supply to the affected part. The last stage is often quite painful. It can happen in response to very small falls in temperature. The ends of the fingers are the usual sites, but in severe cases the hands and forearms may be affected. The hands may be cold in most situations but this worsens in cold weather.

Treatment

This is disappointing conventionally and most people are told to learn to live with the condition. Smoking can make it worse and the avoidance of cold is helpful in stopping the worst attacks. Some people develop symptoms with minimal precipitating factors. Drugs are of no value and cervical sympathectomy is sometimes performed. It is of limited and only temporary help although there are very unpleasant side-effects, including lack of sweating and flushes in the upper limbs.

Holistic management

In energetic terms, this is a condition involving a constitutional lack of heat in the interior and so treatment should be directed at this. It is a chronic illness with debility and lack of energy generally and so efforts should be made at strengthening the person as much as possible. It is important for people to keep warm and protect themselves from the effects of external cold as much as possible.

In terms of Chinese medicine, this usually corresponds to a deficiency of the Yang particularly of the Kidney and this explains why the symptoms appear in cold conditions. Tonification of the Yang will lead to relief. This can be by means of acupuncture and moxibustion but herbs and diet are also important methods to warm the interior. If there is associated autoimmune disease then the problem is clearly more severe and treatment will be prolonged.

Obliterative disease

This is a narrowing of the arteries of the legs due to the development of atheroma. It is the same process as occurs with most cases of ischaemic heart disease. Ninety per cent of those with this condition are male and over 50 years of age. There is a definite association with smoking, as there is with all the diseases of an atheromatous nature in the cardiovascular system.

Symptoms

Intermittent claudication is the term applied to the typical cramp-like pain which occurs in the calves on exercise and which is relieved by rest. People with this condition state that there is a fairly regular limit to the amount of exercise that can be undertaken (compare angina pectoris). There are decreased or absent pulses in the feet and lower legs. The muscles may be wasted due to the lack of blood supply. The skin shows cyanosis and pallor or it can have a reddish dusky appearance. If you press on the toe, for example, it will take a long time for the blood to return to the area when you remove your finger. This is indicative of the sluggish circulation. Hair loss is common in the lower limbs. Oedema will develop if the problem worsens and ulcers may eventually appear, or even gangrene in extreme cases.

The prognosis is dependent on the severity of the generalised disease and what changes the person makes to their life-style. The problems in the legs are only the local manifestation. Eighty per cent of people with this condition die from cerebrovascular disease, namely cerebral haemorrhage, thrombosis or embolism manifesting as stroke.

Investigations

The diagnosis is obvious from the history but investigations may be performed to delineate the extent of obstruction and as a preliminary to surgery. Angiography, involving the injection of dye, will reveal the site and degree of arterial obstruction.

Treatment

A graduated series of exercises can lead to some improvement in the tolerance level. It is vitally important to stop smoking since high levels of carbon monoxide in the blood after smoking will only lead to less oxygen reaching the already compromised tissues. Loss of excess weight is helpful. Conventionally, high blood pressure and raised cholesterol levels are treated. Drugs may be used to attempt to increase the circulation in the legs but they are of dubious value.

Vasodilators are the most common agent used but clearly there are problems in trying to open up an artery that is relatively rigid. Alcohol is often the most effective vasodilator. Foot hygiene is essential as any infection in the feet can lead to serious consequences.

Surgical procedures are sometimes undertaken if the symptoms are not controlled. If there is a single block in a fairly large artery then it may be possible to remove it. However, most people have diffuse disease and so the only surgical operation is that of lumbar sympathectomy. This involves cutting the sympathetic nervous supply in the lumbar region in the hope that the arteries in the legs may dilate more. It is of variable effectiveness.

Holistic management

In terms of Chinese medicine this is Stagnation of Qi and Blood in the channels of the legs. There are several underlying causes of this including external injury, Cold and Damp invading the channels and internal Fire due to smoking, alcohol intake or emotional suppression. Treatment can definitely alleviate the symptoms but success is also dependent on the changes initiated by the person. Gentle exercise and giving up smoking are essential. It is important to view this as part of a generalised problem as there will be organ disease as well. General warming is helpful dependent upon the energetic diagnosis and people should be advised to wrap up warmly in cold weather. Appropriate advice is needed about minimising cold food in the diet and taking warming soups and stews especially in the colder months.

Buerger's disease

This is not as common as obliterative disease. It seems to be a particularly severe form of obstructive arterial disease, which mainly affects young men who smoke excessively. There are similar symptoms as described above but they are more severe. The pathological process is unclear in conventional medicine. There is evidence of inflammation in the arteries and spasm because of undue sensitivity to nicotine may also be a factor.

ISCHAEMIC HEART DISEASE

This is a category of disease that is characterised by chest pain. In conventional medicine, the cause is seen as a reduction of blood flow through the coronary arteries. The heart muscle receives an inadequate supply of blood for its needs and a cramping pain is felt in the chest. The common association is with atherosclerosis. In clinical practice, some people have severe symptoms with little obstruction by atheroma and others, whose arteries are severely affected, have no symptoms. The predisposing factors involved in the development of heart disease are emotional states such as loneliness and separation. This is why heart disease is more common in men. Women find it easier to be connected to others and share experiences. Men tend to be more isolated and out of touch with their feelings. Interestingly, as women strive to emulate men in business, the incidence of heart attacks in women is increasing.[9]

The number of cases of ischaemic heart disease will double for each decade of increase in age. The general tendency is for it to affect younger people but there are also associations with diabetes mellitus, myxoedema, familial hypercholesterolaemia, smoking and high blood pressure. In the case of these conditions, people are affected at a younger age and more severely.

Under the age of 45 years the ratio of men to women is 6:1. As women pass through the menopause it is often quoted as leading to an increase in incidence. However, the increase in frequency reflects no more than increasing age. Menopause has no effect on the rate. It therefore makes no sense to give female hormone replacement treatment to women in an attempt to prevent heart attacks. Oestrogen and progesterone actually *increase* the likelihood of thrombosis and so obstruction to coronary artery blood flow.

There are two clinical syndromes associated with ischaemia. These are angina pectoris and heart attack (myocardial infarction).

Angina pectoris

This is the result of an inadequate blood supply to the muscle of the heart. The common cause is due to ischaemia as outlined above but it may also be due to severe anaemia. The situation that arises is similar to the cramp felt in the legs with undue exercise.

Symptoms
The main symptom is pain in the chest, which comes on with effort and emotional stress particularly in the cold or after a meal. Rest relieves the pain.

There is a remarkably constant limit to the amount of exercise before symptoms appear and people typically state that they can only walk 100 yards, 250 yards or whatever before they feel the pain. The pain is variously described as pressing, heavy, gripping, like a tight band around the chest, raw or burning. It is not usually described as sharp, stabbing or like a knife. It is felt retrosternally in the centre of the chest and often radiates to the neck, back, lower jaw, epigastrium or inner aspect of the arms. The left arm is more often affected than the right.

There is varying intensity from mild to severe. There is associated sweating and pallor. Increasing severity of pain, recurrent pain with decreasing periods of relief or pain occurring at night suggests that heart attack may be imminent (so-called crescendo angina). Certainly pain lasting more than 30 minutes is almost certainly a heart attack. Nitrates (vasodilators) will relieve the pain. Palpitations are a common association with the attacks of pain. Other symptoms include tiredness, shortness of breath on exertion and flatulence.

Clinical examination is often normal and diagnosis can be made on the basis of the symptoms. The presence of such symptoms does indicate fairly advanced disease of the heart and only 30 per cent of people with this condition survive 10 years.

Investigations

Most routine investigations including the resting ECG are normal. An exercise ECG[10] reveals ST depression and is positive in 75 per cent of *severe* cases. It is more often normal in women. Coronary angiography[11] may be done to find the presence and degree of arterial blockage prior to surgery.

Treatment

The symptoms are the main indication as to the progress of the disease. In cases where they are increasing in severity, exercise tolerance is reducing or where there is an acute onset a heart attack may be imminent. In others, where there is a stable exercise limit then this danger is much less.

Conventionally, drugs are the mainstays of treatment along with advice about losing excess weight and stopping smoking. The removal of cigarettes can lead to improvement in any condition due to ischaemia because of the level of carbon monoxide in the blood of smokers. This obviously reduces the quality of any blood that does reach the organ involved.

The conventional treatment of angina pectoris is listed in Table 7.6. Such a list is helpful to the holistic practitioner since it gives hints as to the severity of the condition in a presenting person. For example, if a person who comes for treatment is taking nitrates (symptomatic and prophylactic), together with betablockers then this is a relatively severe case. If, in addition, the person were waiting for investigation with a view to surgery then this would indicate a further stage of severity.

Holistic management

I have treated people with Chinese medicine and it is possible, with appropriate changes in lifestyle, for people to improve even when taking large doses of drugs. These can be reduced as improvement begins and stopped altogether in certain cases.

Surgery is an extremely expensive procedure and is greatly invasive. The term heart bypass is a useful one because this is the effect of the surgery – it bypasses the problem. Then it either returns at some later date requiring the same operation or the imbalance enters another organ or level.

Trials have been published showing that other methods including dietary change, exercise and visualisation are more effective than conventional methods in treating severe heart disease.[12] It would seem that the only reason that they are not taken up enthusiastically by the conventional profession is because these ideas do not fit easily into the accepted medical model.

Treatment (mildest to strongest)	Comments
Nitrates • symptomatic • prophylactic	Nitrates are vasodilators and so decrease the pressure in the circulation so that the heart has to work less. They relax the coronary arteries and so increase blood flow to the heart.
Betablockers	These are commonly used and block the effect of adrenaline, reducing the heart rate and the amount of work done by the heart. There is no effect on production of adrenaline so betablockers are essentially 'anaesthetic' in their action – they block awareness of how people feel. They may be prescribed for anxiety and more so since the realisation of the addictive properties of tranquillisers. They may be given to children for school phobia. This is potentially very dangerous as these drugs affect the heart. Long-term they are weakening and later you would expect to see syndromes of fatigue or heart failure. They are also used to treat tremor, migraine and hypertension. There are several betablockers and all share similar names, e.g. propanolol, atenolol, sotalol. They have common effects, including tiredness, cold extremities, slow pulse, cardiac insufficiency, wheezing, impotence and depression. Sudden withdrawal can lead to a heart attack as the heart becomes exposed to, and unprotected from, the full force of circulating adrenaline.
Calcium channel blockers	Calcium channel blockers have similar effects to betablockers and are of a similar strength. They reduce muscle contractions by interfering with calcium exchange. Other effects include slow heart rate, peripheral oedema, nausea, rash, headache, and jaundice.
Surgery • Angioplasty • Coronary artery bypass	Surgery is offered when symptoms are not relieved by drugs. Angiography is done first and if the function of the heart is adequate then one of two operations are possible. In angioplasty, a catheter is passed into the coronary artery to the atheromatous blockage. A balloon at the end of the catheter is inflated to break down the atheroma. It has a risk of causing heart attack (2-4 per cent) that may be fatal. One third of people re-obstruct within 6 months[13] and need a repeat operation. The major operation is coronary artery bypass, which has been performed for about 30 years. It is the most costly single surgical procedure in the US. A length of saphenous vein from the leg is removed and is used to bypass the coronary artery blockage. There is mortality from the operation of around 2 per cent and symptom relief in around 80 per cent. There is some debate in conventional circles as to whether the operation prolongs life.[14] There is a significant morbidity post-operatively related to the immediate problems of a wound in the leg and the chest. There can be chest pain for months after surgery. Other problems include severe tiredness, which may persist for many months and severe depression. This can be extreme in its manifestation and reflects the deep significance of the heart and chest. The lungs are typically associated with grief and the heart with joy and it takes no great leap of the imagination to see how physical manipulation of this area may disturb the energies to the extent that depression results. The picture in such cases is one of extreme grief and it can be difficult to find relief.

Table 7.6: Treatment of angina pectoris

Case one

A man of 54 years came for treatment with tight pains in the centre of his chest on exertion. The pains radiated to the inner aspect of the left arm and into the back. He could only walk 100 yards before the pain appeared and then would have to stop and rest. These symptoms were much worse in cold weather. He had had a heart attack some 6 months before and was found to be anaemic. This was presumed to be the cause of the heart attack although no cause was found for the anaemia. His work was very stressful and he was currently unable to work. His medication was:

- ranitidine 300 mg each night – used in the treatment of gastric and duodenal ulcer
- atenolol 100 mg daily – betablocker
- glyceryl trinitrate 1 mg when required for pain – symptomatic nitrate vasodilator
- isosorbide dinitrate 20 mg three times daily – prophylactic nitrate vasodilator
- ferrous sulphate one three times daily – iron supplementation.

He was due to have investigations with a view to bypass surgery in the next few months. This is clearly a serious case as evidenced by comparing the information here with that in Table 7.8. I discussed the importance of reducing fatty and sweet foods and eating a whole-food diet at regular intervals throughout the day and taking regular gentle exercise. I gave him information about the bypass operation explaining that its purpose is to relieve pain rather than prolong life. I suggested that he could wait and see how the treatment progressed before making a decision.

He received regular acupuncture treatments and started to notice more energy with an ability to walk further before developing chest pain. After this initial improvement he stopped the ranitidine, as there was never any evidence of an ulcer. He also stopped the iron supplements as they irritated the bowel. As he continued to improve he was able to reduce his betablocker gradually over some months. It must never be stopped suddenly since this may cause a heart attack. He moved onto the isosorbide dinitrate finally and after about 1 year of treatment was able to walk 5 miles with no problems, rarely had any chest pain and felt well. He had decided to give up his previous stressful occupation.

During the course of the treatment he was called for coronary angiography investigation. He decided to go, as he wanted to know how severe any blockage in the coronary arteries was. After the investigation he had some tiredness and increased chest pains for about 4 weeks before it settled down. There was evidence of two blockages in his coronary arteries – one severe and one mild. He was told that he would need a bypass operation by his surgeon, although his physician said that he did not require surgery. He decided to defer the operation as he was doing well with the acupuncture.

This case reveals that holistic treatment is a perfectly valid option for heart disease even if it is severe at the time of presentation. There is often a divergence of conventional opinion and in my experience surgeons usually advise surgery (just as physicians usually advise medicines, acupuncturists acupuncture, herbalists herbs and so on!). As the person improves it is possible to reduce medication although this must be done slowly[15] over several months. It is essential to monitor the person's symptoms closely whilst this is done.

In terms of Chinese medicine, angina pectoris usually corresponds to Heart Qi or Yang deficiency. There may be some Stagnation of Heart Blood that develops as a result of this deficiency or as a consequence of long-term emotional stagnation that disturbs the mind.

Betablockers have common side-effects as mentioned above. They would seem to deplete Heart, Liver, Spleen, Lung and Kidney Yang. In people whose Yang is already markedly depleted, there may be the appearance of Water Overflowing as the Yang then fails to dominate the Yin. An example of this is the precipitation of cardiac insufficiency.

In cases of Lung Yang or Qi deficiency the use of betablockers may initiate wheezing and some people die due to collapse of Lung Yang. It is interesting to note that betablockers are used in painful conditions such as migraine and angina pectoris. In the case of migraine, it is effective in those cases due to Liver Yang Rising or Heat in the Gall Bladder/Stomach. This effect on Liver Yang explains how betablockers relieve tremors. In the case of angina pectoris, the effect would be due to a general weakening of Yang so that Stagnation syndromes are no longer apparent. In the long-term, you would expect to see more cases of cardiac insufficiency, caused by previous betablocker use that has weakened the Heart Yang – see Case two on Page 164.

Nitrates are vasodilators and this is a Yang action. They produce effects such as sensations of heat, throbbing headache and facial flushing. They particularly affect the Heart and Liver.

Another way of describing angina pectoris is to say that there is too much energy in the chest due to stagnation. If this energy can be regulated then the symptoms will be alleviated. Heart attack is merely a more severe form of this stagnation with consequent collapse of Yang (shock).

Case two
A man of 69 years came for treatment of his chest pains. He had been diagnosed as suffering from angina and had first developed chest pains some 20 years before attending the clinic. This was at a time of great difficulties in his personal life. His main symptoms when I saw him were pains in the centre of his chest that came on with exercise. He would get a little out of breath and have to stop and rest. The pains would then ease. Strong emotions would also bring on the pain. He always felt tired and his spirits felt low. His medication was:

- atenolol 100 mg daily
- bendrofluazide with potassium chloride one daily
- fluvastatin one daily
- isosorbide dinitrate one three times daily
- glyceryl trinitrate spray when he needed it.

I made a diagnosis of Heart Blood Stagnation and Heart Qi Deficiency. I treated him with acupuncture and Chinese herbs. It is important in such cases, particularly when complicated by the use of several medications, to assess the patient carefully and select gentle treatments at the beginning. With care, such cases can be managed successfully and the patient can gain much benefit. His energy improved fairly quickly and he felt livelier after one treatment. His exercise tolerance slowly increased and he was able to walk further with less pain following each visit to the clinic. After 6 months of treatment he noticed that he would occasionally forget to take his atenolol, which is always a good sign that people are beginning to feel better. He would need his atenolol later and later each day with no ill effects. His treatment continues and I would expect that he would be able to reduce some of his medication within the next 3 months if he feels confident. His progress is likely to continue with more energy and decreased levels of pain.

Heart attack (Acute myocardial infarction)

This is the death of heart muscle due to an inadequate blood supply. The usual cause is obstruction of the coronary artery due to atherosclerosis as outlined above. The condition may occur suddenly or after a history of angina pectoris. It is the most common cause of death in the Western world although it was rare before 1910. In the UK, there are 300,000 cases per year of whom half die immediately. Ten per cent more die in hospital and up to 20 per cent more in the subsequent two years. Half of the initial *survivors* are alive after ten years.

Some people have little evidence of an actual blockage and the assumption is that spasm of the coronary artery is responsible. This is especially likely to occur with extreme stress or violent activity. The squash court is a familiar venue for such occurrences.

Symptoms
There is pain in the chest that may be of a similar nature to that of angina pectoris – See Table 7.9 – although stabbing pain is more likely with this condition. It is severe and may come on at rest or wake the person at night. Rest does not relieve it. It lasts for anything between 30 minutes and 2 days but may be less severe in the elderly. Palpitations are common. There is great anxiety during the attack and fear of death may be extreme. Heart attack may be fatal and if the person survives then it will probably be the closest they come to death without dying.

Some anxiety may develop in the post-attack phase with people becoming worried about the least activity because of the fear of another attack. Such 'cardiac neurosis' can be very debilitating but can be minimised by appropriate exercise and reassurance.

There are associated signs of shock. The person is pale, cold, and sweaty with a low blood pressure and rapid, thready pulse. If there is associated cardiac insufficiency, and there is some in virtually all cases, there may be cough, breathlessness and so on as seen in this condition.

Gastrointestinal symptoms are common particularly nausea and vomiting. There may also be diarrhoea and flatulence. The existence of such symptoms may lead to a diagnostic confusion with indigestion.

Pericarditis may develop in the days after the attack. In one quarter of severe cases there is also deep venous thrombosis because of the decreased mobility leading to sluggish circulation.

When considering the outcome of heart attack, it is clear that there is a great mortality rate. The greatest risk is in the first two hours after the attack and as time passes more and more survive. Half of the deaths that occur do so in the first 2-3 hours and three quarters in the first 24 hours. There is an increased likelihood of death if a second attack occurs within a short time of the first. Two thirds of people with this condition are alive after 5 years and over half live 10 years.

Symptom	Angina pectoris	Heart attack
Chest pain – severity	Variable	Severe
Chest pain – modalities	Worse for exercise, cold, meals, emotion. Better for rest or nitrates	Not better for rest or nitrates
Chest pain – duration	Few minutes	15 minutes or longer
Associated symptoms	Pallor, slight sweating	Cold, clammy, nausea, vomiting

Table 7.7: Comparison of angina pectoris and heart attack

Investigations
The ESR is raised to 70 mm and there is an increase in the white cell count.

Cardiac enzymes are increased as they are released at the time of the damage to the heart muscle. Creatine kinase (first 24 hours), aspartate aminotransferase (formerly serum glutamic oxaloacetic transaminase–24-48 hours) and lactic dehydrogenase (3-4 days) are all raised. Tests for these are usually performed daily for the first three days and the first test is often normal.

The ECG shows typical features[16] but may take 48 hours to become apparent. They include Q wave development, ST segment depression or elevation and T wave inversion. Q wave development is a permanent feature of the ECG and provides past evidence of a heart attack. Several people have such ECG evidence yet with no history of chest pain. This group forms 20 per cent of the total number of heart attacks counted in the statistics.

Treatment

This is primarily hospital-based with the use of intensive care or coronary care units although there is some debate as to whether such treatment is advantageous.[17] One could argue that travel to hospital at such a vulnerable time for the heart in a speeding ambulance, the stress of hospital admission, the constant observation and general urgent atmosphere may be harmful. Certainly, the major problem is the development of abnormal cardiac rhythms, which may be fatal. Some people are treated, post-heart attack, at home, if the attack is mild and there are no complications.

In hospital, people are closely observed with continuous ECG monitoring. The main treatments are supportive with pain relief, circulatory support to minimise the development of shock, use of anti-arrhythmic agents and treatment of any complicating cardiac failure.

Thrombolytic treatment may be used within the first 24 hours to dissolve the thrombosis. This is not used if there has been recent surgery or injury, a stroke within the previous 2 months, in pregnancy, with a systolic blood pressure of more than 200 mm or if the patient is taking anticoagulants. The main drug used in streptokinase. There is a 1 per cent risk of stroke with such treatment and 0.7 per cent chance of a major haemorrhage.

After the immediate post-attack stage, there is gradual mobilisation with some exercise 2 days after the heart attack. Then full mobility is attained after a week to 10 days. After about 3 months the person should be back to their normal level.

People may be given betablockers for 3 years in the belief that this may prevent a further heart attack.[18] Aspirin (150 mg daily) is administered for life[19-20] and ACE inhibitors may also be given for life if there is evidence of impairment of left ventricular function. If people develop angina pectoris subsequently, the treatment is as indicated for that disease.

Holistic management

Heart attack is a more extreme form of ischaemia than angina pectoris and so the comments I made there are relevant also. With heart attack, however, the situation is more serious and most people will be treated in hospital. There are clearly advantages to be gained from holistic treatment before admission if there is time or whilst an in-patient. This would be especially helpful to prevent and treat arrhythmias, which are so common. When I was training in acupuncture in China, it was an integral part of the management of people with heart attack in the hospital. Treatment in the post-heart attack phase will take a similar form to that of angina pectoris. It is important that you know the features of chest pain and particularly how to recognise a serious condition.

In terms of Chinese medicine, heart attack usually corresponds to Stagnation of Heart Blood with Collapse of Yang.

DIFFERENTIAL DIAGNOSIS OF CHEST PAIN

In all cases of pain there are questions to ask in order to elicit as much information as possible. This will ensure that the diagnosis is as accurate as possible. There are considered to be nine questions to ask about pain. These are:

Main site

The most important question to ask is, 'Where is the pain?' Try to ascertain the precise area of discomfort.

Radiation

The pain may be felt in places in addition to the primary site. This is typical of certain conditions and certain processes.

Character

It can be difficult to describe the particular quality of pain but certain conditions are associated with characteristic types, e.g. burning, stabbing, aching. Some people merely describe pain as being severe but with encouragement will offer terms to describe quality. It may be necessary in some cases to suggest a list of several choices from which one is selected.

Severity

Pain can be of any severity according to the cause or it can vary from person to person. The pain of heart attack, for example, is usually particularly severe.

Duration

Ask how long the pain has been present, not only this attack but also the whole process. Is this a recent event or have there been repeated attacks in the past?

Frequency

How often does the pain recur?

Question	Cardiac (angina pectoris or heart attack)	Oesophageal (reflux oesophagitis)	Pulmonary (tracheitis)	Pulmonary (pleuritic pain)	Musculo-Skeletal (chest wall pain, e.g. injury)
Main site	Central chest	Central chest	Central chest	Axilla/scapula	Any site
Radiation	Jaw, neck, inner aspect of arms (L>R), back	From epigastrium up to throat	None	None	None
Character	Tight, burning, gripping, heavy	Burning	Sore, scratchy	Sharp	Sharp
Severity	Variable	Mild	Mild	Variable	Variable
Duration	Variable	Several minutes	Several days	Several days	Several days
Frequency	Recurrent	Recurrent	One attack	One attack	One attack
Timing	See modalities, possibly nightSH	Night	None	None	None
Modalities[21]	< exercise, meals, cold, emotion, > rest, nitrates	< meals, lying down, bending, > sitting up, nitrates	< coughing, > supporting chest	< coughing, respiration, > shallow breathing, supporting chest	< coughing, respiration, > shallow breathing, supporting chest
Associated symptoms	Sweating, palpitations, pallor, nausea, vomiting	Nausea, vomiting, acid regurgitation	Cough, sputum, fever	Fever, cough	Painful and tender area on the chest wall
Conventional diagnosis	Angina pectoris, heart attack See Pages 98, 102	Reflux oesophagitis See Page 231	Acute bronchitis See Page 126	Pleurisy See Page 140	Injury to chest wall

Table 7.8: Differentiation of chest pain

Time of occurrence
At what time does the pain appear?

Modalities
This term is applied to situations that make the pain worse or better. It is better to ask an open question first such as, 'Does anything relieve or worsen the pain' before moving onto more closed questions in an attempt to confirm a particular diagnosis.

Associated phenomena
Note any symptoms that appear with the pain. These may be nausea, cough, sputum and so forth.

From questioning in a careful and orderly way most cases of chest pain can be diagnosed. Confusion can occur from the history, as with differentiating some cases of angina pectoris from reflux oesophagitis but precise history taking will minimise this. The most important questions are site, radiation, modalities and associated symptoms. These four are the most helpful in the differentiation of disease states.

Table 7.8 is a summary of the commonest types of chest pain. It can be seen that cardiac and oesophageal chest pain have some similarities as do pleurisy and musculoskeletal problems. The latter case may have a history of injury. Such pain may develop after an episode of coughing and this can confuse the issue slightly. The most important thing is to take a careful history and especially take heed of site, radiation, modalities and associated symptoms.

Cardiac insufficiency

This is also known as cardiac or heart failure and these terms may be confused with heart attack, which has been described previously. Cardiac insufficiency is preferable as it implies that there is insufficient blood leaving the heart for the needs of the body. It is a relative term and does not mean that the heart has stopped or failed completely. There is a weakness of the cardiac muscle. As a result there is less blood pumped out of the heart into the arterial system and a consequent build-up of blood in the venous system. Therefore, symptoms are worse on exertion, at the end of the day or in the presence of other disease such as respiratory problems.

It occurs in about 10 people per 1000 over the age of 65 years. It is frequently a serious condition with only 50 per cent of people alive five years after diagnosis. Treatment makes no difference to this prognosis and the use of powerful diuretics is associated with great tiredness and the development of kidney failure.

The main symptom of cardiac insufficiency is oedema - see Page 22. It is useful to study cardiac insufficiency by looking at left ventricular and right ventricular types separately. In reality, the picture is usually a mixed one. The combination of left and right-sided failure is known as congestive cardiac failure.

Left heart (ventricular) insufficiency

This is the most common type and is usually due to a weakness of the left ventricle. The mechanics of the disease is weakness, either due to the prolonged effort of pushing against an obstruction or due to inadequate blood supply to meet the needs of the heart. This may follow a long history of high blood pressure, poor blood supply to the heart muscle (as in long-standing ischaemic heart disease or, less commonly, heart valve disease).

As left ventricular function becomes insufficient for the needs of the body, less blood is ejected and there is a resultant build up of pressure in the left atrium. Increased left atrial pressure is then passed onto the pulmonary circulation. Increased pressure in the pulmonary veins results in the 'leaking' of fluid into the lungs – pulmonary oedema. The main symptoms of this condition are as a result of this process.

Symptoms
In left ventricular insufficiency, the oedema is not obvious as it collects in the lungs. There is cough and breathlessness especially on exertion and when lying flat (orthopnoea). In more severe cases the person wakes in the night at around 12-1a.m. Breathlessness forces them to sit up or even get up to gasp at an open window. There may also be a cough or wheeze. Pinkish frothy sputum may be produced. This picture is known as cardiac asthma or paroxysmal nocturnal dyspnoea.

Other symptoms include palpitations, tiredness, faintness, pain in the chest, sweating. The person looks cold, pale and cyanosed. The symptoms are made worse by effort, emotion and respiratory problems. The lack of blood to the extremities results in nocturia, muscle fatigue that is worse with exertion, cold and pale extremities and peripheral cyanosis.[22]

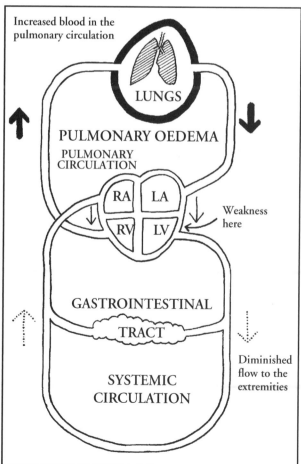

Figure 7.2:
Diagrammatic representation of left ventricular insufficiency

Right heart (ventricular) insufficiency

This is less common than left-sided insufficiency. It usually results from chronic lung disease where the heart has to work harder to push blood through the pulmonary circulation. It may develop secondary to the pulmonary oedema of left heart failure. In right-sided insufficiency, the right ventricle ejects less blood and so the increased pressure in the right atrium is passed backward to the hepatic and systemic veins.

Symptoms
Oedema is found peripherally. There is swelling of the ankles, which is worse at the end of the day and after exercise. The oedema affects dependent parts as a result of the effect of gravity. The feet, ankles and lower legs are the usual sites but in a person who is confined to bed the sacrum needs to be checked. The oedema is pitting in type. Weight gain and scanty urination may be apparent before the noticeable development of oedema because around 10 lb of fluid needs to be retained before it becomes clinically apparent. Other fluid accumulations can be manifest as pleural effusions or ascites. Deep venous thrombosis is a risk because of the reduced rate of flow in the veins of the legs.

Distended veins are apparent especially in the neck due to the increased pressure in the right atrium. In health, the neck veins are collapsed when the person is upright and distended when horizontal. If you see the veins distended in the upright position or when the person is reclining it indicates raised pressure. In this disease venous distension is due to weak heart muscles leading to increased pressure in the venous system. In other situations it may be due to obstruction by tumour.

There is enlargement of the liver leading to tenderness and pain in the right hypochondrium. Eventually jaundice may develop. Fluid may leak out into the peritoneal cavity and lead to ascites. Gastrointestinal symptoms such as nausea and vomiting are common although the drugs used for cardiac failure can be implicated here. Other symptoms include palpitations, breathlessness, pallor, tiredness, pain in the chest, sweating and cyanosis (due to insufficient blood entering the pulmonary circulation).

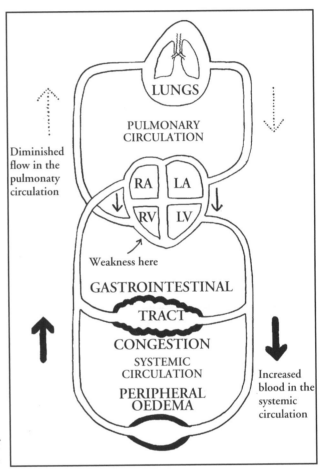

**Figure 7.3:
Diagrammatic representation of
right ventricular insufficiency**

A comparison of left and right heart insufficiency is summarised in Table 7.9. In clinical practice, it is usual to see a combination of these.

Symptoms	Left heart insufficiency	Right heart insufficiency
Oedema	Pulmonary – breathlessness, orthopnoea, cough with pink, frothy sputum, paroxysmal nocturnal dyspnoea	Peripheral – swelling of ankles, lower limbs, sacral oedema if in bed
Palpitations	Yes	Yes
Gastrointestinal symptoms		Nausea, vomiting, anorexia, right hypochondriac pain, jaundice
Symptoms due to decreased blood leaving the heart	Cold extremities, tiredness, cyanosis, sweating	Breathlessness

Table 7.9: Comparison of left and right heart insufficiency

Investigations

A chest X-ray is done to check the size of the heart and an ECG may reveal evidence of ischaemia. Echocardiography, cardiac catheterisation with radionuclide angiography are also done. Twenty-four hour ECG monitoring checks for arrhythmias and serum atrial natriuretic peptide (ANP) levels are performed.

Treatment

The conventional approach is primarily by means of drugs although people will also be given advice about diet, exercise and to stop smoking. If there is a recognised cause such as heart valve disease this may be treated surgically. Other treatment may be instituted through the diet such as reduction of sodium to around 1-1.5 g daily. This may reduce the amount of water retained in the body. Added salt is stopped and salty foods are avoided. Any high blood pressure or raised cholesterol levels will be treated. Vaccination against influenza and pneumococcal pneumonia is recommended although the conventional texts state that there is no evidence that these measures are of any help.

Treatment (mildest to strongest)	Comments
Digoxin	This was originally derived from foxglove, a plant that has the function of making the heart beat stronger. It is given in drug form as a purified chemical and in relatively high dosage and it is easy to produce toxic effects especially in the elderly. It is the only prescribed drug that increases the force of heart contraction – cardiotonic. The toxic effects are more likely to develop in cases of potassium depletion and special care has to be taken when people are given diuretics and digitalis together
Diuretics • low potency • medium potency • high potency	Diuretics are commonly used and can be divided into three groups. High potency ones are used in acute situations or when there is severe oedema. They invariably lead to the loss of potassium so should be given with supplements. Regular checks of blood urea and electrolytes should also be made but this is rarely done in clinical practice. Medium potency and low potency diuretics are correspondingly weaker in their actions
Vasodilator	Vasodilators are used in more severe forms of cardiac failure although, increasingly, may be given early. They may dilate arteries, veins or both depending upon the actual drug given. They do nothing to remedy the cause of the problem, that is, weakness in the heart. They merely move blood from one side of the circulation to the other. If cold limbs and tiredness are a problem due to lack of blood supply to the extremities, arterial dilators are given. This has the effect of placing more blood in the periphery and so there is an increase in peripheral oedema. If peripheral oedema is a problem, venodilators are given. This has the effect of opening the veins so that more blood sits inside the veins. Therefore, the heart has to do more work and symptoms such as cold limbs and tiredness become more marked. A significant number of people cannot take such drugs because of the side-effects produced. Examples include prazosin, hydralazine and amlodipine
ACE inhibitor	ACE inhibitors are given in some cases. They act by causing vasodilatation due to their inhibition of vasoconstrictor substances. Their effects are similar to the vasodilators mentioned above
Cardiac transplantation	This may be an option for end-stage cardiac failure or in younger people. If there is careful recipient selection then 1-year survival is 85 per cent and 78 per cent at 3 years

Table 7.10: Drugs used in the treatment of cardiac insufficiency

Holistic management

It is unusual to see people with cardiac failure in the clinic. This may be because they do not know that holistic medicine may help or perhaps because of the relative severity of the condition. In terms of Chinese medicine, this condition is usually due to Heart and Kidney Yang deficiency with Water overflowing. These are more Deficient conditions than usually associated with angina pectoris and this difference is reflected in the prognoses of the two conditions.

The essential point of treatment is to tonify the Yang by means of warming foods, specific treatment and the avoidance of cold foods. Adequate rest is important but regular, gentle exercise can strengthen the function of the heart.

Digoxin, as it is derived from a herbal remedy, is probably the appropriate energetic remedy in some cases but causes problems because of the dosages used. It would appear to tonify Heart Yang and lead to control of Water so that the oedema lessens.

Diuretics act by causing the kidneys to let go of water and so do nothing to treat the cause. They are cold in nature and long-term use leads to damage to Kidney Qi and Yin deficiency. It is common after some years to see a situation where there is Yin deficiency yet fluid accumulation, so the person still has oedema with thirst and dry mouth.

HOW TO RECOGNISE SERIOUS CONDITIONS OF THE CARDIOVASCULAR SYSTEM

Diseases of the cardiovascular system are common in our society and the symptoms listed below are extremely common. It is important to know how to recognise if a symptom arises from a serious situation. You can use Table 7.11 below as a guide to refer to when faced with a person who has one or more of these symptoms. I make no mention of disease labels in the column on the right, as I would not expect you to be able to diagnose conventionally. Seriousness can be assessed merely by reference to symptom pictures. However, you will be able to recognise that there are clinical appearances that would be diagnosed as a particular disease. For example, if you look at chest pain and its seriousness, you will see that this is the appearance of heart attack.

Symptom	Comments
Chest pain	Severe Long duration (over 20 minutes) At rest With vomiting With rapid pulse, low blood pressure, sweating and pallor Increased frequency of attacks Occurring at night
Breathlessness	Severe Acute Progressive With confusion With cyanosis Pulse rate > 120 per minute Paroxysmal attacks occurring at night
Palpitations	Pulse rate > 120 per minute Pulse rate < 50 per minute With chest pain With oedema With loss of consciousness
Oedema	Acute Unilateral Severe Progressive With cardiac symptoms With renal symptoms
Cyanosis	Central – tongue Peripheral – lips and extremities (unless due to cold)
Loss of consciousness	On exercise
Cough	With pink frothy sputum
Distended veins	In an abnormal site, e.g. neck when sitting up, over the chest or abdominal wall

Table 7.11: How to recognise serious conditions in cardiovascular disease

DISEASES OF THE LYMPHATIC SYSTEM

Introduction

In conventional medicine, the lymphatic system has two main functions. It drains excess fluid from the intercellular spaces and returns it to the cardiovascular system. It also has a function in the production and maturation of lymphocytes and so plays an important role in the deeper workings of the immune system. There is a close relationship between the lymphatic system and the blood, which is reflected, in their similar function of fluid movement. To study lymphatic system disease it would be helpful to be able to:

- List the main structures of the lymphatic system
- State the main groups of lymphatic glands in the body
- Describe the areas of the body that are drained by these main glands
- Describe the function of the lymphatic glands as related to the immune system – lymphocyte production and development.

There are certain diseases affecting the blood, for example, that have associated lymphatic gland enlargement and certain lymphatic system diseases that may exhibit changes in the blood. The diseases of the lymphatic system can be classified as in Table 7.12.

There are interesting interconnections between these illnesses. Removal of the tonsils, a common treatment for recurrent tonsillitis increases the risk of Hodgkin's disease by a factor of three. Glandular fever may be the precursor, some years later, of Hodgkin's disease (and other cancers according to homoeopaths). Some people develop syndromes with or without lymphatic gland enlargement but do have some blood changes and there is doubt about the diagnosis – could it be leukaemia or lymphosarcoma or something else?

Mild case
Acute inflammatory disease, e.g. tonsillitis
Chronic inflammatory disease, e.g. glandular fever
Lymphoma
• Hodgkin's
• Non-Hodgkin's
Lymphosarcoma
Leukaemia
Severe case

Table 7.12: Classification of lymphatic system diseases

A clinical situation may help to explain what I mean. Someone came to see me who had developed an acute fever with sweating and malaise. It lasted for several weeks and there was no firm conventional diagnosis. After a series of blood tests it was concluded that he might have lymphoma. There was no lymphatic gland enlargement but one was removed from his neck to investigate its appearance. After this operation his fever returned to normal and his symptoms subsided. The biopsy was negative but further study of the blood tests had led to a diagnosis of leukaemia. He was to attend for chemotherapy the next week. Before he received his first course of treatment, he had repeat blood tests performed that were now normal. He was then told that he did not have leukaemia. The diagnosis given was of probable glandular fever or a related viral illness for which he required no treatment.

This strange story does not reveal that conventional doctors misdiagnosed the case. What it does show is that as the level of imbalance changes then so do the symptoms and the investigations will show different results. In terms of Chinese medicine, he had an attack of Heat, which had descended deep into the body. This had resulted in fever and malaise. As it descended deeper it disturbed the blood and revealed abnormal blood results. The operation on his neck gland had the effect of bleeding him, which is an old treatment for fevers and still used by practitioners of Chinese medicine. Bleeding relieves heat and so his condition improved. Subsequently, the blood tests had returned to normal and the doctors, no doubt, were confused about the course of events.

Heat descending into the body can, therefore, result in symptoms such as fever, lymphatic gland enlargement and eventually organ damage. If the blood is affected then symptoms such as bleeding occur (leukaemia), convulsions (meningitis) or hallucinations (delirium). The actual pattern seen will depend upon the person, the preceding state of health and the particular circumstances.

Lymphatic gland enlargement

There are four main conditions to consider here. You can get a good idea of the situation from the clinical appearances. Biopsy is often performed in people with persistent lymphatic enlargement of a localised nature especially if one of the more serious causes is suspected. The main thing to consider is whether the problem is acute or chronic and whether the enlargement is localised or generalised. The main situations can be summarised as in Table 7.13.

Localised		Generalised	
Acute	Chronic	Acute	Chronic
Local inflammation,[23] e.g. tonsillitis, skin infection	1. Local inflammation which is chronic, e.g. tuberculosis, fibroadenosis of the breast, malignancy[24] 2. Secondary malignancy[25]	Glandular fever	Lymphoma[26], leukaemia[27]

Table 7.13: Differentiation of lymphatic gland enlargement

Table 7.13, highlights widely differing causes of lymphatic gland enlargement. It is important to ask about duration of the swelling, progression, associated symptoms and, in the case of localised enlargement, to check on the area drained. In this way an assessment about severity can be made. A discussion about lumps – benign and malignant is on Page 78.

DISEASES OF THE BLOOD

Introduction

In conventional medicine, the blood is seen as a collection of cells and fluid, which have a physical function. In terms of Chinese medicine, Blood is Yin and Yin is to do with receptivity, sensitivity and the emotions. There is a close relationship between the function of the Blood and our emotional state. There is a rather old term, sanguine, which means optimistic and confident. It was applied to one of the humours of Greek philosophy, which corresponds to blood. Exsanguination is loss of blood. If the Blood is lost or becomes weak or disturbed, people feel generally sad and may have specific symptoms such as anxiety or depression. This may be the cause of post-natal depression where the Blood has been depleted by pregnancy and childbirth. The situation will be exacerbated by blood loss at the time of delivery. Conversely, long-term worry, anxiety and depression will damage the Blood. I describe a case of a person with anaemia below that illustrates these connections.

In Chinese medicine, Blood has a function of cooling and moisturising. If the Blood is weak there can be symptoms such as feelings of heat, flushes, dry skin, thirst and general dryness, constipation, tingling, numbness, tremors and muscle or joint aches and pains. It is the Yin aspect of the body, that balances the Qi or Yang aspect. Disturbances in the Blood can correspond, in conventional medicine, to anaemia, psychological disorders, multiple sclerosis, Parkinson's disease, arthritis and so forth. This is a much wider idea of Blood than the conventional one.

The manufacture, storage and function of Blood in energetic medicine depends primarily upon the functions of the Spleen, Heart, Liver and Kidney. Disturbances in any of these organs can lead to Blood imbalances.

Conventional diseases of the blood may be classified as in Table 7.14. The more superficial levels of the blood involve the red blood cells. Deeper disease will affect white blood cells and the worst situation here is total collapse of the blood where no cells of either type are produced – pancytopenia.

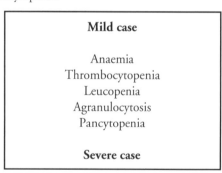

Table 7.14: Classification of blood disease

ANATOMY AND PHYSIOLOGY

The blood in conventional medicine is seen as comprising of fluid and cells. The fluid, plasma, is a transport medium for nutrients and waste products. The cells are of different types and deal with transport of oxygen (red blood cells), immune system function (white blood cells) and prevention of haemorrhage and abnormal clotting (platelets). There is a connection with the bone marrow where the cells are manufactured, and the kidney, which secretes a hormone that stimulates red blood cell production. To study disease of the blood it would be helpful to be able to:

- List the main constituents of blood
- Explain how they are produced and factors which influence this
- Describe the functions of plasma, red blood cells, white blood cells (5 types) and platelets.

ANAEMIA

This is a common condition and is seen in the UK mainly in children under 5 years of age, pregnant women, social classes 4 and 5[28] and the elderly. It is considered to be present when the level of haemoglobin in the blood is decreased. This is a laboratory definition but I would consider the symptom picture to be most important to holistic practitioners.

The type is differentiated in conventional medicine according to the appearance of the red blood cells – small, normal or large. Each of these appearances tends to be related to a particular causation. For example, iron deficiency anaemia is associated with red blood cells that are paler and smaller in size.

The classification below takes account of the site of abnormality, e.g. inadequate intake, inefficient production. It is important to bear in mind that several factors operate in chronic disease. Treatment would need to be directed at all of them to be effective. Those in italics are the most important in outpatient practice.

Impaired production of haemoglobin and red blood cells

Iron deficiency anaemia: the main causes are inadequate intake, malabsorption or excessive loss of blood. Such anaemia is commoner therefore in women who menstruate. The most common situations are poor diet, gastric disease, intestinal malabsorption, parasites, pregnancy, menorrhagia and haemorrhage. The appearance of anaemia in a person in middle life with no previous problems suggests the possibility of a hidden blood loss. The condition that must be considered is cancer of the colon as blood loss here can be unrecognised.

Folic acid deficiency anaemia: the main causes are pregnancy, diet, malabsorption and drugs such as phenytoin, primidone, methotrexate and trimethoprim.

Vitamin B_{12} deficiency anaemia: the major cause is pernicious anaemia which is a disease of autoimmune origin affecting the stomach leading to reduced secretion of intrinsic factor - essential for Vitamin B_{12} absorption. Other situations include gastrectomy, intestinal malabsorption and poor dietary intake.

Vitamin C deficiency anaemia: this occurs due to dietary deficiency or after bleeding.

Thyroxine deficiency anaemia: reduced secretion of thyroxine leads to a reduced red blood cell production.

Protein deficiency anaemia: the structure of red blood cells is made of protein and so may be deficient in malnutrition or intestinal malabsorption.

Bone marrow disease

If bone marrow function is disordered in some way there is a reduction in some or all of the cells produced there. Diseases include:

- aplastic anaemia
- leukaemia
- myelomatosis.

Excessive destruction (haemolysis) of red blood cells

In severe cases there is the appearance of jaundice. If the red blood cells are broken down quicker than their usual 120 days life span, the circulating level of haemoglobin is reduced. Causes include:

- autoimmune conditions
- infection or toxin
- overactive splenic function
- drugs, e.g. sulphonamides.

Defective haemoglobin production

There are uncommon causes of anaemia where abnormal types of haemoglobin are produced. The important situations clinically are thalassaemia and sickle cell disease. It is out of the remit of this book to discuss these but they are important in their particular racial groups. Sickle cell disease affects those of African origin and thalassaemia affects several groups but particularly those of Mediterranean descent.

General symptoms of anaemia

These are indicative of interference with the normal functioning of haemoglobin and the red blood cell and are common to all anaemia, whatever the cause. There is tiredness and pallor. The pulse may be rapid with palpitations, shortness of breath, light-headedness, fainting, anxiety or depression. Some people complain of floaters in the field of vision. Fever is present in severe cases.

Iron deficiency anaemia may also present with spoon-shaped fingernails (koilonychia) and dysphagia.

Vitamin B_{12} deficiency anaemia may also present with a smooth, sore tongue and an enlarged spleen. There is a typical nerve condition – sub acute combined degeneration of the cord – that leads to pins and needles, ataxia, muscular weakness and eventually paralysis. It is classified as a type of neuropathy.

Complications

Complication	Symptoms to look for
Left ventricular insufficiency	Breathlessness, cough with frothy sputum, palpitations
Right ventricular insufficiency	Peripheral oedema, palpitations
Angina pectoris	Central chest pain on exertion radiating to neck, jaw, inner aspect of arms but especially the left

Table 7.15: Complications of anaemia

Investigations

These will vary according to the suspected cause or they may all be done at once to investigate anaemia of unknown cause.

Full blood count will reveal a reduced haemoglobin level and changes in red blood cell colour and shape. Iron deficiency anaemia is characterised by red blood cells, which are paler and smaller than normal. In folic acid and Vitamin B_{12} deficiency anaemia the red blood cells are larger than normal. Serum iron, folic acid and Vitamin B_{12} may be reduced depending upon the cause.

Treatment

The correct treatment of anaemia in conventional medicine hinges upon the diagnosis. If there is a lack of a specific factor then this is given as a supplement. In clinical practice this means replacement of iron, folic acid or Vitamin B_{12}. Dietary advice will be given to maximise intake of the relevant factor.

Iron is particularly found in liver, green vegetables, eggs, meat and milk. Foods such as green vegetables, liver and kidney are rich in folic acid. Vitamin B_{12} is particularly found in animal products such as meat, fish, eggs and milk. Vegans, therefore, have to be careful about their intake of this vitamin.

Other causes of anaemia are more difficult to treat and the success is largely dependent upon the severity of the original condition.

Although most anaemia cases are due to a multiplicity of factors, people are given iron on the assumption that this 'is good for anaemia'. As described above, the causes are many and varied. It is not enough in most situations to only consider iron intake.

Holistic management

Anaemia is common and the common situations leading to it are dietary lack (either quantity or quality), blood loss and chronic disease. Most cases are treated conventionally with iron although this should be reserved for those with proven iron deficiency. Iron is hot energetically and usually causes constipation as it dries the motions. In some people who have Spleen deficiency, perhaps with Damp accumulation, there may be diarrhoea instead. It is a harsh drug and disturbs absorption of other minerals such as zinc. I think that it is better to obtain iron from foods such as liver or green vegetables. Herbal remedies are excellent at strengthening the blood. In chronic cases be aware of the relationship between the blood and the emotions mentioned above. Flare-ups of the emotions may have to be dealt with carefully along the way.

The causes of anaemia in conventional medicine are fine as far as they go but the one important factor that is missing is energy. It is possible to have an adequate diet in terms of nutritional components but if the energy of the digestion, for example, is depleted then the body will not be able to make blood. Holistic medicine gives further insights into the causes and treatment of anaemia.

In terms of Chinese medicine, the counterpart of anaemia is usually Blood deficiency. The precise symptoms depend on the particular organ mainly involved. In Heart Blood Deficiency there is palpitations, anxiety, insomnia, and dream-disturbed sleep which may be diagnosed as neurosis in conventional medicine. In Liver Blood Deficiency there are symptoms of blurred vision, numbness and tingling which may be diagnosed as a central nervous system disorder such as repetitive strain injury or multiple sclerosis.

Case one

A woman of 35 years came for treatment after she had a ruptured ectopic pregnancy some 4 months before. She had lost so much blood that she received 9 pints of transfused blood. Since then she had developed symptoms of weeping, palpitations, general shaky sensation and tiredness. Her blood count was now 12.8 g which is almost normal but it was the emotional symptoms which were the most difficult. In addition to any problems with the blood there was also the sense of loss due to bereavement.

She was reassured when I explained how these symptoms were interconnected and related to the loss of blood. She was treated with Chinese herbs to strengthen the Blood and given advice as to diet. Her basic constitution was quite sound and she improved within a couple of months. Her energy returned and the emotional symptoms resolved.

In cases of more chronic Blood deficiency, it will take a long time to resolve any emotional state. I find that a combination of acupuncture and Chinese herbs together with counselling or psychotherapy is a potent combination for health. The person is supported as well as having the opportunity to resolve old emotional patterns.

Leucopenia

This is a low white cell count and may occur on its own or as part of aplastic anaemia. It is due to factors such as infection, toxins and drugs. It is a common feature of cancer treatment with chemotherapy.

Agranulocytosis

This is a lack of granular white cells and is severe. Its causes include radiation and drugs such as gold, phenylbutazone, chloramphenicol, thiouracil, imipramine, cancer chemotherapy and sulphonamide antibiotics. It may worsen and involve all the elements of bone marrow and then become aplastic anaemia (see below).

Symptoms
There is fever with sore throat as there is a reduction in white cells to fight infection. Septicaemia may result.

Treatment
This is similar to that of aplastic anaemia.

Aplastic anaemia (pancytopenia)

This is a collapse of bone marrow function leading to anaemia, leucopenia and thrombocytopenia. The commonest causes are direct damage to the bone marrow by radiation or by drugs such as sulphonamide antibiotics, gold, chloramphenicol, cancer chemotherapy and immunosuppressants.

Symptoms
These are the classical triad of pallor and tiredness due to anaemia, sore throat due to infection (as a consequence of leucopenia) and bleeding or bruising (due to thrombocytopenia). It is clearly a serious condition and 50 per cent die within 1 year.

Treatment
There is little treatment available other than stopping the drug and supportive transfusions. In some there may be the option of bone marrow transplantation.[29] All people who take drugs with this side-effect must be told to report a sore throat, as a blood count will be necessary.

HOW TO RECOGNISE SERIOUS CONDITIONS OF THE BLOOD AND LYMPHATIC SYSTEM

It is important to know how to recognise if a symptom arises from a serious situation. You can use Table 7.16 below as a guide to refer to when faced with a person who has one or more of these symptoms. I make no mention of disease labels in the column on the right, as I would not expect you to be able to diagnose conventionally. Seriousness can be assessed merely by reference to symptom pictures.

Symptom	Comments
Pallor	Severe With fainting With marked light-headedness or dizziness
Bruising	Severe Spontaneous
Bleeding	Severe Persistent Recurrent With pallor, sore throat and lymphatic gland enlargement
Lymphatic gland enlargement	With pallor, bleeding and sore throat Progressive Moderately enlarged

Table 7.16: How to recognise serious conditions of the blood and lymphatic system

SUMMARY

Disease of the cardiovascular system is common.

Most of this disease will be chronic and degenerative in nature.

The main cause of heart disease in the West is disturbance of the emotions.

Serious heart disease can be clearly identified in most cases by attention to the symptom picture.

Holistic methods of treatment are very effective for cardiovascular disease especially when incorporated with visualisation and relaxation techniques.

Diseases of the blood are frequently associated with emotional changes.

It is wise to know the indications of a serious condition thoroughly.

---

[1] All organs which are capitalised, e.g. Blood, Heart, Kidney indicate that I mean the energetic view of that organ and not the narrowly defined physical structure of Western science.

[2] An excellent source for information about the energetic organ systems of Chinese medicine is, *Between Heaven and Earth* by Beinfield and Korngold (Ballantine, 1991). I mention the main points here to perhaps shed some light on a wider view of the organs. Homoeopaths may recognise remedy pictures in these descriptions as these are merely another way of describing the same energetic entity.

3 It is interesting to note the similarities between the ideas of Chinese medicine and those of homoeopathy. The homoeopathic remedy Aurum metallicum (gold), for example, reveals symptoms of depression, hopelessness, negativity on the mental level and many heart complaints, including retrosternal oppression with breathlessness on the physical. Gold is the most precious metal and the Heart is the precious organ that houses our mind, our consciousness.

4 The mortality from ischaemic heart disease in the UK was studied for the years 1979-83. It was highest in those born in the Indian subcontinent and especially young Indian men. In others cases there was increased mortality amongst Irish, Scottish and Polish-born immigrants. *BMJ* 1991;302(6776):560-4.

Such differences can be due to complex reasons. It is certainly true that most immigrant groups tend to be isolated within the wider community. Racist attitudes serve to further isolate and alienate them. These factors may partially explain why heart attack rates in Northern Ireland and Scotland are amongst the highest in the world and certainly far in excess of those in England.

5 The presence of ischaemic heart disease in middle age is related to poor socio-economic conditions in childhood rather than any so-called risk factors at the time. *BMJ* 1990;301:1121-3.

Deaths from cardiovascular disease in general are related to infant mortality rates rather than current factors. *British Journal of Preventative and Social Medicine* 1977;31:91-5.

People with heart attacks have been found to have an above average death rate in their siblings, tend to come from larger families and are more likely to have had fathers who were unemployed. These factors in childhood have long-term effects on the heart. *Lancet* 1986;i:1077-81.

A study of people who were born in Hertfordshire, UK in 1911 revealed a lower death rate in those who weighed more at birth and were being breastfed at 1 year. The differences in death rate were very large. *Lancet* 1989;ii:577-80.

6 This is forced expiration against a closed glottis.

7 A trial of flecainide and eucainide had to be discontinued in March 1989 because there was a higher death rate from arrhythmias in the treated group. *Lancet* 1991;20(337):969.

8 Diabetes mellitus produces unconsciousness by means of raised blood sugar levels – hyperglycaemia. Hypoglycaemia which may also produce unconsciousness is a consequence of the treatment of diabetes mellitus by insulin or oral medication. This distinction is explored fully in Chapter 15 – Endocrine system.

9 The incidence of ischaemic heart disease is highest in the 'developed' world and commonest amongst the poor in those countries rather than the rich.

10 There have been found to be a high number of false positive results with exercise ECGs. That is, an ECG which is abnormal but with no disease. Only about 5-10 per cent of those with heart disease have a positive test and so some centres resort to coronary angiograms in asymptomatic people to determine who has heart disease and who does not. *BMJ* 1987;295:620.

11 There have been estimates of the 'appropriateness' of investigations and treatments in conventional medicine. These are done because there are many such investigations and treatments that have not been assessed by means of double blind clinical trials. This is despite the assertion of the medical profession that these are necessary before procedures are used widely. Such estimates revealed that coronary angiography is deemed appropriate in 49 per cent of cases and coronary artery bypass in 55 per cent. *Lancet* 1990;335:1317.

12 A landmark trial was carried out in the US partly funded by the National Institute of Health. Dr Dean Ornish, an associate professor at the University of San Francisco developed a programme of diet, relaxation with visualisation and exercise. Eighty-two per cent of the treated group improved within a year as evidenced by symptoms and high-tech cardiac investigations. The people in the control group continued to have conventional drug treatment and deteriorated in almost half of cases. As Dr Ornish states it is the presence of loneliness and separation which is responsible for the genesis of heart disease. *Lancet* 1990;336:129-33.

13 *Eur Heart Journal* 1992;13(12):1626-31.

14 The long-term effects of coronary bypass surgery are open to debate. There have been conflicting trial results with three major trials comparing medical and surgical treatment. Two revealed no difference whilst one was equivocal. Conventionally, it is said, '...but there is a general acceptance that surgery improves prognosis in the highest risk groups.' If they are 'effective' this only seems to be so in cases of severe disease where there is blockage of the left main coronary artery or distally of the three main coronary arteries. There have been no double-blind controlled trials of their effectiveness. Long-term some 80 per cent of bypasses are blocked 10 years later when a saphenous vein is used. It is more effective to use the internal mammary artery. A study published in 1979 by Dr Eugene Braunwald of Harvard Medical School showed that 12 out of 23 cases had significant improvement in symptoms although angiography revealed that the bypasses had obstructed. *Will to be Well* by Neville Hodgkinson (Rider, 1984). A survey at the University of North Carolina revealed that 83 per cent of people were unemployed some some 2 years later. Over 50 per cent had impaired sexual function. A large number had poor self-images.

15 *The Prescribed Drugs Guide – A Holistic Perspective* by Dr S Gascoigne (Jigme Press, 2001) gives detailed advice on the management of prescribed drug withdrawal.

16 This is rather technical information and is provided for the sake of completion to those who are interested in such matters.

17 The mortality rate after heart attack is dependent upon the speed of access to full resuscitation measures. If this is available, then survival is increased. If not, hospital admission for those with cardiac insufficiency and arrhythmias is made a priority. Otherwise home is a valid option and it is certainly far cheaper.

18 The use of betablockers does seem to reduce the possibility of a further heart attack although only by a small degree. There are a large number of side-effects and they are depleting to the general energy of the body. This may lead to more serious conditions of the heart such as cardiac insufficiency.

19 The use of aspirin after a heart attack seems only to help those with unstable angina, i.e. severe chest pains after small amounts of exercise or at night. It is considered that 75 mg per day is the optimum dose to ensure adequate thinning of the blood whilst producing a low incidence of side-effects. *Lancet* 1990; Oct. 6th: 827. Conversely, a trial in the UK showed that long-term aspirin had no effect on the incidence of stroke or heart attack. *BMJ* 1988; 296: 313-6.

20 A letter in the *Lancet* of Feb. 24th 1990 suggested that the use of aspirin given at the onset of chest pain of a heart attack made no difference to mortality. If it is to be of use then it needs to be used long-term in cases of angina pectoris. This will lead to a risk of blood disorders and digestive disturbances such as indigestion and vomiting blood as well as analgesic nephropathy. The replacement of a heart disease by kidney failure is, of course, suppression.

21 For ease I use the following convention – > means better for and < means worse for.

22 Cyanosis is a blue appearance of the skin due to an inadequate amount of oxygen in the blood. In conventional medicine, it is differentiated into central (tongue) and peripheral (lips and extremities). Central cyanosis is due to cardiac or pulmonary disease. Peripheral cyanosis is due to cardiac disease or may occur in normal people with sluggish circulation particularly in cold weather.

23 There will be the appearances of inflammation in the local area (as described in Chapter 3 Pathological Processes) with lymphatic gland enlargement in the group of glands that drain that area. The term lymphadenitis is applied to this situation.

24 Lymph glands may become enlarged when draining an area containing a malignant tumour but they may merely be affected by an inflammatory process. Enlargement in this case then does not always mean that they are involved in the malignant process.

25 The appearances of glands will be dependent upon whether the underlying process is benign or malignant. This is discussed in detail in Chapter 6 – Cancer.

26 The lymph glands are described as being rubbery on palpation and larger than is the case with diseases such as tonsillitis or glandular fever.

27 There will be the associated symptoms of leukaemia, which are bleeding, pallor (due to anaemia) and sore throats (due to increased likelihood of infection).

28 The association of social class with disease seems to be a particularly British institution. When I speak to people from mainland Europe they comment on its strangeness. My personal view is that disease is clearly associated with certain lifestyles, e.g. respiratory disease is more common in miners but this is a consequence of their work rather than their social class. Medical labels are frequently used as a form of social control and when combined with comments about class can only lead to more stereotypical behaviour on the part of the medical profession. Consequently, I avoid using social classification throughout this book.

29 Bone marrow transplantation is indicated for bone marrow disease where there is little, or no, cellular production after chemotherapy treatment of leukaemia. There is a mortality rate of 25 per cent from this procedure alone which increases with age or if there is infection. The original disease may increase this rate depending upon the case and the person.

8 RESPIRATORY SYSTEM

INTRODUCTION

The respiratory system is much more than the mere physical act of breathing. Added dimensions to understanding the respiratory system can be gathered from holistic medicine. Table 8.1 reveals the associations made in Chinese medicine. It is a common experience that grief and loss may lead to lung conditions such as bronchitis or pneumonia. This is readily explained by understanding the energetic connections.

Association	Comments
Rules Qi[1]	Qi is translated as breath or wind[2] – a wider meaning than in conventional thought
Descending & dispersing	The energy of the Lung goes down and out – as in the direction of the bronchial 'tree'
Container of Phlegm	Phlegm may collect in the Lung after production by the Spleen[3] It is important to treat the Lung and the Spleen when there is sputum in the chest, sinus problems and nasal discharge
Dominate the Water passages	The Lungs control movement of water in the body, particularly the upper body. There is no mention of this conventionally but it explains the tendency to upper body oedema in chronic lung disease
Rules the exterior of the body	Protection of the outer levels of the body against pathogenic influence. This has major role in the immune system
Paired organ is Large Intestine[4]	Disease of the lung may be reflected in the bowels. Constipation may be due to a lack of Lung energy, smoking stimulates the action of the Large Intestine, colonic irrigation may weaken Lung energy
Opens into the nose	The nose is considered to be the opening of the respiratory system
Dominates skin	Skin disorders, e.g. eczema may be due to a Lung imbalance. Eczema and asthma often co-exist or alternate
Colour – white	This is the colour of grief. In the West, death is frequently suppressed and denied leading to an association with black. Black is the colour of the Kidney, which is the deepest organ and associated with fear. Lung disease may cause a white nose or face
Taste – pungent	Excess pungent (acrid) foods, e.g. chillies, black pepper, garlic may harm the Lungs
Season – autumn	The energy of autumn is harvesting and reaping, collection and maturation, a time of making ready for the coming winter which is quiet and cold
Element – Metal	The nature of metal is not holding or letting go. The Lungs and Large Intestine reflect this function of elimination. Disturbance of the Metal element may cause difficulty in letting go and thus feelings of grief, loss or constipation
Time – 3am to 5am	Energy of the Lung is full and flourishing. Practising breathing exercises, Qi Gong and meditation are particularly beneficial at this time. Coughs with phlegm, e.g. whooping cough are more common at this time
Emotions – grief, sadness	This is connected to ideas of letting go. If this is incomplete or interrupted then excessive grief or loss may result
Mental aspect	Compassion, vulnerability, sensibility and sensitivity

Table 8.1: Holistic view of the Lung

ANATOMY AND PHYSIOLOGY

The respiratory system can be divided into upper and lower areas. The upper portion contains:
- nose
- sinuses
- naso-pharynx
- larynx.

The lower portion contains:
- trachea
- bronchi and major airways
- bronchioles
- alveoli
- alveolar-capillary membrane
- pleura (lining lungs and chest wall.

The essential function of the respiratory system is the maintenance of a normal level of oxygen and carbon dioxide in the blood. In addition, there are structures to filter and warm air as it enters the lungs. If there is interference with the functional unit of the lungs – the alveolar-capillary membrane – breathlessness will occur. It follows, therefore that if a person complains of breathlessness, this is an indication that the lung is affected at a deep level. To study respiratory system disease it would be helpful to be able to:

- identify the surface anatomy of the lungs
- identify the structures contained in the respiratory system – nose, pharynx, larynx, trachea, bronchi, bronchioles, alveoli, pleura, diaphragm, and pulmonary blood supply
- describe the functions of these structures
- describe the mechanisms of inspiration and expiration (especially with regard to gaseous exchange)
- explain the carriage of oxygen and carbon dioxide in the blood
- describe the control mechanisms of respiration.

CLASSIFICATION OF RESPIRATORY DISEASE

The most straightforward way of classifying diseases of the respiratory system is to consider those that affect the upper and the lower respiratory tracts. The seriousness of a disease can be assessed according to its chronicity, its depth and the rate of its progression – Table 8.2.

Mild disease
Common cold
Influenza
Sinusitis
Tonsillitis
Scarlet fever
Laryngitis
Acute bronchitis
Pleurisy
Pneumothorax – depends on severity
Allergic rhinitis
Pneumonia
Asthma – depends on severity
Bronchiectasis
Pulmonary embolism
Chronic bronchitis and emphysema
Tuberculosis
Cancer of the lung
Severe disease

Table 8.2: Holistic classification of respiratory disease

UPPER RESPIRATORY TRACT DISEASE

Upper respiratory tract infections in general, and the common cold in particular, offer an opportunity to discuss disease according to the principles of energetic medicine without becoming unduly distracted by infecting organisms such as bacteria and viruses. The energetic view of such diseases is that they manifest on the external surfaces of the body. They are therefore an indication that the energy of the person is relatively strong.

Conventional medicine considers that an infectious agent causes these diseases, usually a virus of which there are many types. It is more beneficial for holistic practitioners to differentiate such diseases according to their symptom picture. In energetic medicine, the causes are not organisms but changes in the energetic balance. In the case of upper respiratory tract disease, this is frequently the result of climatic influences – cold, heat, wind, damp, dryness and summer heat. Treatments are used to remove these 'temporary guests' from the body.

People with acute upper respiratory tract infections can be divided into three groups depending upon the precise symptom picture, which is a direct correlation with the strength of their energy. The stronger their energy then the stronger the symptom picture – Table 8.3.

Person's energy	Conventional label	Comments
Strong	Common cold	The description (below) does not match those in conventional texts
Weak	Common cold descending	Weak Qi causes the pathogenic factor to descend into the Lungs
Weak	Influenza	Weak Blood leads to symptoms in the muscles, i.e. aching

Table 8.3: Upper respiratory tract disease classified according to person's energy

Common cold – strong energy

This is the commonest of all upper respiratory tract infections. Conventionally, it is associated with a virus, of which there are many. The incubation period is considered to be between 1 and 5 days. Immunity is short-lived and specific only for that particular virus. The syndrome I describe here occurs in people with strong energy. It is an unusual manifestation, as most people today do not have sufficient energy to produce these symptoms.[5]

The view in Chinese medicine is that when a pathogenic influence such as wind or cold enters the body, the defensive energy tries to prevent further entry and closes the pores. There is then a struggle between the energy of the pathogenic influence and the energy of the person. The stronger the person's energy is the greater the symptoms will be.

Because the pores are closed there is high fever with no sweating. There is stiff neck and occipital headache as this is where the pathogenic influence enters the body. The person is averse to cold temperature. The Lungs are affected and so there are symptoms of a tickling sensation in the nose and sneezing. The throat is dry and sore, the head feels 'stuffed' and there is a profuse, watery nasal discharge. Symptoms last one to two days.

Common cold – weaker energy

The symptom picture is somewhat different to the above because the person's energy is not so strong. The Qi is not able to close the pores and sweating occurs with a lower fever. The complexion is pale and there is aversion to cold. There is fever with chills and the chills predominate. Tightness in the chest with phlegm indicates that the pathogenic influence has descended deeper into the body. There may be diarrhoea and scanty urination for the same reason. In severe cases there may be shortness of breath and this picture would be more akin to severe acute bronchitis.

Influenza

This is associated with a virus. It occurs in epidemics and occasionally pandemics. There are three viruses, A which is the main one, B and C. Immunity is short-lived and type specific. Major epidemics occur every few years. The epidemic of 1918/19 killed 20 million people, more than had died during World War I and confirms the observation that such a disease attacks the weak and debilitated. The incubation period is 1-3 days long.

Symptoms

These are more systemic than those of the common cold. Malaise is usually extreme with pains and aching in the back and limbs. Fever exists with chills but fever is predominant. The skin is greyish and the person is often thin. There is irritability. There is little or no sweating. There may be headache, sore throat and a dry cough, which can last for several weeks. Debility and depression is common with these symptoms and they can be prolonged leading to post-viral syndrome.

Recovery takes place within three to five days but it can take longer to regain full activity. Most people with this condition will not be able to go to work for at least a few days.

Upper respiratory tract infection – general comments

Respiratory complications are more common in people with pre-existing disease, e.g. chronic bronchitis, diabetes mellitus, asthma or in the old and frail. Clearly, the weaker the energy then the more likely are complications. Influenza, for example, regularly leads every winter to deaths especially in the elderly and debilitated. Post-influenzal depression and weakness may be severe. It lasts 1-2 weeks but in some may merge with ME-like syndromes.

Complications

Complication	Symptoms to look for
Sinusitis	Pain in the face especially under the eyes, yellow nasal discharge, and headaches
Tracheitis	Retrosternal pain, dry cough, pain worse for coughing
Acute bronchitis	As above with cough and yellowish sputum
Pneumonia	Cough with brownish sputum, breathlessness
Post-attack debility	Prolonged attack, debility, tiredness, depression
Post-influenzal encephalomyelitis	Occipital headache, neck stiffness, photophobia

Table 8.4: Complications of upper respiratory tract infection

Treatment

This is largely symptomatic and consists of bed rest and paracetamol. There are many proprietary medicines available for the relief of symptoms, mainly fever and the nasal symptoms. Medications such as nose drops may damage the mucous membrane of the nasal cavity. It is preferable not to use them, but to rest and to use simple natural remedies. If sustained and adequate rest is not taken then post-attack debility may occur as the pathogenic influence remains in the body.

Antibiotics are given for the complications of upper respiratory tract infections. The vaccine for influenza changes from year to year according to the predominant virus. It reputedly gives 70 per cent protection. Conventionally, vaccination is recommended for people with diabetes mellitus and chronic lung, cardiac or renal disease. In an epidemic, health service workers are vaccinated. There are the usual immediate problems after vaccination (such as fever and debility) and long-term, adverse effects on the vital force. In conversations with people who care for the elderly, it is clear that influenza vaccination has a great effect on vitality. Those who receive the vaccination seem to have more episodes of ill health during the winter.

Holistic management of upper respiratory tract infection

It can be seen from the above descriptions that what is usually labelled a common cold is nothing of the sort. Any mucus discharge or cough tends to be labelled in this way. If there were no signs of an acute exterior syndrome (such as fever and/or chills or occipital headache) it is unlikely to be a cold.

Mucus collections in the body due to an internal, chronic condition often discharge through the nose or lungs. Conventional practitioners would invariably give such people antibiotics. With an understanding of depths of disease it is possible to differentiate. The antibiotic use can only lead to further depletion of energy, more mucus formation and consequences for the immune system as a whole. Suppression of the symptoms at this stage will exacerbate the chronic condition. Simple supportive measures are the best way to approach this situation.

In the case of an acute condition, there may be no need to treat in cases where the condition is resolving by itself. However, it is helpful to treat someone if their energy is depleted and the symptoms either begin to progress into the interior or become 'stuck' at the exterior level.

In terms of Chinese medicine, these diseases fall into the category of External Pathogenic Invasion. The precise pathogenic factor involved is determined by the symptoms. Cold, damp, wind, dryness and heat may all invade the body and cause problems. Essentially, Wind-heat is present if fever predominates and Wind-cold is present if chills predominate. Wind-heat occurs in those of strong constitution or if the Blood is deficient and Wind-cold occurs in those with Qi deficiency.

The usual conventional drug, aspirin, is derived from willow bark and pretty close to the appropriate energetic remedy. This drug will relieve fever by releasing the exterior of the body, opening the pores, dispersing the energy and causing a sweat. It is warm in nature. It works to relieve the pain of arthritis by the same means. Unfortunately, long-term usage weaken the Blood and the Kidneys. This and related drugs, the non-steroidal anti-inflammatory agents, are the cause of a significant number of cases of analgesic nephropathy. This is drug-induced kidney damage, which may lead to kidney failure. There are variable numbers of people with kidney failure resulting from analgesic use, particularly aspirin and non-steroidal anti-inflammatory drugs. In Australia, for example, this is 20 per cent of kidney failure cases. They are freely available as over-the-counter remedies and there are regular accounts of the damage these drugs can do to the kidneys.[6]

Case one

A woman of 48 years was seeing me regularly for chronic low back pain. In between visits she called me to say she had symptoms of a 'cold'. She had developed pain in her face with a fever, sore throat and sneezing. This had been treated with antibiotics and now she was feeling worse. She was tired, sneezing and still had a cough (producing green phlegm). She described the pain in her face and cheek as sharp and stabbing in nature.

I made a diagnosis of Wind-cold Invasion with Qi Deficiency due to the use of the antibiotics. She had an underlying Kidney Yang Deficiency that was the cause of the low back pain – her chronic condition. I treated her with acupuncture to clear the Wind and the Cold from her body. This had a good effect and she felt better within one day. Her cough settled, her energy improved and the pain in her face had gone. This is an example of an External Invasion in someone with slightly weak energy. The antibiotics had made her more tired and her lungs had become affected. Further antibiotics would have only complicated the case further and, in any case, not cleared the External Invasion.

Sinusitis

This is inflammation of the sinuses which are air-filled cavities in the head. They form part of the respiratory system and have a function in warming and moistening inhaled air. They are affected due to an upper respiratory tract disorder such as the common cold, allergic rhinitis or where mucus is a predominant symptom. The mucus tends to collect in the sinuses and may flare up from time to time as an inflammation. In some people there is an allergic component.

Symptoms

The symptoms are centred around the head and nose. There is blocked nose and nasal discharge, which is usually yellow or green, and a frontal headache. The symptoms can be severe with extreme facial pain or headache in some, particularly if the mucus is thick. The sinuses are tender on pressure. There may be a feeling of 'muzziness' in the head especially in the mornings.

Complications

Complication	Symptoms to look for
Nasal polyps	Chronic nasal obstruction. The polyps may be visible in the nostril
Laryngitis	Hoarse voice, dry and sore throat
Tracheitis	Retrosternal pain, cough, pain worse for coughing
Acute bronchitis	As tracheitis with progression to cough with sputum which is yellowish
Local abscess	Fever, severe local pain
Cerebral abscess	Fever, headache, signs of central nervous system disease such as paralysis, visual disturbances, speech disturbances

Table 8.5: Complications of sinusitis

Investigations

X-ray of the sinuses may show them to be filled or partially filled with fluid (mucus).

Treatment

The conventional treatment of sinusitis is of variable effectiveness. Analgesics are frequently used. Decongestants such as ephedrine and xylometazoline are examples of the sympathomimetic group[7] of drugs and are used to dry up secretions. They are stimulant in nature and as the effect is suppressive any reduction of dosage may result in a flare-up of symptoms. This can be interpreted as another attack and another course of treatment instituted so that the person becomes locked into a cycle of continuing drug-use. Antibiotics are often prescribed for severe attacks and for nasal discharge that is yellow or green in colour - see comments on Page 142. Corticosteroids may be given for local use such as fluticasone propionate spray.

Surgical treatments include sinus washout, which is a singularly unpleasant procedure. Local anaesthetic is used and a probe inserted into the maxillary sinus. Water is washed round the sinuses to remove mucus. This operation is of short-term benefit only as the cause of mucus production is not addressed. Polyps are removed surgically. Both operations are often repeated until either the person wearies of the process or the condition is suppressed, usually into the lungs.

Holistic management

In terms of Chinese medicine this usually corresponds to a combination of Lung Qi deficiency, Spleen Qi deficiency and Damp-accumulation that collects in the sinuses. Alternatively, Fire in the Liver and Gall Bladder may ascend to the head. An acute flare-up is often a result of a Wind-cold invasion attacking the Lungs.

In energetic terms this is a relatively minor condition as the Lung Qi is strong enough to hold the imbalance in the upper respiratory tract. This is why persistent suppression is hazardous as it weakens Lung Qi and may eventually drive the Damp deep into the Lungs.

The Damp (mucus) is produced by the Spleen and so dietary advice is paramount. The general advice for someone with Spleen Qi deficiency is covered in Chapter 13 – Gastrointestinal system. Exercises to strengthen to Lung Qi are helpful, as is specific treatment for the particular individual.

Tonsillitis

This is inflammation of the tonsils and is associated with either a bacterium or a virus. There is no difference clinically between the two types of inflammation and to routinely prescribe antibiotics makes no sense at all. A throat swab will delineate the bacterium (if any) present in the throat but these may also be found in people with no symptoms. A severe tonsillitis with pain in the throat that lasts for longer than normal may be glandular fever. Enlargement of the adenoids may be associated.

Symptoms

Children are more commonly affected than adults. The main symptom is sore throat, which in mild cases may be diagnosed as pharyngitis. Here there is redness of the soft palate and back of the throat. There is associated difficulty in swallowing and fever. The lymph glands in the neck are swollen and tender. In true tonsillitis, the tonsils themselves are enlarged and red, with white or usually yellow material on their surface. The tongue is coated and the person feels generally ill.

Investigations

In normal clinical practice, there is usually no investigation performed. A throat swab can reveal evidence of bacteria.

Complications

Complication	Symptoms to look for
Otitis media	Pain in the ear, discharge from ear in severe cases
Acute glomerulonephritis	Pain in the loin, haematuria, and oedema
Rheumatic fever	Palpitations, malaise, joint pains, skin rashes
Quinsy (tonsillar abscess)	Pain in the throat (rather than soreness), severe tonsillar swelling on one side

Table 8.6: Complications of tonsillitis

Treatment

Symptomatic treatment is all that is required particularly as only 30 per cent of sore throats are associated with bacteria. Penicillin and related drugs should not be used if glandular fever is a possibility because a rash will result. In clinical practice, antibiotics are frequently given and if attacks are recurrent they may be used each time. If attacks are severe or frequent enough to affect the child's health, hearing or breathing, tonsillectomy[8] will be performed. The specific advice is to have tonsillectomy if there are five or more attacks of tonsillitis in one year, three or more attacks in two years, severe attacks or tonsillitis not responding to treatment. There are doubts about the effectiveness of tonsillectomy and there has never been a trial to determine its usefulness. It does reduce the incidence of throat infections for the first two years after the operation only and there is no effect on the numbers of days lost at school by children.[9]

Holistic management

In terms of Chinese medicine, this is usually due to Heat in the Lung or Stomach, which flares up into the throat when there is an acute attack of Wind-cold or Wind-heat. It is important to treat constitutionally between attacks in order to minimise the chance and number of repeat attacks. To remove the tonsils, an essential part of the immune system is to weaken the general immunity. Some children have problems in the stomach or lungs after tonsillectomy as their earlier line of defence has been removed. Holistic treatment on a regular basis is an effective option to prevent such an operation. As with any problem in the throat, it is useful to think of this area and its role in communication. The throat chakra is where energy becomes blocked if speech is suppressed or emotion is held. I discuss this connection in Chapter 15 – Endocrine system – in relation to goitre and thyroid disease.

Some people get recurrent attacks of sore throat, which are not associated with tonsillar enlargement or discharge. If it is mild in its manifestation then it is almost certainly not tonsillitis. Energetically, Kidney or Liver energy can flare up to the throat and cause mild discomfort, dryness, soreness and redness. This may also be treated conventionally by antibiotics. Such an event is, however, not an acute attack affecting the tonsils but a manifestation of deeper organ imbalance.

Scarlet Fever

This is an acute tonsillitis due to streptococci in association with the typical rash. The incubation period is 2-7 days.

Symptoms

These are mostly mild although in the past the disease has been a great problem. It seems to have undergone quite a change in the last 50 years so that now most cases are minor and this is reflected in the diminutive name 'scarlatina'. The alteration can be interpreted as a weakening of the general energy of the population, since sufferers are only able to produce a weaker symptom picture. The conventional explanation is that it is the organism that has become weaker.

There is an acute onset of high fever. Vomiting commonly occurs also. On examination the tonsils are very red with swelling. There may be yellow discharge from the tonsils. There is associated lymph gland enlargement. A fine red rash appears within 24 hours as a fine red rash. It soon becomes generalised although it is more marked at the flexures such as the elbow, axilla and groin and it is less marked around the mouth – the classical circumoral pallor.

The tongue also undergoes typical changes also with white fur on the first day. On days 2 and 3 the papillae are seen to be larger than usual and the coat starts to peel at the tip and sides – 'white strawberry' tongue. On days 4 and 5 the peeling continues until the tongue is clean, red and shiny – 'red strawberry' tongue.

Complications

Complication	Symptoms to look for
Acute glomerulonephritis	Loin pain, haematuria, oedema
Rheumatism	Pain and swelling in the joints
Rheumatic fever	Palpitations, pain in chest, tiredness

Table 8.7: Complications of scarlet fever

Investigation

The characteristic organisms are found on a throat swab. The presence of rising antibody levels confirms the diagnosis. There is no clinical difference between a tonsillitis caused by streptococci and one caused by viruses. In the case of scarlet fever, the presence of the rash is often enough to confirm the diagnosis. It is useful to be aware that many throat swabs in people with no symptoms may also show streptococci.

Treatment

Penicillin is always given and quickly eradicates the bacteria from the throat and renders the person non-infective within 24-48 hours.

Holistic medicine

This condition is not common these days but can be dealt with in the same way as tonsillitis. Treatment in the acute phase will minimise the occurrence of complications. Complications are when the pathogenic heat descends into deeper levels in the body.

Allergic rhinitis

There are similarities between symptoms of this disease and those of the common cold. Allergic rhinitis is chronic in nature in that it recurs and indicates a deeper pathology. It is considered to be due to a hypersensitivity reaction of the nasal mucosa to specific substances and is characterised by the appearance of upper respiratory symptoms when in contact with a variety of stimuli. It is diagnosed when the symptoms are present for at least an hour a day on most days. It is regarded as either seasonal (classic hay fever) or perennial (i.e. symptoms appear more regularly).

The pollens of grasses, flowers, trees and, very commonly, nettles, cause the seasonal types. Contact with oilseed rape is becoming a common problem especially in the UK. These are the 'hay-fevers' you see in the summer and can affect up to 20 per cent of the population. Around 20 per cent of these may also have respiratory symptoms and be diagnosed as asthmatic. The perennial types are caused by many factors (often undiscoverable). House dust and house dust mite are common causes as are moulds and the products of hydrocarbons such as traffic pollution leading to poor air quality, perfumes, sprays, etc. Animals such as cats, dogs and horses lead to reactions also.

Symptoms

Frequent, sudden attacks of sneezing with a profuse watery nasal discharge and nasal obstruction are the usual features. They last a few hours and are often associated with itching, watering and red eyes. There may be itching of the roof of the mouth. In the perennial types the attacks are more continuous and less severe. More chronic cases are characterised by nasal obstruction rather than the acute symptoms of sneezing with watery discharge.

There may be a feeling of heat especially in the head. There may be cough with wheezing. These cases may be labelled asthma.

Investigations

Diagnosis is mainly from the symptom picture. A skin prick test may be done. A serum immunoglobulin E test may reveal an antibody against a specific allergen.

Treatment

Conventional medicine is at a bit of a loss when it comes to the treatment of many allergic disorders and this is no exception. Avoidance is emphasised although this is of variable effectiveness. It may be difficult to determine the exact trigger and in many people there are multiple factors. The general health is also important here as allergic reactions are more common when the sufferer is stressed, overtired or subjected to several allergens at once.

Treatment (mildest to strongest)	Comments
Antihistamines	The usual prescription for any allergic disorder. They are most effective for sneezing, less so for nasal discharge and have little effect on nasal obstruction. Tiredness and drowsiness are common. Astemizole and loratidine have been associated with fatal cardiac arrhythmias. Others include terfenadine and cetirizine
Decongestants – local	Sympathomimetic agents are commonly used if there is a great problem with a runny or a blocked nose. Discharges from the body are a method of elimination. Stopping up a discharge by external means such as drugs or surgery prevents this route and the consequences can be severe. In the case of nasal problems the likely result is the development of lung disease such as asthma or bronchitis
Decongestants – oral	Examples include xylometazoline and oxymetazoline. The drugs, themselves, may lead to increased nasal symptoms of discharge and obstruction. Increasing the dosage to control these can only lead to more difficulties. The best conventional practice is to only use for a short time
Anti-inflammatory drugs	These include sodium cromoglycate and nedocromil sodium. These were always considered to stabilise the mast cell membranes to stop the release of histamine. They also have a direct anti-inflammatory action. Also used in asthma and bowel disorders due to food intolerance
Corticosteroids – local	Examples are beclomethasone spray and fluticasone propionate spray. They reduce inflammation in the nose and so the amount of discharge and obstruction. Systemic effects do occur such as shortness of stature and suppressed immune system
Corticosteroids – oral	The most powerful in their effect – see Page 180. They may be given as short courses of 2 weeks such as prednisolone 10-15 mg daily

Table 8.8: Treatment of allergic rhinitis

Prevention

Attempts are made to 'desensitise' people to the allergen by a series of injections of increasing strength of the relevant allergen. This approach can cause anaphylactic shock and have led to sudden death in people. Injections are now only given in hospital, where resuscitation equipment is to hand. The same criticism can be applied here as in the case of vaccination. The deliberate injection of the offending antigen into the blood stream is potentially harmful. The body tries to prevent this by producing symptoms in the nose, throat and eyes. Bypassing protective layers in an attempt to 'treat' the condition puts the patient at risk. In any case, such treatments frequently are of minimal effectiveness.

Holistic management

In energetic terms, although the acute manifestations are due to an external factor, the chronic cause is due to an internal condition. The acute attack is due to Wind-cold or Wind-heat Invasion due to Deficiency of the Lung and Kidney. In my experience there may also be some degree of Damp-heat Accumulation, which flares up into the Lungs when conditions are right. Some people may have Liver Blood deficiency as is evidenced by eye symptoms. Many people report that there is a poor association with pollen counts. More important factors are diet, levels of emotional stress and the climatic factors of heat and damp.

The most effective approach to take is to begin treatment before the pollen season in the case of the seasonal type and there may not be much improvement the first year. Emphasis outside of the season should be placed on resolving the underlying imbalance. It is generally considered by holistic practitioners that only by the second or third summer after treatment has begun will you notice the main benefits of treatment. There are cases, however, where improvement is much quicker.

Case one

A man of 34 years came for treatment of rhinitis. He would develop sneezing, blocked nose, fullness in the head, impaired hearing and a cough with green phlegm. He had suffered with these symptoms for almost 20 years and they would come on every summer as well as with dust or in damp weather. With these symptoms he would also feel very tired and occasionally would develop glandular swelling in his neck. He was taking a proprietary decongestant medication several times each day. I made a diagnosis of Lung Qi Deficiency, Kidney not Grasping Lung Qi and Phlegm-heat in the Lung. I treated him with acupuncture only.

His cough improved fairly quickly after two treatments but he would still feel stuffed in the head with fullness. If this persisted he would feel tired and his cough would return. I continued to treat him over the course of several months and his improvement continued. As he improved he gradually reduced his medication. In such cases, sudden withdrawal can lead to a severe flare-up of symptoms particularly if the medication has been taken over many years. Slow withdrawal does lead to an exacerbation of symptoms but usually much milder and for a shorter duration. After five months of treatment he felt well with good energy. He would have a slight flare-up of symptoms if he was exposed to large amounts of dust. He continues to be well some 18 months later.

Laryngitis

This is an inflammation of the larynx. It is usually a consequence of an upper respiratory infection, which has descended into this area. It may be herald deeper symptoms (e.g. cough, sputum and breathlessness).

A variant is acute laryngotracheobronchitis, which leads to a croupy (barking) cough in children. In severe cases this may lead to cyanosis and stridor (see terms at end of Chapter).

Symptoms
There will be the symptoms of the original condition with the development of hoarse voice. This may become so severe that the person may only be able to emit a scratchy whisper. It lasts for several days and then begins to recover. Complete recovery is the rule.

It may be recurrent in singers, smokers and those who use their voices excessively, e.g. public speakers. The symptom of hoarseness may be the first sign of a tumour of the vocal cords. In this situation, the hoarseness is long-lasting (more than 3 weeks). In this case it is important for the vocal cords to be examined by an ear, nose and throat specialist (otorhinolaryngologist).

Treatment
This is merely symptomatic including resting the voice. Underlying causes such as smoking need to be addressed. Public speakers and singers may benefit from voice training.

Holistic management
The comments I made with regard to upper respiratory tract disease are applicable here. In terms of Chinese medicine, it is usually part of the picture of an attack of Wind-cold or Wind-heat descending into the Lungs. As mentioned in the description of tonsillitis, Liver or Kidney energy may affect the throat. Hoarse voice may be part of such an energetic pattern.

LOWER RESPIRATORY TRACT DISEASE

Diseases in this part of the respiratory system necessarily indicate that there is a more serious imbalance in lung energy. If the Lung Qi is strong, the symptoms are held in the superficial levels. Diseases of the lower respiratory tract occur in those people who have weak Lung energy or as a result of suppressive treatment. As you treat such diseases, you may see the reappearance of symptomatology in the more superficial levels.

Acute bronchitis

This is an acute inflammation of the trachea and bronchi and is usually associated with viruses. Bacteria are more common in smokers and those with chronic lung disease. It can develop after upper respiratory problems in which instances it is an example of the pathogenic influence descending into the lungs. It may also occur in people with chronic bronchitis as an acute exacerbation of the chronic condition. Predisposing factors are cold, damp and foggy weather, dusty atmospheres and smoking.

Symptoms
The symptoms of the original condition are present which then develop into a dry, irritating cough with retrosternal discomfort. This is the cough of acute tracheitis where the pain is sore and scratchy, it is felt behind the sternum and the person will sit up to cough and hold the chest. There is tightness in the chest with a low fever. Breathlessness is unusual unless there is an associated chronic lung disease when wheezing may also occur.

Sputum is scanty, white and thick at first. It then develops into more copious, yellow or greenish sputum. There is usually a fever. Most people recover in four to eight days without any problems.

Investigations

There is an increase in the white cell count (neutrophils). Chest X-ray is normal.

Treatment

Antibiotics are usually given as indeed they are for any discharge that is yellow or green in colour. It is often said that acute bronchitis lasts around 7 days without the use of antibiotics and 1 week with them! Steam inhalations are helpful to relieve cough and soreness.

Holistic management

In terms of Chinese medicine this usually corresponds to Phlegm-heat Retention in the Lungs. It may be a consequence of an acute pathogenic influence or of an internal condition where Dampness and Phlegm collects in the Lungs. The use of antibiotics will clear any Heat but does nothing about the underlying Phlegm condition and will actually make that worse, as the Lung and Spleen Qi will more depleted. The correct treatment of upper respiratory tract infections such as common cold and influenza is important in order to prevent or minimise the occurrence of acute bronchitis.

Case one

A woman of 52 years came for treatment of her chest symptoms of 5 months duration. She had a tendency to 'catch colds' which would be followed by chest symptoms. Her main symptoms were tiredness, cough with greyish green phlegm and tightness in the chest. I made a diagnosis of Phlegm-heat Accumulation with underlying Lung Qi Deficiency. I treated her with acupuncture. After the first treatment her cough and phlegm were much better and her energy was improved. She continued to come twice more at the end of which her chest was clear, her energy was fine and she felt well. Her basic health was good as evidenced by the rapid improvement. It would have been preferable if she could have continued a while longer with treatment to strengthen her Lung Qi. She attends the clinic about once a year now whenever she feels low or tired. She occasionally gets a cold which goes to her chest but this clears quickly. Conventionally, she would be treated with antibiotics which may clear the green phlegm but would leave her feeling tired and more vulnerable to the next passing 'cold' or weather change. Antibiotics are generally unnecessary and it is perfectly safe in most cases for people either to stop them immediately they begin treatment or as soon as their symptoms start to improve.

Case two

This case is an example of how to treat chest symptoms in a child. Although it was diagnosed 'bronchiolitis', there are many similarities with the above description of bronchitis. In children it is the small airways bronchioles, rather than bronchi, that are affected.

A two-year-old boy came for treatment of bronchiolitis, which was being treated with salbutamol syrup. The cough was worse at night and after 2 hours sleep he started wheezing. Often the cough would lead to vomiting of stringy, white mucus. The boy had a delicate stomach and the syrup and repeated antibiotics he was prescribed often brought on vomiting. He had frequent, greenish stools. His mother felt that, compared to her first child, he was aggressive, strong-willed and short-tempered. He enjoyed breaking things. He fell over frequently, as if his balance or co-ordination was 'a bit off.' Recently he had developed lumps on his right wrist, which had produced a green discharge. This had not been treated conventionally and had resolved by itself. It was suggested to cut out orange juice and cow's milk from his diet (as they are both mucus forming) and using goat's milk and watered down apple juice instead. He was prescribed Ant tart 30c as it fitted the case well on all levels. A month later he came for a follow-up. His father said that he had been 'perfect since the remedy. He is different, happier …just better all round.' The cough, wheezing and vomiting were all completely gone. He no longer took any medication. He was taking a regular one-hour nap and this meant he was less irritable. He had stopped breaking things. He was steadier on his feet. He had had another eruption on his back that had discharged and then cleared. He had halved the number of bowel movements per day (from six to three). His speech was improving and he seemed more interested in learning new words.

Pneumonia

In conventional medicine, pneumonias are classified according to the causative organism, which is usually bacterial. It is more common in people with HIV infection. Table 8.9 classifies pneumonia according to the clinical appearances and so is more useful for the holistic practitioner.

Type of pneumonia	Associated organisms	Comments
Lobar	Pneumococcus, Mycoplasma (occasionally)	Affects 'healthy' adults. Strong symptoms reflect the relatively strong level of energy. Despite the dramatic nature of the symptoms this condition is less serious than bronchopneumonia (see below)
Bronchopneumonia	Mycoplasma, *Haemophilus influenzae, Chlamydia psittaci,*[10] *Staphylococcus aureus, Legionella pneumophilia,*[11] *Pneumocystis carinii*[12]	Affects debilitated people and may be a terminal event. Mild, vague symptoms reflecting the depleted energy

Table 8.9: Classification of pneumonia according to clinical appearances (mild at top, severe at bottom)

Lobar pneumonia

This, as its name suggests, is usually restricted to one lobe of the lung and is fairly localised. It is an illness of young, 'healthy' adults. The usual causative organism is the pneumococcus – a type of streptococcus – Table 8.9.

Symptoms
There is sudden onset of fever with chills and shivering. The temperature is high at about 40°C (104°F) and remains high. The face is flushed. The pleura is usually involved and so there is a typical pleuritic pain – a sharp pain in the axilla or around the scapula that is worse on respiration and coughing. A dry cough is present at the beginning followed within a few days of reddish (rusty) coloured sputum. There is breathlessness. There is often an attack of herpes simplex ('cold sores') on the lip.

Most people are given antibiotics and there will be an improvement in the condition within 48 hours. Before these were available there would be a 'crisis' around the seventh day when the fever would remit and the person would either start to recover or their condition would deteriorate.

Investigations
Clinical examination of the chest shows the typical signs of pneumonic consolidation which is a solidifying of the lung tissue due to inflammation and fluid collection. There is dullness to percussion over the affected area together with a pleural rub and coarse crackling (audible by stethoscope) over the affected area. Chest X-ray will reveal shadowing over the affected lobe of the lung due to the inflammatory process. It returns to normal some 4-6 weeks after the pneumonia has settled. The white cell count is raised with the ESR over 100 mm.

Complications
Lobar pneumonia usually ends in resolution and the person recovers. Complications of lung abscess and empyema are rare.

Treatment
This is universally with antibiotics to which the organism is sensitive. In a case of lobar pneumonia in a young, fit person recovery is usually complete.

Holistic management
Before the advent of antibiotics, homoeopathic and herbal remedies were the only way that people could obtain help. The homoeopathic texts abound with examples of people who recovered in a few days with the appropriate remedy. There is no reason to suppose that this cannot be the case today. However, there are factors to take into account such as the level of support the person has at home and the actual condition of the person. Since few of us currently have access to residential care difficulties arise when caring for people who are too ill to be treated on an outpatient basis. People with early signs of pneumonia can be treated and this will probably remove the need for antibiotics. Assess carefully the condition of the person, give the appropriate treatment and review the case regularly. If the person's condition starts to deteriorate then a reappraisal is essential. You must be familiar with how to recognise a serious condition.

In terms of Chinese medicine, pneumonia usually corresponds to Phlegm-heat congesting the Lungs. The cause of this in the acute phase is Wind-heat or Wind-cold attack but there will be an underlying Lung imbalance as a predisposing factor.

Bronchopneumonia

This is a more generalised disease and is associated with organisms which are normally present in the respiratory tract or which are usually successfully resisted. It occurs in the very young, the elderly and the debilitated. This is clearly more a case of weak defensive energy and this type of pneumonia is seen after other respiratory infections. In this category would be included diseases such as Legionnaire's disease, pneumonia occurring in people with AIDS and so forth.

Symptoms

These are much more vague than with the classic picture of lobar pneumonia. For example, the fever is mild with malaise, aching in the head and limbs and, perhaps, low spirits. The person will feel generally unwell and after a couple of days a dry cough will appear with the typical pain of pleurisy. After a few days, phlegm is produced which is yellow or green. These symptoms are in keeping with the view that intensity of symptoms is a reflection of the strength of the person's energy and weak people exhibit very few symptoms.

In the case of people with AIDS or other severe disease, pneumonia may only be recognised by the existence of breathlessness. The person may be too weak to produce a cough or sputum. The acute onset of confusion, particularly in the elderly, may be the first indication of pneumonia.

Investigations

Chest examination shows only minimal signs such as an area of decreased air entry with crepitations or occasionally bronchial breathing and dullness on percussion. The chest X-ray reveals diffuse shadowing over the bases of both lungs reflecting the more widespread nature of the disease.

Complications

Complication	Symptoms to look for
Chronic 'infection' – persistent inflammation	Persistent cough, sputum and breathlessness
Lung abscess	Symptoms of pneumonia worsen and persist, large amounts of foul sputum
Empyema	This is pus in the pleural cavity. People are severely ill with high fever
Cardiac insufficiency	Oedema, breathlessness worse for lying and at night

Table 8.10: Complications of bronchopneumonia

Treatment

This is with the antibiotic appropriate for the causative organism. Many people continue to have chronic respiratory problems. In some people who develop such pneumonia when they are debilitated, the pneumonia would normally be a terminal event and antibiotics may prevent death. The person then partially recovers to succumb at some later date from another attack of pneumonia or perhaps cardiac insufficiency.

Tuberculosis

I have included this disease as it is of some importance to homoeopaths who regard suppressed tuberculosis, in the person's medical or family history, to be an important cause of disease. It is true that there are similarities between tuberculosis and cancer and we may have replaced one disease by the other. Both diseases are often associated with wasting and there are areas of the body that are affected by destructive lumps.

Tuberculosis is a specific type of respiratory problem, which is unusual in the UK but is becoming commoner. There are currently 7000 new cases per year in the UK and these are not declining in numbers. It can affect virtually any organ and tissue in the body.

It is considered to be due to infection with the tubercle bacillus. In the West, it is the human type that is more common and is spread through droplets (cough, sneeze). In less 'developed' countries you see the bovine type, which is spread, through drinking contaminated milk. In the UK there is a system of accrediting herds as being free of tuberculosis. Therefore, it does not enter the milk supplies. In addition, most milk is still pasteurised as a hangover from the days when tuberculosis was present in cattle.

It is a disease of poor conditions of housing, sanitation and food. This is why tuberculosis is now increasing in the West. Over the past several years there has been a general increase in poverty, particularly in inner city areas and amongst more deprived social groups. The death rate was already declining steadily before the introduction of the relevant legislation governing public health and there is no evidence that any difference to the pattern of the disease has been made by either vaccination or antibiotics – Table 8.11.

Year	Death rate/10000	Event
1812	700	
1882	370	Isolation of TB bacterium by Koch
1910	180	Opening of first sanatorium
1945	48	Antibiotics not yet widely available

Table 8.11: Fall in death rate from tuberculosis prior to antibiotic use[13]

Primary tuberculosis

This is the first infection. It mainly shows itself as enlargement of certain lymph nodes. It is frequently asymptomatic although some people develop a vague illness with cough and wheeze.

Symptoms
In the primary form there is a small affected area in the lung with enlarged local lymph nodes. There is a small shadow on X-ray as well as evidence of lymph gland enlargement. The Mantoux reaction[14] is positive. General symptoms are minimal and around 95 per cent of people will recover on their own. Many people have had such events in the past and are unaware until a routine chest X-ray reveals it. Occasionally, this condition may lead to bronchiectasis, tuberculous bronchopneumonia and tuberculosis in other sites such as bone, joints, kidney and so on.

Post-primary tuberculosis

This is a subsequent infection with the tubercle bacillus or, more likely, a reactivation in someone with a depleted immune system.[15] It is invariably pulmonary in site and usually in the upper lobes. The infected area breaks down, a cavity forms in the lung and infected sputum is produced. Infection may occur in other parts of the lung from this sputum. Pleurisy may develop if the periphery of the lung is involved and blood is coughed up when blood vessels are eroded.

The rate of progression of the disease is variable and clearly depends on the strength of the individual person. In some there is slow deterioration and the healing process of fibrosis and calcification may in fact arrest the illness. In others there is a steady, and at times rapid, progress into ill health and death.

Symptoms
In the early stages there may be minimal symptoms and coughing blood can be the first sign. Typically there are night sweats, fever, tiredness, progressive weight loss and loss of appetite. There is cough with sputum which may be white, yellow/green or bloody. There may be a dull ache in the chest. Later, the fingers may take on a clubbed appearance in severe cases. There may be a prior history of catching colds frequently. Eventually the person will waste hence the old name of consumption. There may also be the symptoms of tuberculous infection elsewhere such as the larynx (laryngitis), trachea (tracheitis) and ileum (ileitis). Supraclavicular lymph gland enlargement is common.

Investigations
Chest X-ray shows signs of shadows in the upper lobes, fibrosis and possibly cavities. Chest x-ray can show changes in people with little or no symptoms. Bacteriological examination of the sputum reveals the causative organism – *Mycobacterium tuberculosis* – although culture takes 4-8 weeks to show results with a further 4 weeks to determine antibiotic sensitivity. Biopsies of the pleura and lymph glands may be performed to help confirm the diagnosis. Fibreoptic bronchoscopy can be used to obtain sputum for culture and to biopsy the pleura or lymph nodes.

Treatment
Conventionally, this is with combinations of antibiotics usually rifampicin, isoniazid and pyrazinamide. They are generally given for 6 months and up to 2 years in cases of bone TB. Ethambutol or streptomycin are occasionally used. Rifampicin given with isoniazid is a common combination. They are given for at least 6 months and usually for 1 or 2 years and in combinations so that two or more drugs are usually given together. Attention is made to general health such as adequate diet, rest and convalescence although not as much emphasis is placed on this as in the days of sanatoria. Vaccination by means of the BCG[16] is recommended for all children who are Mantoux negative.

Holistic management
It is not likely that people with tuberculosis will present for holistic treatment. They usually seek conventional advice. There are treatments that exist in Chinese medicine and homoeopathy. In terms of Chinese medicine, tuberculosis corresponds to two main patterns. It may be due to Deficiency of Yin where Fire damages the fluids. The other type is due to Deficiency of

Yang especially of Lung, Spleen and Kidney. Both of these syndromes may also be responsible for what may be diagnosed in conventional medicine as cancer. This would seem to underline a possible connection between the two diseases.

Case one

A girl of 4 years of age came for treatment following 8 months conventional treatment of a tubercular gland. She had a nasty keloid scar on the left side of her neck where the skin had been wide open and had wept dark green pus for six months. Her mother was very distressed and said since the treatment she felt she had 'lost' her daughter, as her temperament and behaviour was so changed after it. She hated to try anything new or go anywhere unfamiliar. She was very aggressive towards her mother, slapping her and finding fault with what she did. The mother would have to offer 3 or 4 cups and be shouted at until she found the 'right' one.

Her teeth and bones had become weakened. She had to have many cavities filled and had recently suffered a greenstick fracture of the arm. Her appetite and sleep were poor. Her stools were loose and she had a lot of flatus with them. She had frequent bouts of diarrhoea and vomiting with high temperatures and a rash on her stomach, these lasted three days and left her shaking with thirst from dehydration. The girl said very little during the consultation except for twice saying that she was afraid of birds.

She was given Calc arsenicosum 30c. She improved steadily over the following months and repeated the remedy when symptoms returned or stopped improving. In less than one year she was back to normal.

Sarcoidosis

This is a multiple system, inflammatory disease that has many characteristics in common with tuberculosis. When I was at medical school and studying respiratory diseases, I always felt that they were the same disease but one had bacteria and the other did not. I now find that energetically this is the case.

There are collections of inflammatory tissue that are most often in the lungs, but may collect in any organ. The cause is unknown in conventional medicine. It mainly affects young people and is more common in women. It occurs in the UK at the rate of 19 cases per 100,000. It is more severe in African Americans than in Caucasians.

Symptoms

Sarcoidosis may affect many organs and the clinical picture is dependent upon the exact sites involved. The lungs are a common site. The symptoms are similar to those of tuberculosis and may include tiredness, weight loss, lymphatic gland enlargement and fever. There will be a cough with or without sputum. A dull ache in the chest may be present.

In 10 per cent of cases the skin is involved with the occurrence of erythema nodosum. This is the appearance of painful lumps on the shins. They fade to a bruised appearance over several weeks. Other causes of erythema nodosum include sulphonamide antibiotics, oral contraceptives, inflammatory bowel disease and streptococcal infections. Other skin problems in sarcoidosis include chilblain-like areas and nodules.

Around one quarter of people develop an anterior uveitis. Conjunctivitis may also occur in people with sarcoidosis. The eyes may be dry due to decreased tear production. The central nervous system is involved in only about 2 per cent of cases but the effects, weakness, tingling and numbness, can be severe.

Investigations

Chest x-ray is the usual method of diagnosis. Lung biopsy may be obtained via bronchoscopy. Lung function tests reveal decreases in function.

Treatment

Corticosteroids may be given especially if the symptoms are severe or vital tissue such as the eyes or nervous system are affected. Certainly these drugs will be used if there is no spontaneous improvement some 6 months after diagnosis. This is despite the fact that '...no controlled trials that have proved the efficacy of such treatment, it is difficult to withhold corticosteroids when there is continuing deterioration of the disease'.[17] Prednisolone is given at the rate of 30 mg daily for 6 weeks then 15 mg on holistic days for 6-12 months. Otherwise there is little which can be offered conventionally. In some cases, there is resolution of the disease particularly in those with only localised lung disease. Recovery occurs in 60 per cent of the mildest cases but only 30 per cent of cases where there is more widespread lung involvement.

Holistic management

This is a severe condition, which would benefit from a multiple approach similar to that taken with the treatment of cancer – please see Chapter 6 for details. In terms of Chinese medicine, it usually corresponds to the same patterns as described under tuberculosis. Corticosteroids may help the symptoms in the short-term but eventually the person's health will be worse as the medication erodes the vital energy.

Case one

A man of 40 years came for treatment after being diagnosed with sarcoidosis. His main symptoms were a chronic daily cough with yellowish or greenish sputum. He would wheeze regularly, his energy was low and he tired easily. He was having check-ups every 6 months at the hospital and although they had suggested that he might need corticosteroids in the future he was currently not on medication. I made a diagnosis of Phlegm-heat in the Lungs with underlying Lung Qi Deficiency and Kidney Yang Deficiency. His illness had come on some 6 months after an emotional shock and it was clear that he was still feeling the effects of this.

I treated him with acupuncture and Chinese medicine and within two months his cough was much better, his energy had improved and his wheezing was much less. I treated him for over a year and he continued to improve. The following Spring he had an exacerbation with increased cough, low energy and lots of phlegm. This coincided with the anniversary of the original emotional shock some 5 years previously. The hospital put him under a lot of pressure to take corticosteroids and also chloroquine. He declined to take them mainly because he was concerned about the risk of side-effects. His treatment continued and he began to improve again. He is now well with no cough, occasional phlegm and his energy is much better.

Bronchiectasis

This is an unusual condition of chronic infection in the lungs where there is persistent dilatation of the airways. It is rare nowadays. It begins with an obstruction to an airway that causes secretions to collect in the air passages. Infection supervenes and the inflammatory and infective process leads to widening of the bronchioles and smaller bronchi. Usually a small segment of lung tissue is involved distal to the obstruction although in extreme cases there can be most of the lung is affected. The presence of large amounts of infected material in the lungs leads to the classic symptoms of this condition.

It usually occurs after an acute childhood respiratory infection, which is why there is emphasis placed on the prevention of whooping cough. Obstruction of an airway, e.g. by peanuts or other inhaled object, carcinoma, pulmonary tuberculosis and the thickened secretions of cystic fibrosis can lead to distal infection, which becomes chronic unless the obstruction is relieved.

Symptoms

The main feature is of copious amounts of sputum. This is coughed up each day and amounts to several cupfuls. The sputum is yellow or green in acute attacks in mild cases. There is offensive breath. Haemoptysis (blood in the sputum) can occur as the infective process erodes into blood vessels. Breathlessness, cyanosis and finger clubbing are seen in severe cases.

Investigations

Chest X-rays and CT scan are widely used in diagnosis. Bronchography is rarely performed nowadays. Sputum culture reveals any infecting bacteria. Sinus X-rays reveal evidence of sinusitis in around one third of people. Serum immunoglobulins are done as 10 per cent have evidence of immune deficiency. Sweat electrolytes are determined if cystic fibrosis is suspected.

Treatment

Daily physiotherapy using postural drainage is the main measure utilised by conventional medicine. It is essential to clear sputum out of the chest and antibiotics are administered for acute exacerbations. Bronchodilators are useful in some people and inhaled or oral corticosteroids are believed to slow the progression of the disease. Surgery may be an option if the area of bronchiectasis is clearly defined and small although this is rare.

Holistic management

This is a chronic infective condition where there are large amounts of infected material in the lungs. There are problems of general debility as well as the issue of lung symptoms. Any measure, which will lead to a reduction in the amount of infected sputum, is important. Here postural drainage is useful and should be continued regularly. A diet that lessens mucus production will also help. Specific therapy, such as tonifying breathing exercises, will help clear and strengthen the lungs. You would expect cases such as these for a considerable length of time and 'cure' may not be something to realistically expect. However, there is a lot that can be done especially in the area of self-help with regard to diet, exercise and breathing. By helping the general health the infective area should become less active and acute flare-ups (where infection 'spills over' into other areas of the lung) should be less frequent.

WHEEZING DISEASES

Introduction

Wheezing is a specific musical sound produced by the small airways of the lung when they are narrowed. This narrowing may be:

- the result of spasm of the muscle surrounding the airways
- mucus partially obstructing the airways
- disease that damages the lung tissue.

Wheezing may be diagnosed as asthma but this is merely one possibility so I have chosen to discuss the three diseases of asthma, chronic bronchitis and emphysema together with ideas gathered from holistic medicine. You will then have a clear idea of the common patterns of chest disease characterised by wheezing and how they can be differentiated. I prefer to differentiate asthma and the other wheezing diseases according to their clinical appearances. Therefore, the descriptions I give below may not completely match those given in conventional textbooks.

Asthma

This is common and becoming more so with the general deterioration in the immune system and the increasing levels of atmospheric pollution. It is uncommon in 'developing' countries. In the UK some 10-15 per cent of people between 10 and 20 years are affected with a total number of cases of over 2 million, 1 in 10 of these being children. The disease consumes 8 per cent of the NHS drug budget. Asthma may be severe and can kill although it was rarely fatal before 1900. It affects some 3-5 per cent of the US population (14-15 million people) including almost 7 per cent of those under 18 years of age. In 1990, asthma cost $6 billion in the US. There are around 3 deaths per 100,000 cases in some countries now and the mortality rate is increasing. In the US in 1982 there were 13.4 death per million population and 18.8 per million in 1991. This increase in death rates has been more marked in other countries including the UK, Canada, Germany and Australia. There have been many suggested causes for this increasing death rate but a persistent source of discussion is the use of beta-agonist inhalers. These are discussed fully below.

Asthma is characterised by episodic attacks of reversible wheezing and breathlessness. The key term here is 'reversible'. The airways of the lungs are constricted by muscular spasm – bronchospasm – and this can come and go. The transient nature of the spasm and its response to bronchodilators accounts for the reversibility.

The disease is divided conventionally into extrinsic and intrinsic types. Extrinsic asthma is usually first seen in childhood and there is often a family history of allergies. This occurs in the so-called atopic type of individual. The person may also have other conditions such as eczema, hay fever or migraine. Ninety per cent of people have positive skin tests to inhaled allergens. The intrinsic type is seen in adulthood and there is not such an emphasis on allergy either in the family or personal history. This type has more in common with the clinical picture that I describe under chronic bronchitis. Overall, there are more children affected with asthma than adults and it occurs more commonly in males than females.

Symptoms

There is tightness in the chest, which develops before the wheezing. The difficulty with respiration and wheezing is always described in conventional texts as being worse on expiration. In fact clinical practice shows that it depends upon the individual and expiration *or* inspiration may be the most troublesome. As the wheezing develops there is breathlessness. The severity of attacks varies from mild episodes (only wheezing) to severe episodes with breathlessness.

A cough is common. It is usually dry and worse at night. A nocturnal cough may be the first indication of asthma. Any sputum produced is scanty and white but may be yellowish. The yellowish appearance is almost always due to allergy, not infection. Eosinophils, the white blood cells produced in allergic situations, impart a yellow colour to discharges.

There is a rapid pulse, which can be quite high. At a level of 120 per minute it indicates a severe attack and at 140 per minute a life-threatening situation.

Attacks are episodic and will occur at intervals dependent on the particular person and the presence or absence of precipitating factors. Acute attacks of wheezing can be precipitated by several factors including allergens,[18] exercise, emotion, dust, fumes, cold environment, respiratory infection and, importantly, drugs particularly aspirin, non-steroidal anti-inflammatory drugs, betablockers,[19] acetylcysteine,[20] betahistine and the female sex hormones (found in oral contraception and hormone replacement therapy). Tranquillisers, sleeping tablets and morphine derivatives including codeine may suppress respiration to a dangerous degree in people with asthma and should not be used.

At the end of an attack more sputum may be produced when the bronchospasm releases. It may take the appearance of 'casts' – mucus plugs that have taken on the outline of the bronchiolar wall.

Emotional symptoms are the norm in attacks of asthma with anxiety and fear (particularly of suffocation). People may feel that they are taking their last breath.

Investigations

Chest X-ray is a common first test and is unremarkable except for showing hyperinflation of the lungs. Lung function tests can show the amount of bronchospasm present in a quantitative way. An easy test is the peak flow meter, which measures the force of expiration. This may be used to monitor progress during treatment. More complex lung function tests may also be done. It is preferable to decide upon treatment on the basis of symptoms and use such tests as a guide. Medical treatments such as corticosteroids may be given solely on the basis of an investigation revealing reduced airflow even with no or minimal symptoms.

Skin hypersensitivity tests are performed in cases of suspected allergy. These are notably unreliable since a positive response on the skin has a poor correlation to respiratory symptoms. A white cell count may reveal a raised eosinophil count.

Treatment

The main aim in conventional medicine is to prevent wheezing and to minimise long-term lung damage. Medical practitioners are keen to use treatments regularly and long-term in an attempt to achieve this result. Corticosteroids are increasingly likely to be used as a first choice even in children.

Precipitating factors (if known) are avoided and exercise is helpful to strengthen the lungs.[21] Physiotherapy and breathing exercises are underused in the context of general practice.

Allergic cases may be given courses of desensitising injections – see Page 125. They are more hazardous in cases of asthma because of the risk of precipitating a severe attack. Deaths have occurred due to overwhelming allergic reaction – anaphylaxis.

Treatment (mildest to strongest)	Comments
Sodium cromoglycate	This is taken as an inhaler three or four times daily. Its stabilises the membrane of the mast cell and stops the release of histamine in an allergic reaction. It is intended to prevent wheezing in the presence of an allergic stimulant but it can also relieve wheezing once it has begun
Bronchodilators • inhaled • nebulised • oral	There are several bronchodilators on the market with similar adrenaline-like effects. They are moderately effective as dilators of bronchi but have problems with cardiac effects such as tremor and rapid pulse and the lungs start to rely on the stimulant effect. It is generally better if people take it when necessary and not 'just in case'
Corticosteroid • inhaled • oral • injected	Corticosteroids are used at diagnosis in most cases these days. They are administered orally in severe cases or inhaled in less severe cases. The inhaled form will certainly have fewer side-effects than the oral form but it is still suppressive and you will need to take the same general approach to corticosteroids as outlined on Page 180

Table 8.12: Treatment of asthma

People with a severe attack of asthma will be admitted to hospital. They will be given oxygen as well as intravenous bronchodilators and corticosteroids. Bronchodilators may also be given in nebulised (i.e. fine spray) form. In relatively severe cases these may be prescribed for home administration.

Antibiotics are invariably prescribed in an acute flare-up of asthma, despite the fact that there is rarely evidence of bacterial infection. In my days as a hospital doctor, I had the opportunity to work for 6 months on an asthma ward. We never used antibiotics in an acute flare-up and they were considered to be unnecessary. The correct management, conventionally, is to use a combination of bronchodilators and corticosteroids.

Chronic bronchitis

The formal definition is of a daily cough, productive of sputum for 3 months a year, for at least 2 years. It leads to around 30,000 deaths per annum in the UK. Smoking and air pollution may lead to the accumulation of mucus in the lungs and are linked to chronic bronchitis. Recurrent chest infections are also a factor in people with chronic bronchitis.

Symptoms

In the early stages, it is merely a morning cough with sputum, as is seen in many smokers. Breathlessness with wheezing develops as the lung is increasingly affected. The cause of wheezing here is mucus collections, spasm of bronchi and destruction of lung tissue by the inflammatory process. The key feature to distinguish this situation from asthma is that in chronic bronchitis the wheezing is usually more constant and bronchodilators are of variable benefit.

The sputum is usually white but, typically, there are episodes of yellow sputum with perhaps increased breathlessness and cough. Haemoptysis is an occasional associated symptom. This may occur due to a rupture of small blood vessels as the coughing damages them. It usually takes place during an acute exacerbation of the chronic condition. Such an event is more common in the winter months or in cold, damp weather. It is more likely to occur if the person smokes or if the atmosphere is smoky or dusty. Each acute infective episode will further damage the lungs and so there is a gradual deterioration in lung function. The end result is either respiratory failure or cardiac insufficiency.

The term 'blue bloater' has been used to describe people with chronic bronchitis. They may be overweight and as the disease progresses there is the development of oedema. Due to the interference with pulmonary function, there may be blueness (cyanosis). The general appearance is of dampness, mucus, sluggishness and coldness.

Investigations

The chest X-ray in this condition is usually normal and so is only of use if the existence of another condition, such as cancer, pneumonia or lung collapse, is suspected. Lung function tests in an acute episode are often abnormal and ECG examination will reveal the presence of right ventricular enlargement.[22] Sputum may be taken for culture of the infective organism and its sensitivity to antibiotics determined.

Treatment

This disease is considered to be incurable in conventional medicine and so people are advised to minimise the rate and the amount of lung damage. The most important advice is to stop smoking and be in clean air whenever possible. Antibiotics are used for acute exacerbations. The long-term management includes the use of bronchodilators if wheezing is a major problem, although they are of variable effectiveness. Physiotherapy to the chest aids the removal of secretions and breathing exercises strengthening the chest are of definite benefit.

Emphysema

Emphysema is the term used to describe abnormal distension of tissues with air. This can occur in several sites but here we are talking about pulmonary emphysema. The distension occurs in the alveoli and there is gradual destruction of lung tissue leading to the development of enlarged air spaces – Figure 8.1. The distension occurs because the lungs are dry and lacking in moisture.

Smoking is the commonest association. The disease is to be feared by smokers because of its severely debilitating effects. The occupations that may lead to emphysema are those involving dust such as coal mining, quarry workers and those involving heat (e.g. glass blowing).

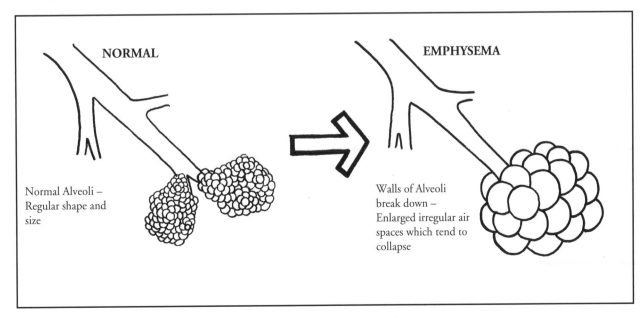

Figure 8.1: Emphysema and changes in lung stucture

Symptoms

The main symptom is breathlessness. It can be severe and is responsible for severely restricting activity. The process of alveolar wall destruction described above leads to a great reduction in the area of lung tissue available for gaseous exchange. There is associated wheezing which in this case is due to destruction of lung tissue and so tends to be constant.

Upper chest breathing develops and a barrel-chested deformity is seen. Accessory muscles of respiration are used, e.g. sternocleidomastoid, intercostals. The expiratory breath is done through pursed lips and leads to the description of such people as 'pink puffers'. There are rapid, puffing respirations and the person is usually pink and thin. People do not become cyanosed as in chronic bronchitis since the rapid respirations washes carbon dioxide out of the blood.

Complications

Complication	Symptoms to look for
Right ventricular insufficiency	Peripheral oedema, palpitations, nausea, anorexia
Pneumothorax	Sudden worsening of breathlessness, pain and reduced movement on the affected side of the chest
Respiratory failure	Increasing breathlessness, confusion

Table 8.13: Complications of emphysema

Treatment

Emphysema is seen as being progressive and incurable in conventional medicine. Oxygen is administered if there is severe breathlessness and disability. An acute infective situation is treated with antibiotics. Smoking is advised against as this only leads to further lung tissue destruction. Breathing exercises are useful to try to improve the function of the lung. Bronchodilators may be given in some cases but there is little relief as the narrowing of the airways is due to a destructive process.

Symptom	Asthma	Chronic bronchitis	Emphysema
Wheeze	Episodic	Variable	Permanent
Cough	Dry, scanty sputum	Profuse sputum	Dry
Body type	Children, usually thin	Overweight, 'blue bloater'	Thin, 'pink puffer'
Bronchodilator response	Yes	Variable	No

Table 8.14: Comparison of the diseases of asthma, chronic bronchitis and emphysema

Holistic management

It is recognised in conventional circles that in cases of asthma, fresh air is better treatment than drugs with the former improving lung function by 30 per cent and latter by only 5-10 per cent. Fresh air also reduces drug use by 60 per cent. Despite this, most people will be taking some form of medication.

Whenever you see a person with wheezing it is important to come to an energetic diagnosis. In Chinese medical texts, the term asthma is used to describe all conditions characterised by difficult breathing and so the meaning of the term is not the same as its use in conventional terms. In energetic medicine, it is clear that asthma is made up of several discrete entities. One key question is whether the wheezing and breathlessness is worse for expiration or inspiration. Expiratory difficulty indicates a disharmony in the Lungs and inspiratory difficulty is due to a Kidney disharmony.[23]

Conventionally, descriptions of asthma, chronic bronchitis and emphysema are related to several syndromes in Chinese medicine. Asthma commonly corresponds to Lung Qi Deficiency and Kidney Not Grasping Lung Qi. The Chinese medical counterpart of chronic bronchitis is commonly Spleen Qi Deficiency with Damp-cold Accumulation and Lung Qi Deficiency. Emphysema usually corresponds to Lung and Kidney Yin Deficiency.

Breathing exercises are extremely helpful for strengthening the chest and lungs and should be given to every person to practice at home.[24] Gentle exercise such as swimming, walking or cycling is very beneficial and can be recommended. With these measures many people can benefit and you will probably find that the dose of drugs can be reduced or stopped completely.

Bronchodilators are related to the chemical ephedrine. This is related to adrenaline and shares many effects. These latter two are grouped together as sympathomimetics. Ephedrine is derived from the herb ephedra (Chinese – *Ma Huang*). In Chinese medicine, this herb is always used in a balanced formula with other herbs to release the exterior and induce a sweat. It is warm in nature and is used in External Pathogenic Invasion, which affects the Lungs.

Its action is to disperse Lung Qi and relieve symptoms such as cough and wheezing. In an acute situation this may be the appropriate treatment. In conventional medicine, it is used in a purified form, in high dosage (compared to herbal dosages), for chronic conditions and for many years. The results of this will be weakness of Lung Qi, Lung Yin Deficiency and ultimately Kidney Yin Deficiency. This explains the common observation that bronchodilators are ineffective for emphysema as it is already a case of Lung Yin Deficiency.

Asthma is a potentially serious condition depending upon the severity of the attack. In the 1950s, adrenaline itself was used to treat asthma but it was discovered that the mortality rate from asthma was related to the number of prescriptions of adrenaline inhalers. They were withdrawn from the market and the drugs used now are milder in their action. There are still some doubts about their safety however and fenoterol, a common bronchodilator, was banned in Australia and New Zealand in 1990.[25] It is still widely used in the UK and USA. Salbutamol is a related drug as is the recently approved salmeterol. This latter drug is under suspicion as several patients have been found dead holding their inhalers. Several studies have confirmed the risk of dying from asthma if using beta agonist inhalers. These include Sears *et al* who found that patients did better if they took their inhaler when necessary rather than regularly. Spitzer *et al* in Canada found an increased risk of death in those who used fenoterol or albuterol. Studies in Japan[26] have confirmed this.

It would seem clear, from knowledge of Chinese medicine, that long-term use of such drugs will deplete the Lung Qi to such a point that it may collapse. This is particularly likely to happen when a sudden strain is placed on the person such as stress, sudden allergic load or an infection. As the Lung and Heart Qi are closely related in the chest, any drug that depletes Lung Qi is also likely to deplete Heart Qi. Certainly bronchodilator use causes palpitations in some people. They are strong drugs and need to be approached with care.

Corticosteroids are widely used for asthma. They are being prescribed as a first line treatment in increasing numbers. I discuss their energetic actions more fully on Page 180. They are hot in nature, stimulate Lung Qi strongly and dry Phlegm and Dampness in the Lungs. Sudden withdrawal must be avoided as the Lung Qi is in danger of collapsing. Gradual withdrawal whilst holistic treatment is progressing is definitely possible.

In chronic bronchitis, there is a collection of mucus in the lungs worse in damp and cold weather. Smoking heats and dries the lungs thereby helping to relieve the symptoms of cough and phlegm. Smoking may be the *result* rather than the *cause* of the underlying imbalance. This may be the reason why smoking is associated with this disease. If you are cold and wet (mucus) then smoking, which is heating, dries up the secretions and warms the energy.

Case one
A boy of 9 years came for treatment of his asthma. It had started with a cough and occasionally wheezing when he was 4 years old. He had a regular cough with no phlegm. He was generally well. I made a diagnosis of Spleen and Lung Deficiency and treated him with acupuncture and Chinese herbs. His medication was a corticosteroid inhaler (taken regularly twice daily) and a bronchodilator (taken when he needed it for cough or wheezing). He responded well to treatment which is a frequent observation with children. He was able to reduce his corticosteroid inhaler after one month of treatment and was off all inhalers after 3 months. He remains well 2 years later.

Case two
A woman of 54 years came for treatment of her asthma. She had developed this some years previously and her main symptoms were breathlessness, wheezing and cough with a little white mucus in the mornings. She was on corticosteroid and bronchodilator inhalers (regularly four times daily). She had just finished a course of oral corticosteroids some 2 months previously for a flare-up in her symptoms. I made a diagnosis of Kidney Yang Deficiency and Kidney not Grasping Lung Qi. I treated her with acupuncture and Chinese herbs. She made a remarkable recovery and in a short period of time felt much better, her wheezing and cough eased and she felt much better in herself. She was able to reduce her medication gradually and had stopped all inhalers within 3 months. She remains well 5 years later.

Case three
A woman of 63 years came for treatment of her asthma. Her main symptom was cough with white phlegm. She had had four courses of antibiotics in the 3 months before attending the clinic. Her chest symptoms always eased off slightly after an antibiotic and then would return. She had had these symptoms for the past 2 years since pneumonia, which had followed an attack of influenza. I made a diagnosis of Lung Qi Deficiency, Spleen Qi Deficiency with Damp-cold Accumulation. I treated her with acupuncture and Chinese herbs.

After the first treatment, she noticed that a lot of phlegm was produced but this left her breathing easier and her cough was less severe. One of the difficulties of recurrent antibiotic usage is that phlegm remains in the lung to interfere with the breathing and leads to flare-ups from time to time. With subsequent treatments, her energy continued to improve, her energy was stronger and her cough settled.

Case four

A man of 72 years came for treatment of his emphysema. He had been a smoker for 55 years and was now smoking only five cigarettes daily. He suffered with breathlessness to the point where he would have to rest going upstairs, aching in his left lower chest and wheezing on expiration. He had no cough or phlegm. His bowels were sluggish and he would pass stools of small pieces, like 'rabbit droppings'. He would get headaches whenever he was breathless and after physical exertion. His medication was:

- lisinopril 15 mg daily
- salmeterol and ipratropium nebuliser daily
- salbutamol inhaler 2 puffs twice daily
- oxitropium inhaler 2 puffs twice daily
- beclomethasone inhaler inhaler 100 mcg 2 puffs twice daily
- paracetamol 500 mg with codeine 30 mg 2 four times daily
- alprazolam 0.25 mg twice daily
- theophylline 200 mg twice daily

He had recently finished a course of corticosteroids. I made a diagnosis of Lung Qi and Yin Deficiency with underlying Kidney Yin Deficiency. I treated him with acupuncture and Chinese herbal medicine. In such a case of long-standing illness with fairly severe symptoms complicated with many conventional medications, it is important to proceed slowly and carefully. Sudden changes in medication are to be avoided and as the patient improves small adjustments can be made. The first priority however is to treat appropriately and wait for improvement to occur.

After one treatment his bowels improved, he felt better in himself and he had had no headaches. Over the course of the next few weeks and months he continued to improve and his chest felt generally easier. He was less breathless and wheezy. He had one episode in hospital for a chest infection when the weather suddenly became cold and damp but he resumed treatment with me when he returned home. He had a trip abroad during this time and he was surprised, as were his conventional doctors, that he was well enough to go and was fine whilst he was away. His treatment is continuing.

Case five

A boy aged 8 came for treatment. He had used inhalers for his asthma since the age of 6. He had been taking beclomethasone 50 mcg (two puffs – morning and evening) and salbutamol syrup 3 times daily. He had suffered from occasional accelerated heart rate whilst on the inhalers and didn't like taking them. A combination of garlic perles and a holiday by the sea had recently helped him to come off them. He still had an unproductive cough that came on one hour after going to bed (at about 9pm). When the cough was very bad he would vomit and continued to vomit without any relief until he was retching bile.

Ipecac is well known as the remedy for incessant vomiting without relief and vomiting related to coughing. There was confidence that Ipecac would be a good prescription, which it was, up to a point. Whenever the boy had an acute episode it was relieved very quickly by Ipecac 30c, but overall he did not improve much and worsened as the winter came. The potency was changed to a 200c, but this made little difference.

At this stage the case was reviewed and although details of the family medical history had been taken, it was checked again with his mother. She was asked if there was a possibility of anyone having suffered from TB. She gasped and pointed to a huge scar on her own neck. 'How did I forget that?' she said. At the age of five she had had a tubercular gland removed from her neck and had been in hospital for some time. He was prescribed Tuberculinum 30c and thereafter the results were infinitely better. The cough became less bothersome and phlegmy and would only last a few minutes and he was in very good form. His mother said: 'It seems to have really finished it off'.

CANCER OF THE LUNG

This is the most common primary malignant tumour and a major cause of disease. Each year in the UK there are 35000 deaths from lung cancer. It was rare before the 1940s. Over half of cases will occur in people over the age of 65 years. Over three times more men are affected than women.

There has been a well-documented connection made between cigarette smoking and lung cancer. In fact, 1 in 10 smokers

The Clinical Medicine Guide *A Holistic Perspective*

develop this disease and smoking is more likely to lead to heart disease and stroke. Certainly, continual irritation of the lungs with cigarette smoke and air pollution are risk factors. Other factors include radiation, contact with chromium, arsenic, asbestos and petroleum products.

Secondary cancers can also develop in the lung particularly with cancer of the kidney, prostate, breast, bone, gastrointestinal tract, cervix and ovary. They are usually multiple in number.

Symptoms

There is almost always a history of smoking. The key features indicating cancer are short history and progression of symptoms. In the case of lung cancer, there is a persistent cough, haemoptysis on several occasions and the recent development of other symptoms such as breathlessness. Pain is less common than usually believed although around 1 in 4 people have pain at diagnosis. Pain due to cancer is invariably dull and constant in nature. It does not change with respiration or movement. If pain is due to the invasion of bone by secondary deposits it can be severe. There may be symptoms of a general nature such as anorexia and weight loss.

There may well be signs of the spread of the disease at the time of diagnosis. These include lymphatic gland enlargement in the supraclavicular region on the affected side, hoarse voice[27] and distended veins in the neck and chest.[28] Secondaries in the liver, bone, brain and skin may give rise to pain, nodules or symptoms specific to that organ.

Diagnosis

Chest X-ray will show the tumour in most cases (although it fails to pick up cancers less than 1-2 cm in size). CT scans reveal more detail and are useful in identifying the stage of the cancer as are MRI scans. Sputum examination may reveal the presence of cancerous cells. Fibreoptic bronchoscopy may be used to obtain sputum samples for cytology and to take biopsy material. Transthoracic fine-needle aspiration biopsy is used to obtain biopsies were the bronchoscope cannot reach. This is associated with a pneumothorax in 25 per cent of cases and haemoptysis in 5 per cent.

Treatment

It is said conventionally, that surgery 'offers the only cure'. Certainly, only 15-20 per cent of cases at the time of diagnosis are operable, as it has spread too far by that time. Of these who have surgery, only 30 per cent survive 5 years.[29] Over 90 per cent of people diagnosed with lung cancer die within 5 years. Radiotherapy and chemotherapy are generally considered to be merely palliative. Radiation is given in high doses to those who are relatively fit and in cases of slow growing squamous cancer. Radiation pneumonitis (cough and breathlessness) occurs in 15 per cent. Chemotherapy is most helpful in cases of small-cell (oat cell) cancer where survival rates are now 10 months rather than 2 months.

Holistic management

The issues involved for the holistic practitioner in the treatment of cancer are discussed on Page 84.

PNEUMOTHORAX

This is the presence of air in the pleural cavity. The resultant clinical appearances are due to compression of the lung on the affected side, with collapse of the lung occurring in severe cases. The air is the result of a connection either with the outside (as via a perforating chest injury) or with the internal air spaces of the lung. The latter can be the result of an injury or due to rupture of air spaces (as in emphysema or asthma). I mention this condition, not because it is common (it is in fact quite unusual) but because of the importance to acupuncturists.

Spontaneous pneumothorax can occur in young people under 40 years. It is six times more likely in men than women They are usually tall and thin. Otherwise, pneumothorax can be as a complication of lung diseases (such as asthma, emphysema, tuberculosis, and pneumoconiosis) or the result of a perforation injury (such as by fractured rib, knifing or the insertion of a needle may pierce the lung.

Symptoms

There is the sudden appearance of pain in the side of the chest that is affected and breathlessness. If the pneumothorax is large, there is pallor and rapid pulse. The severity of the clinical picture is variable depending upon the amount of air in the pleural cavity and the general condition of the person. Those with pre-existing lung disease may be severely affected and death can occur. There may be breathlessness and in severe cases, cyanosis and confusion. Occasionally the air in the pleural cavity can continue to build up through a valve-like mechanism. Such a *tension* pneumothorax is characterised by increasing breathlessness and more discomfort. These cases are a medical emergency.

Diagnosis

Chest X-ray confirms the diagnosis.

139

Treatment

The air is drained from the pleural cavity by means of a tube inserted through an intercostal space. This necessitates a stay in hospital of several days.

Holistic management

The main issue for holistic practitioners is for acupuncturists. They must be aware of back and chest points that overlie the lungs – Table 8.15. This is particularly important in thin people and those with hyperinflated lungs (such as occurs in emphysema and asthma). It is impossible to perforate the lung if a needle is inserted correctly in terms of depth and angle.

Point number	Point name	Point number	Point name
Lung 1	Zhongfu	Urinary Bladder 11	Dashu
Lung 2	Yunmen	Urinary Bladder 12	Fengmen
Large Intestine 16	Jugu	Urinary Bladder 13	Feishu
Large Intestine 17	Tianding	Urinary Bladder 14	Jueyinshu
Stomach 12	Quepen	Urinary Bladder 15	Xinshu
Stomach 13	Qihu	Urinary Bladder 16	Dushu
Stomach 14	Kufang	Urinary Bladder 17	Geshu
Stomach 15	Wuyi	Urinary Bladder 18	Ganshu
Stomach 16	Yingchuang	Urinary Bladder 43	Gaohuangshu
Stomach 18	Rugen	Urinary Bladder 44	Shentang
Spleen 17	Shidou	Urinary Bladder 45	Yixi
Spleen 18	Tianxi	Urinary Bladder 46	Geguan
Spleen 19	Xiongxiang	Urinary Bladder 47	Hunmen
Spleen 20	Zhourong	Urinary Bladder 48	Yanggang
Spleen 21	Dabao	Pericardium 1	Tianchi
Heart 1	Jiquan	San Jiao 15	Tianliao
Small Intestine 14	Jianwaishu	Gall Bladder 21	Jianjing
Small Intestine 15	Jianzhongshu	Gall Bladder 22	Yuanye
Kidney 22	Bulang	Gall Bladder 23	Zhejin
Kidney 23	Shenfeng	Gall Bladder 24	Riyue
Kidney 24	Lingxu	Liver 14	Qimen
Kidney 25	Shencang	Extra point M-BW-1	Dingchuan
Kidney 26	Yuzhong	Extra point N-CA-8	Ganshi
Kidney 27	Shufu	Extra point M-BW-12	Yishu
		Extra point N-CA-7	Xiongdaji

Table 8.15: Acupuncture points overlying or adjacent to lung tissue

PLEURISY

This is inflammation of the pleura. The two pleural layers rub together and this leads to the classic pain of this condition. With a stethoscope you can hear a coarse crackle – the pleural rub.

The inflammation may be a localised affection of the pleura or part of a wider problem, e.g. pneumonia or pulmonary embolism. The main thing to consider is whether the pleurisy has occurred following an upper respiratory tract infection. These cases are relatively straightforward. More serious situations are present if more severe respiratory symptoms are associated with it.

Symptoms
The primary feature of pleurisy is pain in the chest. This is sharp in nature and commonly felt in the axilla or around the scapula. It is worse for movement, coughing and respiration. There may be a low-grade fever and a dry cough. The differential diagnosis of chest pain is on Page 103. The main differentiation is from musculoskeletal conditions.

Complications

Complication	Symptoms to look for
Pleural effusion – fluid in the pleural cavity	Pain disappears but there is the development of restricted breathing, breathlessness
Empyema – pus in the pleural cavity	Similar symptoms to the above but with fever, malaise

Table 8.16: Complications of pleurisy

Treatment
Antibiotics are invariably given although the majority of associated infections are viral. Rest and painkillers are advised. Investigations such as chest X-ray and tomography will be performed if a serious underlying cause is suspected.

Holistic management
In most cases this condition is mild and self-limiting. There is more cause for concern if breathlessness or haemoptysis is present.

PULMONARY EMBOLISM

This is an obstruction of the pulmonary artery by a clot, which has usually become detached from a deep vein thrombosis.

Symptoms
These are of sudden development due to the underlying process. If a large artery is obstructed then sudden death may result. In milder cases there is appearance of breathlessness, pleuritic chest pain and haemoptysis. There may also be fever. Most people are acutely ill and require hospitalisation for pain relief.

Investigations
An ECG is normal in most cases apart from an increase in heart rate. In severe cases there may be tall P waves with evidence of enlargement of the right ventricle. A chest X-ray may be normal in the early stages but later shows, in severe cases, a wedge-shaped area of affected lung. More sophisticated techniques such as radioisotope scans and angiography will confirm the diagnosis. The diagnosis can usually be made, however, on the basis of the history.

Treatment
This is similar to that of deep venous thrombosis particularly with regard to anticoagulation.

Holistic management
The main issue for holistic practitioners is around the use of anticoagulants – see Page 96.

REVIEW OF SYMPTOMS

Cough
This is exceedingly common and many people suffer from it at some time or another. It may be such a feature of someone's life that they can deny a cough even when you hear it during the consultation. It will have passed out of awareness because it has been around for so long. Conventional medicine sees cough as important in terms of three factors:

1. *The degree of disturbance to the person*
If the disturbance is great then suppressants will be given for dry coughs and expectorants for a productive cough. There is little evidence to suggest that either are effective and certainly not more so than honey and lemon as a hot drink or a steam inhalation. This is the view of most respiratory specialists. Most proprietary cough medicines contain lots of sugar and suppressants are usually based on codeine or its derivatives. Codeine is methylmorphine and as such will produce addiction if taken for long periods and will also cause constipation and drowsiness. Expectorants usually contain anti-histamines and/or amphetamine-like compounds, e.g. ephedrine which dries mucus but can lead to agitation and insomnia. Suppression of any cough may be harmful as it is a natural defence mechanism aiming to discharge problems from the body although there is no fault with taking soothing, non-toxic substances. Honey is a lubricant and so will aid dry coughs. It is, however, mucus forming and should not be taken in large quantities if there is expectoration.

2. Presence or absence of bacterial infection

Any cough or sputum that seems to indicate a bacterial infection will be treated with antibiotics. If sputum is white (mucoid) no bacterial infection is considered to be present. If it is yellowish (mucopurulent) or greenish (purulent) bacterial infection is assumed. Conventionally, these drugs should not be given unless there is bacteriological evidence for infection but the routine is to give antibiotics on the supposed clinical evidence. The other reason for waiting for bacteriological evidence is that the wrong antibiotic may be prescribed. The organism responsible may be resistant to the particular drug prescribed and only laboratory investigation will reveal the correct drug to be taken.

This reflex attitude to the colour of the sputum leads to large quantities of antibiotics being prescribed during winter episodes of upper respiratory tract infection whether or not they are actually indicated. It is worth noting that green or yellow sputum can be seen in certain allergic disorders such as asthma where it is due to the presence of eosinophils and it cannot be differentiated on naked-eye appearances from sputum where bacteria are present.

In energetic terms the colour of the sputum is to do with the amount of Heat present. White means Cold, yellow means Heat and green indicates more Heat.

3. Presence of serious underlying disease

There are some people with cough who have severe pathology. These cases will be investigated with at least a chest X-ray.

Sputum

The colloquial term for this is catarrh or phlegm but you must always check with people what they mean by various terms. Medically, mucus describes the substance produced from the respiratory system and sputum refers to mucus that is coughed up. Conventionally, the distinction is of sputum that is white, yellow or green.

Mucoid sputum is white or colourless and is due to an overproduction of bronchial mucus. Purulent sputum is yellowish or greenish and may indicate a bacterial infection (see above). The consistency of sputum can be helpful in aiding the diagnostic process and should be enquired about.

Tendency to catch colds

This is a symptom that is not given much emphasis in conventional circles but is very important from the point of view of holistic medicine. It gives an indication of the effectiveness of the defensive system in warding off attack from the outside in general and the strength of the lungs specifically.

Haemoptysis

This is the appearance of blood in the sputum ranging from faint streaking to obvious blood. You should ensure the blood is of respiratory origin (bleeding gums, nose or mouth may lead to confusion).

The symptom of bleeding, wherever it occurs, should always be viewed seriously. It is sensible to consider making an assessment of the source of the bleeding. If the symptom is associated with an acute bronchitis in a young person then perhaps there is no cause to worry. However, the situation in a 55-year-old smoker who perhaps coughs blood on several occasions is a different proposition. In the case of haemoptysis, only 40 per cent of cases have a demonstrable cause in conventional medicine.

Chest pain

Dull, constant pain in the chest pain can be indicative of serious disease such as lung cancer. In general, pain of this type is seen in people with severe conditions where the energy is quite weak. In conventional terms it is often associated with cancer. It is more worrying to see pain of this type than sharper pain that changes in response to posture, respiration and so on. Chest pain is also discussed on Page 103.

Breathlessness

Breathing is a complex act and related to many areas of body and mind. Emotional disturbances are often reflected in changes in the breath. Some psychotherapeutic procedures, especially the newer bodywork therapies, utilise the breath to release emotional, mental and physical energies. The Hindu word *prana* may be translated as breath and is the ayurdevic equivalent of Qi in Chinese medicine. This translation indicates the link between these energies and the mind.

This area is accessible through some schools of psychotherapy and some religious traditions. Unskilful use of the breath by practitioners, particularly utilising hyperventilation, can lead to the release of emotional states, which can overwhelm the person. Such a catharsis can present powerful emotions into the person's conscious mind and lead to severe problems. Transformative practices are much gentler and allow people time to adjust to altered states.

Cyanosis

This indicates a severe situation unless it is the extremities in cold weather (poor circulation).

Wheeze

This is a high-pitched musical sound, which is heard during respiration. It may be present during inspiration, expiration or both. It is an indication of an obstruction to the airflow in the smaller airways of the lungs. The main point to consider is the degree of interference with respiratory function. Breathlessness is the key issue to take into account when presented with someone who is wheezing.

Stridor

This is obstruction of a major airway and is a crowing noise mainly heard during inspiration. It is seen in cases of obstruction (e.g. an inhaled object) and in some infectious disorders of childhood, e.g. whooping cough.

Finger clubbing

This is thickening at the base of the fingernails. It may also be seen in the toes. There is normally an angle between the nail and the finger at the nail bed. This disappears in finger clubbing. In extreme cases the end of the finger or toe becomes bulbous. It occurs in several diseases and including tuberculosis, bronchiectasis, lung abscess, empyema, lung cancer, congenital heart disease, liver cirrhosis and inflammatory bowel disease.

In terms of Chinese medicine, it is due to Phlegm, which collects in the ends of the digits as the flow of Qi is obstructed.

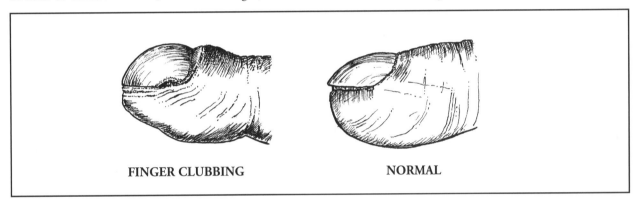

FINGER CLUBBING   **NORMAL**

Figure 8.2 Diagram of appearance of finger clubbing

HOW TO RECOGNISE SERIOUS CONDITIONS OF THE RESPIRATORY SYSTEM

Symptom	Cause for concern
Cough	Persistent With blood With breathlessness
Chest pain	Constant Dull
Breathlessness	Severe Acute Progressive With confusion With cyanosis Pulse rate > 120 per minute Paroxysmal attacks occurring at night
Haemoptysis	Recurrent Older person, Smoker
Sputum	Copious Green/yellow Blood stained Frothy
Wheezing	If accompanied by breathlessness (see above)
Tendency to catch colds	Not serious
Nasal discharge	After head injury
Blocked nose	Not serious
Sneezing	Not serious
Stridor	Always
Cyanosis	Central – tongue Peripheral – lips and extremities (unless due to cold)
Hoarseness	Persistent (more than three weeks)
Finger clubbing	Always

Table 8.17: How to recognise serious conditions in respiratory system disease

Diseases of the respiratory system are common in our society and the symptoms listed here are extremely common. It is important to know how to recognise if a symptom arises from a serious situation. You can use Table 8.17 as a guide to refer to when faced with a person who has one or more of these symptoms. I make no mention of disease labels in the column on the right, as I would not expect you to be able to diagnose conventionally. Seriousness can be assessed merely by reference to symptom pictures. However, you will be able to recognise that there are clinical appearances that would be diagnosed as a particular disease. For example, if you look at breathlessness and its seriousness, you will see that this is the appearance of a severe asthma attack.

SUMMARY

The lung is known as the 'tender organ' as it is vulnerable to attack by external climatic factors.

The respiratory system can be divided into an upper and lower part. The depth and rate of progression of symptoms is directly related to the state of the person's energy.

Many respiratory conditions are treated with antibiotics, which are overused and frequently unnecessary from a conventional viewpoint.

Chronic lung diseases are common, especially in cold, damp and polluted climates. Holistic medicine is an effective option for dealing with them.

In cases with mucus collections, it is useful to remember that this substance has emotional overtones. What I mean by this is that mucus is Yin, as are emotions. Emotional states may manifest as such or be held in the body. Mucus is a typical way in which they may be stored. An example of this is when people stop cigarette smoking. They may develop emotional discharges of vulnerability, weeping, feeling sensitive and so on or develop a cough with mucus. Such releases of suppressions may, therefore, present in several ways and it is important for the practitioner to recognise this.

---

[1] All organs that are capitalised, e.g. Blood, Lung, Kidney indicate that I mean the energetic view of that organ and not the narrowly defined physical structure of Western science.

[2] As is the Ayurvedic *prana* and the Tibetan *rlung.*

[3] Aspects relating to the Spleen are covered in detail in Chapter 13 – Gastrointestinal system.

[4] Aspects relating to the Large Intestine are covered in detail in Chapter 13 – Gastrointestinal system.

[5] As I discussed in Chapter 5 - Infectious Disease, the manifestation of symptoms and their sites depends upon the strength of the person's energy. In people, who have very strong energy they will not manifest even acute disease. They remain well whatever the situation or climate. This is rare! However, people who have very weak energy do not manifest acute disease as their energy is not strong enough to generate such symptoms. When they are ill, they develop a chronic illness. The art of medicine is to differentiate these two groups – at first sight they appear to be similar in that acute disease is rare or non-existent.

[6] Dangers of analgesics being sold as over-the-counter medication – *Geriatr Nephrol Urol* 1999;9(1):3-4.

Encouraging the use of other analgesics particularly in the elderly as they are particularly at risk of side-effects which include gastrointestinal tract haemorrhage, renal failure and worsening of cardiac insufficiency – *J Am Acad Orthop Surg* 1994;2(5):255-260.

Low dose aspirin (commonly used in people with cardiovascular disease) as a cause of continuing decreased renal function – *Arthritis Rheum* 2000;43(1):103-8. Nephrotic syndrome due to the use of diclofenac – *Wien Klin Wochenschr* 1999 111(13):523-4.

[7] The sympathomimetics are those chemicals which 'mimic' the sympathetic nervous system. Adrenaline and noradrenaline (epinephrine and norepinephrine in the US) are the main examples of this group but others include ephedrine, pseudoephedrine, phenylpropanolamine, phenylephrine. They are stimulatory in action and have related effects to other groups of drugs such as antidepressants, bronchodilators, appetite suppressants and amphetamines.

[8] The numbers of tonsillectomies performed have declined in recent years with a corresponding increase in the number of operations for grommet insertion to drain fluid in the middle ear – see Chapter 19 – Children's Health for more details.

[9] A review of tonsillectomy for recurrent throat infection. *British Journal of General Practice* 1998;48:1331-5.

[10] An organism present in birds, particularly parrots.

[11] The organism of Legionnaire's disease.

[12] The organism affecting people with severely depleted immune system such as those with AIDS or receiving immunosuppressive corticosteroid or cancer chemotherapy medication.

[13] Data extracted from *Medical Nemesis* by Ivan Illich (Penguin, 1991) and relates to New York.

[14] The Mantoux reaction is an intradermal injection of tuberculin protein. If there is a reaction, the person is considered to be positive. Those who are negative are given BCG whilst those who are positive are checked by chest X-ray. A common test which is based on the same principles but simpler to administer is the Tine test.

[15] Studies have shown that tuberculosis is more likely to occur in those people who have suffered a loss or bereavement recently. *Emotional Factors in Pulmonary Tuberculosis* by David M Kissen (London, 1958) and *Diseases of Civilisation* by Brian Inglis (Paladin, 1981).

[16] BCG is the Bacille Calmette-Guérin vaccination which has been given in the UK since 1954.

[17] *Clinical Medicine* Edited by Kumar and Clark 4th Edition (W B Saunders, 1998).

[18] Salbutamol bronchodilators can produce allergic wheezing attacks and deaths have occurred.

[19] Some betablockers are denoted as being cardioselective, that is, they are reputed not to affect the lungs. This is not true and it is dangerous for any person with a history of wheezing to take betablockers. Deaths have resulted from such a prescription.

[20] This is a constituent of cough medicines.

[21] One study showed that blowing up a balloon 10 times a day was as effective a treatment in the long-term as bronchodilators.

[22] In cases of chronic lung disease, there is increased strain on the right side of the heart which has to push blood through the diseased organ. This is the reason why respiratory disease is a cause of right-sided cardiac insufficiency.

[23] One of the energetic functions of the Kidney is to grasp Qi from the Lungs. If the Kidney cannot do this there will be respiratory symptoms such as wheezing, breathlessness and cough.

[24] Yoga exercises are particularly helpful. A double-blind study revealed that after yoga breathing exercises there was an increased resistance to allergic factors. *Lancet* 1990;335:1381-83.

Yoga breathing exercises have the effect of increasing lung function. *Indian J Physio Pharmacol* 1992;36(2):105-8.

Yoga breathing exercises led to a significant improvement in lung function, decreased symptoms and decreased drug requirements in children with asthma. This beneficial effect was present some 2 years later. *J Asthma* 1991;28(6):437-42.

[25] It has been suggested that the increasing illness and death rate associated with asthma may be related to the use of such drugs. They have an effect on opening up the airways but also have a suppressive anti-inflammatory mechanism in the lungs. This may have the effect of causing increased levels of inflammation in lung tissue. *Lancet* 1991;337:717-20.

Also see a discussion of the adverse effects of bronchodilators in asthma – *Br J Clin Pharmacol* 1992;33(2):129-38.

[26] *Lancet* 1998;351:1406-7.

[27] The recurrent laryngeal nerve dips into the chest and up again to supply the larynx. If the cancer presses on the nerve it can lead to a hoarse voice. The causes of some symptoms in conventional medicine require some detailed knowledge of anatomy or physiology. I have kept these to a minimum but I mention them for the sake of completion and to connect with conventional textbooks.

[28] Pressure on the superior vena cava, the main vein draining blood from the head and neck, may slow blood flow or prevent it. The appearance is of many distended veins over the chest wall and a congested appearance to the upper body.

[29] The use and meaning of 5 year survival rates by conventional medicine is interesting. They are usually seen as being the same as 'cure' in the conventional sense of the word. I treated a woman once who had a malignant melanoma diagnosed and removed surgically. She was well for 4 years and 11 months and then developed symptoms of secondaries. Another month and she would have been classified as a 'cure'. This is why you have to be very careful with statistical statements of survival and 'cure' rates. What is of over-riding importance is the quality of life of the person taking account of individual circumstances regarding life-style, emotional state and relationships.

9 URINARY SYSTEM

INTRODUCTION

In conventional medicine, the kidney primarily deals with water regulation and electrolyte balance. There are additional functions of acid-base balance, maintenance of blood pressure, stimulation of red blood cell production and vitamin D metabolism. This is clearly a dynamic process that involves retaining essential substances and allowing unwanted materials to be excreted.

In clinical practice the kidney is likened to a passive filtration system and from this view arises the concept of 'flushing', taking large quantities of water. With conditions such as urinary infections or kidney stones, people are advised to drink 5 or 6 pints of water (minimum) each day.

This view denies the existence of energetic factors and sees the kidney merely as a physical filter. The energy will be swamped if excessive amounts of fluid are taken. Long-term this will lead to depletion of kidney energy and the development of urinary symptoms such as tiredness, frequent urination, backache and oedema. In conventional physiology, there is acknowledgement that the processes of water and electrolyte balance are active and dynamic. This is not recognised by conventional clinicians.

The information in Table 9.1 reveals the associations that are made through knowledge of vitalistic principles. The comments on the right of the Table are to explain these associations. The information in this Table is derived from Chinese medicine and will be most familiar to its practitioners. However, the underlying energetic principles are common to all methods of holistic medicine and so there will be glimpses of recognition for other practitioners.

Association	Comments
Stores Jing	Jing is a fundamental substance of Chinese thought and is associated with birth, reproduction and maturation. On a narrow, physical level it may be likened to ideas of genetics in Western science
Root of Yin and Yang	This has no counterpart conventionally. The Kidneys[1] are the basis of Yin and Yang for the whole body. Long-term disease leads to depletion of Kidney Yin or Yang or both. The decline in constitutional energy over the past few generations can be viewed in one way as a general decrease in Kidney function
Rules Water	This is a Yang (Fire) aspect of the Kidney. People who retain fluid and become overweight easily may have Kidney Yang deficiency. Large intakes of water cause fluid retention due to Kidney Yang damage
Rules Bones	In conventional medicine, the kidney influences vitamin D metabolism. Vitamin D affects calcium metabolism and thereby bones
Rules grasping of Qi	The Kidneys pull Qi down from the Lungs and aid in respiration. Some lung disorders such as asthma, therefore, may be due to a Kidney imbalance. This has no counterpart in conventional medicine
Generates Marrow, Fills up the Brain	This is an interesting connection. The Chinese understood that the Kidneys have a role in making marrow, and thence Blood, centuries before this was understood in conventional medicine. In addition, the Brain is described as the 'Sea of Marrow' and so Kidney function is reflected in thought, memory and concentration
Paired organ is Urinary Bladder	This is comparable with the conventional view that the bladder stores urine produced by the kidney
Opens into the ear	Many ear problems are considered to be due to Kidney imbalance in Chinese medicine. In conventional medicine it is recognised that administration of certain drugs in kidney disease may cause deafness
Colour – black	This is the colour of Yin, Water (see below). It also corresponds to the deep unconscious
Taste – salt	Each major organ has an associated taste. In this case excess salty food can damage the Water element
Season – winter	The energy of winter is quiescent, drawn deep within the body, descending. This can be compared to the kidneys in that they are hidden deep within the body, difficult to palpate[2]
Element – Water	The Element correspondence reveals the connection of Chinese medical theory to nature. Each Element is connected to the others to provide, in health, a harmonious balance
Time – 5-7 p.m.	The 'time' of an organ is when its energy it at its maximum. Most people die in the early hours of the morning – time of deficient Kidney symptoms. Asthma caused by a Kidney weakness is worse at 5 am
Emotions – fear	This association explains why extreme fear can affect the Kidneys. There may be increased urination, for example, at such times
Mental aspect	Intellect, intelligence and wisdom, insight and quality of intelligence. Will power and ambition depend upon Kidney function

Table 9.1: Holistic energetic view of the Kidney[3]

ANATOMY AND PHYSIOLOGY

There are several facts of anatomy and physiology that it is useful to know prior to studying pathology. I have included the male organs of testes and prostate since their function, in Chinese medicine, is dependent upon Kidney energy. In women, disorders of menstruation, fertility and childbirth are often related to the function of the Kidney (as well as other organs) but all these are discussed separately in Chapter 17 – Pregnancy and Childbirth and Chapter 18 – Women's Health.

To study disease of the urinary system it would be helpful to be able to:

- State the main structures of the urinary system
- Identify the main features of the kidney
- Describe the appearance of the basic functional unit of the kidney – the nephron
- Discuss the function of the nephron
- Describe the endocrine functions of the kidney – erythropoeitin and red cell production, Vitamin D metabolism, renin-angiotensin and maintenance of blood pressure
- Identify the main features of the testes and prostate
- Discuss the functions of the testes and prostate.

CLASSIFICATION OF URINARY SYSTEM DISEASE

The conventional classification of kidney disease is confusing since it changes every few years. This reflects the confusion in conventional circles as to the physiology of the kidneys. The reasons for this are discussed above.

Table 9.2 reveals the main differentiation between infective and inflammatory kidney disease. I discuss these in detail below and how to analyse the relative severity of each complaint. The main thing to consider is the site of the problem. If the disease affects the deeper organs such as the kidney, then it is clearly more serious than disease that affects superficial areas such as the urethra. When comparing infective versus inflammatory conditions, it is helpful to note that complaints involving bacteria indicate stronger energy. Therefore, acute glomerulonephritis is more serious than acute pyelonephritis, because the sufferer is weaker.

Mild disease		
Inflammatory (non-infective)		**Infective**
		Sexually transmitted disease • gonorrhoea • non-specific urethritis
		Prostatitis (including prostatic enlargement)
		Cystitis
		Acute pyelonephritis
Acute glomerulonephritis		
Proliferative: aka nephritic syndrome aka Ellis Type I aka Bright's disease	Minimal lesion/membranous: aka nephrotic syndrome aka Ellis Type II	
Renal stones		
Cancer		
		Chronic pyelonephritis
Chronic glomerulonephritis		
End-stage kidney disease		
Severe disease		

Table 9.2: Classification of renal disease

INFECTIVE DISEASE OF THE URINARY SYSTEM

This is a major category of disease of the urinary system. Such disease is very common and occurs in the kidney, ureters, bladder or urethra. The urinary system may be divided at the level of the bladder into the upper and lower urinary tracts (cf. the respiratory system. Most lower urinary tract infections will not lead to infection in the upper urinary tract. Infection in the deeper levels of a system only occurs if the energy of that system is markedly disturbed. If the energetic state of the person improves then the disease will move out into more superficial areas. I would emphasise that organisms are not the cause of such disease but merely an associated occurrence. Strong symptoms, with a clearly identified organism, indicate that the energy of the person is relatively strong.

Gonorrhoea

This is classified as a sexually transmitted disease. It is associated with a bacterium, *Neisseria gonorrhoeae*, and has an incubation period of 2-10 days. It is mainly an affection of the mucous membrane of the genital tract, rectum, pharynx and eyes.

The incidence increased rapidly in the 1970s as a result of greater sexual freedom and the decline in use of barrier contraceptive methods. The risk of infection is different in males and females. Sixty to 80 per cent of women in contact with an infected man will develop gonorrhoea. This is in contrast to 20-30 per cent of men who contract the disease when in contact with an infected woman. Such male–female discrepancies in infection rate are also noted with HIV. It seems that the *penetrating* partner is less likely to develop infection than the *penetrated* partner – male or female. There are large numbers of cases in the West and especially so in the United States. In 1985, there were 1 million reported cases in the US (with an estimated similar number going unreported). There were 35 million cases world-wide in 1990.

Symptoms
The main symptoms in men are severe dysuria (likened to passing broken glass), frequency of urination and a yellow urethral discharge. A minority (10 per cent) experience only mild symptoms, or none at all. This asymptomatic figure rises to 50 per cent amongst women.

In women, the lower cervical canal is affected together with the urethra and rectum in 50 per cent of cases. Vaginal discharge is the common symptom with frequency of urination and dysuria. For this reason, the illness may go unrecognised by women.

There may be systemic symptoms of fever, muscle aches and pains, a diffuse rash of redness or pustules and a general feeling of ill health. The pharynx is involved in a significant proportion of cases where there has been oral contact.

Investigations
These are performed if the diagnosis is clinically suspected. Swabs and culture are done using special media on which to grow the organism.

Complications

Complication	Symptoms to look for
Urethral stricture (narrowing) – this is rare now and was due to the use of caustic treatments	Urinary frequency, urgency, poor stream, dribbling urination
Epididymitis (males)	Swelling and pain in the testis
Prostatitis (males)	Urinary frequency, dark and strong smelling urine, dysuria, suprapubic tenderness, fever
Pelvic inflammatory disease (females)	Lower abdominal pain, fever, and vaginal discharge
Neonatal conjunctivitis – born to infected mothers (rare)	Redness of the conjunctiva, yellow discharge
Proctitis	Pain in rectum, discharge, and itching
Arthritis	Joint pain (often a single joint), fever, malaise, purplish macular rash

Table 9.3: Complications of gonorrhoea

Treatment
This is with penicillin although some strains are resistant to this now. Large doses of antibiotics are given for the complications of gonorrhoea. Repeat cultures are taken until they are negative. Another aspect is the tracing of contacts and the offering of treatment to them.

Non-specific urethritis (NSU) – Non-gonococcal urethritis (NGU)

This is also known as non-gonococcal urethritis and is classified as a sexually transmitted disease. It was first recognised in the 1970s when people who had been treated for gonorrhoea returned with similar symptoms but no evidence of the gonococcal bacterium. The organism that is associated with this condition is an unusual one, *Chlamydia trachomatis*. It is also isolated from women with pelvic inflammatory disease. It is an interesting organism in that it is classified as being somewhere between a virus and a bacterium. In the UK, in men, urethritis is more often non-gonococcal than gonococcal.

Symptoms

These are the same as gonorrhoea but milder. The urethral discharge is less yellow and profuse than that of gonorrhoea.

Investigations

These are the same as for gonorrhoea.

Treatment

This is with oxytetracycline, as the organism does not respond to penicillin.

Complications

These are the same as those of gonorrhoea.

Holistic management of gonorrhoea and non-specific urethritis

This is the one situation in the UK that is governed by law. The Venereal Diseases Act of 1916 means, in effect, that gonorrhoea and syphilis must be treated by conventional medicine. Contact tracing by clinics is also an important aspect of management. There is no harm in treating someone at the same time as conventional practitioners but it is important not to put yourself in the position of threatening your practice.

In energetic terms, it is clearly suppressive to treat these conditions by means of antibiotics. An insight into ailments that may occur on deeper levels following conventional treatment may be gleaned from the following account of the homoeopathic remedy, Medorrhinum,[4] which is made from the discharge of a gonorrhoeal infection:

'A powerful and deep-acting medicine often indicated for chronic ailments due to suppressed gonorrhoea. Chronic rheumatism. Great disturbance and irritability of nervous system. Pains intolerable, tensive; nerves quiver and tingle. Children dwarfed and stunted; sour smelling. Chronic catarrhal conditions in children. Nose dirty, tonsils enlarged, thick yellow mucus from nostrils; lips thickened from mouth breathing. State of collapse and trembling all over. Often restores a gonorrhoeal discharge (as per direction of cure). Intensity of all sensations. Oedema of limbs; dropsy of serous sacs. Disseminated sclerosis. Affects the mind; nerves; mucous membranes. Profuse acrid discharges, causing itching. Fishy odours of the secretions. Offensive odour of the body, esp. children and women. Many different kinds of pains; stiffness, aching, soreness. Trembling all over [subjective]; intense nervousness and profound exhaustion. Numbness; formication, internal. Arthritic; rheumatic pains. Diseases of the spinal cords, even organic lesions ending in paralysis. Enlargement of the lymphatic glands all over the body; & heat and soreness. Loss of power in the joints; joints feel loose. Burning. Small, very sore aphthae; blisters. States of collapse; wants to be fanned all the time. Tumours, cancer, scirrhus, etc.; & history of sycosis. Body smells badly to her, can't be washed away. Must walk bent from pain in groin. Said to be the mother of pus and catarrh. History of early heart disease in the parents.'[5]

In terms of Chinese medicine, the syndromes which correspond to disorders in this area are similar to those listed under the urinary disorders in general on Page 156.

Prostatitis

Prostatitis is an inflammation of the prostate. It is commonly a secondary development to a urethritis, usually of a sexually transmitted origin. It may also occur without evidence of infection but with identical symptoms. This latter type is of unknown cause in conventional medicine.

Symptoms

There may be acute or chronic attacks. The acute types have stronger symptoms but most cases seen in the clinic are of the chronic variety, which is described here. There are episodes of perineal pain with dysuria, frequency of urination, urgency and nocturia. Systemic disturbances are common with fever, general malaise and tiredness. There are acute flare-ups from time to time, perhaps related to dietary factors, sexual activity, overwork and stress.

Treatment

Antibiotics are invariably prescribed despite the poor penetration of the drugs into the substance of the prostate. Relapses are almost universal. Non-steroidal, anti-inflammatory agents are used in many situations especially if there is no evidence of infection. Conventionally, there is no long-term relief and some people may be given low dose antibiotics continuously for years.

Holistic management

In terms of Chinese medicine this usually corresponds to a condition of Dampness and Heat which collects in the Lower Jiao due to weak Kidneys. Such an event is also associated with the function of the Spleen. There may also be a degree of Liver Qi Stagnation as the Liver Channel traverses this area.

Cystitis

This is inflammation of the bladder. It is rare in men and common in women where it is frequently associated with gynaecological symptoms. There are a variety of theories as to why this condition is more common amongst women. They all revolve around the germ theory of disease causation, despite the fact that a significant number of cases have no demonstrable organism.

There are three main ideas discussed in conventional texts. Firstly, the area around the urethra is heavily colonised with bacteria, although this is true in both sexes. Secondly, the urethra of women is shorter than in men so infection can pass up it easier. I would think that *any* length of urethra is adequate and this may be a reference to the penis-envy theory of psychological thought. Lastly, if the bladder is not emptied properly, i.e. totally, there is residual urine that may serve as a reservoir for the growth of bacteria. It is suggested in some texts that women do not empty their bladders completely. The implication, of course, is that either there is an inherent design fault causing a loss of function or that women wilfully do not empty their bladders completely. These ideas reflect the, sometimes sexist, attitudes of conventional medicine and lead to treatments that are ineffective.

Symptoms

Many women (50 per cent) have the following symptoms at some point in their lives but usually as a single attack (90 per cent of attacks are not repeated). The main symptoms are urinary frequency, dysuria and suprapubic pain. There is an intense desire to pass urine even if the bladder is empty (strangury). The urine may be of a strong colour, cloudy and with an unpleasant odour. Haematuria occurs in some. There is suprapubic tenderness on examination of the abdomen. There may be associated fever and chills although these symptoms are more typical of acute pyelonephritis.

In about half of cases there is no culture of bacteria. This is called the 'urethral syndrome' and is ill understood in conventional medicine for reasons stated above.

Around 1 in 20 pregnant women have evidence of bacteria in their urine and so all women who are pregnant have urine cultures as part of their antenatal care. The presence of such bacteria may be associated with pyelonephritis later in pregnancy, pre-eclamptic toxaemia and anaemia.

Investigations

The correct management includes urinalysis with culture and determining the sensitivity of any organisms to antibiotics. On examination, the urine will contain bacteria and possibly pus cells. Dipsticks are available to detect nitrites, which are produced by bacteria, but they are unreliable. Blood tests reveal a raised white cell count.

Recurrent attacks of lower urinary tract infection (three or more in women or one episode in men and children) may be further investigated first by means of intravenous excretion urography. Other investigations include plain abdominal X-rays, ultrasound and DMSA scanning – dimercaptosuccinic acid used in a radioactive form (^{99m}Tc DMSA). This investigation may be used in children. These are performed to detect predisposing factors such as structural abnormalities or kidney stones. Urinary tract infections are common when there are congenital defects of the kidney. From an holistic point of view this makes sense as a congenital structural defect means there must be a preceding energetic imbalance.

Treatment

Antibiotics are the mainstays of treatment and these may be given long-term. It is preferable to determine the presence of bacteria and their sensitivity to antibiotics before prescribing drugs but this is rarely done in clinical practice. Cultures should be repeated at the end of treatment to check that the bacteria have disappeared. There are some situations, particularly in the elderly, when there is 'asymptomatic bacteriuria'. This is the presence of bacteria in the urine with no symptoms. The correct conventional response is to observe since there is generally only a problem when there are symptoms. The same is true of women with asymptomatic bacteriuria unless pregnant. General advice includes drinking large amounts of fluid each day to 'flush' out the kidneys. People are advised to urinate frequently.

Pyelonephritis

This disease is at the level of the kidney and indicates a deeper, more severe situation. There are still the relatively strong symptoms associated with the presence of organisms but now revealing that the substance of the kidney is affected.

Acute pyelonephritis

This may occur secondary to infective disease in the urethra or bladder, which has ascended into the upper reaches of the urinary tract. This may be due to associated factors that are mechanical (catheterisation, obstruction to urinary flow by kidney stones, prostatic enlargement or urethral stricture), systemic (diabetes mellitus) or drug-related (after use of analgesics/non-steroidal anti-inflammatory agents). Some people develop pyelonephritis without any associated factor.

Symptoms
There is sudden onset of fever with chills, loin pain and vomiting. The person feels ill. The inflammation affects most of the urinary tract. There are also symptoms of frequent painful urination of small amounts of urine and painful desire to pass urine with nothing there (strangury) due to associated cystitis. Haematuria occurs in severe cases.

Investigations
The general approach is the same as described above for cystitis. A full blood count reveals increased numbers of white cells. Urinalysis is positive for protein and perhaps blood. Urine culture provides evidence of bacteria in many cases including their sensitivity to antibiotics.

Treatment
This is invariably by means of antibiotics, which may be given without evidence from urine culture.

Complications
These are rare unless there is a structural abnormality of the kidney or chronic disease such as diabetes mellitus.

Complication	Symptoms to look for
Chronic pyelonephritis	Loin pain, frequent urination, tiredness, possibly dysuria
Renal papillary necrosis	Worsening symptoms, high fever, haematuria, the person is ill, deteriorating condition
Perinephric abscess	Fever, one-sided loin pain, recent history of urinary infection
Kidney abscess	Fever persists or relapses

Table 9.4 Complications of acute pyelonephritis

Chronic pyelonephritis

This is persistent pyelonephritis. It may occur in people who are not strong enough to throw off an acute attack. Other factors include obstruction in the urinary tract (also multiple sclerosis as it leads to reduced urinary flow), the presence of stones, diabetes mellitus or analgesic/non-steroidal anti-inflammatory agent use.

Symptoms
These are more vague than in the acute type, recur at intervals and tend to persist. The main symptoms are ill health, tiredness and frequent urination. Loin pain is universal and there may be episodes of dysuria.

Investigations
These are as for acute pyelonephritis.

Complications

Complication	Symptoms to look for
Hypertension	Headaches, tinnitus, dizziness
End-stage kidney disease	Anorexia, nausea, vomiting, tiredness and others

Table 9.5: Complications of chronic pyelonephritis

Treatment
This is as for acute pyelonephritis.

INFLAMMATORY DISEASES OF THE KIDNEY

Inflammatory conditions of the kidneys not associated with infection are probably more common than is generally realised. Although the categories below are the definitive gross forms as recognised by conventional medicine, milder degrees do exist.

Glomerulonephritis

This is inflammation of the functional unit of the kidney. It indicates a generalised affection at a deep level within the kidney. In conventional medicine, the underlying process is known to be related to the immune system, where antibodies are formed that damage the kidney. This is an example of an autoimmune disease.

The precise cause for this dysfunction of the immune system is not known in conventional medicine although there are various substances that act as triggers. Some are external and some are internal – Table 9.6. In the case of infection as listed in this Table, it is not that the infection directly affects the kidney, but more that the immune system attacks the infecting organism and it is this reaction which involves the kidney.

There are two major clinical presentations of glomerulonephritis – nephritic syndrome and nephrotic syndrome. The exact terminology changes with time – Table 9.2 is a clear classification.

Infections	Streptococcus, staphylococcus – also causes boils, abscesses, viruses of glandular fever, hepatitis, measles, mumps. Other infections such as malaria
Malignant disease	Cancer of any type
Drugs[6]	Antibiotics, captopril, gold, hydralazine, interferon, lithium, mesalazine, non-steroidal anti-inflammatory agents but particularly ketoprofen, penicillamine, phenytoin, practolol, probenecid, quinidine, rifampicin

Table 9.6: Known causes of glomerulonephritis

Nephritic syndrome (Acute proliferative[7] glomerulonephritis)

This was formerly known as Bright's disease. It may also be known as Ellis Type I nephritis. There is a classic picture of tonsillitis (streptococcal bacterial infection) that some 1-3 weeks later leads to the development of kidney symptoms. It is not that the infection directly affects the kidney. Rather that the body produces antibodies against the bacteria which also damage kidney tissue. This accounts for the delay in symptoms since the number of antibodies has to reach a certain level in the blood.

Symptoms
Children are affected commonly. There is the acute development of haematuria, proteinuria and scanty urination. There is mild fever, general malaise, abdominal pain, nausea and vomiting. Since fluid is retained there is oedema and high blood pressure (which may give rise to headaches). The oedema classically occurs first on the upper body such as around the eyes, face and hands. Later as it worsens it is seen in the legs. There may be convulsions in severe cases.

After a period of 4-7 days, there is usually full recovery with profuse urination and the disappearance of oedema.

Investigations
Urinalysis is positive for protein and blood. Red cell casts will be seen also. Full blood count reveals a mild anaemia. There is increased blood urea and ESR. In those who do not have an uncomplicated recovery (see below), annual checks of blood pressure and serum creatinine are advised.

Prognosis
There is 'complete'[8] recovery in 90 per cent of cases and this is especially true of children. The least favourable prognoses are in adults and in those without the specific trigger of tonsillitis. Even in this 'recovered' group, 20-50 per cent have mild raised blood pressure and impaired kidney function tests for some years. Others may have persistent haematuria and proteinuria for 2 years.

Less than 5 per cent have scanty urination for more than 9 days. These have more severe kidney damage. The remainder develop a rapidly progressive picture with persistent proteinuria. This develops into end-stage kidney disease in months or years.

Treatment

There is no specific conventional treatment for this condition. The main aim is to prevent serious symptoms, as recovery is the usual event. Uncomplicated and mild cases may be monitored at home but more severe attacks need to be dealt with in hospital. In extreme situations the use of dialysis is indicated. Penicillin is given if there is residual evidence of tonsil infection. The administration of antibiotics is widely advocated for tonsillitis and the possibility of glomerulonephritis is stated as an indication. There is no evidence that the use of such drugs makes any difference to the occurrence or severity of post-streptococcal glomerulonephritis.[9]

Nephrotic syndrome (Minimal lesion/membranous[10] glomerulonephritis)

This is a more severe type of acute glomerulonephritis. Any age may be affected rather than the predominance of children seen with nephritic syndrome. The trigger for the development of antibodies is unknown.[11] It is as if the body spontaneously produces antibodies, which attack the kidney tissue. This unprompted autoimmune response would indicate the more serious nature of the condition.

Symptoms

There is slow onset of symptoms. Protein is lost in the urine for some time before oedema develops. The cause of oedema in this case is low protein levels in the blood (hypoproteinaemia). The oedema is general in site. Fluid collects in the abdominal cavity (ascites) and causes discomfort and abdominal swelling. There is pallor and the continued loss of protein leads to ill health and increased infections.

Investigations

Twenty-four-hour urinary loss of protein exceeds 3-5 g/day in adults and may be as high as 40 g/day. The serum albumin is low. Serum urea and creatinine are estimated as a check on renal function. Urine examination reveals red blood cells and red cell casts. Renal biopsy is performed in some cases when it is suspected that treatment with corticosteroids is applicable. Young children are given corticosteroids anyway, unless there is high blood pressure or blood in the urine, as it is assumed their cases will respond. Biopsy is not done in those cases known to be caused by diabetes mellitus, metal toxicity, drugs and so forth.

Prognosis

In cases of the membranous type, around one third have gradual deterioration of kidney function leading to end-stage kidney disease within 15 years.

In the case of the minimal lesion type, most children stop losing protein in their urine after the acute phase but this is much less likely in adults.

Treatment

The use of antibiotics and improvements in general management has resulted in a decrease in the mortality rate over the years. The use of corticosteroids has never been shown to improve survival rates. Despite this, they are frequently administered particularly in membranous glomerulonephritis as this group of conditions has a relatively high relapse rate. They may have some symptomatic effect but long-term outcome is unaffected and side-effects are an additional burden.

Medium potency diuretics are administered to reduce the level of the oedema. Immunosuppressants such as cyclophosphamide, chlorambucil or azathioprine may be given in addition to corticosteroids in those with frequent relapses. Cyclosporin may be given long-term to suppress the immune reaction. Its use has to monitored closely as it is damaging to the kidneys. If the glomerulonephritis is secondary to an autoimmune disorder or diabetes mellitus, the prognosis depends upon the severity of the original disease.

Chronic glomerulonephritis

This develops from acute glomerulonephritis, which may or may not have been recognised. The type of acute glomerulonephritis is the nephrotic syndrome rather than the nephritic syndrome. End-stage kidney disease is the usual conclusion of this process.

Symptoms

Chronic glomerulonephritis is a severe dysfunction and its clinical picture merges with that of end-stage kidney disease. There is progressive loss of kidney function with proteinuria, abnormal urinary sediments and diminishing kidney size.

Treatment

This depends upon the clinical picture. Some cases have the features of nephrotic syndrome whilst others have more in common with end-stage kidney disease.

End-stage kidney disease

This is the final stage of degeneration of kidney function. It is placed in the context of kidney disease in Table 9.2.

Symptoms
The clinical picture is due to increasingly severe biochemical abnormalities. There are disturbances of water, mineral and acid-alkaline balances. Abnormalities are seen in levels of calcium, magnesium phosphate, potassium and sodium.

There is a general feeling of ill health with malaise. Nausea, vomiting and gastrointestinal bleeding are common. The person feels tired, irritable, depressed with insomnia and agitation. Twitching and restlessness of the legs are frequent associations. There is generalised itching which may be severe. Tingling and muscular weakness are experienced in the limbs. Loin pain is seen in everyone with this condition.

In the cardiovascular system, there is increased atherosclerosis, lipid (fat) levels are raised, and blood pressure is high. There may be pericarditis as evidenced by sharp chest pain with palpitations. Anaemia is universal leading to pallor and adding to the feelings of tiredness. Infections are more likely in people with end-stage kidney disease.

Treatment
This is initially symptomatic with control of protein intake and the treatment of infection and hypertension. The end result is renal failure and dialysis, or transplantation is the last resort.

Holistic management of urinary disorders

In terms of Chinese medicine the conditions usually associated with these symptoms are Damp-heat in the Bladder (Damp-heat in the Lower Jiao) or Excessive Heat in the Small Intestine.[12] Urinary disorders with urinary frequency, urgency and pain are classified as Lin syndrome with five subtypes. There are Stone Lin (kidney stones), Lao Lin (chronic prostatitis), Milky Lin (diseases characterised by turbid urine), Heat Lin (acute infection of the urinary tract) and Blood Lin (tuberculosis, cancer or other tumour of the urogenital system, acute urinary infection).

The general principle of all the urinary disorders is that they indicate a systemic imbalance. The reasoning for such a statement is that an internal organ[13] is affected, episodes are usually recurrent and they are triggered by factors that lead to a flare-up of the underlying condition. The triggers are those things that, in terms of Chinese medicine, generate Heat, Dampness, Liver Qi Stagnation or Kidney depletion – Table 9.7.

The most beneficial approach to urinary system disease is one that takes all the factors in Table 9.7 into account. It is important to think about education, information, relaxation, the resolution of emotional issues, diet and habits such as clothing and hygiene. I describe cases below that illustrate some of these.

There is a phrase in common usage, 'pissed off' or in American English 'pissed', which suggests irritation or resentment. It is not surprising to note that the emotions closely associated with the bladder in Chinese medicine are suspicion and jealousy. In homoeopathic medicine, the remedy Staphysagria has suppressed anger and resentment as a strong guiding symptom. It may be given for complaints of shame and mortification, for invasion by penetration. It is also indicated in cases of 'honeymoon cystitis' where sexual activity has led to the symptoms of cystitis. It is much more useful to look at symptoms from this perspective so that a deeper understanding of aetiology is gained which leads to more effective treatment. Men do not have the same symptoms as they are rarely 'invaded' in a similar manner. I have treated a number of women with recurrent symptoms of cystitis or burning pains in the vagina and there is almost always a history of a traumatic event (often sexual or emotional), preceding this clinical picture.

Trigger factor of urinary disease	Comments
Alcohol, dehydration, irritants – perfumes, douches, 'feminine hygiene' products, spices, emotional stagnation including anger, irritation, being 'pissed off'	These generate heat, which can lead to inflammatory reactions in the bladder and urinary tract
Dairy products, greasy and fatty food	These lead to the formation of Dampness (mucus), which collects in the pelvic organs
Sugar	This generates Dampness (mucus) as well as leading to Heat[14] stagnation
Cold weather,[15] fear/shock, sexual activity[16]	These tend to deplete Kidney energy and this adversely affects the functioning of other organs dependent on this energy[17]
Constitutional factors	The constitution relies upon Kidney function. The strength of this has much to do with inherited factors
Drugs – prescribed or social	The effect of these will depend upon their energetic quality. For example, antibiotics that are generally Cold and Damp in nature will deplete Kidney energy and lead to the collection of Dampness

Table 9.7: Important factors in the development of urinary disease

Case one

A man of 35 years of age came with pains in the knee after playing squash. It had been a recurrent problem over the past 6 months. On further questioning, he had a history of low back pain, recurrent attacks of dysuria, frequent urination with cloudy and smelly urine over the previous 3 years. His doctor had diagnosed it as prostatitis. He had two attacks of non-specific urethritis in the year prior to his first bout of prostatitis. He had always received antibiotics for his acute flare-ups.

In terms of Chinese medicine, his diagnosis was Damp-heat Accumulation in the Lower Jiao with underlying Kidney Yang Deficiency. The Kidney governs the lower back and knees. I gave him advice about his diet to reduce the foods that lead to Dampness and Heat as well as to eat those which strengthen the Spleen (digestion).

I discussed relaxation with him as he had some stresses at home and his job was a high-powered position in the insurance world. He occasionally had flare-ups of his prostatitis symptoms along the way but these were managed by Chinese medicine rather than resorting to more antibiotics. In a woman, this imbalance would have led to recurrent vaginal discharge, pelvic inflammatory disease or similar congestion.

It is an important part of the process to support people so that they can begin to have faith in the restorative abilities of their own body. Eventually, they will depend less on conventional treatments such as drugs that can only worsen the underlying, chronic condition.

Case two

This case connects with several areas including Chapter 10 – Musculoskeletal system. A woman of 55 years came for treatment of her joint problems. She had swelling, stiffness and pain in her hands, feet, elbows and knees. She felt generally hot with sweating. She urinated twice each night and had frequency of urination some eight times or more during the day. Her urine would leak involuntarily on straining or physical exercise. Her energy was very low. Her skin was itchy and dry.

Her past medical history revealed a uterine prolapse followed by hysterectomy and bladder repair. A bladder repair is designed to reduce the amount of weakness at the bladder neck and so minimise leakage of urine and frequency. They are of variable effectiveness.

In terms of Chinese medicine, her diagnosis was Kidney Yang Deficiency with Blood Deficiency. Her pulses were extremely weak on her first visit and reflected a much-depleted state of health. Her symptoms of heat, dry and itchy skin and joint discomfort were a consequence of the Blood Deficiency. Blood moistens, cools and nourishes and so heat may appear if it is lacking, as well as symptoms in muscles and joints. The Kidney Deficiency was responsible for the urinary symptoms.

The aim of treatment was to gradually strengthen Kidney Yang and Blood. Her symptoms gradually improved over the next few months. She was working hard but her joints improved quite quickly. Her nightly urination declined to once and the frequency in the day became less. There was little leaking.

She was prescribed a homoeopathic remedy by a homoeopath and developed pain in her left loin radiating to the groin, bloated abdomen, alternating constipation and diarrhoea, painful urination and cloudy urine. These were bowel and bladder symptoms. She also experienced emotional symptoms similar to those she had some years before around the time of her hysterectomy. This release of old emotional states is typical of treatment by holistic medicine as the process of cure progresses. It is important to continue treatment, to deal with these flare-ups in a non-suppressive manner, to offer support to the person as they are experiencing these changes and to reassure them that this is a normal part of the healing process.

After a week or so of these symptoms, they settled. She ended with treatment soon after as she was generally very well. There were few symptoms in any area and she managed a busy work schedule.

Case three

A woman of 39 years came for treatment of her urinary symptoms. She would have frequent attacks of dark and strong smelling urine, which had become worse in the past 4 months. There was nocturia four times each night although no burning pain on urination. All investigations were normal but there were now few occasions when her urine was normal. She would feel generally toxic and her bowels were sluggish, with movements only every 2 to 3 days. She was very concerned about her health and particularly whether she would develop a chronic kidney disease. I made a diagnosis of Damp-heat in the Lower Jiao secondary to long-standing Blood Deficiency and Kidney Yang Deficiency. I treated her with acupuncture and Chinese herbs for several months and although her general condition was improved and emotionally she began to feel more settled, her urinary symptoms did not change much. I encouraged her to seek other support and she began to see a counsellor to work through several long-standing emotional issues. It was only after treating her for some 2 years that her urinary symptoms began to subside. Her emotions were much more balanced and she began to notice the connection between her psychological state and her urine. The urine would darken and become more smelly if she felt upset or worried. She continues with treatment but her urine is now generally normal, she feels well and she is functioning much better on many levels.

Case four

Three years ago, a boy aged 5 years came for treatment. He was adopted and little was known about his natural parents. Since 3 years old he had had repeated kidney infections with pain and crying out after urination, night fevers, bed-wetting and restlessness. He had been treated with antibiotics three times. A scan and a reflux test both came back as no abnormality detected. His appetite was poor. He looked immaculate. He was extremely neat and wearing very smart clothes. He didn't want to speak to the homoeopath and his adoptive parents did nearly all the talking.

'He's slow to make a decision...even which cereal he wants in the morning...then he's sorry if it causes an argument.' (His indecision annoys his mother.)

'He is very particular about clothes. He likes 'cool clothes' with designer labels.'

'He's better when there are lots of people around. He hates feeling he's being observed or the attention is on him.' (This is why he finds the consultation difficult.) He hates anyone (doctors or us) looking at his genitals ...he's very private.'

His mother says: 'He didn't want to go to school. It was a wrench, (initially).' The boy speaks for the one and only time 'I just want to be with Mam and Dad'.

'He cannot bear anyone to touch his toes. His feet just jump. He feels like he is being tickled when he is only being touched. He likes his boots really tight.'

This child was paralysed by indecision even in the simplest of choices. In his father's words: 'He wants to be good, but he really can't make a decision'.

He wants to be 'good' and this is obvious from his neat appearance. He likes to play, but if he gets dirty then he wants to clean himself up soon after. He is not at ease with himself.

He likes to have his boots laced very tightly. I found out only recently from a social worker that this is a common trait amongst children who are in care, fostered or adopted. They are also very reluctant to take their shoes or boots off. His wanting the boots tight was a sign of his insecurity that was echoed by the reluctance to be separated from his mother and father.

Thuja has the following symptoms:

- Urination, pain at close of
- Thoughts: inconstancy of
- Irresolution, indecision: changeable

- Looked at: cannot bear to be
- Feet, Sensitive, oversensitive: sensual impressions, to

In the *Materia Medica,* Gray gives this description of Thuja:

'Present a manufactured image to the world which is calculated and formed from childhood. During childhood they had the experience [or delusion] of being neglected or abused. The message the child gets is that they can never be good enough'. (Perhaps he had a deep memory of being given up by his natural mother.)

'They feel unlovable. Because they feel they can never be loved they make an extra effort to be liked. They look around to see what is most popular, how they walk, dress, what they do, etc., to see what is successful. Then they go about imitating this systematically and scientifically, copying what they think works in the world and by adulthood they have the perfect image.'

After the first remedy (Thuja 30c) he had a nosebleed and came out in a lot of itchy spots. Thereafter, his indecision improved markedly and his urinary symptoms cleared. His feet became much less sensitive and he began to wear his boots in the trendy loose style! When his symptoms return (which is now rare) he repeats the remedy.

His mother says he is in great form and that they are getting on extremely well. However she is now having difficulties in her relationship with her adopted daughter.

Case five
A 56-year-old farmer came for treatment. He seemed very anxious and was accompanied by his wife, who sat in throughout the first consultation. His energy had always been low, even as a teenager. In his early twenties he had a bad shock when his father fell through a loft, breaking his hip. As a result he had to take over the farm.

Two months later he was diagnosed with nephritis with severe swelling of the ankles and eyeballs. He was told by the doctors he had only 6 months to live. When he proved them wrong they told his wife 'You have a miracle for a husband!'

In his thirties he inherited a farm from an uncle. He and his wife had to care for this uncle (and aunt) who were both disabled. It was a difficult time, he felt his new neighbours were hostile and his wife was also expecting their first child.

After an upsetting incident, where he was cheated at the cattle market, he had to be readmitted to hospital for 2 weeks with nephritis and within a month had a severe relapse. For the next 2 years he was on steroids, although he had now stopped these. He was told that his only chance of recovery lay in a transplant.

Since childhood he had felt 'too weak' and timid for this world. He believed he was being persecuted and this made him frightened. This fear presented not only as a mental state, but had come through to the physical level as very severe, at times life-threatening, kidney pathology. This had left both kidneys badly damaged, but particularly the left.

The homeopathic remedy China matched his case very well. It has the following symptoms:

- Mind, delusions persecuted, tormented, wronged
- Irritability, with weakness
- Kidney ailments in general: left
- Nephritis
- Pinching pain in the foot. (Hahnemann)
- Energy, wanting< 7-8pm
- Sleep, restless.

The remedy (China 30c) worked well. He came to his next appointment alone. His irritability was much less and every month he reported a gradual and steady improvement in all his other symptoms. He found he no longer needed to take afternoon naps. His self-confidence increased and he no longer felt persecuted. He began to socialise more. After 6 weeks he was able to come off his sleeping pills and his sleep 'was sound as could be'. He said: 'I can feel my whole system changing…I've put on weight and feel much stronger. There's less tension and I'm easier in myself'.

INCONTINENCE

This is the involuntary passage of urine. There are several causes in conventional medicine. The condition causes many problems for people, not the least of which are embarrassment and inconvenience.

Stress incontinence

Small amounts are passed upon straining, laughing, exercise and so forth. It occurs more commonly in women than men and is more likely with increasing age. It is unusual in women who have not had children. It is due to a weakness in the pelvic floor muscles.

Retention-overflow

This is characterised by dribbling, pain in the pelvis and a palpable bladder. The bladder is full and urine leaks out intermittently. This type is seen in urinary outflow obstruction as with prostatic disease, with drugs such as anticholinergics, antidepressants, and opiates and after the administration of anaesthetic agents.

Confusion

This may lead to urination due to lack of awareness. A variable volume is passed depending upon the contents of the bladder.

'Spastic'

This term is applied to spasm of the bladder causing large volumes of urine to be passed sporadically. Urgency is a characteristic. This type may be due to the simple fact that the person cannot get to the toilet in time due to mobility problems. Do not always assume that urinary disease is present. Improvement of the person's mobility will improve the incontinence. Others in this category include spinal cord disease such as prolapsed intervertebral disc or spinal tumour and multiple sclerosis.

Enuresis is a term that is reserved for incontinence in children. It is the involuntary passing of urine at night when asleep. The existence of incontinence during the day suggests a kidney or bladder condition. It is mainly a disorder found in boys and affects 10 per cent of boys aged 4-11 years. There are estimated to be 500,000 cases in Britain between the age of 6 and 16. As a group they also have signs of decreased muscle tone, co-ordination problems and EEG abnormalities. It is considered to be a sleep disorder and so is treated by the antidepressant, imipramine. This is an attempt to alter depth of sleep and has little effect. There is the added danger of poisoning by overdose as well as addiction due the effects on the psyche of long-term prescription.

Less harmful are behavioural methods such as an alarm bell. This is connected to a mat under the sheet so that the bell sounds if the child wets the bed. Intranasal desmopressin,[18] antidiuretic hormone, is used in some cases although the manipulation of pituitary hormones to treat bed-wetting seems a little excessive. Enuresis can be difficult to treat and is frequently related to psychological factors. It may be necessary to address the family as a whole as well as the individual child.

Holistic management

In terms of Chinese medicine, enuresis is to do with the function of the Kidney, Spleen, Lungs and Bladder. There may be Deficiency of Kidney Yang, weakness of Spleen Qi or an affection of the Lung in its function of dominating Water passages. This can be considered as either a Before Heaven Qi or an After Heaven Qi problem. If the Before Heaven Qi is imbalanced then it may be that a factor in the parents or during pregnancy is more important. If the After Heaven Qi is imbalanced then you may consider more environmental factors such as diet and emotional issues in the family. As with all conditions of childhood, there may be complex familial issues at play.

Case one

A boy of 6 years came for treatment of his bed-wetting and behavioural difficulties. He would wet the bed every night but this would stop when his behaviour was more difficult. On occasions, he would get very angry, aggressive, shout and kick. This would be worse after eating junk food. His bowels were usually loose, yellowish and explosive. He would generally have urinary urgency and frequency. I made a diagnosis of Spleen Qi Deficiency, Damp Accumulation and a Heart-Kidney imbalance. I treated him with Chinese herbs initially with good effect. Within a month he was only wetting the bed twice each week, his bowels were normal and he was somewhat calmer. He would still react after eating foods containing a lot of sugar or additives. He continued to improve with treatment and although he would have an occasional setback with a run of wet beds for a few days, he was generally dry. His behaviour settled and he is now a happy and normally boisterous 9 year old.

HYPERTENSION

This is raised blood pressure and is a common situation in the Western world. Blood pressure in the West and indeed many societies rises with age and this is a consequence of several factors regarding life-style. Excess intake of salt, stressful living patterns, being overweight, lack of exercise and the presence of chronic degenerative disease all contribute to what is seen as a 'normal' pattern of rising blood pressure. In traditional societies such as South Sea Islanders and some nomadic groups there is no such rise and the same level is maintained throughout life.[19]

In conventional thought, raised blood pressure is seen as leading to heart disease and stroke and so it is treated whenever it is diagnosed. Drugs are the mainstays of treatment. Treatment with drugs is considered to be for life.

The blood pressure reading consists of two figures (e.g. 120/80 mm Hg). The top figure relates to cardiac systole (i.e. when the heart contracts), the bottom figure to cardiac diastole (i.e. when the heart relaxes). The diastolic reading is the important one since this is the pressure when in a state of relaxation. If it is high for persistent periods of time it indicates a general heightened state of tension in the system.

Conventionally, hypertension is diagnosed if the blood pressure is consistently above 160/95 mm Hg although this would seem to be a low figure for someone over the age of 65 or 70 years. Mild hypertension is said to be 140/90 – 159/99 mm Hg, moderate is 160/100 – 179/110 mm Hg, severe is 180/110 – 209/119 mm Hg and crisis hypertension is said to be a systolic of more than 210 and or a diastolic of more than 120. The systolic pressure is less important in terms of diagnosing hypertension.[20]

Blood pressure varies with many factors and one reading means very little. It needs to be taken over several days and allowance made for factors such as exercise or stress. The correct size of cuff must be used for the size of the arm or false results will be obtained. Certainly, people can be monitored over 6 months before a final diagnosis of hypertension is made.

In conventional medicine, the majority of cases (90 per cent) have no known cause and this is known as primary or essential hypertension. There are relationships to stress levels,[21] genetic factors, being overweight, alcohol and salt intake. This explains why blood pressure levels are consistently higher in the West than in traditional cultures.

Secondary hypertension is where there is demonstrable disease of the kidneys (chronic glomerulonephritis and pyelonephritis, endocrine disorders such as Conn's syndrome and Cushing's syndrome, pre-eclamptic toxaemia of pregnancy) or an effect following prescribed drugs (female sex hormones, carbenoxolone, vasopressin and occasionally mono-amine oxidase inhibitor antidepressants when taken with cheese, wine or some other contraindicated food).

Symptoms

In conventional medicine, there are considered to be no symptoms unless the level of blood pressure is very high. This is not the whole story and many people take their medication only when they 'feel' their blood pressure is high. The exact symptom picture will vary with the individual but it is common to see headache, dizziness, tinnitus, and eye symptoms such as dry or red eyes, irritability or anger.

A severe variant is called malignant or accelerated hypertension. Malignant in this context indicates a progressive problem, not a cancerous process. If it is not treated then 90 per cent of this group die within one year. The levels of blood pressure are very high with severe headaches, red face and eyes, blurred vision, tremors, proteinuria and haematuria.

Complications[22]

These must be differentiated into those that are due to the long-term effects of raised blood pressure and those that may occur in the short-term due to the actual level of blood pressure at the time.

Complication	Symptoms to look for
Cardiac insufficiency	Palpitations, breathlessness, cough with pink frothy sputum, peripheral oedema
Accelerated or malignant hypertension	Very high blood pressure, blurred vision, red face, tremor, throbbing headaches
Cerebral haemorrhage (stroke)	There may the symptoms of accelerated hypertension prior to the event. Headaches, paralysis or weakness of limbs and face on one side of the body, loss of consciousness at the onset of the attack

Table 9.8: Short-term complications of hypertension

Complication	Symptoms to look for
Heart attack	Central chest pain radiating to the arm, palpitations, vomiting, pallor
Stroke	Paralysis or weakness of limbs and face on one side of the body
Peripheral arterial disease	Cramping pain in the calves on exertion relieved by rest, cold feet, absent or diminished pulses in the feet
End-stage kidney disease	Proteinuria, tiredness, loin pain, anorexia, nausea, vomiting (see above)

Table 9.9: Long-term complications of hypertension

Investigations

In general, there are no investigations performed if the level of raised blood pressure is slight, there is no previous history suggestive that this is a case of secondary hypertension and the age of the person is over 40 years. If the blood pressure responds easily to treatment this is confirmation that the diagnosis is almost certainly primary hypertension (i.e. of unknown cause).

Investigations will be performed in cases where it is suspected that there is an underlying cause. These include chest X-ray, ECG, urinalysis, serum cholesterol, urea and electrolytes.[23] Examination of the retina may show changes to the blood vessels typical of hypertension. These are graded into four levels indicating mild to severe damage.

Treatment

The mainstay of treatment is with drugs but there are some moves towards a more holistic approach.[24] Certainly there will be general advice about reducing excess weight, stopping smoking, taking of regular exercise and reducing salt and alcohol intake. Salt intake in the West is around 14 g per day, which is over four times the amount compatible with health. There is some debate about the level of 'healthy' drinking of alcohol and there is advice about how many units[25] of alcohol are safe. My personal view is that since alcohol is a toxin, any intake is potentially a problem but some people may benefit from the relaxing effects. Most trials involving the calculation of these amounts have come to the conclusion that moderate drinking protects against certain diseases. This does not take into account that some people do not drink alcohol because they are ill. The incidence of diseases related to drinking (such as cirrhosis of the liver and some psychological disorders) is directly related to the amount of alcohol drunk and the ease of availability in society.

An intake of alcohol less than 20 units for men and 13 units for women per week is considered to be without risk to health. Up to 36 units for men and 24 units for women per week is considered to be unlikely to lead to health problems. This seems to me to be a large amount that in my experience, needs to be reduced if people are to maintain their health. Thirty-six units of alcohol for a man translates to 18 pints of beer per week. This level of drinking is likely to damage the energy of the Spleen (digestion), Kidney and Liver.

The drugs used in the treatment of hypertension are summarised in Table 9.10. Combinations are commonly used in an attempt to reduce the incidence of side-effects and to increase the desired effect. The most common prescription seen is the combination of a diuretic and a betablocker. A vasodilator is added to these if there is an inadequate response. Other combinations are diuretic and ACE inhibitor, diuretic and centrally acting alpha agonist, diuretic and alpha-1 adrenergic blocker.

Treatment (mildest to strongest)	Comments
Diuretic	Please see Page 107
Hypotensive agent • Centrally acting alpha agonist, e.g. clonidine, methyldopa	Clonidine may also be used in lower doses for menopausal flushing and migraine. Sudden withdrawal may cause a marked rise in blood pressure. Methyldopa was introduced in the 1960s and is less commonly used now. It is particularly likely to cause postural hypotension.
Hypotensive agent • Calcium channel blocker • Betablocker	Please see Page 100
Angiotensin-converting enzyme (ACE) inhibitor	Please see Page 107
Vasodilator • Alpha-1 adrenergic blocker, e.g. prazosin, indoramin • Alpha and betablocker, e.g. labetalol	Please see Page 107

Table 9.10: Treatment of hypertension

Holistic management

In terms of Chinese medicine, there are several energetic diagnoses associated with hypertension. The usual syndromes are related to Kidney and Liver imbalances (Kidney Yin Deficiency with Liver Yang Rising is a common one). Others include less deficient syndromes such as Stagnation of Liver Qi and Liver Fire Blazing. Spleen Qi or Yang Deficiency with Damp Accumulation may also lead to high blood pressure.

The main groups of drugs are diuretics and hypotensive agents. Diuretics are cold in nature and make the Kidney let go of Yin (urine). Long-term they damage Kidney Qi and lead to Yin Deficiency. The predominant clinical picture will depend upon the original condition of the person and how long they have been taking the diuretics.

The hypotensive drugs in general can be considered to have similar effects to betablockers. They are an excellent example of this group and are discussed in detail in Chapter 7 – Cardiovascular system.

You can see from this that the effect on the person will depend upon the original condition. For example, if the cause of high blood pressure is Kidney Yin Deficiency with Liver Yang Rising, betablockers will reduce blood pressure as it destroys Yang. If, however, the cause of the problem is Spleen Qi Deficiency with Damp Accumulation, then betablockers will make the person ill. They may feel more tired, cold and lethargic. With knowledge of the energetics it is possible to understand the response to drugs.

Case one

A man of 55 years came for treatment. He had been diagnosed with high blood pressure some 10 years previously and had been on medication ever since. This consisted of:

- Labetalol 200 mg twice daily – alpha and betablocker
- Indapamide one daily – diuretic
- Allopurinol half a tablet daily – reduces uric acid levels in gout.

He had a past medical history of prostatitis, cystitis and gout. His highest blood pressure had been 170/125 mm Hg before he started his medication. He had low energy, irritability, and loose bowels when tired. In terms of Chinese medicine, his diagnosis was Spleen and Kidney Yang Deficiency with Damp-heat Accumulation. His past medical history revealed that the Damp-heat would collect in the bladder and prostate and occasionally flare-up in the big toe. Allopurinol in its side-effects can *cause* high blood pressure. There are frequently occasions when you study combinations of prescribed drugs you will see that they may interact or one drug may cause the original condition for which the person is receiving treatment.

He was very nervous about the prospect of reducing his tablets and it is important in such cases to wait until the person is happy to do so. They need to gain confidence in the treatment and the ability of his body to effect changes. I treated him for 10 months before he started to discuss the question of reduction. He was then keen to try.

It is essential that any reduction is slow and blood pressure is monitored during the process. His blood pressure on his initial visits had been 130/95 to 150/100 mm Hg. This settled over the months of treatment and was 120/80 mm Hg when he began to reduce his medication. He had stopped his allopurinol in the early weeks as it may cause high blood pressure.

He reduced his medication to 200 mg morning and 150 mg evening. This led to a rise in his blood pressure to 140/85 mm Hg. This is to be expected and it is important to wait for this to settle before continuing. He reduced his drugs by 50 mg a day each time it was appropriate and waited for things to settle down in between. After some months, he felt he had more energy and was generally well.

He continued to reduce his medication until 4 months later he was able to stop them completely. It takes several further months to gain the full benefit of being without them.

The main cause of this man's blood pressure was a busy, stressful job with a history of overwork. With the treatment and discussions about relaxation and exercise, he was able to become more balanced in himself and the need for his drugs became less.

There is no problem with reducing blood pressure medication so long as the following issues are considered:

- the person taking the drugs must be happy about drug reduction
- an initial improvement in the person's condition must be seen
- monitoring of blood pressure must be done
- any reduction should be slow
- wait for stabilisation before further reductions in dosage
- do not worry unless there is a rise of more than 30/20 mm Hg or symptoms such as headaches, blurred vision, red eyes, dizziness, tinnitus after a reduction.

Case two

This case illustrates the hazards of hypertensive drugs over a long period of time. A woman of 75 years came for treatment after a right-sided stroke some 3 months previously. She had some remaining weakness in her right arm and leg. She had suffered from palpitations for years. She was tired easily with little energy. Her appetite was poor. Her concentration and memory were poor. Her medication at that time was:

- atenolol 25 mg daily
- digoxin 0.2 mg daily
- aspirin 100 mg daily

I made a diagnosis of Heart and Kidney Yang Deficiency and treated her with acupuncture and Chinese herbs. The cause of her condition was the use of betablockers for the previous 10 years when she had been prescribed them for high blood pressure. She had been taking 100 mg of atenolol daily for all that time. With Chinese medical treatment, she slowly improved with increased levels of energy and increased appetite. She would occasionally develop palpitations but these gradually decreased in frequency and severity and eventually disappeared. Some 2 months after beginning treatment she saw a cardiologist who wanted her to take Warfarin (an anticoagulant) and powerful anti-arrhythmic drugs. She declined as her condition was improving and she did not want to repeat the difficulties she had run into before with prolonged medication.

It is now 2 years since her treatment began, she is generally well with no palpitations, good mobility and although she still has some memory and concentration difficulties, she lives alone and manages quite well. Such a case as this reveals the consequences of long-term treatment with anti-hypertensive medication. Although the blood pressure may be controlled, long-term there can only be deterioration of health and the occurrence of other, frequently more severe, disease.

KIDNEY STONES

Stones in the urinary system usually form in the kidney. They do not cause symptoms unless there is an associated inflammatory condition or they move into the ureter. Bladder stones were common in the 18th century. It was possible to earn a respectable living as a lithotomist – one who removes stones.

The stones are formed from the normal constituents of urine and usually occur first in the pelvis of the kidney. They may exist there for some time unnoticed and causing no symptoms. They are more likely in the following situations:

- hot climates where the urine is more concentrated
- high blood level of calcium, e.g. corticosteroid use, sarcoidosis, overconsumption of vitamin D
- excessive intake of calcium

- with infective conditions of the urinary system
- increased blood levels of uric acid (e.g. gout, leukaemia). Less than 5 per cent of kidney stones are of this type.

Symptoms

There are three consequences of stones in the kidney. Firstly, they may be asymptomatic. Stones do not lead to symptoms unless they move or if there is associated inflammation.

Secondly, the person may pass small amounts of 'gravel', which cause some pain for a brief period of time. The pain will be a much milder form of classic renal colic described below.

Thirdly, there may be severe symptoms of renal colic (also known as ureteric colic), which are due to spasms in the ureter as the stone is passing through the urinary system. The pain begins in the loin on the affected side and radiates round and down into the groin. It may also be felt in the thigh to the knee. The pain may come and go for several hours or days. Associated symptoms occur such as restlessness, vomiting, sweating and pallor. The stone may be small enough to be passed in the urine when there may be dysuria. Blood in the urine is common although it may only be discovered on urine testing.

Some people have stones, which grow so big that they cannot pass into the ureter. These are usually associated with chronic urinary tract infections such as pyelonephritis. The stones act as a focus for organisms to live and organisms provide a focus around which stones form. There may be associated infection in some and so there will be the added symptoms of fever, chills, dysuria, and cloudy and strong smelling urine.

Investigations

Urinalysis shows blood, protein, and pus cells. Cystoscopy may be performed to enable catheterisation of the affected ureter to attempt removal of a blocked stone. Plain X-ray reveals the stone in 90 per cent of cases as it usually contains calcium. Intravenous pyelogram will detect any blockage to urine flow.

Complications

Complication	Symptoms to look for
Acute pyelonephritis	Loin pain, fever, dysuria, frequent urination
Obstruction to urine flow in affected ureter	Increasing fever, severe pain in the loin, the person is ill

Table 9.11: Complications of renal stones

Treatment

The person with kidney stones is advised to drink large amounts of fluid – in the order of 3 litres per day. Avoidance of calcium rich foods is recommended in cases due to excess calcium levels. Any infection will be treated with antibiotics.

Surgical treatment is reserved for those situations where the stone is too big to pass and is associated with chronic infection. In some, a stone is small enough to pass into the ureter but too large to complete its passage into the bladder. This situation may lead to urinary obstruction in the affected ureter with potentially dangerous consequences for the kidney.

Stones may be removed using a cystoscope, through an incision over the kidney (percutaneous nephroscopy) or by breaking them up using ultrasound (extracorporeal shock-wave lithotripsy). The latter situation is the most helpful because it is much less invasive and holistic treatment can be administered to prevent a recurrence.

Holistic management

The acute picture of renal colic will almost always be treated in hospital because of the degree of pain. The chronic condition is amenable to constitutional treatment by holistic medicine. If removal of the stone is required then breaking by ultrasound (see above) is the preferable method. Most people have no demonstrable biochemical abnormality, so there is no conventional advice that is clearly and logically indicated.

In terms of Chinese medicine, this condition usually corresponds to long-term Dampness and Heat, which forms a stone from body fluids. This may obstruct the flow of Qi and interfere with urine flow.

CANCER OF THE KIDNEY

This makes up 10 per cent of all cases of cancer. There are several types but the commonest is termed renal cell carcinoma.

Symptoms

The classical presentation is of haematuria, loin pain and a palpable abdominal swelling but this is only seen in 20 per cent of cases. In 60 per cent, there is only haematuria. Painless haematuria must always be taken seriously

Investigations

Performing intravenous urography, computerised axial tomography and ultrasound makes the diagnosis.

Treatment

At the time of diagnosis, 50 per cent of people with cancer of the kidney have evidence of spread to local or distant sites. Secondaries occur in the adrenal glands, lymph glands, lung and long bones. The comments I made in Chapter 6 – Cancer with regard to treatment are relevant here.

CANCER OF THE BLADDER

This is twice as common in men. It presents with similar symptoms to cancer of the kidney.

Symptoms

The main presentation is of haematuria, frequency of urination and dysuria without evidence of infecting organisms. These symptoms reflect a degree of bladder irritation from the cancer. The cancer takes the form of warty growths on the bladder lining. They tend to be localised and grow slowly in 80 per cent of cases. If there is distant spread then this tends to be to the lymph nodes, lung and bone.

Investigations

Cystoscopy and biopsy make the diagnosis. Computerised axial tomography of the chest and abdomen together with bone scans are an integral part of the staging process.

Treatment

This is by local removal via cystoscopy with regular check-ups. If there is recurrence, intra-bladder chemotherapy washouts will be used.

Case one

A man of 57 years came for treatment with exhaustion and general lassitude. He had been diagnosed with high blood pressure some years before and was on regular medication. He had an episode of haematuria some 6 months before attending the clinic that had been diagnosed by cystoscopy as a bladder tumour. He had had several cystoscopies since then at intervals of 1 month or 6 weeks. Each time he had some bladder tumours excised but they would grow back by the next time. He was due to a cystocopy 6 weeks later and he wanted to have treatment to help him prepare. His surgeon had told him that he would almost certainly need a partial cystectomy (bladder removal), which would necessitate restructuring the ureteric opening into the bladder. This is fairly major surgery and would necessitate a stay in hospital of some 4 weeks.

I made a diagnosis of Kidney Yin Deficiency with Liver Yang Rising and treated him with acupuncture and Chinese herbs. He made a good response and felt generally better with more energy. He felt emotionally much stronger and less bothered by stressful events. After the 6 weeks of treatment he had a repeat cystoscopy fully expecting to wake up from the operation with various tubes attached to him. His surgeon told him that his bladder was the best he had ever seen it and he only had needed to cauterise a small area of tumour growth. His treatment continues and he will have further check cystoscopies but at much longer intervals than previously.

MALE GENITAL DISORDERS

Benign enlargement of the prostate

This is more common over the age of 60 years and is rare before 40 years. The prostate gland enlarges which obstructs the flow of urine as it leaves the bladder. The cause is unknown in conventional medicine but it is noticed that it is rarer in those of African or Asian races and never seen in eunuchs. Despite this latter situation, I have never known removal of the testes to be advocated as a preventative measure! This is surprising when one considers the suggested treatments of gynaecological symptoms and breast cancer.

Symptoms

The classic clinical features are those of urinary outflow obstruction. They are frequency of urination, difficulty in beginning to urinate, nocturia, urgency, poor urinary stream and dribbling at the end of urination. People may develop acute retention of urine. Treatment with diuretics may precipitate this event.

Some people may have impaired kidney function and there will the signs and symptoms of chronic kidney disease with anaemia.

Differential diagnosis

There are several causes of obstruction to the flow of urine and they include:

- cancer of the prostate (see below)
- urethral narrowing due to gonorrhoea (stricture)
- neurological disorders – see Chapter 14 – Central Nervous System (especially multiple sclerosis, intervertebral disc prolapse).

Investigations

Rectal examination is performed to feel the size and shape of the prostate. A benign enlargement is smooth. Urine culture is done to determine if urinary infection is present. Kidney function tests of serum urea and creatinine give an idea of renal function. Further tests of the kidney include plain X-ray and ultrasound. Cystoscopy is always done. The main aim of these investigations is to determine if there is damage to the upper urinary tracts by the backpressure of urine as a result of the obstruction to flow. Blood test for serum urea, creatinine and prostate-specific antigen are performed as the latter is raised in cases of prostatic cancer.

Treatment

The primary treatment is by the operation of prostatectomy, which is done either via a urethral or abdominal approach. The former is the more common one as it has a lower mortality rate, results in less ill health post-operatively and hospital stays are shorter. It is common for people to have bowel difficulties that are long-term and take the form of a weakness in evacuation.

In terms of Chinese medicine there are several syndromes that may be seen. The most common ones are Deficiency of the Spleen and Kidney and Damp-heat Accumulation in the Lower Jiao.

Cancer of the prostate

This makes up 7 per cent of all cancer in men. The incidence of prostatic cancer increases with age until at the age of 80 some 80 per cent of men have evidence of some malignant cells in the prostate. Most of these are minor and only discovered by chance or at post-mortem examination.

Symptoms

The symptoms are similar to those for benign enlargement of the prostate, which are detailed above. However, since the underlying process is malignant the symptoms appear more quickly and are progressive over a period of weeks and months.

The cancer spreads to lymph glands, pelvis, lumbar spine, femur, thoracic spine, ribs, lung and liver in decreasing order of frequency.

Investigations

These are the same as performed in benign enlargement with the addition of a transrectal ultrasound and a needle biopsy of the prostate. On rectal examination there is a hard, irregular prostate. An ultrasound scan can reveal the size of the prostatic enlargement. A biopsy will be performed to determine the exact nature of the cells and to confirm malignancy. If secondaries are present the serum acid phosphatase level will be increased. Isotope bone scans and X-rays of bone may be performed to detect secondaries. Prostate-specific antigen levels in the blood are raised.

Treatment

Prostatectomy is performed if the cancer has not spread. If secondaries are present the testes will be removed (orchidectomy) combined with hormonal treatment. This is by means of oestrogens or antiandrogens.

Case one

A man of 69 years came for treatment of his prostatic cancer. He had a Prostatic Specific Antigen (PSA) test in the early 1990s at a level of 8.2. He had a needle biopsy of the prostate that showed cancer of the prostate in one small section. He was advised to have a radical prostatectomy, which he declined and he pursued a holistic method of treatment primarily with homoeopathy. When I saw him, his symptoms were not progressing but neither were they subsiding. He had nocturia five times each night, urgency, dribbling urination, frequent urination during the day and the need to return to pass urine fairly soon after urinating. He had continual phlegm in his throat and had a tendency to sticky discharges from his ears and nose. His energy was generally low. I made a diagnosis of Kidney Yang Deficiency and Damp-heat Accumulation and treated him with acupuncture and Chinese herbs.

Progress was slow and although sometimes he would feel generally better, his urinary symptoms would remain the same. After 6 months or so of treatment he said, 'I have not felt this well in ages'. His sticky discharges are beginning to ameliorate and his treatment continues.

Orchitis

This is inflammation of the testis and is mainly secondary to mumps in post-pubertal men. It rarely leads to sterility and it never interferes with sexual function.

Symptoms
There is the onset of fever with chills, headache and lower abdominal pain. The affected testis is painful and tender. The symptoms subside after 5 days.

Treatment
Cases resolve spontaneously and so analgesics are the only treatment required.

Epididymitis

This is inflammation of the epididymis. It is almost invariably a consequence of an infection in the urinary tract and this may be gonorrhoea or non-specific urethritis. There may be associated cystitis or prostatitis.

Symptoms
There is pain and swelling of the affected side with redness of the overlying scrotum. There is malaise and low grade fever.

Treatment
This is invariably with antibiotics although it is a chronic disease, and like prostatitis, relapses easily.

Torsion of the testis

This is twisting of the testis within the scrotum. It is serious because the blood supply to the testis is obstructed.

Symptoms
It occurs in males under the age of 18 years. There is an extremely rapid onset of severe pain in the affected testis, which becomes swollen. The symptoms rapidly worsen. There may be previous episodes of testicular pain.

Treatment
This is a surgical emergency and if the problem is not corrected within 4 hours the testis dies.

Impotence

This is an inability of the penis to become erect and this can be total or partial. Conventionally, it is divided into organic (i.e. structural causes) and functional (i.e. psychological causes). In practice, there is often a combination of influences with few cases due to purely physical disease.

It may occur due to disease of the nervous system (secondary to diabetes mellitus or a spinal cord problem) and severe endocrine disease (such as under- or overactivity of the thyroid gland). The other thing to consider is peripheral arterial disease leading to poor blood circulation in the lower part of the body. All these situations are rare but may be blamed as an acceptable physical reason. This commonly tends to be true for conditions in men where emotional factors may be difficult to face.

Psychological factors are extremely important and there is often the added issue of 'performance anxiety' where the man worries whether he can produce an erection at the appropriate time. Erections during sleep would seem to confirm that the problem is psychological rather than physical.

A common situation is the effect of prescribed drugs, which may cause impotence. Alcohol and cannabis are the well-known 'recreational' drugs that lead to inability to produce an erection. The prescribed drugs that may do this are included in Table 9.12.

Areas affected	Drugs
Cardiovascular system	Betablockers, diuretics, adrenergic neurone blockers, vasodilators
Psychological	Lithium, phenothiazines, opiates, benzodiazepines, barbiturates, antidepressants
Central nervous system	Anticholinergics, anti-Parkinsonism drug
Immune system	Cancer chemotherapy, immunosuppressants
Gastrointestinal system	Cimetidine/ranitidine

Table 9.12: Drugs causing impotence

In terms of Chinese medicine, impotence usually corresponds to Kidney Yang Deficiency with or without damage to the Qi of the Heart and Spleen.

Premature ejaculation

This is very common and probably more common than generally realised. It is difficult to define but is ejaculation by the male before the 'appropriate' time. Kinsey in his well-documented report on sexual matters in the USA reported that 75 per cent of men ejaculate within 2 minutes of penile insertion. In severe cases of premature ejaculation, it can occur before insertion of the penis. It is very much seen as due to psychological factors. These must be addressed if there is to be any improvement in the symptom.

In terms of Chinese medicine, this symptom is seen as part of the picture of Deficient Yin and Excess of Yang, Sinking of Qi, or Disharmony between Kidney and Heart. The principle here is that there is an excess of Yang compared to Yin so that the fluid of semen is lost prematurely.

Infertility

Male factors in infertility are discussed together with female factors in Chapter 18 – Women's Health.

REVIEW OF SYMPTOMS

Pain

Pain in the loin or low back pain is a common indicator of kidney disease. Conventional medical texts often consider low back pain to be a condition of the back whereas energetic medicine may see this as a Kidney imbalance. In my experience, virtually all cases of chronic low back pain are associated with a weakness of Kidney energy and treating only the back will not lead to long-term relief.

Ureteric pain is felt radiating from the loin round to the inguinal region and sometimes into the thigh to the knee. This is in the distribution of the first and second lumbar nerves.

Urinary disturbances

Frequency may be seen during the day, or if at night is known as nocturia. It can be an early symptom of many urinary conditions or of systemic conditions such as diabetes (mellitus or insipidus).

The normal urinary volume is 800-2400 ml in 24 hours. It varies according to intake and other losses such as sweat and respiration. Polyuria is an increased urine volume and is not necessarily the same as urinary frequency, which is passing urine more often.

Dysuria is used to describe pain or discomfort when urinating. This can be felt either in the bladder (in cystitis) or in the urethra. It may be severe with gonorrhoea.

Urinary disturbances such as urgency, frequency, poor flow, terminal dribbling are due to obstruction to the flow of urine and implies a problem with the urethra, bladder neck or prostate in men.

Haematuria

This is blood in the urine and the precise colour depends upon the amount of blood present. A trace of blood will not be apparent in the urine unless urinalysis is performed. Larger amounts may be seen as a smoky appearance in the urine and eventually reddish urine occurs. Blood in the urine at the beginning of urination indicates that the source is distal to the bladder; blood mixed with urine indicates the source is any part other than the urethra.

Oedema

Swelling of the tissues by fluid was discussed in Chapter 7 – Cardiovascular System. Kidney disease may lead to oedema, which is typically seen in the eyelids and upper part of the body although eventually it will be widespread.

HOW TO RECOGNISE A SERIOUS CONDITION OF THE URINARY SYSTEM

It is important to know how to recognise if a symptom arises from a serious situation. Use Table 9.13 as a guide to refer to when faced with a person who has one or more of these symptoms. I make no mention of disease labels in the column on the right, as I would not expect you to be able to diagnose conventionally. Seriousness can be assessed merely by reference to symptom pictures.

Symptom	Comments
Pain in loin	Severe
Pain in abdomen	Severe Persistent With abdominal rigidity With guarding With rebound tenderness
Pain in urethra	Not serious
Anuria	Always
Oliguria	Severe Persistent Without clear reason such as hot climate, decreased fluid intake
Haematuria	Painless
Enuresis	Severe especially if with incontinence in the day
Frequent urination	Severe Progressive Short history
Dribbling	Severe Progressive Short history
Urgency	Severe Progressive Short history
Pain in the testis	Rapid onset of severe pain under the age of 18 years
Swelling of the testis	Progressive No signs/symptoms of a urinary tract infection[26]

Table 9.13: How to recognise serious conditions in urinary system disease

SUMMARY

The conventional view of the kidney is of a physical sieve.

The holistic view of the kidney as revealed by the insights of Chinese medicine is that is it the root of energy for the other organs in the body. The strength of the kidneys is very important in health and connected to vital aspects of life such as constitution, longevity and reproduction.

Many people have symptoms of kidney disease but are not so severely affected that disease labels such pyelonephritis or glomerulonephritis can be applied.

[1] All organs which are capitalised, e.g. Blood, Heart, Kidney indicate that I mean the energetic view of that organ and not the narrowly defined physical structure of Western science.

[2] It is interesting that the conventional classification of kidney keeps changing and there are many aspects of physiology which are still not understood. This is a reflection of the nature of the kidneys. They are hidden from view and are the deepest level of the physical body.

[3] An excellent source for information about the energetic organ systems of Chinese medicine is *Between Heaven and Earth* by Beinfield and Korngold (Ballantine, 1992). I mention the main points here to perhaps shed some light on a wider view of the organs. Homoeopaths may recognise remedy pictures in these descriptions as these are merely another way of describing the same energetic entity.

[4] There are several homoeopathic materia medicas available including *Materia Medica of Homoeopathic Medicines* by S R Phatak (Foxlee Vaughan, 1988). Medorrhinum is the remedy made from cases of gonorrhoea and may be indicated in cases of suppressed gonorrhoea. This may manifest as an infection in the person or there may be an indication of this particular susceptibility in the family history.

[5] Frans Vermeulen's *Concordant Materia Medica*.

[6] *Davies Textbook of Adverse Drug Reactions',* Edited by DM Davies (Edward Arnold, 1998).

[7] The term 'proliferative' applies to the cellular changes seen in the kidney cells. These changes are usually related to the nephritic syndrome but may cause nephrotic syndrome (see after). Whatever the term used for cellular changes, it is the clinical syndrome which is important.

[8] This is the conventional description although there may be a continuance of dysfunction in some.

[9] *Cecil Textbook of Medicine,* Edited by Russell L Cecil, J Claude Bennett and Lee Goldman (W.B. Saunders, 2000).

[10] The terms 'membranous' and 'minimal lesion' apply to the cellular changes seen in the kidney cells. These changes are usually, but not always, related to the nephrotic syndrome. Whatever the term used for cellular changes, it is the clinical syndrome which is important.

[11] In some it may be as part of an autoimmune disease (see Chapter 10 – Musculoskeletal system), diabetes mellitus, prescribed drugs (see Table 9.7), industrial metals such as mercury and cadmium or allergic reactions.

[12] Energetically, the Small Intestine is paired with the Heart and is at the same level as the Urinary Bladder, and so anxiety and worry may lead to the symptoms of cystitis via this connection.

[13] Although the symptoms may arise from the bladder or prostate, for example, this whole area is governed energetically by the function of the Kidney.

[14] For students of Chinese medicine it is necessary here to clarify my meaning. White sugar is Cold in energy and leads to the generation of Heat because the Cold causes Stagnation. This is more so in those with strong Qi. Brown sugar and malted products are Warm in nature and so lead to less problems although excess sweet taste from any source tends to deplete Spleen (digestive) energy.

[15] You may have heard comments from folk medicine of not walking in bare feet on a cold floor otherwise 'you will get a chill in your kidneys'. This is because the Kidney channel starts in the sole of the foot and cold can penetrate to travel up to the Kidneys.

[16] Sexual activity is not necessarily or inherently depleting of Kidney energy. There are methods for men and women of conserving energies during sexual intercourse. This belongs to the tantric aspect of spiritual traditions such as Buddhism, Hinduism and Taoism. The aim is to use the energy generated during sexual practice for higher spiritual practices. At the level of health, information about techniques in what could be called sexual yoga of the Chinese tradition can be found in the books of Mantak Chia. There are several including *Taoist Secrets of Love – Cultivating Male Sexual Energy* (Aurora, 1984).

[17] These are the organs in the lower part of the body and include the large intestine, bladder, prostate and the reproductive organs of the male and female.

[18] In clinical trials only 31 per cent of children are dry on such treatment. This is little better than placebo.

[19] A survey over 20 years of the blood pressure of nuns in a secluded monastic order revealed that their blood pressure did not change. This was in contradistinction to a control group whose blood pressure increased. *Hypertension* 1988;12(4):457-61.

[20] The systolic figure is roughly 100 plus the person's age.

[21] It has been noted that the current level of blood pressure and the risk of high blood pressure are strongly related to the weight at birth and the weight of the placenta. This was a survey done in Preston, England. *BMJ* 1990;301:259-62.

[22] It is stated that the treatment of blood pressure leads to a reduction in problems later. Numerous trials have shown that such treatment is beneficial but only in terms of stroke. There is no change in mortality reduction from all causes and as conventional medical textbooks state, '... a very large number of people have to face the inconvenience, risks and side-effects of treatment to save one life.'

[23] Urea and electrolytes (U and E's) is a common preliminary blood test to check on renal function and to monitor treatment such as diuretic therapy. The electrolytes include chloride, bicarbonate, sodium and potassium.

[24] There have been trials showing that non-pharmacological methods have a role to play in treating hypertension. These have not filtered into routine practice because they do not fit easily into the conventional medical model.

A trial using a type of Buddhist meditation (Dhammakaya) led to a reduction in serum cortisol, increases in serum total protein and reductions in blood pressure and heart rate. *Physiol-Behav* 1991;50(3):543-8.

Another paper describes the non-drug measures for the treatment of hypertension and the existence of many well-controlled studies. It makes the point that if these are used widely then there may well be a fall in the incidence of complications from hypertension and halt the progression to moderate or severe hypertension. *Cardiovasc-Drugs-They* 1989;3(6):847-52.

[25] One unit is half a pint of average strength beer, a single UK measure of spirits, one glass of sherry or one glass of wine. One unit contains the equivalent of 8 g of absolute alcohol.

[26] This is the presentation of cancer of the testis.

10 MUSCULOSKELETAL SYSTEM

INTRODUCTION

The musculoskeletal system is responsible for movement and structure. Hierarchically, it is deeper than the skin yet more superficial than the organs. An important proviso is that some conditions of the musculoskeletal system are generalised in nature and reflect deep internal disturbances. These are the autoimmune diseases.

Autoimmune diseases are characterised by the presence of antibodies attacking the body's own tissues. There are many and varied types including those discussed here. Others include diabetes mellitus, Addison's disease, thyroid disease and pernicious anaemia. In terms of seriousness, these disorders indicate a deep imbalance in the body. The blood is disturbed[1] (as revealed by the presence of antibodies), the body is attacking itself and the diseases affect deep, internal organs as well as the surface of the body. Autoimmune diseases are becoming more common, which is an indication of the worsening health of the general population.

It is interesting here to consider diseases of this type in relation to other disturbances of the immune system (in its narrower conventional sense, i.e. disturbances on the level of the antigen-antibody).

Disease	Comments
Allergy, e.g. hay fever, asthma	Over-reaction to an external factor, e.g. pollen, dust
Autoimmune diseases	Over-reaction to an internal factor, e.g. kidney tissue in glomerulonephritis, connective tissue in rheumatoid arthritis
Cancer	Lack of reactivity to abnormal cells leading eventually to their appearance as tumours
AIDS	Complete collapse of the immune system resulting in severe infections by organisms not normally pathogenic

Table 10.1: Disturbances of the immune system

Whenever a system is imbalanced, the first reaction is overproduction or over-activity. As the energy in the system declines there is replacement of over-reaction by exhaustion. An example of this is thyroid disease. The first signs of disease are of hyperthyroidism. After some years, with or without treatment, the natural history of the disease is for hypothyroidism to become evident. In Table 10.1, allergy and autoimmune disease represent over-activity. These are situations where the immune system is too active. It fiercely attacks external or internal factors. It is clearly more harmful to attack internal tissues and so the autoimmune diseases represent a more serious threat than allergic responses.

If a person's energy is more imbalanced and correspondingly weaker, there is not enough energy to produce strong reactions. Cancer is where abnormal cells, which are constantly being produced in healthy people, are not recognised as such. They grow to produce detectable tumours. AIDS is the end-state where there is no reactivity and strange organisms invade with little or no response. Interestingly, when people with cancer become healthier, they may notice symptoms such as joint swelling and stiffness suggestive of an inflammatory arthritis. Allergic reactions also develop.

In Chinese medicine, the Blood is considered to be responsible for moistening, cooling and the nourishment of muscles and joints. Damage to the Blood may be manifest by symptoms such as muscle pain, stiffness, joint swelling and pain which may be labelled arthritis by a conventional practitioner. It has been known for many years that overuse of a joint and injury may lead to the development of osteoarthritis. Recently, it has been observed that over-exercise, particularly to extreme by athletes, results in impaired functioning of the immune system, increased susceptibility to viral infections and general symptoms of debility. There is a close relationship between emotions and Blood –see Page 110. Stressful activity, overwork, worry and emotional turmoil all contribute to harming the Blood and to the development of autoimmune disorders. Meditation and relaxation are powerful methods to improve immune system function.[2] Similarly, excessive muscular activity (particularly when associated with sweating) will increase the risk of Blood disturbances and the appearance of musculoskeletal diseases.

The common symptoms of disease of this system include pains, stiffness and swelling in the joints and muscles, weakness of the muscles, muscle wasting (in severe cases) and joint deformities. They are extremely common, especially in climates that are cold and damp. They make up a significant proportion of the workload of a holistic medicine clinic.

ANATOMY AND PHYSIOLOGY

There are several facts of anatomy and physiology that it is useful to know. I consider that most courses in these subjects are over detailed and reflect orthodox thinking rather than the particular needs of the holistic practitioner. To study disease of the musculoskeletal system it would be helpful to be able to:

- list the structures comprising the musculoskeletal system
- describe the functions of the musculoskeletal system
- discuss the mechanism of muscular contraction and its relationship to nervous tissue.

CLASSIFICATION OF MUSCULOSKELETAL DISEASE

The important differentiations are based upon the clinical picture. In musculoskeletal diseases this is between those where inflammation is a predominant feature and those where it is not –Table 10.2.

Inflammatory	Non-inflammatory[3]
Autoimmune disease • Rheumatoid arthritis • Systemic lupus erythematosus • Polyarteritis nodosa • Scleroderma • Ankylosing spondylitis • Systemic sclerosis • Dermatomyositis • Polymyalgia rheumatica Gout	Osteoarthritis Other musculoskeletal conditions • Tennis elbow/golfer's elbow • Bursitis • Nerve compression • Repetitive strain injury • Frozen shoulder

Table 10.2: Classification of musculoskeletal disease

AUTOIMMUNE DISEASES

This term is applied to a group of diseases where the immune system attacks the body's own tissues. The site of the symptoms determines the name of the disease. This section considers those diseases that affect the musculoskeletal system.[4]

There are several autoimmune disorders listed and I discuss treatment of them all in the section dealing with rheumatoid arthritis rather than unnecessarily repeat information. The treatments of the autoimmune disorders are similar except that in diseases other than rheumatoid arthritis, corticosteroids are used early and in very high dosages. I have summarised holistic management at the end of this section and my comments can be applied equally to all similar diseases.

Rheumatoid arthritis

This is a chronic, inflammatory, destructive and deforming polyarthritis. It is systemic in nature and affects a wide range of tissues. It affects 3 per cent of people in the West and three times more women than men. It usually begins at about 30-40 years of age. It is worse in damp and cold climates. The cause is unknown according to conventional medicine although an autoimmune process is recognised. There is often a search for an infective origin and this idea recurs from time to time.

Symptoms
There are pains in the joints, which often feel hot and are stiff and swollen. There are the classic appearances of inflammation – pain, redness, swelling, heat and loss of function.

Pain is brought on by movement, initially, then appears after resting. Early morning joint stiffness occurs later. The main joints affected are the small joints of fingers and toes particularly the proximal interphalangeal and metacarpophalangeal joints of the hands and the equivalent joints in the feet. The distal interphalangeal joints are not usually involved. Other joints affected are the wrists, elbows, shoulders, knees and ankles. The hip is involved in severe cases. Pain and stiffness are common in the neck and there may be symptoms in the temporomandibular and sternoclavicular joints.

There is a progression of pain, muscle spasm and joint destruction. Muscle pain is widespread with weakness and wasting. Common symptoms in the extremities are weakness, tingling and numbness as a result of a combination of nerve entrapment, tendonitis and inflammation of the nerves themselves. As the inflammatory process increasingly affects the tendons, they may rupture adding to the deformity and disability. Eventually there is joint instability, limited joint movement and deformities. Subcutaneous nodules occur in 20 per cent of people, mainly at pressure sites such as the elbow around the olecranon.

Rheumatoid arthritis is a generalised disease and there is anorexia, weight loss and lethargy. The lymph glands are enlarged generally. Raynaud's phenomenon is common. The eyes may be dry and red and secretions in general are reduced. There may be dry mouth. Sjögren's syndrome is the term applied to such symptoms. Bone density decreases and osteoporosis may become evident on X-ray or bone scan. The blood shows evidence of anaemia, which is of the type seen in chronic disease.

Prognosis

After 10 years of the disease the following are seen:

* complete remission – 25 per cent
* moderately impaired – 40 per cent
* severely disabled – 25 per cent
* severely crippled – 10 per cent.

These figures show the severity of the disease but remember that it is the conventional prognosis. If people are seen early and treated effectively by means of holistic medicine, the prognosis will be less serious.

Investigations

The diagnosis is usually clinically obvious but blood tests will be used to support this. Rheumatoid factor is found in 70 per cent of people with rheumatoid arthritis. It is interesting to note that rheumatoid factor may also be found in people with no evidence of joint problems. A full blood count will reveal anaemia. X-rays will show joint destruction in the later stages of the disease.

Treatment

There is no cure in terms of conventional medicine. The aim is to reduce, as much as possible, the degree of inflammation in the hope that this minimises the long-term damage. This is attempted by means of drugs – see Table 10.3. If the inflammatory process fails to be controlled with aspirin or non-steroidal anti-inflammatory agents then more powerful agents are used. All of these take between 6 weeks and 6 months to act and produce their full effect. The prescribing practitioner should monitor their use closely.

In the acute phase the person is told to rest and the joints may be splinted. Physiotherapy is initiated once the inflammation has subsided. This is to help preserve muscle strength and bulk.

Treatment (mildest to strongest)	Comments
Aspirin	Aspirin is the drug of choice to treat inflammation but only 50 per cent of people can tolerate it because of the side-effects. It is given in high dosage of two tablets every 4-6 hours
Non-steroidal anti-inflammatory agents	Non-steroidal anti-inflammatory agents are related to aspirin and are commonly prescribed for all types of joint pains. They are acidic in nature, (as is aspirin) and all have similar side-effects. They burn the stomach leading to indigestion, poor appetite, nausea and vomiting. In severe cases they may cause upper gastrointestinal tract bleeding. There are several people who die each year from such problems. This whole group of drugs is widely used for rheumatoid arthritis and for any general musculoskeletal problem even where there is little or no evidence of inflammation
Sulphasalazine	Sulphasalazine is a combination of aspirin and a sulphonamide antibiotic. It is also used in the treatment of ulcerative colitis. It may lead to blood disorders including agranulocytosis, aplastic anaemia, anaemia, leucopenia and thrombocytopenia
Gold	Gold is one of the few treatments to survive from the alchemical days of medicine. Its use continues whilst the use of substances such as mercury, lead and arsenic has lapsed. It is given either orally or injected and it takes several months for any alteration in symptoms to take place. It may cause kidney damage
Chloroquine	Chloroquine is a derivative of quinine – the malarial treatment. It may damage the eyes when used for long periods of time. It is less commonly used than the others in this group
Penicillamine	Penicillamine may lead to kidney damage or autoimmune diseases such as systemic lupus erythematosus and myasthenia gravis
Corticosteroids	Corticosteroids are frequently given for this disease. They relieve symptoms by reducing inflammation yet do nothing to the underlying cause, which is, in any case, unknown in conventional medicine. A common formulation is prednisolone for all the autoimmune diseases. The dosage[5] of prednisolone may be defined as: • low dose – 1 mg daily • medium dose – 5 mg daily • high dose – 10 mg or more daily In acute disease, particularly with systemic lupus erythematosus or polyarteritis nodosa, 100 mg daily may be given in the early stages. This is reduced as the symptoms are controlled but long-term administration of 10 mg or more daily is not unusual. They are powerful drugs and physiologically arise from the adrenal glands. They suppress adrenal activity. With long-term use, sudden withdrawal is dangerous, as the adrenal glands will not be able to supply sufficient corticosteroids to maintain life – see Addison's disease. It is considered that reduction must take place at a rate of no more than 1 mg per month. Therefore, if someone is taking 10 mg per day it may take almost one year to get them off prednisolone, provided that there are no large flare-ups to contend with. In practice, it can be quicker than this but care is needed because the adrenal glands have to recover their function
Immunosuppressants	These are used for severe cases where corticosteroids fail to control the symptoms. They are powerful in their effects and suppress the immune system in the same way as chemotherapy treatment for cancer. Such drugs include azathioprine, cyclophosphamide and cyclosporin. A more commonly used drug of this type is methotrexate which may become the next drug of choice amongst rheumatologists. Side-effects are severe and include liver damage, cirrhosis, damage to bone marrow and thence to production of white blood cells and platelets and pneumonitis which can be fatal

Table 10.3: Drugs used in the treatment of rheumatoid arthritis

Surgery is used in several situations. In the acute phase, the synovial membrane may be removed (synovectomy) from the joint. This is only done if the disease is unresponsive to drugs. In the later stages of the disease, joint replacement may be an option for the hips, knees, elbows and fingers. Of these, the hip is the most amenable to replacement.

Rehabilitation has a major place to play in the conventional treatment of rheumatoid arthritis. Many people have great problems with joints after some years of the disease. Modification of the home, the use of walking aids and specially designed tools all have a part to play in easing difficulties with mobility.

Systemic lupus erythematosus (SLE)

This is a systemic disease, which affects most of the connective tissue of the whole body. It is particularly common in the US and Far East. Women are affected nine times more than men and it usually first presents in teenage years or the twenties. There may be a history of migraine and depression.

Symptoms
The initial presentation is of fever with joint pain, swelling, redness and heat. Malaise and tiredness is marked. It may be indistinguishable from an acute onset of rheumatoid arthritis. It is common for the skin to be affected. There is redness of the face and cheeks in a butterfly distribution. Urticaria, sensitivity to light and purpuric spots may all be seen. Alopecia is present in over 50 per cent of cases. There may be psychological symptoms such as depression or even dementia.

Systemic symptoms such as anorexia and weight loss are common. Multiple organ systems are involved – Table 10.4. The presence of kidney disease indicates the worst prognosis.

Organ involved/disease	Symptoms to look for
Raynaud's phenomenon	Coldness of fingers and hands, precipitated by cold, classic appearance of whiteness, blueness and then redness
Pericarditis	Sharp chest pain, palpitations
Pleurisy	Sharp axillary or scapular chest pain worse for breathing
Myocarditis	Chest pain, palpitations, tiredness
Pneumonitis	Cough, breathlessness
Glomerulonephritis (present in over half)	Loin pain, oedema, high blood pressure

Table 10.4: Associated symptoms of systemic lupus erythematosus

Investigations
The ESR is typically very high. Rheumatoid factor is positive in 50 per cent of cases. Kidney biopsy reveals a typical appearance.

Treatment
Corticosteroids are given to damp down the immune reaction especially in the acute phase. Aspirin and non-steroidal anti-inflammatory agents are given for symptomatic relief. These drugs may cause skin sensitivity to light, which is one of the symptoms of the original disease. In severe cases immunosuppressants may be used.

About 5 per cent of people with SLE die within 5 years of diagnosis. For most people there is a chronic course of symptoms that come and go, but are usually present. They are controlled by corticosteroids to a variable degree but side-effects are universal because of the dosages employed. There is less joint destruction than occurs in rheumatoid arthritis.

Polyarteritis nodosa

This usually affects middle-aged men and is uncommon. There is widespread involvement of small arteries so that blood flow to many organs is diminished.

Symptoms
There is acute onset of fever with rapid heart rate, malaise, pains in the muscles and joints. Weight loss is common. It is virtually indistinguishable from an acute onset of rheumatoid arthritis. Later, as kidney damage develops, there is high blood pressure and abnormal kidney function tests. There may be heart and lung involvement with breathlessness, palpitations, oedema and chest pain. Numbness and tingling are experienced in those with central nervous system involvement. It is the effect on the kidney that is the most important prognostic indicator. Kidney disease is the usual cause of death.

Investigations
The ESR is raised markedly but biopsy of liver or kidney is the usual method of definitive diagnosis.

Treatment

This is with corticosteroids often combined with immunosuppressants such as azathioprine. Most people with this condition survive less than 5 years after diagnosis.

Scleroderma

In this autoimmune disease, the skin becomes swollen and hardened. The lungs, oesophagus, heart muscle and kidneys are also involved.

Symptoms

The main manifestations are on the skin. Three times more women are affected than men and it usually begins at a young age. Thickened, waxy patches affect the skin and these enlarge with time or come and go. If they disappear then this area is darker than surrounding skin. If large areas develop then restriction of movement may occur with severe skin thickening, pains in the muscles and joint stiffness.

Treatment

There is nothing, conventionally, that will change the long-term outcome of the disease, although corticosteroids may be given for symptomatic relief.

Ankylosing spondylitis

This is an inflammation affecting the spinal column. Ninety per cent of cases occur in males and the common age of onset is 20-40 years.

Symptoms

The classic presentation is of pain and stiffness in the back. The sacro-iliac joints are commonly affected first. As there is an inflammation there may be fever and malaise also. The whole vertebral column is affected. The symptoms increase in severity until the whole spine becomes stiff and rigid. Joints (especially in the lower limbs) may also be involved in the process and become swollen and stiff. Breathing may be painful and shallow due to the chest wall being affected. Inflammation of the iris (iritis) is seen in 20 per cent of cases giving rise to redness in the eye.

Examination of the spine reveals loss of the normal lumbar curve and an exaggerated kyphosis of the thoracic spine.

Investigations

The ESR is raised. X-rays of the spine almost always show abnormalities. Early radiological examination shows thickening of bone and erosion of sacro-iliac joints. Later there is fusion of the sacro-iliac joints with calcification in the spinal ligaments.

Treatment

Corticosteroids may be given but it is generally accepted that they make no difference to the outcome and will only result in the addition of side-effects to the clinical picture. Symptomatic treatment with aspirin and non-steroidal anti-inflammatory agents is given. Sulphasalazine may be prescribed long-term. Radiotherapy may be administered to the spine to reduce the inflammation. Physiotherapy is used to try and reduce the degree of stiffness and impaired function.

Systemic sclerosis

This is an autoimmune disease, which mainly affects the skin. It is three times more common in women than men. It tends to begin under the age of 50 years.

Symptoms

Multiple organs and tissues are affected in this disease. The skin becomes hardened and swollen. There is subsequent restriction of movement particularly in the hands and fingers. In the face, there is fixing of the expression and sharpening of the nose. Muscular aches and pains are common.

Raynaud's phenomenon occurs in around 75 per cent of cases. These symptoms may develop some years before the diagnosis of systemic sclerosis is made.

Oesophageal involvement leads to heartburn, dysphagia and indigestion. Diarrhoea and abdominal distension also occurs. Affection of the lungs causes breathlessness. Palpitations reveal cardiac involvement. Dry eyes due to Sjögren's syndrome are the norm. This is a common feature of many autoimmune diseases.

As with all the autoimmune disorders, the kidneys are affected in severe cases. This will lead to frequent urination, loin pain and tiredness.

Investigations
The ESR is raised since it is a non-specific indicator of inflammation. Rheumatoid factor is positive in 30 per cent of cases. Antinuclear antibodies are more commonly positive. Anaemia is common and is due to multiple factors.

Treatment
This is only symptomatic. No treatment, even corticosteroids or other immunosuppressants, makes any difference to the course of the disease. The disease tends to be severe in its manifestations and only 50 per cent of those who have it are still alive 5 years after diagnosis.

Dermatomyositis

As its name suggests, this disease affects skin and muscle. It is characterised by muscle weakness and there are inflammatory changes in the muscle and skin. It is related to polymyositis, which primarily leads to muscle symptoms.

Symptoms
There is weakness and wasting of the muscles especially of those around the shoulders, hips and pelvis. The muscles are painful and tender. Joint pains, swelling and stiffness are common. This may resemble the appearances of rheumatoid arthritis but long-term joint destruction does not occur. Difficulty in swallowing and speaking is seen in over 50 per cent of cases. The symptoms of Raynaud's phenomenon and Sjögren's disease are frequent accompaniments.

Skin rashes are common. These include reddish/blue discolouration over the exposed areas. Redness of the eyelids is classically seen. These appearances, with muscle weakness, indicate that dermatomyositis is the diagnosis. Malignant disease is a common development especially of the lung (in men) and ovaries (in women).

Investigations
Serum creatine phosphokinase is raised and indicates that muscles are involved. Electromyography (EMG) shows typical changes. Muscle biopsy will give the definitive diagnosis.

The ESR is raised. There is anaemia and the white cell count is raised. Test for rheumatoid factor is often positive.

Treatment
This is by means of corticosteroids although it has little effect in chronic cases. Immunosuppressant drugs such as azathioprine or methotrexate may be given in addition.

Polymyalgia rheumatica

This is an affection of the muscles and the inflammatory process may also involve the temporal artery – temporal or cranial arteritis. It is this complication that is potentially hazardous to sight. Polymyalgia rheumatica usually first develops around 60-70 years of age and three times more commonly in women than men.

Symptoms
There is the sudden onset of pain and stiffness in the muscles, particularly of the shoulders, hips and pelvis. The neck and lumbar spine is a common site for pain and stiffness. The symptoms are typically worse in the mornings on getting out of bed. There may be systemic symptoms such as weight loss, anorexia, malaise, and tiredness. Fever is common but mild.

There may be an associated headache, which is localised to the temple. There is tenderness in this area and the temporal artery may be thickened and tender. In severe cases there may be no pulsation felt over the cranial artery. It is this complication that is hazardous as it may lead to sudden and irreversible blindness.

Investigations
The ESR is very high at around 100 mm per hour. Anaemia is common. Serum alkaline phosphatase is raised. Temporal artery biopsy is done in some cases but the diagnosis is usually obvious clinically.

Treatment
This is by means of corticosteroids, which reduce the inflammation and ESR. This treatment is continued for at least 2 years and may be resumed if there are relapses. After 4 years the disease has disappeared in virtually everyone. Corticosteroids are given to everyone with polymyalgia rheumatica, as there is a slight risk of blindness. If there is temporal arteritis then this risk is greatly increased.

Holistic management of autoimmune disease

There is a close relationship between the musculoskeletal system and Blood in its energetic sense. The other organ, which is frequently involved, is the Kidney as it dominates bone, produces Bone Marrow and is the root of all the body's energies. This is an interesting association as the main treatment for these conditions is with corticosteroids, which anatomically come from the adrenal glands situated on top of the kidneys.

In terms of Chinese medicine, such diseases are often Bi Syndrome (usually of the Hot type) with mainly underlying Kidney Yang Deficiency and Blood Deficiency. There may be other organ imbalances to consider in addition. All these diseases tend to be severe and difficult to treat. Diagnosis will be hampered by the almost invariable presence of corticosteroids or other powerful drugs. You would expect treatment to be prolonged.

Case one

A woman of 30 years presented for treatment with generalised pains in the joints. She had been involved in a road traffic accident some 3 months previously when she had sustained marked bruising over her right hypochondrium and abdominal wall from the safety belt. Some 4 weeks after the accident, she developed pains in the chest, which were worse when breathing, stiffness in the muscles and joints, hot swellings of the joints, nausea, fever, night sweats and general malaise and tiredness.

Her symptoms worsened to the point where she could hardly move and she had to be admitted to hospital. After some days a diagnosis of polyarteritis nodosa was made and she was given:

- prednisolone 100 mg daily
- azathioprine 125 mg daily

Her symptoms quickly improved and at the time of her consultation with me she had some residual tightness and discomfort in the chest, weak legs, hot and swollen wrists. Her appetite was normal now and she slept well. Her dosage of prednisolone had been reduced to 60 mg daily. She came for treatment because she wanted relief of her symptoms and to come off her drugs. Her consultant had specifically told her that the drugs had no side-effects. However, she had met people who had taken corticosteroids long-term and realised that she was likely to develop problems, particularly at the dosage she was prescribed.

The dosage of corticosteroids reflects the strength of inflammation in this case. As she had been on the medication for some 2 months now it was not sensible to reduce quickly. I impressed on her that the appropriate time to start drug reduction would be when she started to improve. If she reduced them too soon then the original clinical picture might return.

In terms of Chinese medicine, her diagnosis was Damp-heat Stagnation, which was confirmed by a pulse quality, which was full and slippery. Her tongue was pale and swollen, which is contradictory, as it would be expected to be red with a thick, yellow greasy coat. This was because of the effect of the corticosteroids, which I discuss later. The accident was clearly the trigger because of damage to the Blood, particularly Liver Blood given the site of the injury. A predisposing cause was taking the oral contraceptive, which tends to lead to Blood disturbances particularly Stagnation. Also, she had a history of a kidney 'infection' when aged 7 years necessitating hospital admission. Prior to and after the car accident she was under a lot of emotional strain at home.

I gave her an acupuncture treatment and five packets of herbs to release the Stagnation and protect the Blood. She returned some 2 weeks later. She told me that after her last visit she had decided to stop the prescribed drugs and flushed them down the toilet! She felt very shaky and nauseous for a week but this then settled. She now had very few symptoms with some aching in her neck and wrists. Her general weakness had subsided and there were no swellings.

Over the course of the next few months, I concentrated on correcting her underlying Kidney and Blood imbalances. After 6 months of treatment she was well with no problems.

This case illustrates several important points. Her initial reaction to the injury illustrated a pre-existing susceptibility at a fairly deep level. However, the strong nature of her symptoms, the acute onset and her rapid response to treatment reveal a basically strong constitution. This was responsible for her clearly taking charge of her medication. Two months of medication is not long enough to lead to significant suppression of adrenal function and if the holistic treatment is correct there will be little in the way of a flare-up.

This brings me onto the question of the energetic action of corticosteroids. There is some discussion as to whether they are Cold or Hot in nature as they are commonly used for inflammatory conditions. The key is to look at what happens if the body does not produce its own supply or if long-term prescribed corticosteroids are withdrawn rapidly. The clinical appearance is that of Addison's disease. There is low blood pressure, low temperature, general slowing of the body functions and eventually coma and death. This corresponds to a collapse of Yang picture in Chinese medicine and so corticosteroids would be the counterpart of a Rescue Yang formula. They are Hot in nature and primarily affect the Lung, Spleen and Kidney Yang. They are strongly moving and release Stagnation syndromes such as Bi Syndrome. They will rescue the Yang Deficiency with Water Overflowing of severe cardiac insufficiency. In the long-term they will lead to depletion of Blood and Yin especially of the Liver and Kidney. In the acute phase, because the Heat is due to Stagnation, the clinical symptoms and signs of Heat will disappear. This is why this woman's tongue was pale rather than the expected red with a thick yellow coat. In long-term use Heat will be much more evident as the fluids become damaged.

Since these drugs are Hot and strongly moving, they tend to disperse the Yang of the Lung, Spleen and Kidney. This explains the typical side-effects of oedema, especially of the upper and middle parts of the body. The Lung is responsible for the water passages through its dispersing and descending function and the Spleen transforms and transports. Interference with these two organs leads to oedema.

There is increased appetite due to Stomach Heat, there is wasting of the limbs due to the damage to body fluids and muscles, diabetes mellitus can develop as the Yin is consumed, heating of the Heart can lead to mental disturbances and psychotic manifestations in some. The effect on Lung Yang explains the relief obtained from wheezing in asthma. Long-term, of course, there will be Kidney Yin and Yang Deficiency as this organ is weakened.

The strongest effects are with oral corticosteroids but there are similar results with all prescriptions – inhaled, enemas, nasal, topical on the skin or eye drops.

Case two
This case is more revealing of the long-term results of corticosteroid prescriptions. A woman of 56 years came for treatment. She had been diagnosed as having systemic lupus erythematosus some 38 years previously. Her current medication was:

- prednisolone 10 mg and 7.5 mg daily on alternate days.

Her symptoms began after an episode of low back pain and she rapidly developed a similar clinical appearance to those described in Case 1 above. She was one of the first people to receive corticosteroids in the UK in the late 1950s and she had remained on them ever since. Whenever she tried to reduce them there would be a flare-up of joint pain, redness, swelling and heat.

Her main symptoms now were pain and cracking in the joints, which were worse after exercise, pain in the epigastrium with acidity in the chest, diarrhoea several times each day, nocturia four times each night, dryness of skin, hair, mouth and eyes. She had bleeding gums and teeth that would suddenly become loose and drop out. She had palpitations. Occasionally, she would experience hot feelings on the surface of the body with severe icy coldness inside. At these times she would feel exhausted and these had occurred every few weeks over the past 10 years or so.

In terms of Chinese medicine she had marked Blood and Yin Deficiency of Liver and Kidney, Heat in the Stomach and Yang Deficiency of the Spleen and Kidney. There was some evidence of Damp-heat Stagnation in the joints but this only became obvious when she reduced her corticosteroids. Her tongue was very red, thin and dry which revealed the damage to body fluids as caused by the prescribed drugs. This case shows much more clearly the Hot nature of corticosteroids and their long-term effect.

It is sometimes said that there is little point treating such people as their energy is too severely depleted. Whilst it is true that this woman had been greatly weakened by the drugs, it is rarely the case that nothing can be done. No attempt must be made to reduce the corticosteroids since her energy is weak and unless improvement begins, it is in danger of collapsing especially if reduction is rapid. The episodes of heat on the exterior and cold on the interior is typical of a condition called True Cold False Heat where lack of Fire internally leads to Yang floating to the surface. It is indicative of a severe Yang deficiency.

I treated her with acupuncture and herbs trying to strengthen her Qi and Blood gently to begin with. She improved gradually and more so than I had originally anticipated. She has a strong spirit and despite her long years of corticosteroid therapy was remarkably well. Many people in a similar situation are very ill with more problems. Her digestion improved, as did her nocturnal urination. Her general energy picked up and she would occasionally develop discharge of green mucus from the nose with mild fever and sweating. This was indicative that her energy was improving to the point where it can 'throw out' internal toxins.

She continued treatments for some months and was able to reduce her corticosteroid medication. She would experience some tiredness when this happened and mild flare-ups of joint pain and swelling. Her general health was also much improved. If she could have had holistic treatment 38 years previously then she would have been saved the debilitating effects of a long-term corticosteroid prescription. It is not appropriate to continue powerful, acute treatments for a long time. They need to be replaced by more gentle, balanced methods.

Case three

A woman of 51 years came for treatment. She had been diagnosed with scleroderma some 15 years previously. She had been fairly well since that time. In the few months before attending the clinic, she had been feeling very tired. She often had a feeling of pressure in the upper oesophagus like a pressure. This would be worse when she was tired. She was constantly feeling chilly, her bowels were generally constipated and she would commonly have a burning feeling in the epigastrium passing up to the chest. She had to be very careful with her diet or she would easily develop epigastric discomfort and belching. Her only medication was omeprazole for indigestion.

I made a diagnosis of Spleen Qi Deficiency, Kidney Yang Deficiency, Damp-cold Accumulation and Blood Deficiency. I treated her with acupuncture and Chinese herbs to good effect. Her energy picked up well and her digestion improved markedly. She always had to be careful about the food she ate and eating out or poor quality food would always give her indigestion. Her treatment continues but in the 12 months she has been receiving treatment, she has felt much stronger, is more able to live a busy life and her physical symptoms have, by and large, subsided.

Case four

A woman came for treatment of rheumatoid arthritis, which had begun 35 years earlier after the birth of her only child. She was 64 years old but looked much older and was very pale, almost ghostly. In her early 20's she had had severe back pain and foot pain, which was treated with steroid injections. The rheumatoid arthritis started in her right big toe joint then spread to both ankles. In her late 40's, her knee was drained and treated with cortisone. Two years later she broke both her tibia and fibula. In her early 60's, she had a knee replacement. She said that she was told after the diagnosis that she would end up in a wheelchair, to which she replied: 'I won't'. She had also had gold injections into the knuckle area and some alternative therapy in the past, but no classic homoeopathic treatment.

She did avoid the wheel chair, but her shoulder had no power and was painfully sore. Her left arm and right wrist were swollen, painful and stiff. Her right elbow was loose and it was hard to hold up her forearm (she had to use her other hand to support it). Her fingers were hard to bend and needed constant exercise. She had severe, sharp neck pain, when turning her head. Her hips were starting to trouble her. All these were treated with aspirin. Her balance was poor. She could predict when it would rain because she felt stiff and very low in energy. She was terribly prone to colds and flu-like symptoms.

A striking aspect of her story was her strong desire to be of service to others and the feelings of guilt and unworthiness when she became unable to fulfill this purpose. She had great faith in humanity and lacked interest in material possessions. She was given Hydrogen 30c.

One month later there was definite amelioration of all symptoms, her sleep was more restful, her energy had doubled and her balance improved. Her joints had begun to creak, which was new. After 2 months she developed skin eruptions under her right arm and on her chest, these cleared within 1 month and then similar eruptions appeared on the ankles. She continued to make steady progress with more freedom of movement and less pain. 'Everyday I'm not suffering as much.' She repeated the remedy if she caught a cold or felt low. Three years later she continues to be well.

GOUT

This is an inflammatory arthritis, which, in conventional medicine, is due to an excess of uric acid in the blood. Crystals are formed in joints, which leads to symptoms. Uric acid is a breakdown product of purine. Increased levels occur due to drugs such as frusemide and thiazide diuretics or dietary factors. Foods with a high protein content, e.g. meat and alcoholic drinks increase uric acid levels. Middle-aged men are more commonly affected.

Symptoms

This condition is extremely painful and most of us have an image of an elderly, irritable man with a heavily bandaged foot suffering from gout. The pain of gout is so severe in most cases that any contact is excruciating. The commonest joint affected is the first metatarsophalangeal joint but others may include ankles, hands, knees and elbows in an asymmetrical pattern. There is usually an associated fever. In chronic cases, there may be joint deformity due to damage by crystal deposits. Collections of uric acid, tophi, may be found in the cartilage of the ears.

Investigations

The serum uric acid level is raised, as are the ESR and white cell count.

Treatment
This is by means of drugs to reduce the inflammation such as aspirin and non-steroidal anti-inflammatory agents. Dietary advice is given to reduce the amount of uric acid in the blood and drugs may be administered to do the same. Such medication is long-term and those commonly used are sulphinpyrazone, probenecid and allopurinol.

Holistic management
This is essentially the same as for the general inflammatory conditions described above. Gout usually affects one or few joints and in terms of Chinese medicine corresponds to Damp-heat Accumulation, which affects the Spleen and Liver (hence its usual site over the Liver and Spleen channels in the foot). It is important to take diet into consideration and to avoid or reduce foods that generate Damp and Heat. These include excessive sweet food, greasy food, spices, alcohol, red meat, citrus fruit and whitebait.

OSTEOARTHRITIS

This is a degeneration of the joint cartilage with growth of new bone and connective tissue within the joint. Inflammatory changes are minor and secondary to this process. Eighty per cent of people over the age of 65 years have x-ray evidence of osteoarthritis yet only 25 per cent have symptoms. It is more common in women than men. There are more symptoms if the weather is cold and damp. The risk of this condition is increased if the joint is affected by a previous fracture, in cases of overuse such as professional sports people or manual labourers or if there has been previous damage to the joint, e.g. inflammatory arthritis, trauma.

Symptoms
This disease mainly affects the spine, load-bearing joints of hips and knees and the first metacarpophalangeal joint. There is the gradual onset of joint pain with aching. Pain is worse for movement and better for rest. Stiffness is common and may be worse after resting for some time or in the mornings.

There is cracking in the joint and the muscles surrounding the joint may be tender. These muscles may waste in long-term cases. There may be joint swelling due to (effusion) increased amounts of fluid in the joint. Bony swellings appear on the hands over the distal interphalangeal joints. In some cases they are red, hot, swollen and painful but this inflammation settles to leave hard swellings.

Investigations
There are typical appearances on X-ray of narrowing of the joint space, bone formation (osteophytes) at the edges of the joint, thickening of the adjacent bone and the presence of loose debris in the joint. Blood tests are normal.

Treatment
There are many treatments available for osteoarthritis yet none are completely satisfactory in terms of symptom relief. General advice will include reducing excess weight, change of occupation and physiotherapy. Prescribed drug use is common. Aspirin and non-steroidal anti-inflammatory agents are given despite the lack of any degree of inflammation in most cases.[6] Corticosteroids are injected locally into the joint rather than given systemically. Repeated use weakens the joint and may lead to further joint damage and deterioration. This is particularly true in weight bearing joints. Surgery is offered as a last resort if there is great discomfort and disability.

Holistic management
In terms of Chinese medicine, osteoarthritis usually corresponds to Bi Syndrome (frequently Cold and/or Damp). There is frequently an underlying syndrome such as Blood Deficiency. This is why such symptoms appear in people who have overused their joints through physical activity. The Blood is weakened and so cannot nourish the muscles and joints.

Treatment may be effective in some people if just the joint is treated. In others it is important to nourish the Blood at the same time. Physical therapies such as massage are helpful as an adjunct to such treatment. I find a combination of massage and acupuncture to be particularly effective. General advice to take regular *gentle* exercise and for a healthy whole-food diet is important. Reduction of weight, if excessive, is useful to take the strain off affected joints particularly in the lower part of the body.

Case one
A woman of 62 years came for treatment with feelings of exhaustion. She would feel dizzy on standing and these symptoms would be worse in the mornings. She had a lot of pain in her right hip and right ankle, which had been diagnosed as arthritis. The pain would be severe at times and the joints would feel hot and stiff. She needed to take regular non-steroidal anti-inflammatory drugs to ease the pain in her joints. Her eyes were often gritty and sore. Her bowels were sluggish and she would miss days or occasionally have no motion for up to 1 week. I made a diagnosis of Spleen Qi Deficiency and Blood Deficiency particularly of the Heart and Liver. I treated her with acupuncture and Chinese herbs.

In such a case, any improvement in joints occurs secondarily to any improvement in general energy levels. Within 4 weeks, her energy was much better and her hip was fine with no pain. She would have pains across the tops of both her feet where they would feel hot. Over the next few months, her general energy continued to improve, her hip didn't trouble her again but her feet caused her increasing levels of discomfort.

After 5 months of treatment, she decided to stop her drugs as they were not really helping and her stomach was often uncomfortable due to their side-effects. She went through a difficult period of pain in her feet. Her ankle settled but she was so uncomfortable at times that she was unable to go dancing, which was her great love. She continued with treatment, her energy continued to be good and over the course of a couple of months the pain shifted further down her feet to lie mainly under the metatarsal heads.

I continually encouraged her that treatment was helping and that eventually I expected that her feet would settle. Sure enough, some 12 months after her original visit, her feet were fine and she was able to resume dancing. At times she would still have some tiredness and dizziness but this was now clearly related to overwork or emotional upsets. She now attends for treatment only when she begins to feel tired and is well.

OTHER MUSCULOSKELETAL CONDITIONS

There is a wide range of conditions that are usually labelled as inflammatory, i.e. they have the suffix of –itis, but do not fit comfortably into a categorisation of rheumatoid or osteoarthritis. There are terms used such as rheumatism, fibrositis and so forth that are often used imprecisely in cases of muscular and joint aches and pains. Investigations are invariably normal and treatments such as physiotherapy, prescribed drugs and exercise are of variable effectiveness. Injected corticosteroid preparations may be given but it is common to find that people have chronic problems. At times their activity may be severely limited. It is not possible to list all the conditions that exist but I do mention the most common:

- Tennis elbow
- Golfer's elbow
- Prepatellar bursitis (housemaid's/clergyman's knee)
- Olecranon bursitis (student's elbow)
- Carpal tunnel syndrome
- Repetitive strain injury
- Frozen shoulder
- Fibrositis
- Achilles tendonitis
- Morton's metatarsalgia
- Osgood-Schlatter's disease
- Plantar fasciitis
- Sacroiliac strain
- Trigger finger.

Tennis elbow/Golfer's elbow

This is a tendonitis due to over activity, which, despite its name, is often not sport related. Tennis elbow affects the lateral epicondyle of the humerus and golfer's elbow the medial epicondyle. Any repetitive activity may lead to its development and they are common in housewives and manual workers. The common activity is a twisting action of the forearm as for example using a screwdriver or opening jars. I have seen tennis elbow in herbalists who have the occupational hazard of having to open dozens of jars each day.

Symptoms
There is frequently pain up and down the arm and the muscles around the shoulder may be affected. There may be weakness and the muscles and tendon over the affected epicondyle are acutely tender.

Treatment
Non-steroidal anti-inflammatory agents may be used but corticosteroid injections are common.

Holistic management
As with osteoarthritis, the key to treating this condition is to assess the condition of the energy and Blood. If it is a sole occurrence in an otherwise healthy person, treatment of only the elbow may be sufficient. If there are other aches and pains or there is evidence of Deficiency of Blood generally[7] perhaps with insomnia, palpitations, anxiety or worry then local treatment must be combined with constitutional remedies. This is a common situation in women who may have Blood Deficiency or in people who have over exercised.

In those who have received corticosteroid injections, treatment tends to be prolonged with more aggravations along the way. This is because these drugs weaken the tendon and it takes time to heal.

Bursitis

A bursa is a small sac or pouch lined with synovial membrane. They are present around joints. Inflammation in a bursa may arise because of repetitive injury as in housemaid's knee, clergyman's knee, student's elbow and so forth or can be part of a more widespread disorder such as rheumatoid arthritis.

Symptoms
The affected area is swollen, hot, tender and perhaps reddened. Movement will be limited. There may be an association with a recurrent type of activity.

Treatment
Injection of corticosteroid locally is the usual method of treatment.

Case one
This case, although not specifically diagnosed as bursitis, is a common situation in children and adolescents who are growing quickly. A boy of 12 years came for treatment of weakness and pain below the kneecaps. He found it hard to keep up with others and stumbled often. The pain was sudden and shooting and worse on the right. His ankles felt tight and would crack. He found it difficult to write well. He also suffered from nightmares about a particular teacher, who had been abusive to him. He would wake screaming. He had headaches where he felt his forehead was swelling in and out. His energy was low and he felt the cold easily. He often had nocturnal enuresis.

His description of the pain in his legs and head exactly fitted a remedy called Taraxacum that is made from Dandelion, incidentally Dandelion gets its name from the French 'dans de lit', which refers to the folklore that they make you pee in the bed. It is also an excellent remedy for night terrors. He was given a dose of 200c.

A month later he said that his legs were stronger and looser. The pains were gone and so were the headaches. He was sleeping very well and had had no nightmares or bed-wetting. He felt good all over. His mother said he was able to run and write much better. He repeated the remedy regularly as needed and 4 years later continues to be well.

Nerve compression

The classic example of nerve compression is carpal tunnel syndrome. The clinical appearance has similarities with that of repetitive strain injury (RSI) described below.

Symptoms
There is tingling and pins and needles in the hands, wrists and occasionally into the arm. Despite its supposed cause in conventional medicine, i.e. pressure on the median nerve in the wrist, there are frequently symptoms up the arm. Weakness of the muscles of the hands and forearms is common. In severe cases there is wasting.

Treatment
This is directed at the area in the wrist where the nerve passes through a fibrous tunnel. Local corticosteroid injections are common but surgery is used in long-standing cases. In my experience, the conventional treatments are of variable effectiveness and many people may have the symptoms after surgery with the addition of a scar.

Repetitive strain injury (RSI)

This is a common problem amongst people whose work entails a repetitive action. It tends to be under diagnosed and its existence is still denied by some conventional authorities. It may be seen as being psychological in origin by some conventional doctors. It can also be called chronic (work-related) upper-limb pain syndrome.

Symptoms
There is tingling, pins and needles and even numbness in the affected areas. These are usually the hands and forearms. The symptoms occur after prolonged activity such as typing, writing and so forth. There is also weakness, which can interfere with function to a great degree. In severe cases, little activity may precipitate the symptoms.

Treatment
This is by physiotherapy and non-steroidal anti-inflammatory agents but these are of variable effectiveness. It is important to

consider the work situation especially with regard to length of continuous activity, posture, height of chairs in relation to work surfaces and so on.

Case one

This is a good example of how to deal in general with musculoskeletal problems of this type. A woman of 28 years came for treatment of her repetitive strain injury. She is a teacher and for the past 3 years has had symptoms in her upper limbs. These developed after writing a lot of reports for school. She had had varying degrees of trouble over the preceding 3 years but the symptoms had been constant for the 8 months prior to coming to see me.

She had burning and stabbing pains with tingling over the shoulders, extending into the arms and hands. They came on after using her hands and arms and she had recently found that minor degrees of activity could precipitate symptoms. She also had visual floaters, insomnia and pre-menstrual breast soreness with irritability. She was occasionally constipated with abdominal cramps. She was taking a non-steroidal anti-inflammatory agent daily, with little change in symptoms.

In terms of Chinese medicine, this is a case of Liver Blood Deficiency. She needed constitutional treatment and I gave her herbs to strengthen her Liver Blood. She responded quickly and had much less pain in her shoulders and arms. Her sleep was still disturbed but she felt better in herself. After several months of treatment she was able to use her arms and hands with no discomfort although prolonged exercise would cause minor degrees of tingling.

This case reveals why treatments such as physiotherapy and local corticosteroid injections are of variable effectiveness, particularly in chronic conditions. It is essential to consider the underlying state since the symptoms will be relieved only when this has improved. I find that physiotherapy is most effective in acute injuries, as it is strongly moving in terms of Qi and Blood. For chronic conditions, it is generally more beneficial to use treatments that take the constitution into account. People with a chronic condition due to weakness of Qi and Blood may, in fact, be made worse by physiotherapy (or indeed local acupuncture treatment). This is because the energetic pathways on the surface are forcibly opened without there being adequate supplies of Qi and Blood in the interior to respond to such opening.

Frozen shoulder

This, as its name suggests, is a 'freezing' of the shoulder joint. It is common in people who have restricted activity or perhaps after a stroke when the affected side cannot be moved. It is usually one-sided.

Symptoms

There is pain and stiffness in the affected shoulder. There is marked limitation of movement and this causes problems with dressing, brushing hair and the like. The limited movement may be in one particular direction, (e.g. extension, flexion, abduction, etc.). This is of significance in Chinese medicine as it indicates the channels affected.

Treatment

Prevention is helpful so exercise of the shoulder in cases of reduced activity is helpful. In established cases, physiotherapy, non-steroidal anti-inflammatory agents and local corticosteroid injections are used with variable effectiveness.

OSTEOPOROSIS

This is a decrease in the density of bone, which occurs as part of the ageing process. It is a problem with the substance of bone rather than the calcium structure. Calcium supplements, therefore, have no part to play in either its prevention or its treatment. It is more common with lack of activity, low body weight, smoking, corticosteroid medication and in women after the menopause.

Symptoms

There are usually no symptoms and the diagnosis is made by X-ray or bone scan. In conventional practice, the diagnosis may be made because of joint pains and stiffness. These are *not* symptoms of osteoporosis. The prescription of hormone replacement therapy (synthetic oestrogen with or without synthetic progesterone) may lead to the disappearance of such symptoms. This is merely because such hormones have a corticosteroid effect of relieving inflammation.

In some people there may be fractures with the lumbar and thoracic vertebrae, the neck of femur, upper end of humerus and lower end of radius being the most common sites. With vertebral collapse there may be pain, backache, loss of stature and kyphosis.

Investigations

X-rays reveal a less dense bony structure. Bone scans with radioactive isotopes show the same changes. There are raised levels of alkaline phosphatase.

Treatment

There is little treatment that is available once osteoporosis has developed. Some people spontaneously improve. Fractures are treated if and when they occur.

Prevention is a fashionable topic at the moment with increasing prescriptions given of hormone replacement therapy – Page 370.

Holistic management

The main difficulty here is the large number of women who are prescribed hormone replacement therapy. Ideally it is given for specific indications but in many situations it is difficult to see a clear reason. Its correct use, conventionally, can be summarised as treating symptoms during the menopause and to prevent osteoporosis. Conventional practitioners may use osteoporosis and the fear of its development to 'persuade' women to take HRT. Osteoporosis is part of the normal ageing process although it may be more severe in some situations. To prescribe a powerful drug to everyone on the basis that they *may* develop a disease is potentially hazardous. This approach takes no regard of the time, money and effort spent on prescriptions, monitoring its use and dealing with the side-effects.

Women who smoke, have a family history of osteoporosis, are of a light build, under-exercise and have received corticosteroids are at more risk. Most of these factors can be addressed by changing life-style. In terms of Chinese medicine, the condition of bone is related to the function of the Kidney. As the Kidney function declines later in life, the bone may be affected. It would make sense to protect Kidney function early in life and to strengthen this organ as much as possible. Individualised constitutional treatment with Chinese medicine or homoeopathy is an effective means of doing this. Nutritional supplements are advocated by some and have a protective effect.

HOW TO RECOGNISE A SERIOUS CONDITION OF THE MUSCULOSKELETAL SYSTEM

Symptoms of the musculoskeletal system are rarely hazardous to life. However, there may be an underlying process that is potentially damaging and it is important to know these, unusual, situations.

You need to be concerned by any symptom that is severe, acute and with strong systemic features. Also, a single joint that acutely becomes hot, swollen and painful may indicate an infective arthritis, which rapidly damages the joint.

SUMMARY

Musculoskeletal conditions are extremely common and form a large part of the caseload of an holistic medicine clinic.

The most effective treatment will be a combination of physical therapy such as massage, gentle exercise with strengthening treatments such as acupuncture, homoeopathy or herbs.

Autoimmune disease is characterised by systemic involvement as well as joint and muscle symptoms. These are deep diseases and treatment is usually prolonged.

---

[1] Comparisons can be made here with energetic ideas of Blood, which were introduced in Chapter 7 – Cardiovascular System.

[2] I have already referred to the effect of Buddhist meditation on circulating corticosteroid levels. Also see *Mind as Healer, Mind as Slayer* by Pelletier (Allen and Unwin, 1972) particularly Chapter 6 – Meditation and Chapter 7 – Autogenic Training and Visualisation.

[3] Inflammation is either not evident or plays a minor part in the disease.

[4] Autoimmune diseases of the musculoskeletal system affect the connective tissue substance (collagen) of the body. They are therefore named collagenoses.

[5] In the case of other corticosteroids, which may be prescribed, it is important to compare the dosages with those given here.

[6] The use of non-steroidal anti-inflammatory agents accelerates joint deterioration. *Lancet* 1989;Sept2:519. With an understanding of their energetic action it can be seen that this is due to a sustained and increasing depletion of the Blood so that the joints and muscles become undernourished.

[7] See anaemia in Chapter 7 – Cardiovascular system for a discussion of the symptoms of Blood Deficiency as this term is understood in holistic medicine.

11 DERMATOLOGY

INTRODUCTION

When I was about to go to University to study medicine, my general practitioner told me to specialise in dermatology if I had the opportunity. He said that he had missed such a chance himself and regretted it ever since. When I asked him why, he replied that it was because there are plenty of people with skin problems, lots of private practice and no-one ever gets better. At the time I was surprised by his apparently cynical attitude. Later, with the benefit of experience I saw that this was, indeed, the conventional view. Rashes may come and they may go but in the end they are usually chronic in nature. The conventional treatments help to some extent but no-one pretends that it is a cure.

It was when I was in general practice myself that I saw the effect of holistic medical treatments. I had treated a young boy with eczema and asthma, using conventional medication, with little relief. After some months, his mother brought him to see me and he was the best he had ever been. He had received acupuncture over the intervening period with steady improvements. After my training in acupuncture, but especially in Chinese herbal medicine, it became clear to me that treatments exist which are powerful yet gentle and effective and this is especially so for skin diseases.

Skin disease is variable in its response to any form of treatment. This is because it may be either a problem that is merely on the surface of the body or it may reflect a deeper underlying imbalance. In cases where the skin rash is superficial, perhaps only affecting the palms or hands, the response to treatment can be dramatic and rapid. This is in line with Hering's Law of Cure where disorders on the lowermost and outermost parts of the body are the least severe. In cases where there is a marked internal imbalance, treatment may be long and involved. However, it is rewarding for the individual if they persist with treatment as relief of skin symptoms can have important effects in areas such as employment, confidence, physical activity and so on.

ANATOMY AND PHYSIOLOGY

There are several facts of anatomy and physiology that it is useful to know. I consider that most courses in these subjects are over detailed and reflect orthodox thinking rather than the particular needs of the holistic practitioner. To study dermatological disease it would be helpful to be able to:

- describe the structure and functions of the skin.

The skin is sometimes thought of as being an inert protective covering which does little more than line the outside of the body. There could be nothing further from the truth. Skin is a living dynamic organ with interesting connections with the interior of the body. Anyone with skin disease knows how quickly it can react to adverse situations. Abnormalities may appear over the course of a few hours (and disappear with equal rapidity). These are not the actions of an inert object.

The energetic view of the skin is that it is connected to the Lung. The Lung dominates Water passages and so is responsible for moisture reaching the surface of the body. Its energy is dispersing and descending and passes out to the extremities of the body. The Blood is necessary for moistening, cooling and nourishing imbalances in the Blood that may lead to dryness, scaling and itching. Internal factors such as Heat, Dampness, Wind and so forth may manifest on the skin. The skin, therefore, may be an indicator of internal imbalances.

In conventional medicine, it is frequently realised that skin disease may indicate internal disease. However, without a view of energetic connections it is impossible to see these symptoms as part of a coherent whole. In addition, treatment is frequently only applied to the surface of the body and in the form of medicaments to suppress inflammation, commonly with corticosteroids. The inflammation may pass deep into the body and cause a worsening of the internal imbalance. For example, removal of an eczematous skin rash by corticosteroid cream frequently results in the appearance of lung disease such as asthma or bronchitis.

The essence of holistic medicine is that it sees the underlying disharmony, balances this and therefore resolves the skin symptoms. As treatment progresses, the skin symptoms may get worse for a short time but the end results are often excellent. The conventional approach is to treat from the outside and although there may be short-term relief, the long-term result is invariably chronic problems – external or internal.

DEFINITION OF TERMS

It is helpful to review the somewhat specialist terminology applied to dermatology.

- Atrophy – thinning of the skin often accompanied by wrinkling
- Bulla – large blister filled with clear fluid
- Crusts – dried secretions
- Cyst – a lump containing fluid which may be thin or thick
- Ecchymosis – small bruise more than 3 mm in diameter
- Erosion – break in the continuity of a surface but shallow than an ulcer
- Erythema – redness
- Excoriation – marks caused by scratching or damage to the skin
- Exfoliation – scaling or peeling of superficial skin layers
- Lichenification – thickening of skin with increase in appearance of skin markings
- Macule – small, flat, discoloured, round spot
- Maculopapule – a combination of a papule and a macule
- Nodule – palpable solid area which may or may not be raised more than 5-10 mm diameter
- Papule – small, raised, round spot less than 10 mm in diameter
- Petechiae – small bruises less than 3 mm in diameter
- Plaque – a group of confluent papules
- Pruritus – itching
- Purpura – bleeding into the skin
- Pustule – small blister filled with yellowish fluid (pus)
- Scale – dry flake of skin
- Sclerosis – hardening of an area of skin
- Telangiectasia – abnormal visible dilation of blood vessels
- Ulcer – break in the continuity of surface tissue. This may be skin or mucous membrane
- Vesicle – small blister filled with clear fluid
- Wheal – localised area of oedema surrounded by redness.

CLASSIFICATION OF SKIN DISEASE

In conventional medicine, skin disease is classified according to its causation or listed in any order if this is unknown. In terms of conventional medicine, the key differentiation is between infective and non-infective skin rashes. The former will receive antibiotics or antifungal agents whilst the latter will, more often than not, receive corticosteroid preparations. Any skin condition of an infective type will become rapidly much worse if corticosteroids are given. Conversely, antibiotic and antifungal preparations have a propensity to cause allergic reactions in people with sensitive skin. The pharmaceutical industry has attempted to get round this problem by combining corticosteroids and antibiotics or antifungal agents in the same preparation. This is hardly subtle medicine but it does cover all the options.

The lists in Table 11.1 are not in any particular order of severity. They will vary according to each individual. There is a summary of skin diseases at the end of this Chapter where they are listed according to their appearance.

Infective	Non-infective
Staphylococcal infections • Boils Streptococcal infections • Erysipelas • Impetigo Fungal infections • Tinea pedis • Tinea corporis • Tinea capitis • Pityriasis versicolor (Tinea versicolor) • Candidiasis Infestations • Scabies • Head lice	Eczema Psoriasis Acne vulgaris Acne rosacea Urticaria Alopecia Vitiligo Tumours of the skin • Warts • Basal cell carcinoma • Squamous cell carcinoma • Malignant melanoma • Kaposi's sarcoma

Table 11.1: Classification of skin disease

ECZEMA

This word comes from the Greek and means 'boiling over'. It is an inflammation of the skin and is known as dermatitis. By convention, dermatitis is applied to those cases that are the result of coming into contact with specific irritants – contact dermatitis. The term eczema is used for those cases that occur without contact and are more to do with internal factors.

There is a relationship between eczema and asthma in that they frequently co-exist in the same person and there may be a family history of both conditions. Other diseases in the family may include migraine and hay fever. Atopy is the term applied to a state of sensitivity to factors such as pollen, foods and so forth. It is estimated that some 10 per cent of the population have some form of eczema and up to 40 per cent experience it at some time in their lives.

Symptoms
There are many forms of eczema and the following is a general description. In the acute phase there is redness, weeping of clear fluid and itching. There may also be vesicles (small blisters) in affected areas. The itching may be so severe that the person scratches until the skin bleeds. After some months or years, the main symptoms are dryness, scaling and itching. The areas most affected are the flexor surfaces of the elbow and knee but in severe cases the whole skin is involved. In chronic cases, the skin may be thickened and dry between affected patches.

In children, it may start at any age with common triggers being vaccination and the introduction of cow's milk. It is important to enquire about events in the life of the child that may have precipitated the illness. It may start on the face, cheek and scalp but invariably there is involvement of the wrists, ankles, and the flexor surfaces of the elbows and knees. Some cases seem to settle down after some years and the rule of 7 years[1] for girls and 8 for boys is a factor. That is, girls may recover at 7 or 14 years of age and 8 or 16 for boys. Almost 50 per cent of cases go on to develop asthma and hay fever. If the eczema is severe then asthma is more likely to develop later.

It is important to take into account factors such as occupation. Hairdressing, engineering and any work that involves contact with irritant substances carry a risk of precipitating eczema. Items that may exacerbate or precipitate eczema include:

- wool[2]
- petroleum products,[3] oils
- cleaning agents used to remove grease and oil from the skin
- metals such as nickel in watches and jewellery
- chemicals contained in deodorants, sprays, perfumes
- 'biological' washing powders, detergents, soaps[4]
- rubber.

If a skin problem is caused by contact there will be a typical area of distribution. It may be on the palms of the hands or in a site where jewellery or a watch has been worn. There will be a clear-cut area with scaling, itchiness and redness.

Dietary factors are important in some, notably dairy products and food additives. Many dietary ingredients may be implicated and individual cases will vary in their sensitivity to these. Eczema has a hereditary component and a child has a 60 per cent chance of developing the disease if both parents are affected. Two important trigger factors are teething in children and times of emotional stress.

Treatment
The conventional treatment of all skin diseases is variable in its effectiveness. It is important to avoid factors that exacerbate the rash and to consider diet. The mainstay of treatment is with corticosteroid applications. Useful general advice includes bathing using a simple, non-perfumed soap. Emulsifying ointment is helpful to moisturise the skin but care should be exercised with those based upon lanolin (wool fat) or hydrocarbons (petroleum products such as paraffin). Allergic reactions are common with both these types and will cause symptoms indistinguishable from the original condition.

Tar based preparations are an old form of treatment which includes sulphur applications. Homoeopaths know that sulphur is one of the strongest suppressers of skin conditions and the tar applications utilise this effect.

Corticosteroids are central to the conventional management of eczema and many other skin conditions. They are mainly administered locally. Oral administration may be given in severe cases. Conventionally the milder forms should be prescribed if at all possible and care should be taken in putting such products on the face. They have a suppressive effect and will not cure. Removal of the creams will lead to a flare-up of the rash that may be worse than the original. The degree of flare-up is dependent upon the health of the person, the strength of the corticosteroid application, the original condition and the duration of treatment.

There are 4 potency levels for corticosteroid applications – Table 11.2.

Strength	Examples
Mild	Fluocinolone 1:10 (0.0025 per cent), 1 per cent & 2.5 per cent hydrocortisone, methylprednisolone
Moderate	0.05 per cent Clobetasone butyrate, 0.05 per cent desoxymethasone, fluocinolone 1:4 (0.00625 per cent), fluocortolone, flurandrenolone, 0.05 per cent alcomethasone diproprionate
Strong	Beclomethasone, 0.1 per cent betamethasone, budesonide, 0.25 per cent desoxymethasone, diflucortolone, fluclorolone, 0.025 per cent fluocinolone, fluocinonide, hydrocortisone 17–butyrate, triamcinolone
Very strong	0.05 per cent clobetasol propionate, 0.3 per cent diflucortolone, halcinonide

Table 11.2: Strength of corticosteroid applications

The use of corticosteroids leads to an increased risk of infection or sudden spreading of the skin symptoms if infection is already present. For this reason, there are many applications that contain a mixture of a corticosteroid with an antibacterial or an antifungal agent. This may, in some instances, lead to their prescription when the precise diagnosis is unknown. There can be confusion between eczema and some fungal rashes. The application of a mixture of drugs may be used to avoid adverse effects. The problem with such a practice is that it confuses the clinical picture, there is no precise diagnosis and the application of antibacterial and antifungal agents on to the skin is associated with a high risk of allergic reactions. This will result in symptoms that are identical to the original condition. Antihistamines may be given for their sedative effect to decrease itching.

Holistic management
In terms of Chinese medicine, eczema is due to a combination of Wind, Heat and Dampness depending upon the actual appearance of the rash. Underlying Blood Deficiency is common, as is Lung Deficiency due to its function of dominating skin. Spleen Qi Deficiency is usually involved in cases with Damp Accumulation.

Case one
A woman of 27 years came for treatment of her eczema. This was generalised, flaky and mainly on her face, arms and behind her knees. It was worse in the heat and she scratched it until it bled. This would relieve the itching. She had eczema as a child until the age of 7 years when it disappeared. It recurred 2 years before she attended for treatment and had been worse in the past 18 months. The eczema was always worse in the sun. She was using mild potency corticosteroid applications.

She often had a feeling of not being able to get enough air into the lungs. There was no wheezing or cough. She would be short of breath occasionally when this sensation was severe.

Her diagnosis in terms of Chinese medicine was Blood Deficiency and Kidney Yang Deficiency Not Grasping Lung Qi. After some months of treatment she felt more able to cope with her symptoms and less depressed. Her general energy was better. Her skin had improved to the point where there were only small patches affected and mainly in the skin creases. Her circulation had improved. The skin problem was moving distally now and was mainly on the legs and arms. This is in line with Hering's Law of Cure.

Her skin would always be much better whenever she went away into the country or to the Alps for skiing. The eczema would return within 12 hours of her return to London. The things to think about in such a situation are diet, water, stress levels and air quality. As the Lung dominates skin, the purity of air and the function of the Lung are closely associated with skin symptoms.

After 6 months of treatment, her skin was generally good. She had occasional patches of dryness. She would have some flare-up with emotional stress but she was much more aware of this.

Case two
A woman of 56 years came for treatment of her eczema. She had developed a skin condition some 10 years earlier. The skin of her feet and hands were dry, scaly, itchy and weeping. The soles of her feet were particularly affected and were hot, red, sore, weeping and peeling. These areas were extremely itchy. Nothing ever made any difference to her skin condition. She had used hydrocortisone cream twice daily for 2-3 years. She had stopped this for 1 week before her visit to me.

In terms of Chinese medicine, this was diagnosed as Damp-heat in the skin. I gave her five bags of herbs and she noticed an improvement within 2 days of taking them. At her second visit some 4 weeks later, she now had no symptoms. Her hands were normal and her feet were slightly discoloured only. There was no weeping, scaling or itching. She came into the clinic with a new pair of shoes – the first for many years! The speed of her response reveals that the pathology was already at the extremity of the physical body – the soles and palms. With holistic medicine this should be fairly easy to treat. This is not the case with psoriasis which is notoriously more stubborn or as in Case 1 where the skin is generally affected with internal symptoms.

Case three

A boy of 10 months was brought for treatment of a skin rash. He had developed chickenpox when he was 2 weeks old (at the same time as his mother). At the age of 3 months he had a diphtheria, whooping cough, tetanus and polio vaccination. He felt hot after this and then developed a dry, scaly area on his scalp. This goes by the name of 'cradle cap'. His scalp would occasionally weep also. He had a repeated vaccination at 5 months and at 7 months. After the last one he developed a fever and wheezing which was diagnosed as a 'chest infection'. He received antibiotics.

This episode was followed by skin problems. He developed a dry, itchy, flaking rash behind one knee and over his face, neck, scrotum, and umbilical area. This had improved with a dairy-free diet, but only slightly. He always had loose bowel motions and a phlegmy cough.

His diagnosis in terms of Chinese medicine was Spleen Qi Deficiency, Lung Qi Deficiency and Damp-heat Accumulation. This is a typical story after vaccination and reveals the often-unrecognised damage caused by vaccination procedures. His health was clearly already compromised as he had chickenpox at the age of 2 weeks. Chickenpox is an attack of Damp-heat and shows why he now has such a condition and an associated Spleen Deficiency.

His improvement after a dairy-free diet points to a Spleen involvement. Dairy products produce Damp (mucus) particularly in the presence of Spleen problems. Their removal will take the strain off the digestion. I gave him Chinese herbs and within 1 month his bowels had started to improve. After 4 months of treatment, his bowels were normal, he was energetic and his skin was almost normal. He had some dry, reddish patches on his feet but this was the only abnormality.

Case four

A woman of 46 years of age came for treatment of her eczema. It was on the palms and fingertips of both hands and her left foot. She had had outbreaks on and off for the past 20 years and these had been treated with hydrocortisone creams. These no longer had any effect, so she had also been taking cortisone tablets for the previous 2 weeks. The skin was desquamating and very itchy and her hands were puffy. She also suffered from headaches, pre-menstrually.

She loved company and felt a little cut off by a recent move. She had a recurrent dream of being abandoned at the top of a hill, which she found very frightening. She was given Pulsatilla 30c (although in retrospect LM1 would have been more appropriate).

She came for regular follow-up visits over the next few months and said she was feeling good. Her energy was better and her headaches infrequent and less severe. Her hands were appalling. The skin was hard and yellow. It was tight, cracked easily and flakes of skin more than 2 inches long fell off. Both hands discharged thick yellow pus.

She was unable to do anything for herself. Water burnt her hands as if it were acid. Her stoicism was impressive. Her perseverance was finally rewarded. At the end of the 6 months she came to see me and her hands were beautiful. The skin was like that of a new born.

Case five

A woman of 53 years came for treatment of her feet. She had very itchy, fluid-filled blisters, with a generalised redness, on the soles of her feet. They were very hot and she had to put her feet out of the bed at night. If she was woken by the discomfort she would run her feet under cold water and this brought relief. Once the blisters had burst she got instant relief. She was generally in good health, although she had some hot flushes. She tended to lack self-confidence and could be anxious, particularly about the well being of close family members.

On the basis of this symptom picture she was given Arsenicum LM1. Her feet steadily improved and eventually cleared entirely. Two years later, she had a nasty shock and suffered from acute anxiety and diarrhoea. The picture, once again, fitted Arsenicum well; she took one dose of 30c and after a short aggravation all these symptoms quickly resolved.

Incidentally, her daughter had an identical condition, which in her case seemed to be stress-related. Arsenicum was also her remedy based upon a full case history and it worked very well clearing the eruption very quickly, probably because her energy was stronger than her mother's. Her son's skin complaints (and personality) were quite different and responded very well to Sulphur.

193

It is clear from these cases that it is important to take all aspects of the person into account. In conventional medicine it is just the skin that is treated. When you are treating a person with eczema there may be a sudden worsening of the skin problem. Such an event should make you think of emotional stress, dietary indiscretion, changes in climate or a reaction to a recent vaccination. These are the classical factors that lead to acute flare-ups.

It can be difficult managing people who also take conventional medication, i.e. local corticosteroid applications. Withdrawal must be slow or a flare-up is likely and you may lose the case. People find it difficult to return if their original symptoms are gradually worsening. This is especially true if areas such as the face are involved. Ask also about other applications since allergies are common to substances with lanolin (wool fat) or those based on petroleum. I find it preferable to advise people to use simple moisturisers in the form of oils or creams. Try to avoid applications with chemical additives.

The correct treatment of eczema can be rewarding for both client and practitioner. Improvement of a skin condition can lead to great changes in people's lives through enhanced self-confidence. Treatment can be prolonged in the cases of internal imbalances and in such cases it is more important to address factors such as diet, stress levels, work environment and so forth.

A note is applicable here about the use of Chinese herbs for skin disease. There is some discussion about them being toxic to the liver and kidneys. This is true to the extent that all medicinal substances in a material dose have a toxic potential, some more so than others. The problems which people have developed have been the result of taking *large* doses of Chinese herbs.

In China, where people are generally of a stronger constitution, large doses are regularly given. If these are then used in the West, people may develop problems. Treatment must be adapted to correspond to the constitution of the person. The *principles* of Chinese medicine have stood the test of time. It is in their *application* that great care must be taken to 'first do no harm'.

PSORIASIS

This is one of a group of skin diseases that are characterised by scaling. It is of unknown cause in conventional medicine. It is uncommon before the age of 15 years and is as common in men as women. It is chiefly a cosmetic nuisance because of its appearance and degree of scaling. The standard treatments of tar or dithranol add to this, as they are messy and time-consuming. The skin becomes overactive and so it thickens, more scales become apparent and there is redness and heat of the affected area. Around 1 in 10 people with psoriasis have symptoms of joint disease.

Symptoms
Areas of skin become thickened, red and scaly. This commonly occurs over the extensor surfaces of the elbow and knee. The patches may vary from almost pinhead size to large areas of the body. I was taught at medical school that psoriasis is never itchy and if a skin rash does itch that it will probably be eczema. This is not true and some people with psoriasis do have itching. The scales on the surface of the rash are white or silvery. There may be severe scaling in some and this can cause embarrassing cosmetic problems. The nails may be pitted, thickened and discoloured. In some cases they separate from the underlying nail bed. The scalp is a relatively common site to be affected.

The appearance of the skin lesions can take different forms in different people. Some have tiny, pinpoint areas (guttate psoriasis), others have thickened, reddish areas overlain with silvery scales (plaque psoriasis) whilst others develop pustules containing sterile yellowish material (pustular psoriasis).

It is a characteristic of all skin disease that damage to an area of skin may result in the appearance of skin symptoms at that site. This is known as the Koebner phenomenon. Scratching or rubbing may lead to the typical scaly rash appearing in that area.

Some people may be severely affected with generalised disease. In this case, there may be difficulties due to loss of heat from the body. Severe cases may require hospital treatment. The disease is worsened or precipitated by emotional stress,[5] associated tonsillitis, treatment with lithium carbonate[6] and betablockers.

Treatment

Treatment (from mildest to strongest)	Comments
Ultraviolet light	Psoriasis commonly improves in strong sunlight
Coal tar	An old treatment that relies upon the sulphur contained in tar. Stains the skin. Messy application. May cause a rash due its irritant effects
Dithranol	A synthetic holistic to tar with the same problems
Low dose tetracycline (antibiotic) orally	Long-term in some cases of pustular psoriasis
Corticosteroid applications	Conventionally this is not useful and may create problems in the long-term. In common usage, nevertheless. Only mild to moderate applications should be used
Corticosteroid orally	See above
Etretinate	Causes foetal damage and so not for pregnant women. Effective contraception must be used. Toxic to the liver
Immunosuppressants, e.g. methotrexate,[7] azathioprine, cyclosporin	Should only be used in severe or life-threatening disease. The main problem is damage to the bone marrow and thence blood cell production. Regular blood tests are needed

Table 11.3: Conventional treatments of psoriasis

Holistic management

In terms of Chinese medicine, this is due to Wind and Damp complicating cases of Blood Deficiency. Other syndromes to consider are Heat in the Intestines and Stomach given the usual distribution over the Yangming channels.

Case one

A woman of 32 years came for treatment of a scaly skin rash on the skin over her shins from the knees to the ankles. This had developed some 7 years previously. This was itchy especially in the heat and it felt generally hot. Her scalp was affected when the rash was severe. She suffered from constipation and only had a bowel movement once per week. This had been the case since she was 5 years old. She had strong symptoms of pre-menstrual tension, particularly irritability. In terms of Chinese medicine, a diagnosis was made of Heat in the Intestines with Liver Blood Deficiency and Liver Qi Stagnation.

I treated her with Chinese herbs as well as giving her advice about relaxation, avoiding heating foods such as spices, alcohol and coffee. It took 2 months of treatment before there was a slight change in her skin and 6 months before a significant change. After 1 year of treatment her skin was almost normal, her bowels were fine and she felt more relaxed generally as well as having fewer problems before a period.

This is typical of psoriasis in that it is slow to respond and it is important for people to persevere. Stress is a common trigger and practising relaxation techniques is very helpful.

ACNE VULGARIS (common acne)

This is experienced by most adolescents of both sexes although males are more affected. The cause of the problem is not understood in conventional medicine. There are various theories about sebaceous gland secretions (sebum) despite the fact that sebum is unchanged even when the symptoms clear in their early twenties.

Symptoms

The conventional idea is that sebum blocks the sweat glands and leads to blackheads and then inflammation. Pustules develop which may leave scars. The face is the usual site but in severe cases the chest and upper back are affected. Some people develop large spots, which may be uncomfortable. The main issue, particularly at this age, is a cosmetic one and almost everyone has some spots at some time during puberty. For some people it is more severe with multiple pustules affecting large areas of skin. There may be areas of redness, which affect similar sites.

Treatment

Treatment (from mildest to strongest)	Comments
Antiseptic washes, e.g. hexachlorophene Abrasive agents Keratolytic agents, e.g. benzoyl peroxide	These are fairly innocuous and at the level of simple hygiene. There are many available and of variable effectiveness
Ultraviolet light	Many skin diseases improve on exposure to sunlight
Antibiotics, topical	This is now entering the level of medicinal effects. Topical drugs are suppressive but less so than those given orally
Antibiotics, oral	Long-term use has the effect of reducing inflammation
Retinoic acid	Vitamin A derivative. It causes liver damage, foetal abnormalities and bone changes
Cyproterone	Anti-androgen. It is occasionally given for acne vulgaris
Oral contraception (females only)	These are discussed in Chapter 18 – Women's Health

Table 11.4: Treatment of acne vulgaris

Holistic management

In terms of Chinese medicine, this is due to the Accumulation of Heat in the Lung, Spleen and Stomach. There is almost always an element of Qi Stagnation, which may manifest as Liver symptoms of irritability, headaches and the like.

Case one

A woman of 33 years came for treatment. She had indigestion, diarrhoea each day and abdominal bloating. She was generally tired and felt irritable and depressed. She had a constant runny nose. She frequently had headaches across her forehead. She had been diagnosed as having polycystic ovaries some 2 years previously.

Her skin was badly affected by large pustular swellings on the face. These would appear at any time but particularly before a period. These had begun when she was 13 years old. Her current medication was:

- Cyproterone 50 mg daily for 10 days after end of her period
- Cyproterone 2 mg with oestrogen for the 3 weeks commencing on the first day of her period

Cyproterone blocks androgen – the male hormones. It is used in high doses of 50 mg daily mainly for male sexual offenders. I had never seen it used before.

In terms of Chinese medicine, the diagnosis was Spleen Qi Deficiency with Liver Qi Stagnation. This was clearly a severe case because of the powerful drugs used and the presence of other indications of Stagnation such as the ovarian cysts. The aim of treatment in this case is to strengthen the Spleen whilst relieving the Qi Stagnation. After some time of treatment then it would be possible to reduce the drugs. She was very nervous about reducing them because of the severity of the facial eruptions. They would appear as boils on the face before her period, large and quite painful.

After some months of treatment, her bowel function was much improved and her remaining skin eruptions subsided. It is important to reduce the cyproterone slowly although the second formulation with the addition of oestrogen must be stopped suddenly to prevent any possibility of breakthrough bleeding.

She reduced the 50 mg dose down to 25 mg and a large red skin eruption appeared under the skin at the side of her nose. This settled with treatment. She then saw her consultant who stopped all her drugs suddenly because she had been having headaches with visual disturbances. The drugs are very strong and he was worried that they were giving her side-effects.

Her skin flared-up quite badly with large pustules on her face and chin, irritability, severe pre-menstrual symptoms and depression. She was treated for several weeks before these started to settle. After some months she felt well, her skin would occasionally flare-up before a period but much less than before and her digestion was much stronger. She continues to be well.

The difficulty with such a case is the degree of heavy drug suppression. It takes time to sort out what is going on and each time the drug is reduced there will be a release of symptoms. This needs to be resolved before moving on. The root of the case can be difficult to see and this will vary according to each person. It is essential to take each level in turn as it presents itself. In this way, progress will be slow but sure and the person will, in the end, be much healthier. In this case, her doctor stopped the medication and this took any question of drug withdrawal out of her hands. On the one hand this was a sudden withdrawal and may have caused severe consequences. Conversely, at least it was possible to treat without the interference of the drugs.

ACNE ROSACEA

This is quite a different disease despite the common use of the term, acne. It is a chronic rash seen on the face. It affects women more than men.

Symptoms
There is a redness of the cheeks, nose and sometimes chin in a 'butterfly' distribution. There are broad patches over the cheeks like the wings of a butterfly with a narrow connecting strip across the nose. There are papules and pimples, which can be severe at times. There may be swelling of the affected skin. Redness of the eyelids and eyes are seen in about 50 per cent of patients. These appearances may take the form of blepharitis, conjunctivitis, keratitis, episcleritis or iritis.

There may be general flushing of the face in response to stressful situations, hot climate, hot drinks, spicy food and alcohol. There may be associated upper gastrointestinal symptoms such as indigestion.

Treatment
General advice will be given to avoid factors that cause flushing.

Treatment (from mildest to strongest)	Comments
Tetracycline	Long-term prescription – compare acne vulgaris
Metronidazole	Long-term prescription of a more hazardous antibiotic. May be used locally
Corticosteroid – local	It is unusual to see oral corticosteroids. Used locally they lead to long-term skin damage
Retinoic acid derivative	Very powerful, causes liver damage, foetal abnormalities, bone changes

Table 11.5: Treatment of acne rosacea

Holistic management
In terms of Chinese medicine, this is considered to be due to Stagnant Blood Accumulation due to injury of the Lungs by Stomach Fire.

URTICARIA

This is a rash, which is similar in appearance to that seen due to contact with the stinging nettle (*Urtica urens*). In conventional medicine the cause is generally unknown. The common things to think about are allergic reactions to drugs and chemicals. Skin and laboratory tests are unreliable.

Symptoms
In the acute phase, there is the appearance of wheals, localised swellings of the skin surrounded by redness. They are itchy. Around the lips and eyes there may be oedema. The attack may last for minutes or hours and the skin then returns to normal. There are many possible causes of such a reaction. It is essentially allergic in nature although many cases are of unknown cause.

Dermatographia is a variant of urticaria where scratching the skin produces the typical wheal reaction. It is possible to gently scratch a name or symbol on the skin and soon there will be oedematous swellings following that shape. Other triggers of such appearances include cold weather, water and sunlight.

Internal causes of this condition are varied and include prescribed drugs especially aspirin and non-steroidal anti-inflammatory agents, opiates, antibiotics, injections of radiological examination dyes, foods, parasitic infestation, blood transfusion and so forth. The list is actually endless as any substance may produce an allergic reaction in the susceptible individual. The above are merely the most common ones or those that are easily recognised.

If the attacks continue for more than 6 weeks or if the symptoms are continuous for this length of time, the term chronic urticaria is used. It is less likely in such cases that a trigger will be found. Attacks in these cases may last for up to a day but some people are more or less constantly affected. It is more likely that oedema of the eyes or lips will be a feature.

Treatment

Any known cause is removed but in many people the urticaria arises for ill-definable reasons.

Treatment (from mildest to strongest)	Comments
Antihistamine – oral	Often causes drowsiness and so is usually given at night. Tranquillisers may also be used
Cimetidine/ranitidine	These drugs interfere with the production of histamine are more commonly seen in the treatment of peptic ulcers
Corticosteroid – oral	May be used in chronic cases
Adrenaline – subcutaneous	In severe cases where there is anaphylaxis[8]

Table 11.6: Treatment of urticaria

Holistic management

In terms of Chinese medicine, this is due to several causes. There may be Damp in the superficial tissues complicated by Wind-heat or Wind-cold. Damp-heat Accumulation in the Stomach and Intestines or disturbance of the Chong and Ren due to irregular life-style may also lead to these symptoms.

Case one

A boy of 8 years came for treatment of an allergic reaction to cats, certain foods (hamburgers, chips, sausages, breakfast cereal and ice-cream) and possibly citric acid. This came in the form of very itchy eruptions like nettle stings that were worse under the eyes and a generalised swelling of the lips, bridge of the nose and eyes. This swelling moved from area to area in no discernible pattern. The eruptions also appeared on his stomach, back, arms and legs. This was treated with daily (sometimes twice daily) doses of anti-histamine. His mother was very anxious about the possibility of his airways becoming blocked as the swelling at times made his face unrecognisable.

He also had a sensation of soreness in the hipbone on the right. This had been getting worse over the previous four weeks, particularly if he ran.

He had had a cough every couple of weeks for the past 2 years and, since the prescribed inhalers had not relieved it, he had stopped taking them. In total he had had over 30 lots of antibiotics for his chest symptoms. These had weakened his teeth.

According to his parents, he tended to be stubborn, but would cry easily if admonished. He was easily startled and upset by loud noises. If something was said during the consultation that he didn't like he covered his ears. He was a solid looking child and he was prescribed Calc carb 30c.

By the next visit over 4 weeks later he had only needed to take five antihistamines instead of the usual 40 plus. The eruptions were itchy, but not painful and not as big as they had been. In accordance with the Direction of Cure, they were concentrated more on the extremities (fingers, hands, arms, feet) and he no longer had eruptions or swelling on the face. He had not coughed or wheezed all month.

At the next visit, 1 month later, he had been drug and symptom free for the preceding 3 weeks and was able to eat all the foods he had previously been allergic to.

ALOPECIA

This is loss of hair and may be of any degree from partial to total. It may be localised or generalised. In severe cases, there is loss of all body hair including eyebrows and eyelashes. It may be part of a skin disease such as tinea capitis or systemic lupus erythematosus. Radiation to the scalp causes permanent loss of hair to the specific area affected. Alopecia areata is a specific type of hair loss described below.

Symptoms

This may be localised or complete and usually affects just the scalp. There may be acute loss of hair. Patches of baldness typically have distinct margins. It is common and occurs as often in men as women. It is related to stressful situations and events. The risk of recurrence is increased in accordance to the degree of hair loss. Thus, the more hair that is lost, the more likely is any recurrence.

Treatment
There is no effective treatment in conventional medicine for alopecia areata. Treatment is given to the underlying skin disease if there is one.

Treatment (from mildest to strongest)	Comments
Irritant substances	Baldness usually persists with the addition of itching, soreness and weeping
Minoxidil	Also used in the treatment of hypertension. Used orally or locally
Local corticosteroids	High potency usually used
Injected corticosteroids (into scalp)	Triamcinolone usually used. Repeated every 4 - 6 weeks. It may cause blindness and lead to long-term systemic effects
Systemic corticosteroids	High incidence of side-effects

Table 11.7: Treatment of alopecia

Holistic management
In terms of Chinese medicine, the function of the Kidney and Blood is related to head hair. This is why alopecia comes on after a shock, as the Kidney is susceptible to fear and fright. Treatment is easier the sooner you see people after the commencement of symptoms. If the alopecia is severe and long-term, treatment will necessarily be more difficult and prolonged.

Case one
A girl of 15 years came for treatment of her hair. She had suffered with alopecia areata for the past 7 months. This was 1 month after starting a new school. She was generally anxious about lots of things including exams and school. She had fears of dogs and the dark. Her sleep had never been good and she often had a lot of unpleasant dreams. She would wake at intervals through the night. She had palpitations after a previous accident and difficulties at school.

In terms of Chinese medicine, the diagnosis was Kidney Yang Deficiency, Liver Blood Deficiency and Spleen Qi Deficiency. I gave her Chinese herbs to strengthen her Qi and Blood. The first thing her mother noticed was that she was much happier. Her hair became stronger and less fell out. She was energetic and after some 3 months her hair was fine.

She had had a bout of alopecia some years before and had recovered. Due to the stressful time she was having she had suffered a recurrence. It would probably get better on its own again but the point of treatment is to make sure that she is stronger than before and the recovery happens more quickly. It also reduces any likelihood of a later relapse.

VITILIGO

This is depigmentation of the skin. It is a common occurrence and indicates an autoimmune process. It is seen in about 1 per cent of the population and is mainly a cosmetic nuisance. There is depigmentation of the skin of the face, neck and knuckle areas. The significance of this condition is that it is associated with underlying conditions, namely diabetes mellitus, pernicious anaemia, Addison's disease, myxoedema and hyperthyroidism.

Some one third of cases may re-pigment spontaneously. In most people the affected areas extend gradually. Treatment may be given in the form of local corticosteroid applications but with little response.

Holistic management
In terms of Chinese medicine, this corresponds to an invasion of Wind and Dampness. It is known as 'white Wind'. There must be an internal disharmony to allow this invasion to occur, particularly in the case of a systemic autoimmune disease.

SKIN INFESTATIONS AND INFECTIONS

Staphylococcal infections

A staphylococcus is a bacterium, which is associated with localised inflammation and the formation of pus. This usually takes the form of boils or abscesses but in people with weak energy it may descend into deeper levels and cause pneumonia, septicaemia and so forth.

Boils

Bacterial conditions of this type, particularly if recurrent, may be associated with underlying disease. This may merely be a vague sensation of tiredness and being 'run down'. The underlying medical condition to consider is diabetes mellitus especially in recurrent boils, multiple boils and carbuncles.[9]

Symptoms
The hair follicle becomes infected with staphylococcal organisms and there is the appearance of localised inflammation with pus formation. This is the characteristic 'spot'. Its technical name is furuncle. It only occurs on skin where hair is found. They are commonest on the neck, axilla, buttocks and thighs. If they become multiple in numbers they may form a carbuncle.

Investigations
Swabs may be taken of sites such as the nose, axillae and perineum. Hospital workers are routinely checked to detect the presence of such bacteria.

Treatment
Oral antibiotics are invariably given to people with boils. These are of little use unless it is at an early stage, there is surrounding redness and there are constitutional symptoms such as malaise and perhaps fever. The use of antibiotics may lead to a reduction in size of the boil but the end result will be that the pus becomes surrounded by a thick wall and increases the likelihood of a recurrence. The body is now prevented from discharging the pus to the surface, which is the natural way of ridding the body of the problem. If the boil has formed pus then the correct conventional treatment is drainage. The boil is lanced and the purulent material allowed to discharge. The routine use of antibiotics in this inappropriate manner can only result in erosion of people's health and the continuance of boils.

If boils are recurrent, emphasis is placed on antiseptic washes and bathing although they are of variable effectiveness as the boil is a manifestation of an inner imbalance.

Holistic management
In terms of Chinese medicine, this is described as being due to invasion of Summer Heat. This is unusual in a cool temperate climate such as the UK. The more likely diagnosis is excessive intake of heating and greasy food leading to Heat in the internal organs. This causes the Accumulation of Poison or Damp-heat, which manifests on the skin.

It is worth making a point here about conditions that are associated with organisms. Of course, we only develop these if we are susceptible, however, it would be advisable to ensure that contact is controlled as far as possible. The people who are most likely to be susceptible are babies; pregnant women and those who take drugs that deplete the immune system. Sensible precautions to reduce contact are welcome but avoid alienating people since most disorders are difficult to 'catch'. If items such as towels or couch covers are in contact with infected areas then these must be adequately cleaned before allowing contact with another person. This is particularly true of the more infectious diseases of herpes infections, erysipelas and impetigo. Anything that perforates the skin must be sterilised.

Streptococcal infections

The streptococcus is associated with inflammation, which is less localised than that of a boil. It is connected to a wide variety of disorders, which include acute tonsillitis, scarlet fever, erysipelas, puerperal fever and wound infections (traumatic or operative). The inflammation does stay localised but spreads into surrounding tissues. In the case of tonsillitis there may be spread into the general circulation to produce rash (scarlet fever), heart symptoms (rheumatic fever) or kidneys (acute proliferative glomerulonephritis).

Erysipelas

This is streptococcal infection of the skin. It can occur at any age but is most severe in the very young and the very old. It often affects the face since the bacteria can live in the nostrils. Legs may be affected in areas of varicose ulceration. Infants are susceptible around the umbilical cord where inflammation may spread to the trunk. Circumcision wounds may also be affected.

Symptoms
These develop quickly with shivering and fever. There is painful swelling of the superficial tissues in the affected area with redness and soreness. The condition spreads rapidly outwards from the first area affected. Blisters may develop in the central area because of the degree of inflammatory oedema.

There are systemic symptoms of toxaemia such as fever, restlessness, insomnia and possibly delirium. The relevant groups of lymph nodes are enlarged. Oedema may be seen in recurrent cases.

Treatment
Penicillin is always given to eradicate the streptococci and reduce the inflammation.

Holistic management
In terms of Chinese medicine, this is due to an Invasion of Wind and Fire.

Impetigo

This is a superficial skin infection, which is streptococcal in some cases and staphylococcal in others.

Symptoms
The typical appearance is of superficial vesicles, which rupture to leave a yellowish crusting area. It mainly affects the face, especially around the chin and angle of the mouth, and is commonest in children. It may spread in some cases but is usually fairly localised.

Treatment
It can be spread by close contact and via towels, flannels and so forth. The main treatment is by means of antiseptic washes. Oral antibiotics are only required if there is widespread disease.

Holistic management
In terms of Chinese medicine, this is due to Heat in the Lung channel and Damp in the Stomach channel, which explains its typical distribution. The Stomach channel crosses the cheek near the angle of the mouth.

Case one
A boy of 8 months, who had been born prematurely, was brought for treatment of his chest. He had a phlegmy cough, felt hot in the head and was sweaty. He had had chickenpox some 4 weeks earlier. I made a diagnosis of Phlegm-heat in the Lungs. I treated him with massage to acupuncture points and gave him a herbal formula to resolve the Damp-heat in the Lungs. His chest recovered well and some 4 weeks later he developed itchy skin generally with some dryish papular patches. These were mainly on his feet and cheeks. He continued with the herbs and over the next few weeks his feet improved. His cheek worsened and his chest remained good. The rash on his cheek was now dry, red and scaly with some crusting. His doctor diagnosed this as impetigo and he received a course of antibiotics.

Subsequently, he developed a dry cough with fever, was generally off colour with no appetite and his skin looked much better – more dry and scaling than crusting. This is the classical picture of a suppression. I treated him in the acute stage of the fever and he improved within half an hour. The next day he was good in himself. Over the next 4 weeks, his rash worsened to become reddened and crusting again. His chest, appetite, energy and bowels were all normal. I encouraged his mother to go with the herbal treatment as he was clearly improving although outer levels may worsen for a short time. I impressed on her the importance of healthy inner levels as an indication of a healing process. Within 4 more weeks, he continued to improve and his skin was normal. He is well some 2 years later. He occasionally reacts to climatic changes with wheezing or a slight cough but this quickly clears. His growth and development are normal and he is very healthy.

Case two
A girl of 6 years came for treatment of frequent outbreaks of impetigo around her right eye. She had had it on and off for 18 months. It had been conventionally treated with steroid creams. She found it difficult to go to sleep on her own. She had a 'giddy feeling' in her stomach and was generally fidgety and restless. She had nightmares about spiders. Her mother said she liked to do dangerous and forbidden things. She also said she was very curious. During the consultation, she drew a stick picture of her family in bright primary colours and they all looked like spiders! She was given Tarantula Hispanica 30c.

She was able to sleep alone and the bad dreams stopped. Her giddy feeling disappeared. Her mother said the remedy made her very calm, which was just as well because she had to deal with quite a physical clear out.

An area on her left foot (corresponding to the Spleen channel) opened up and began discharging pus, as did her left thumb and right elbow. Her right eye filled with pus and swelled closed. She also had swollen glands in her neck. Both the child and the mother were very happy with the situation, as I had told them about the Direction of Cure. Other members of the family were not so pleased with the results! This went on for over 1 week. At the time of writing 1 year later she remains well and has had no major outbreak since.

FUNGAL INFECTIONS

Ringworm

This, despite its name, is a fungal infection. It is given different terms depending upon the site affected. The infection is spread from animals, humans or the environment.

Tinea pedis

This is when the feet are affected. There is inflammation, which can be severe, and secondary infection may develop. It is spread in swimming baths, saunas and showers. This association has led it to be termed 'athletes foot'. Several members of the same family may be affected.

Symptoms
The main areas affected are in between the toes and the soles of the feet. There is redness, scaling, weeping, itching and occasionally blistering. It may spread to the hands, groins (tinea cruris) and perianal area.

Treatment
The older type of treatments include local application of potassium permanganate solution, which is dark purple in colour and correspondingly unpopular. Antifungal agents are commonly used. Griseofulvin is given orally for about 3 months. Local applications are with clotrimazole, miconazole, terbinafine or amorolfine. Other oral treatments include itraconazole and terbinafine.

Holistic management
In terms of Chinese medicine, this is due to Damp-heat in the Stomach and Spleen draining downward into the feet and manifesting on the skin.

Tinea corporis

This is increasingly common as a result of the wide use of topical corticosteroids. It is ringworm affecting the body.

Symptoms
Patches of redness and scaling are seen on the body. There may also be papules and pustules in some cases. The areas are itchy. These are the symptoms of eczema. The main points of differentiation are that eczema tends to worsen and improve in a cyclical nature; people with eczema may have generalised skin symptoms (such as dryness and itching) and the typical eczema distribution (see above). In contrast, ringworm tends to be concentrated in one site.

Treatment
In general, this is treated as tinea pedis above. If the nails are affected then systemic treatment with griseofulvin is given for at least 9 months for fingernails and 2 years for toenails. Itraconazole may also be used. This condition is notoriously resistant to treatment. In some cases the nails will be removed.

Holistic management
In terms of Chinese medicine, this is due to invasion of Damp-heat into the skin.

Tinea capitis

This is rare now.

Symptoms
There are patches of scalp affected by scaling and hair loss. It is much more likely to occur in children. In some there is associated inflammation with weeping and crusting. This more severe type may result in permanent hair loss.

Treatment
The disease spreads from animals and so the source of infection is treated. This is by means of systemic anti-fungal treatments. Griseofulvin is an older drug, which has been largely replaced by itraconazole. Treatment is given for up to 3 months.

Holistic management
This is due to invasion of Wind and may develop as either a white or a yellow appearance.

Pityriasis versicolor (tinea versicolor)

This is caused by a yeast and is common in tropical climates. It has become commoner in temperate climates in recent years. There is scaling and confluent macules on the trunk, upper arms and neck. They may be hyper- or hypo-pigmented, usually the latter.

Treatment
Selenium sulphide shampoo is applied to the body. Otherwise, the antifungal agents miconazole, clotrimazole or econazole are applied locally. In severe cases there may be oral itraconazole or ketoconazole given.

Holistic management
In terms of Chinese medicine, this is described as 'white skin Wind'. It is due to Invasion of Wind into the skin.

Candidiasis

This is a yeast type of fungus, which may cause symptoms in many areas of the body. In this situation it leads to skin symptoms. The fungus, *Candida albicans*, is present in many people with no symptoms. Symptoms occur when the immune system is depleted either as a result of condition (such as diabetes mellitus, pregnancy) or drugs (such as female sex hormones, antibiotics, corticosteroids and cancer chemotherapy). For more details of Candidiasis see Chapter 18 – Women's Health and Chapter 13 – Gastrointestinal system.

Symptoms
Moist areas of the body are more commonly affected, e.g. skin folds, groin, axillae and nappy area in babies. There is the appearance of a skin rash, which bears some similarities to eczema. There is redness, soreness, some scaling although this is slight if there is any wetness and itching.

The nails may be affected (paronychia) and is commoner in situations where the hands are frequently wet. There is redness and soreness of the cuticle and eventually deformity of the nail.

Treatment
It is important to keep the affected area clean and dry. Specific treatment is given by means of antifungal agents. They may be given locally, e.g. nystatin or an imidazole such as miconazole or clotrimazole. Oral drugs may be given, e.g. trizoles such as fluconazole, itraconazole. Some cases may be given a combination corticosteroid and antifungal to reduce inflammation as well as kill the fungus. Ketoconazole is used for cases which are extremely severe and life-threatening since it causes potentially serious liver damage.

Holistic management of fungal infections
This is essentially the same as described for eczema. The appearance is the same and the fungus only attacks the skin because of an underlying susceptibility. To treat the skin with antifungal agents runs the risk of suppressing the imbalance deeper into the body. Constitutional treatment is necessary and this may have to be prolonged to change nail disease.

TUMOURS OF THE SKIN

Warts

These are tumours, which are associated with a virus. They may be spread to susceptible people by contact. This usually occurs in public bathing places such as swimming baths. Once they have appeared, they may disappear spontaneously within 6 months. Up to 30 per cent of cases may do this.

Symptoms
Warts are papular growths on the surface of the skin and may appear in a short period of time. They may be seen in any area but the hands, knees and feet are the commonest sites. In some cases the warts may be flatter and more elongated. These are known as plane warts. On the feet they are termed verrucas and on the soles turn inward due to pressure. They are evident there as flattened, hard areas with a darkish centre. They may give rise to discomfort when walking.

As mentioned in relation to psoriasis, damage to the skin in any skin disease may lead to the appearance of symptoms at that site. This also occurs with warts where damage to warts by scratching, rubbing or conventional treatments often leads to the appearance of more warts in the surrounding area.

Treatment

Warts may disappear spontaneously and so it is often preferable to leave well alone. People may request treatment due to cosmetic considerations or because skin problems are often poorly tolerated in our society. Conventional treatments are aimed at burning the wart with chemicals, carbon dioxide snow or liquid nitrogen. The warts may be surgically removed in some instances. Injections of alpha-interferon or bleomycin (cancer chemotherapy agent) may be used. They are painful and cause permanent scarring.

When warts disappear naturally they leave no scars. The treatments above damage the skin and may leave scars, which may be painful in some cases, particularly on the feet.

Holistic management

In terms of Chinese medicine, the exact cause depends upon the appearance of the warts. They are usually considered to be due to Liver and Blood Deficiency. Flat warts are related to Liver Fire and Invasion of Wind and Heat.

A time-honoured way of removing warts is to have them 'charmed'. This may be by means of rubbing them with potato peel, broad bean pod or other items of food and bury this in the garden. As the object rots then the wart disappears. One method I advised was to draw a circle the same size as the wart. This was to be repeated each day but drawing a slightly smaller circle. After several weeks when the circle had reduced in size to a dot this was to be rubbed out. The warts should then disappear. I was waiting with bated breath to see if it worked but I never saw the person again! Either the warts had completely disappeared or the person thought my suggestion was so strange they decided not to return. I would place wart charming in the same category as visualisation.

Case one

A boy of 12 years of age came for treatment of his stomach pains. He had suffered with epigastric and hypochondrial pains over the previous 4 years. All investigations at the hospital had been normal and he had no conventional diagnosis. His bowels were sluggish and never felt as if they emptied. His general energy was poor and he had missed a lot of school in the year prior to seeking treatment. He had frequent colds which would go down to his chest leading to wheezing and coughing. He had had pneumonia some 5 years previously when he was very ill. I made a diagnosis of Spleen and Lung Qi Deficiency and gave him tonic herbs as well as acupuncture treatment.

He improved quickly, which is often the case with young people. His general energy improved, he had very few pains in his abdomen and his bowels became more regular. After 2 months of treatment, he started to develop some warts over his fingers and also the soles of his feet. He was keen to have treatment for those in his feet as they were becoming uncomfortable. Such an appearance on the skin during the course of treatment for a chronic condition is a good sign of a curative process. He continued with the treatment and within 2 months the warts had disappeared. His health continues to be good.

Case two

A 9-year-old girl came for treatment of warts on her hands. She had nine, including one large one. There were more on the left than the right hand. She also had one under her eye and a verucca on her right foot. She had a tendency to croupy coughs.

She said that she was impatient to be older and when asked why she said: "So I can wear high shoes and kiss a boy". Her mother described her as very sexual and curious. She liked to get lost in supermarkets because it was "cool and adventurous".

She loved loud music and dancing. She spent a lot of time talking to me about colours she liked and disliked. "When I'm angry I love black. When I'm happy I like yellow. When I'm sad I like light blue. When I love the whole world I feel purple". During the consultation she couldn't sit still and wriggled on her chair constantly. She also said: "Sometimes I feel really angry and I have to hit myself".

Taking all of this into account she was prescribed Tarantula Hispanica 30c, which is a spider remedy. It suited every aspect of the case.

The next time I saw her she came in wearing a T-shirt with a web on the front! She sat through the whole follow up without wriggling. After the remedy her warts became very itchy, some got bigger and two new ones appeared. When I asked her if there had been any other changes she said: "I feel more happy". Her cough improved and her fear of the dark completely disappeared. Her appetite had improved and she was having daily bowel movements (before it had been every 2 days). The warts completely cleared soon after this second appointment.

Many people take Thuja to try to clear warts. It is probably unwise to take anything routinely to clear a skin condition, as there is a risk of driving the disease to a deeper level. An accurate constitutional treatment will not only clear the warts but also make the person feel better in themselves.

Genital warts

These are often associated with sexually transmitted disease. They may be penile, vulval or anal in site.

Symptoms
Genital warts are fleshier in their appearance than the simple warts above. They appear quite moist. In women it is the vulva which is usually affected. In men the warts are found around the glans penis. Anal warts may affect both sexes.

There is an association with a whole range of disorders including sexually transmitted disease, cervical dysplasia, pelvic inflammatory disease and so on.

Treatment
They are treated by the application of mildly burning chemicals or by surgery.

MALIGNANT TUMOURS OF THE SKIN

Tumours of the skin are common as it is in constant contact with ultraviolet light, chemicals and external influences and is continually actively regenerating. I shall discuss here four malignant tumours of skin, which are the most important clinically.

Basal cell carcinoma

Also known as 'rodent ulcer' and found mainly on the head and neck. Its frequency is increased with more exposure to sunlight, particularly in a hot climate, and in fair skinned races. Other causes include medical irradiation and arsenic medication.[10]

Symptoms
There is the development of a papule, which grows slowly. Its centre starts to degenerate and an ulcer is eventually formed. A common first complaint is of a 'sore' which will not heal. As they grow commonly on the face it may be cut whilst shaving and this may be the first sign. The cancer tends to invade locally, hence its name 'rodent ulcer'. Secondary spread is extremely rare.

Treatment
This is by means of radiotherapy or local excision.

Squamous cell carcinoma

This is a more invasive type of malignancy, which can spread to distant sites. It is more frequent in skin that has been damaged in the past to the point of scarring, perhaps by chemicals. Sunlight increases the likelihood of such a cancer.

Symptoms
The tumour appears as a hardened lump usually on the ear or lip. There is thickening of surrounding tissue. It may ulcerate.

Treatment
This is by local excision. Radiotherapy may also be applied.

Malignant melanoma

This is much more frequent with the increase in sunbathing and the desire for suntans. It is more common in fair-skinned races. Melanoma is a mole, which is a benign, pigmented area, found in many people. It becomes a problem only if it undergoes malignant change.

Symptoms
If a mole changes in size, shape or colour then malignancy must be suspected. There may be symptoms of itching or bleeding.

Treatment

The outcome, conventionally, depends upon the size of the tumour at the time of diagnosis and the site on the body. If it is less than 1 mm thick, histologically, then the 5-years survival rate is more than 90 per cent and less than 50 per cent if more than 3.5 mm thick. The prognosis is better on the trunk than the face and the limbs than the trunk.

Local excision is the conventional treatment of choice with a wide area of skin taken from around the melanoma. Secondaries are treated with a combination of radiotherapy and chemotherapy which, conventional practitioners admit, make no difference to the outcome.

Kaposi's sarcoma

This is more common now as it is one of the malignancies seen in people with AIDS.

Symptoms
The original symptom is of a discoloured area, which resembles a bruise. This becomes darker and develops into a lump. They may be multiple in sites. They may also occur in the gastrointestinal tract, liver and lymph glands.

Treatment
In people with AIDS such sarcomas are frequently rapidly progressive. Classically, treatment is by means of radiotherapy and chemotherapy but this can only be considered to be symptomatic in such cases.

Holistic management of malignant skin tumours
The discussion in Chapter 6 – Cancer – with regard to malignant disease is relevant here. Most people will probably opt for conventional treatment. People with secondaries from malignant melanoma may present for holistic medical treatment but usually at a severe stage. In terms of energetic medicine, these cancers should be the easiest to produce improvement as they are on the most superficial physical organ. Certainly in discussion with practitioners who treat cancer by holistic methods it seems this is true. This is, of course, at variance with the conventional prognosis, particularly of malignant melanoma.

HOW TO RECOGNISE SERIOUS CONDITIONS OF THE SKIN

Skin diseases are common in our society and the symptoms listed below are extremely common. It is important to know how to recognise if a symptom arises from a serious situation. You can use Table 11.8 below as a guide to refer to when faced with a patient who has one or more of these symptoms. I make no mention of disease labels in the column on the right, as I would not expect you to be able to diagnose conventionally. Seriousness can be assessed merely by reference to symptom pictures.

Symptom	Cause for concern
Vesicles	Haemorrhagic
Bullae	Large
Redness, weeping	Severe Large areas of skin surface
Lumps, nodules	Short history Recent change Progressive Bleeding

Table 11.8: How to recognise serious conditions in dermatology

Summary

Table 11.8 summarises diseases according to their appearance. This will be more helpful if you obtain an illustrated guide to skin disease.[11]

Symptom	Disease label
Crusting	Impetigo
Dryness	Eczema
Exfoliation	Psoriasis
Itching	Eczema, psoriasis, urticaria, tinea, candidiasis, scabies, head lice
Lumps, nodules	Warts, tumours
Plaque	Psoriasis (some types)
Pustule	Psoriasis (some types), acne vulgaris, boils
Scaling	Psoriasis, tinea, candidiasis
Redness	Eczema, psoriasis, acne rosacea, erysipelas, tinea, candidiasis
Thickening of the skin	Eczema, psoriasis
Ulcer	Tumours
Vesicles (blisters)	Eczema, erysipelas, impetigo, tinea, scabies
Weeping	Eczema, impetigo, tinea, candidiasis
Wheal	Urticaria

Table 11.9: Skin diseases listed according their appearances

Skin disease is very common and conventional treatment is relatively ineffective.

Conventional treatments suppress the skin lesions resulting in internal disease at the worst or variable control of the skin symptoms at best.

Holistic treatment of skin disease may result in a worsening before improvement particularly if it has been suppressed. This has cosmetic considerations.

Although the skin is the outermost level of the physical body, it does reflect internal imbalances. If the skin problem is associated with a marked internal imbalance the treatment may take a long time to achieve results.

If the skin problem is relatively superficial, i.e. on the palms or soles and there is little in the way of an internal imbalance, response can be rapid and dramatic.

---

[1] It is considered in Chinese medicine that males go through cycles of 8 years and females 7 years. This is further discussed in relation to the cycles of menstruation and fertility in Chapter 18 – Women's Health.

[2] Lanolin, wool fat, is a common component of creams and ointments and may cause a contact dermatitis which is indistinguishable in its appearance from the original condition.

[3] Petroleum products may cause allergic reactions in the skin and it is helpful to enquire what applications the person is using. These may include paraffin which is used to treat eczema.

[4] It is sensible to use ecological soaps and detergents both in terms of health and to benefit the environment.

[5] A study found that the use of stress reduction techniques such as meditation and imaging led to a marked improvement in cases of psoriasis. *Acta DermVenereol-Suppl-Stockh* 1991;156:37-43.

[6] Lithium compounds are used in the treatment of manic depression.

7 This may cause liver fibrosis and people require a liver biopsy before treatment commences and yearly.

8 Anaphylaxis is a severe allergic reaction characterised by wheezing, breathlessness, cyanosis, low blood pressure, nausea, vomiting and diarrhoea. It is a life-threatening situation.

9 A carbuncle is a collection or group of boils.

10 Arsenic was formerly used to treat syphilis and parasitic infestations.

11 Examples include *A Colour Atlas of Physical Signs in General Medicine* by Zatouroff (Mosby, 1979), *Dermatology – An Illustrated Guide* by Fry (Butterworths, 1984).

12 SPECIAL SENSES

INTRODUCTION

Diseases of the eye are not commonly seen in the clinic. Ear disease is more frequently encountered and many children with acute and chronic ear conditions present to holistic practitioners. Tinnitus and vertigo are also quite common.

The eye and ear are important sensory organs and so it is useful to know what symptoms may appear and in the case of eye disease, particularly, it may be necessary to seek specialist help. The situations where this is most helpful are discussed in the text but it frequently involves those symptoms that suggest a threat to sight.

More commonly, people may come for treatment of a systemic problem and also have symptoms of eye or ear disease. The two may be considered to be unconnected by conventional practitioners.

EYE DISEASE

ANATOMY AND PHYSIOLOGY

There are several basic facts of anatomy and physiology that it is useful to know. I consider that most courses in these subjects are over detailed and reflect orthodox thinking rather than the particular needs of the holistic practitioner. To study eye disease it would be helpful to be able to:

- Identify the structures of the eye
- Describe the functions of these structures
- Explain the mechanism of vision

The common symptoms that arise from eye disease are pain, soreness, redness and visual disturbances (such as blurring, 'floaters' or double vision. There may also be discharge from the eye.

CLASSIFICATION OF EYE DISEASE

In conventional medicine, this is made according to the site of the problem:

- Conjunctivitis
- Keratitis
- Episcleritis
- Scleritis
- Uveitis
- Posterior uveitis (choroiditis)
- Cataract
- Glaucoma

For holistic practitioners it is more useful to categorise these diseases according to their severity and their ability to harm sight – Table 12.1.

Mild disease
Conjunctivitis
Episcleritis
Scleritis
Posterior uveitis (choroiditis)
Cataract
Keratitis
Uveitis (iritis)
Glaucoma
Severe disease

Table 12.1: Energetic classification of eye disease by severity

INVESTIGATION OF EYE DISEASE

These are specialised and carried out by ophthalmologists rather than general physicians. Technical equipment can be used to examine the eye and parts of the eye. Pressure of fluid within the eye can be measured. Eye charts are well known to all as a method of checking visual acuity. All such investigations are non-invasive and would be in Category 1 as defined in Chapter 4 – Investigations. The only exception to this is the use of some eye drops and stains for particular examinations. These are temporary in their effect and of low risk.

CONJUNCTIVITIS

In conventional medicine this is usually considered to be infective in nature – bacterial or viral. Conjunctivitis is more likely in situations of poor hygiene or a dusty environment. A milder, recurrent form is a feature of Reiter's syndrome which is a classical triad of conjunctivitis, urethritis (comparable to non-gonococcal urethritis) and polyarthritis. Allergic reactions may produce similar symptoms although the discharge then is clear or white with associated itching and nasal symptoms.

Symptoms
The main feature is redness that may be mild and only affect small area of the conjunctiva or more extensive. There is discomfort in the eyes, which usually is described as a feeling of grittiness. There is a white, or more commonly yellow, discharge in the eyes. This is often accompanied by sensitivity to light. The symptoms may vary in severity from person to person and some have severe problems with soreness, redness and a profuse discharge. The most extreme cases involve the whole conjunctiva, including the area lining the inside of the eyelids.

Complications
The main complication is chronic conjunctivitis which is characterised by persistence of the redness and discharge, grittiness, and feelings of heat in the eyes.

Treatment
This is invariably by means of local antibiotics although many cases are viral in nature. Advice is also given about bathing the eye and local hygiene.

Holistic management
In terms of Chinese medicine, conjunctivitis is due to Invasion of Wind and Heat. If these factors continue to affect the eye then acute cases become chronic. Overindulgence in alcohol, overuse of the eyes, exposure to wind, poor lighting and inadequate sleep may all contribute to a chronic state. In some, there may be underlying Liver Blood Deficiency.

This condition is rarely serious despite the appearance and the uncomfortable nature of the symptoms. There are very effective treatments available in Chinese medicine, homoeopathy and herbalism, which can remove the need for antibiotics.

KERATITIS

This is inflammation of the cornea, which is associated with either viruses, fungi or, less commonly, bacteria.

Symptoms
There is pain in the eye rather than the soreness of conjunctivitis. Watering is profuse and there is associated discomfort from light. There may be spasm of the eyelid and pupil. Redness is present but usually restricted to the circumcorneal area. It may be possible to see a corneal ulcer, which will have the appearance of a grey circular area on the corneal surface.

Investigations
An ulcer on the cornea or small spots may be seen using special staining methods.

Complications
The main worry of keratitis is impairment of vision and ultimately blindness from scarring of the cornea. Symptoms to look for would include persistence and worsening of symptoms. Any visual disturbances would clearly be a cause for concern. Because of the threat to sight, effective treatment must be instituted without delay.

Treatment
This is invariably with antibiotics or antifungal agents.

Holistic management
The main issue for holistic practitioners is to recognise the more serious nature of this condition when compared with conjunctivitis.

EPISCLERITIS AND SCLERITIS

This is an inflammation of the episclera. It is part of a more general autoimmune reaction and so may be seen in people with rheumatoid arthritis, systemic lupus erythematosus and so on. A more severe variant is scleritis.

Symptoms

In cases of episcleritis, there is a localised area of redness in one eye. There is pain rather than irritation and tenderness on palpation through a closed eyelid. There is no discharge from the eye. Occasionally, both eyes may be affected.

Scleritis, on the other hand, is a more serious problem with more severe symptoms. There is pain in the forehead and sinus area also. The redness is darker than that of episcleritis with white patches. These indicate that parts of the sclera are dying.

Treatment

Episcleritis usually settles on its own within a few weeks. Non-steroidal anti-inflammatory drugs will be given if it persists.

Scleritis is treated with high dose non-steroidal anti-inflammatory drugs and occasionally by means of corticosteroids.

Holistic management

This condition, in its milder forms, is merely uncomfortable and treatment must be directed at the underlying systemic disease. Care must be taken if the more severe scleritis is suspected.

UVEITIS

This is an inflammation of the uveal tract[1] and is a combination of an affection of the iris – iritis (anterior uveitis) and ciliary body – cyclitis. These areas are intimately connected with function of the pupil and so a common symptom is blurring of vision.

Symptoms

There is an acute onset of severe pain, discomfort from light and a mild to moderate degree of blurred vision. It is usually present in one eye. There is redness, which is generalised (as seen in conjunctivitis) but with intense redness in the circumcorneal region. There is watering particularly on exposure to light, but never a yellowish discharge. There is marked tenderness. There are some similarities with the symptoms of glaucoma.

Complications

Cataract may develop some years after attacks of uveitis.

Treatment

This is by means of corticosteroids and in severe cases, immunosuppressants or cytotoxic drugs.

Case one

A man of 40 years came for treatment of his Reiter's syndrome. This is characterised by recurrent attacks of arthritis, conjunctivitis and urethritis. In this case, he would develop uveitis every year usually in the winter. It is considered to be autoimmune in nature. His main symptoms were joint pains for the previous 15 years, which on occasion would be so severe that he could hardly walk. He had received treatment with Chinese medicine in the past, which had helped, but he had received no treatment for the previous 5 years.

His main complaints now were severe back pain worse at night, which would affect his sleep. Movement would alleviate the pain but only after sometimes an hour of walking around. His joints generally would be uncomfortable but particularly his ankles and knees. His energy was generally low and he had feelings of irritability and general dissatisfaction with his life. I made a diagnosis according to Chinese medicine of Liver Blood Deficiency, Kidney Yin Deficiency and Damp Accumulation. I treated him with acupuncture and with herbs over the course of the next 8 months.

In that time, he felt generally better with improved energy, less joint pains and some improvement in his emotional state. Then he developed an acute redness of his left eye, which would happen once a year. His eye was sore and painful, markedly red with blurring of vision. Such symptoms are indicative of a severe inflammation affecting the eye. I treated daily for several days with small improvements each time but it would not hold and after 1 week his visual disturbances were more severe. Blurring with redness are indications of a severe process and I recommended that he attend the local eye hospital. In such a situation, his vision is at risk and this needs to be addressed as a matter of some urgency. He had a short course of corticosteroids and antibiotics, which rapidly settled his symptoms. Since this attack, his treatment has continued and he is looking much more at the underlying psychological issues of his condition. His treatment is ongoing.

POSTERIOR UVEITIS (choroiditis)

This is an inflammation of the posterior part of the uveal tract – the choroid. It is associated with infection, rheumatoid arthritis or gout. There is swelling and consequently disordered function of the retina.

Symptoms
There is usually only blurring of vision due to retinal oedema and damage.

Treatment
Local applications are given to maintain pupillary dilatation as this decreases pressure in the eye. Corticosteroids with or without antibiotics are prescribed depending on the cause.

CATARACT

This is a loss of transparency of the lens, which leads to a distortion of vision especially for distant objects.

Cataract may develop due to various factors. These include:

- drugs. This is known as toxic cataract and may be the result of several drugs including chlorpromazine, ergotamine, corticosteroids (oral and locally in the eye), smoking, alcohol
- ultraviolet B radiation
- diabetes mellitus
- low antioxidant vitamin status[2]
- perforating injury
- eye disease, e.g. uveitis.

Its development without these predisposing causes in later life is known as senile[3] cataract.

Symptoms
There is the gradual development of myopia – shortsightedness. In the case of those with hypermetropia (longsightedness) this tends to improve. Interference with vision becomes more obvious with increasing lens opacity. Eventually only hand movements may be vaguely seen.

Treatment
There is no conventional medical treatment to prevent cataract or its progression. Correction of vision by means of spectacles or contact lenses may be possible in the early stages. It is helpful to reduce the strain caused by reading using good light, large print books and so on. Surgery is the usual conventional treatment and is best reserved for severe cases of sight-impairment where there is interference with daily activities. Anaesthesia may be general or local.

Surgery is the only conventional treatment available if the cataract interferes seriously with vision. Only one eye is dealt with at a time. There must be a delay of several months before treating the second eye. The surgery improves vision for 90 per cent of patients. People usually require reading glasses after the operation. There are three types of surgical procedure available. The commonest is removal of the lens and the front part of the lens capsule. Rarely, the lens and the entire lens capsule is removed. Removal of the lens with implantation of a plastic lens may be performed. Rejection of the implant may lead to episodes of redness, soreness and visual disturbances. Antibiotic and corticosteroid drops are given routinely after the operation.

Eye complications of surgery, which occur in up to 5 per cent, include retinal detachment, uveitis, glaucoma, haemorrhage into the eye (usually minor and occasionally severe) and infection. General complications include cardiac failure, respiratory problems, stroke, diabetes mellitus, uncontrolled nausea and vomiting, acute urinary retention and acute confusional state.[4]

A consequence of modern cataract surgery is opacification of the posterior lens capsule. As the opacification increases, the person begins to notice a decrease in visual function. Laser surgery is usually performed for this. Complications include glaucoma, haemorrhage, retinal detachment and corneal oedema.

Case one
A woman of 47 years came for treatment of cataracts. She couldn't focus properly and said it was like seeing through smoke. Bright light caused a knife-like, yet painless, sensation in her eyes. Her lower field of vision was the worst affected. She was under a lot of stress and was an insulin-dependent diabetic. She was also taking thyroxine. She had a history of gallstones and experienced the colic as also knife-like. She was prescribed Lachesis 30c. This remedy covered many of her symptoms

well, including her vision difficulties.

A month later she was able to undo some strings, something she hadn't been able to do before and she felt her vision was better, but wanted to take a test to be sure. The knife like sensations had gone. Her blood sugar levels were lower. Her sleep was better and she felt calmer. She felt livelier and able to think more clearly.

A subsequent test revealed that the cataracts had gone. Her vision began to deteriorate again about 2 years later and the remedy was repeated.

SQUINT

A squint (strabismus) is an abnormal alignment of the two eyes. This results in an object being seen from slightly different angles by each eye. The consequence is the classical symptom of squint – double vision (diplopia). It is important to differentiate this from blurring and close questioning may be necessary to determine the exact nature of the visual disturbance. True double vision means two separate objects – side by side or one above the other.

There are considered to be several causes conventionally – Table 12.2.

Process	Comments
Paralysis or weakness of one or more eye muscles (paralytic squint)	Injury Central nervous system disease, e.g. stroke, brain tumour Neuropathy, either single or associated with systemic disease, e.g. multiple sclerosis, thyroid disease, myasthenia gravis, diabetes mellitus
Failure of eyes to co-ordinate	This is the type requiring eye exercises and spectacles. In the young, the cause is unknown but the child will rarely complain and soon learns to suppress one image. In older people intermittent double vision might occur when they are under stress or sedation
Alteration in angle of long-standing squint	This is one of the difficulties of treating squints in adults. Squints should be treated in early life before unwanted images are suppressed

Table 12.2: Common causes of double vision

Symptoms
There is double vision as each eye is seeing an object from a slightly different angle. The long-term consequence is suppression of vision in the squinting eye. Some people may develop abnormal head postures to achieve as much reduction in the double vision as possible.

Treatment
This is dependent upon the cause. Paralytic squint is, as its name suggests, due to paralysis of the muscles of the eye. This may occur as part of a local problem with a cranial nerve or due to diseases such as stroke or brain tumour. Treatment will therefore depend upon the total clinical picture.

In young children, squint may develop due to inadequate maturation of binocular vision. The vision in the affected eye may be rapidly suppressed. The most effective treatment is that which is given early. Covering of the normal eye allows the 'lazy' eye an opportunity to recover. Eye exercises are an important part of such treatment. Surgery to the eye muscles may be applied in resistant cases to adjust the angle of vision.

Holistic management
In Chinese medicine, the frequent cause is insufficiency of Qi and Blood supplying the eye. Treatment is aimed at improving these and regulating the muscles of the eyes. Eye exercises[5] are useful for this condition.

Case one
A boy of 2 years came for treatment of a squint which had been noticed some 12 months previously. His left eye turned inward and he would blink frequently. His appetite was not good and his bowels were often loose. I made a diagnosis of Qi and Blood Deficiency and treated him with Chinese herbs. I also recommended points for his mother to massage each day particularly around the eyes.

After 3 months of treatment, his appetite had improved and his bowels were normal. His blinking had stopped and his eyes were generally stronger. His squint was much less noticeable and generally only when he was tired.

GLAUCOMA

This is a rise in the pressure within the eye. If this persists or worsens, the optic nerve can be damaged resulting in visual loss. There are several types of glaucoma.

Chronic simple glaucoma (open-angle glaucoma) develops in the middle-aged or elderly and is unusual before the age of 40. It affects both eyes and there is frequently a family history of the condition. It is also commoner in those with shortsightedness and diabetes mellitus.

Congestive glaucoma (closed-angle glaucoma) is found more often in people with longsightedness. The mechanism of development is not well understood by conventional medicine.

Secondary glaucoma develops as a result of a pre-existing condition. This includes injury, uveitis, and the use of local corticosteroid drops.

Symptoms

In chronic simple glaucoma, there may be virtually no symptoms except an occasional ache. There is an insidious, progressive visual loss, which is mainly peripheral until it becomes severe.

In congestive glaucoma, the onset is more acute. There is discomfort of the eye with associated mistiness of vision and rainbow-like haloes. This may be transient but if prolonged and severe leads to discomfort in the light, watering of the eye and perhaps vomiting. There is marked loss of vision if the pressure remains high and it may result in intractable blindness. Circumcorneal redness is a constant feature. Symptoms are worse in the dark since pressure within the eye is then greater due to the pupil being dilated. The condition may affect both eyes.

Treatment

Chronic simple glaucoma can be treated by several methods. Eye drops of pilocarpine, latanoprost, brimonidine or acetazolamide are commonly used. The betablocker, timolol, can also be used as eye drops. In resistant cases, surgery may be employed. This is either by an operation to drain fluid from the eye or, more commonly nowadays, by laser treatment. Eye drops have to be continued after laser treatment.

Congestive glaucoma is treated in the acute phase by dilation of the pupil as this reduces intra-ocular pressure. Surgery is always carried out at a later date.

The treatment of secondary glaucoma is by means of acetazolamide drops but frequently surgery is performed. Laser surgery or microsurgery can be used to open the drainage channels to reduce intra-ocular pressure. The effects of the surgery usually last less than 1 year.

Holistic management

In Chinese medicine, this is due to depletion of Kidney Yin. This causes Wind and Fire in the Liver and Gall Bladder to ascend disrupting Qi in the channels. It is reasonable to treat people with glaucoma by means of holistic medicine but it is important for monitoring of the intra-ocular pressures to be done. The normal figures are between 16 and 22 mm Hg (millimetres of mercury) with variations up to 3–5 mm that may occur over the day. The highest pressures are seen in the early hours of the morning during sleep.

I have treated people with glaucoma who had pressures up to the high 20's and low 30's and this would seem to be fine. The other things to take into account are the symptoms. It would be a cause for concern if these were marked even with relatively low pressures.

REVIEW OF SYMPTOMS OF EYE DISEASE

Visual acuity

This is sharpness of vision. Its measurement can be a precise guide to the severity of a condition and whether it is changing. The recorded loss of one line on the standard sight-testing chart is indicative of a significant impairment.

A test with a card pierced by a pinhole will show whether or not the blurring is caused by changes in refraction.[6] If these are the cause then the visual acuity will improve when the person looks out through the pinhole placed close to their eyes. This test will determine whether or not spectacles are likely to solve the problem. The common refractive errors are shortsightedness (myopia), longsightedness (hypermetropia) and astigmatism. They can be corrected, more or less, by the use of spectacles and/or contact lenses.

There is a possibility that some purely visual symptoms may be the presenting symptoms of systemic disease. Anaemia, for example, may present with only visual symptoms of floaters and weak vision.

Blurred vision

There are important questions to ask about this symptom:

- does it affect one or both eyes?
- is it constant or episodic?
- is it for near or distant vision?
- is it getting better or worse?

Blurring is the commonest visual symptom and the questions above will help to define its significance. It is helpful to determine the visual acuity since blurring due to shortsightedness improves when looking through a pinhole.[7]

Blurring in only one eye is much more likely to be due to an eye problem particularly if of sudden onset. If it has developed slowly over months or years with no other symptoms then the most likely situation is short or longsightedness. In the elderly, it may also be associated with cataract formation if mainly distance vision is affected, or vascular disturbances if mainly near vision is affected.

If the blurring is of sudden onset over a few weeks or days in only one eye then it is almost certainly not short or longsightedness. It is safest to assume, however, that the situation is potentially serious and urgent unless it suddenly recovers.

Episodic blurring is never a refractive error. In cases of multiple sclerosis the blurring lasts for many days. Migraine usually affects both eyes and occurs for the first time in younger people. More rarely the episode of blurring may be caused by interference with blood supply as in a transient ischaemic attack. This is usually described as a shutter or blind effect.

Floaters and blurred areas

Spots floating about in front of the eyes may be the first sign of failing vision in cases of shortsightedness. They are frequently first noticed during times of tiredness. Floaters are more easily seen against a white background. There is no cause for concern if no further developments occur during the first week or so.

Circulatory disturbances in the retina may cause bouts of 'seeing stars' or flashes, particularly at the edge of vision when tired or stressed. Floaters must be distinguished from the much rarer solitary area of blurring that does not float but moves with the eye without any time lag. This may be described as a piece missing from an object or a blurred spot. It tends to be constantly present. They are more serious than the common floater because they are often progressive or indicative of some other disorder, such as retinal disorders or neurological disease.

Pain

Visual disturbance with pain in the eyes is always serious and advice is urgently needed. The causes of pain in the eye include:

- iritis*
- glaucoma*
- multiple sclerosis
- shingles*
- cranial arteritis*
- in growing eyelash.

Those of most concern are marked with an asterisk*. A painful white eye with no visual symptoms is more likely to be due to a neurological disorder, e.g. trigeminal neuralgia.

Watering of the eyes

This may be due to excessive production of tears. There are several associated situations that include:

- inflammation – conjunctivitis, keratitis, uveitis
- injury – foreign bodies, chemical agents, in-growing eyelashes

- closed-angle glaucoma
- excessive exposure to bright light.

Alternatively, there may be inadequate drainage of tears, which may be associated with:

- eyelid abnormalities
- blocked tear duct.

Watering is common in a white, painless eye in infants, the middle aged and elderly. If there is no associated yellow discharge then it is not serious although it may be long lasting and a nuisance. If watering is the only symptom there is no danger to sight. Watering with discharge is treated as conjunctivitis and people will be given antibiotics.

It tends to clear spontaneously by the age of 9 months in babies. Since treatment involves a general anaesthetic and probing of the duct, it is better to wait for nature to take its course.

In middle age, probing or syringing of the duct is attempted much earlier as there is a worry about complications such as infection or in extreme cases, abscess formation in the duct. Reconstructive surgery of the duct may be necessary.

If the tear duct is open, watering is commonly caused by several possibilities. These include loss of tone in the eyelids or spasm of the lower lid leading to eversion or inversion, particularly in the elderly. This is treated by outpatient surgery.

In younger people (particularly students) excessive watering might be caused by close work and reading. The person usually describes it as watering when reading or trying to read. Eye exercises are helpful in these cases.

Watering associated with pain or photophobia may indicate corneal disease and is more serious.

Dryness of the eyes

This is reduced formation of tears and may be termed, keratoconjunctivitis sicca. It is frequently associated with autoimmune diseases such as rheumatoid arthritis[8] where it is known as Sjögren's syndrome. Such symptoms are common in middle age but little is understood about how these are caused in the absence of visual disturbance. These symptoms tend to be more common in women than men and are almost always bilateral. Some people who suffer sore or irritable eyes have an allergy – sometimes to local eye medication.

Symptoms
There is dryness of the eyes associated with dry mouth. There may be burning in the eye and the sensation of grittiness.

Treatment
These are by means of artificial 'tears' such as methylcellulose eye drops.

Holistic management
In terms of Chinese medicine, this condition usually corresponds to Deficiency of Liver Blood and/or Yin. There are well-recognised treatments available to nourish Yin (fluids) within the body. Progress tends to be slow as these problems are usually deep seated.

Headache

The comments I make here are specifically to do with the eyes but also see Chapter 14. The headache of glaucoma usually occurs only while the blurring of vision is present, and it is seldom severe. It is often also accompanied by aching of the eye. Headaches of visual origin are extremely rare in children aged under 10. They may occasionally be caused by refractive disorders in children.

Dizziness

This is rarely caused solely by an eye problem. It is essential to determine what the person means by this term. Some may complain of dizziness when in fact they mean double vision, which is why careful questioning about the exact phenomena is important – see Page 221. The situations leading to such a symptom may be sudden loss of sight in one eye or sudden loss of visual field (usually in cerebrovascular disease).

Redness of the eye

A red eye does not necessarily mean a more serious situation than a white one. The extent and severity of the redness are no guide to the severity of the condition. It is vision that is important so visual acuity needs to be checked. If a red eye were accompanied by any degree of visual disturbance then, unless the symptoms gradually improve within a few days, it would be wise to obtain an assessment from an ophthalmologist.

Always	Often	Rarely
Acute glaucoma	Corneal disease	Conjunctivitis
Iritis	Herpes zoster (shingles)	Episcleritis, scleritis
		Subconjunctival haemorrhage
		Entropion[9] – inward turning of the eyelash

Table 12.3: Conditions causing a red eye which present a threat to sight

Spontaneous subconjunctival haemorrhage that totally obliterates the white sclera is harmless despite its appearance and carries no complications unless due to trauma. In that case the outcome is dependent upon the degree of injury. In other situations, it will resolve on its own. In terms of Chinese medicine, red eyes may be connected with the syndromes associated with high blood pressure.

Redness in one eye that is hardly noticeable may signal intra-ocular disease and a potential threat to sight. Most of the serious causes of red eye do not affect both eyes at once. One-sided redness is generally more of a danger signal.

True infective conjunctivitis is usually bilateral and not usually a serious disease in Western countries. There is always some discharge, which may only be manifest as making it hard to separate the lids on waking. This distinguishes it from other conditions. Failure of these symptoms to respond may indicate corneal complications such as keratitis, especially if the person has been suffering from a systemic or local virus disease, e.g. herpes simplex, herpes zoster. Permanent visual loss is a real possibility in such cases. The redness and soreness that accompany measles have no special significance. It is important for doctors to distinguish infective conjunctivitis from other forms of red eye because corticosteroid treatment will make infective conditions much worse.

Any of these symptoms occurring in a person with only one useful eye would require a greater urgency about referral than if they still have the use of both eyes.

EAR DISEASE

ANATOMY AND PHYSIOLOGY

There are several basic facts of anatomy and physiology, which it is useful to know. I consider that most courses in these subjects are over detailed and reflect orthodox thinking rather than the particular needs of the holistic practitioner. To study ear disease it would be helpful to be able to:

- identify the structures of the ear
- describe the functions of these structures
- explain the mechanisms of hearing and balance.

The common symptoms that arise from disturbances are pain in the ear (particularly with acute conditions), deafness, noises in the ear and difficulties with balance. Other symptoms include discharge from the ear, tinnitus, vertigo, deformity of the ear, lumps around or on the ear,[10] headaches,[11] facial weakness[12] and double vision.

CLASSIFICATION OF EAR DISEASE

The most appropriate way do this is according to severity and chronicity – Table 12.4.

Mild disease
Otitis externa
Otitis media
Perforation of ear drum
Ménière's disease
Otosclerosis[13]
Severe disease

Table 12.4: Classification of ear disease

INVESTIGATIONS

Examination of the auditory canal and eardrum is done with an auriscope (US – otoscope). It is helpful to learn this skill as it can provide valuable information. Simple problems such as earwax may cause impaired hearing or vertigo. They can be easily diagnosed and treated.

An audiogram is a measurement of hearing. The person is subjected to various frequencies of sound and the results charted. Both ears are tested. It has an invasiveness of Category 1 as defined in Chapter 4 – Investigations.

Ménière's disease

In this condition, there are recurrent attacks of vertigo, which are severe with associated tinnitus and progressive deafness. These three symptoms together are virtually diagnostic of Ménière's disease. The cause is unknown in conventional medicine but there may be a history of migraine.

Symptoms
The most disabling symptom is a sudden attack of vertigo, which is severe, of sudden onset and usually associated with nausea and vomiting. Attacks are recurrent and there is progressive deafness as the auditory nerve is damaged with each attack. Tinnitus of varying degrees and types is experienced. The person has to go to bed for a day or two and can do very little as any movement makes the symptoms worse. The deafness increases progressively and frequencies of attacks tend to decrease as the years go by. The condition can last for years and virtually rule people's lives.

Treatment
This is with antihistamines such as betahistine, cinnarizine or prochlorperazine which may give symptomatic relief. There is little that is available to change the course of the illness. Ultrasound destruction of the nerve may be done in severe cases.

Holistic management
In terms of Chinese medicine, this condition often corresponds either to Phlegm and Dampness in the Stomach interfering with the rising of pure Qi to the head or to Kidney Yin Deficiency with Liver Yang Rising.

Case one
A woman of 53 years came for treatment of her Ménière's disease, which was first diagnosed some 30 years previously. Her main symptoms were poor balance, which was worse before a period, noises in her ears particularly the left (tinnitus) and poor hearing in both ears. She needed to use a hearing aid in her left ear. Interestingly, she told me that when she had stopped smoking some years before, she developed a phlegmy cough for a year, which was followed by tinnitus and loss of balance. She described the tinnitus as a soft, humming sound and low-pitched. It would be high-pitched when her balance was affected. She would have several colds a year, which would develop into a cough with phlegm. I made a diagnosis of Spleen and Lung Qi Deficiency with Damp-cold Accumulation and treated her with acupuncture and Chinese herbal medicine.

Her general energy improved quickly with treatment with prolonged times between episodes of poor balance. Some 2 months after treatment she noticed that her right ear would almost clear for a few days and then would be much quieter. She noticed her hearing was much clearer in that ear.

Two months later, she suffered a severe attack of Ménière's disease with vomiting and diarrhoea. Her balance was severely affected and she would fall after only a few steps. She was reminded of the original attacks of Ménière's disease all those years previously, as this was markedly similar. She then told me that her first attack had been some weeks after her father had been taken ill and died.

This attack settled with treatment and she continued to improve as before this attack. After 9 months of treatment, she was well with much improved hearing. She no longer needed her hearing aid, her balance was generally good although she would be slightly affected once a month. The tinnitus had subsided in one ear and was only slight in the other. Her general energy was good.

Otitis externa

This is inflammation of the auditory canal. There is always increased pain and discomfort on moving the ear and this differentiates the condition from other disorders. There are several forms of inflammation, which vary in intensity. They include:

- those associated with systemic skin diseases, e.g. psoriasis, eczema, contact dermatitis
- 'swimmer's ear'
- bacterial infection.

Symptoms
These depend upon the causes listed above and vary from mild to severe. In the case of systemic skin disease, there is evidence elsewhere of skin abnormalities. There is itching to a variable extent perhaps with scaling. In severe cases there may be weeping with a watery discharge. Conventional treatment is by means of corticosteroid drops.

In 'swimmer's ear' there is mild inflammation associated with evidence of fungal or bacterial infection. There are symptoms, after swimming, of a blocked ear with mild discomfort. This may become painful within the next 24 hours. Conventional treatment is with mixed antibiotic–corticosteroid drops.

In bacterial infection of the auditory canal there is redness, pain, enlargement of pre-auricular and post-auricular lymph glands. The canal is narrowed due to swelling. There may be a low-grade fever of around 38°C (100°F). Conventional treatment is with oral antibiotics.

Otitis media

This is inflammation of the middle ear and is more common in children. It is usually associated with infection, bacterial or viral. It may also arise due to congestion of fluid in the middle ear where infection may have a minor role to play.

Symptoms
There is the acute onset of fever, pain in the ear and decreased hearing. Occasionally, there may be mild vertigo. On examination, the eardrum is red and may be bulging towards the examiner.

Complications

Complication	Symptoms to look for
Mastoiditis	Persistent symptoms of otitis media for over 8–10 days, pain and swelling of mastoid
Serous otitis media – may progress to 'glue ear' in children	Continuing impairment of hearing, crackling sounds in ear, feeling of fullness. The eardrum is opaque, dull and slightly retracted. In 'glue ear' the eardrum has a bluish appearance
Perforation of eardrum – most heal with no complications	Increasing pain in the ear followed by discharge from the ear and relief of pain. The perforation will be visible on examination of the eardrum
Chronic otitis media with perforated drum	Few or no symptoms usually. There may be vertigo in a cold wind. Occasionally yellow discharge from the ear but no pain or fever. The perforation will be visible on examination of the eardrum
Facial paralysis (rare)	Weakness of one side of face with symptoms of otitis media

Table 12.5: Complications of otitis media

Treatment
This is almost invariably by means of antibiotics although some conventional practitioners use only decongestants, e.g. pseudoephedrine (a sympathomimetic). This is based on the belief that the main problem, particularly in children, is of catarrhal congestion in the middle ear and eustachian tubes. There is some debate in conventional circles as to whether the

use of antibiotics leads to more frequent recurrences and persistence of the condition. It is important to avoid flying for at least seven days or the eardrum is at risk of perforation.

'Glue ear' is an uncommon complication of otitis media and, as its name suggests, is due to thickening of fluids in the middle ear. It may lead to damage of the delicate bones in the middle ear and severe hearing loss. 'Glue ear' is treated by means of surgical perforation of the eardrum (myringotomy) and the insertion of drainage tubes (grommets). This treatment is also frequently used in those children who have evidence of chronic mucus congestion with some hearing loss. It may be combined with tonsillectomy and adenoidectomy. Some conventional practitioners now treat such cases with decongestants because surgery to the ear may cause scarring of the eardrum. Scarring is less likely if perforation occurs naturally. Such treatment, of course, does nothing to remedy the underlying problem, which is the production of mucus.

Holistic management

This is easily treated in most people by the application of homoeopathic remedies or herbal formulae. It is unnecessary in most cases to give antibiotics. If the symptoms do not begin to subside within 12 or 24 hours after you have started treatment, review the case and your treatment. The danger of mastoiditis is very much overplayed nowadays and it is perfectly valid to treat otitis media with holistic medicine alongside appropriate monitoring.

Perforated ear drum

There are several causes of perforated eardrum. They include:

- injury, e.g. blow to ears ('boxing' the ears) or direct damage to ear drum, e.g. with perforating object
- complication of otitis media.

Management

This depends upon the cause. Otitis media is treated as described above. Traumatic perforation usually heals spontaneously although direct injury may result in some infection.

Swimming is prohibited with eardrum perforation. If the perforation is small and linear it may heal within 1 week. If the perforation has healed then swimming may be resumed but diving is prohibited for a further 3 weeks.

Flying is no problem in the day or so after perforation as there is no pressure difference between the outside and the middle ear because of the perforation. It should be avoided for 2 to 3 weeks after this as the perforation is healing. Large perforations and those associated with chronic otitis media may be repaired surgically (myringoplasty).

Case one

A girl of 14 years came for treatment of a permanently blocked nose for the previous 4 years. She had previous ear problems since the age of 10 years, which developed after Hepatitis B vaccination. She developed abscesses in her ears with recurrent fevers and had grommets inserted some months previously. Her chest was affected by cold air with wheezing and cough. When her ear was troublesome, she would develop pain in the ears for a few days followed by a clear discharge. Occasionally, a thick red mucoid discharge would be seen from the ear. Both ears were affected but mainly the left. She would have painful periods with diarrhoea as well as feeling pale and faint. I made a diagnosis of Spleen and Lung Qi Deficiency with Phlegm-cold Accumulation and underlying Kidney Yang Deficiency. I treated her with acupuncture and Chinese herbs.

She responded well to the course of treatment with increased energy levels. Her periods settled well with no pain or diarrhoea after one month. Her chest and ears were fine and she went through that winter with no difficulties. Some 8 months after treatment began, she developed a pain in her left ear with a yellow discharge. She had no fever and her chest was fine. There was some discussion with her family about whether antibiotics were necessary. She, herself, felt that the Chinese medicine had the most positive effect on her health and she did not want conventional medication. I continued to monitor and treat her regularly until the acute episode subsided. The ability to examine the eardrum is very helpful in such situations.

In total, she had treatment with me for 16 months and at the end of the time she was well, with no pains in her ears, her chest was fine and she had good energy. I recommended that she see a cranial osteopath, as she had some developmental difficulty with her teeth and an orthodontist had suggested that surgery might be needed soon. Certainly, there is frequently a connection between nose and ear symptoms, teeth development and general cranial development. Cranial osteopathy is extremely effective in relieving such tensions in growing children and removing the need for more severe interventions.

REVIEW OF SYMPTOMS OF EAR DISEASE

Tinnitus

This is any noise such as buzzing or ringing in the ear. There are several causes in terms of conventional medicine including:

- blockage of the auditory canal by wax
- damage to the eardrum
- otosclerosis
- Ménière's disease
- drugs, e.g. aspirin, quinine
- auditory (VIII cranial) nerve disease.

In terms of Chinese medicine, this symptom may be caused by Phlegm from the Stomach or Gall Bladder ascending to the head or Deficiency of Kidney Yin leading to Yang Rising.

Deafness

This is partial or total hearing loss in one or both ears. It is conventionally divided into conductive and perceptive deafness. Conductive deafness is due to a problem with the conduction of sound through the outer and middle ear. Causes include:

- earwax in the auditory canal
- otitis externa
- otitis media
- otosclerosis.

Perceptive deafness is due to a disorder of the inner ear, the auditory nerve or the centres in the brain dealing with sound. Causes include:

- congenital, e.g. congenital rubella syndrome
- Ménière's disease
- prolonged exposure to loud noise
- advancing age.

Vertigo

This has a specific meaning of a sensation of constant movement of the individual or of the environment. It is usually a spinning movement but it may be a feeling that the ground is moving. Causes of vertigo include:

- wax jammed against eardrum (mild)
- acute otitis media (mild)
- fluid accumulation in the middle ear
- labyrinthitis
- Ménière's disease
- multiple sclerosis
- transient ischaemic attacks.

Differentiation is made by the other symptoms that are present. It is important to examine the eardrum. People may report a symptom of dizziness and it is important to identify the precise meaning. There are several possibilities:

- true vertigo (as defined above)
- light-headedness as before a faint. There is no spinning rather a feeling of floating
- unsteadiness which leads to difficulties walking or standing. This may be a minor degree of the two possibilities above
- rarely it may indicate depersonalisation or derealisation as may occur in the psychoses or severe neuroses.

Case one

A woman of 88 years came for treatment. She suffered from dizziness all the time, which was worse if she turned her head suddenly. She had first had this at the age of 21. She had suffered a minor stroke 5 years earlier, but had made a good recovery.

Her medication was:

- captopril 12.5 mg daily for high blood pressure
- digoxin 62.5 mg daily for cardiac arrhythmia
- acetazolamide 250 mg for glaucoma
- aspirin 75 mg daily to prevent stroke.

She had a damaged right eye due to undetected glaucoma and cataracts in both eyes. She felt great anxiety for her family and worried if they came home late. She also had a fear of being burgled. She had a severe gnawing chest pain, extending to her stomach and right shoulder blade. She had a tendency to have diarrhoea especially after red meat or fatty foods. Her symptoms pointed to Arsenicum and she was given 30c of it.

One month later she was able to read again and the shadow in her vision cleared. Her fear of her home being broken into was completely gone and although she still worried about her family, the disturbing dreams she had of them dying were gone. She said she used to fear having a heart attack, but now the chest pain was completely gone and she felt 'great ease'. The vertigo did not respond to the remedy, perhaps it will take longer to clear, as it is such an old symptom.

HOW TO RECOGNISE A SERIOUS CONDITION OF THE EYE AND EAR

It is essential to consider visual symptoms carefully, as they are always potentially graver than non-visual ones. Although discomfort or redness in the eyes seems more serious, it is the disturbance of vision that is more worrying. For this reason, it is important to know how to recognise if a symptom arises from a serious situation. You can use Table 12.6 as a guide to refer to when faced with a person who has one or more of these symptoms. I do not mention disease labels in the column on the right as I would not expect you to be able to diagnose conventionally. Seriousness can be assessed merely by reference to symptom pictures. However, you will be able to recognise that there are clinical appearances that would be diagnosed as a particular disease. For example, if you look at redness and its seriousness, you will see that this is the appearance of the more serious conditions of keratitis, iritis and glaucoma.

Symptoms	Comments
Redness	Circumcorneal, with visual disturbance
Discharge from the eye	Not if alone. Of concern if severe, prolonged and with pain in the eye
Soreness	Not if mild. Of concern if *pain* rather than soreness especially with circumcorneal redness
Visual disturbance	Short history, progressive, with pain, with redness
Blurred vision	Progressive
Pain in eye	With visual disturbance
Spots, floaters	If localised area of blurring
Double vision	Short history
Pain in the ear	Severe, with fever
Discharge from the ear	Long duration
Vertigo	Severe
Deformity of the ear	Severe
Lumps around or on the ear	Severe, if with redness, pain and deafness
Headaches	Progressive, severe with short history, with central nervous system symptoms
Facial weakness	With history of ear pain
Deafness	Short history, progressive
Tinnitus	Progressive

Table 12.6: How to recognise serious conditions of the eye and ear

SUMMARY

Ear conditions are relatively common in the holistic medical clinic. Eye conditions are more often seen as a secondary complaint.

If you are treating children, it is helpful to know how to manage acute ear conditions and how to recognise complications. Other common conditions seen in children are 'glue' ear and recurrent tonsillitis.

Most eye and ear conditions are self-limiting. Know those which may lead to further problems particularly those eye diseases which may threaten sight.

[1] This comprises the iris, ciliary body and choroid. Inflammation of the iris and ciliary body is termed anterior uveitis or iridocyclitis. Inflammation of the choroid is termed posterior uveitis or choroiditis.

[2] There have been suggestions that the administration of Vitamin E, C and betacarotene may prevent or reverse the formation of cataract. Varma, SD. *American Journal of Clinical Nutrition* 199;53(1):335S(11).

[3] The term senile is used as an adjective for any disorder which appears after the age of 60 years.

[4] O'Day, Denis M. *American Family Physician* 1993;47(6):1421(10).

[5] There are well described sets of exercises for use with many types of eye problems including short-sightedness (myopia), squint and so on. For further information see bibliography in Appendix One.

[6] Refraction is a term from physics. It is the change of direction in light rays when they travel from one area to another, e.g. from the air into the eye. In practical clinical terms, an error of refraction is due to abnormal lens function or eye shape.

[7] This is the basis of 'pinhole glasses' which can be part of a natural treatment for eye disorders. The pinholes cut down on peripheral light and improve central vision. Such aids, together with appropriate eye exercises, can be used to treat short-sightedness (myopia), squint and so forth. Please see the Bibliography on Page 387 which lists books describing eye exercises.

[8] Other disorders include systemic lupus erythematosus and inflammation of the thyroid.

[9] A condition where the margin of the eyelid, more often the lower, turns inwards so that the eyelashes touch the eye surface and irritate the cornea.

[10] Lumps on the ear are rare. Causes include injury, frostbite and abscess formation. Lumps around the ear may be lymphatic gland enlargement. I would remind you here of the importance in knowing the main groups of lymphatic glands and the areas they drain. Mastoid enlargement is rare nowadays and is a complication of otitis media.

[11] These are described in Chapter 14 – Central Nervous System.

[12] This is described in Chapter 14 – Central Nervous System.

[13] This is described in Chapter 18 – Women's Health on Page 371 in relation to hormone replacement treatment.

13 GASTROINTESTINAL SYSTEM

INTRODUCTION

Disturbances of the gastrointestinal system are common and many people seek help for disturbances in digestive function. These may manifest as diarrhoea or constipation, disturbed appetite, nausea or vomiting, pain in the abdomen or perhaps excessive wind. Most of the underlying conditions are of relatively minor significance and reflect the close relationship between the digestive tract and the emotions. However, some conditions are more serious and it is important for the practitioner to be able to recognise the symptoms of severe disease.

ANATOMY AND PHYSIOLOGY

The conventional view of the gastrointestinal system is that it is merely a conduit for the passage of food and its digestion. Each part of the system has several and similar functions. These are ingestion, secretion, digestion, absorption, storage and elimination. There is merely a different emphasis in each area. For example, the mouth is mainly concerned with ingestion, some secretion and absorption. The small intestine is mainly concerned with digestion and absorption. The large intestine is mainly concerned with storage and elimination with some absorption.

Before studying disease of the gastrointestinal system you will need to familiarise yourself with its anatomy and physiology. Check that you are able to:

- list the organs of digestion (including the 'accessory organs')
- describe the main structure of these organs
- describe the functions of the digestive system as a whole with particular reference to each of these organs
- explain how the processes of digestion are regulated.

HOLISTIC VIEW OF THE GASTROINTESTINAL SYSTEM

Vitalistic principles presume the existence of energy as the root of any structure. In terms of the gastrointestinal system, its function is not only dependent on the food eaten. It also concerns the energetic quality of food and the energy of the system itself.

The main function of the gastrointestinal system is linked in Chinese medicine to the function of the Spleen. Spleen Qi, together with that of the Stomach, is responsible for the transformation and transportation of food into energy. Other organs use this energy as well as contributing to the formation of Blood and Body Fluids. If Spleen energy is depleted for any reason, then not only is less energy produced but mucus also is produced. This can collect in various areas of the body and cause problems. For example, in the intestines it may lead to bowel disturbances, which correspond to Crohn's disease or ulcerative colitis. Mucus may pass up into the lungs and be associated with conditions such as chronic bronchitis. It may be lodge in the skin and be associated with conditions we know as eczema.

The Liver, as that organ is understood by Chinese medicine, is also important in the regulation of the digestion. Details of these energetic associations are listed in Chapter 14 – Central Nervous System. The Liver is considered to deal with the free flow of energy. Any obstruction to this in the digestive system may lead to symptoms such as belching, flatulence, bloating and abdominal pain. These connections will become more obvious when individual diseases are discussed.

Association	Comments
Governs transformation and transportation	The Spleen deals with food by transforming it into energy (Qi) and body fluid. It separates the pure from the impure, ascends the pure and descends the impure. Weak Spleen Qi leads to inadequate transformation and transportation and so to mucus formation (thickened body fluids) and tiredness (lack of energy)
Controls Blood	The Spleen holds Blood in the circulation and prevents it leaking out of the vessels. Bruising may be a sign of weak Spleen Qi. Vitamin C deficiency producing bruising corresponds here
Dominates muscles and flesh	The health of muscles and flesh are dependent upon the efficiency of Spleen function
Raises the pure Qi	Spleen Qi ascends and is responsible for holding organs in place. Prolapse of uterus, rectum and other organs may be due to weakness of this aspect
Residence of Thought	Overthinking and rumination may weaken the Spleen. Similarly, an imbalance of Spleen energy may affect thought
Paired organ with is Stomach	This connection is self-evident as food enters the Stomach to be processed
Opens into the Mouth	Diseases of the mouth may be due to Stomach or Spleen problems such as mouth ulcers and bleeding gums
Manifests in the lips	The condition of the lips is a reflection of Spleen function
Colour – yellow	The colour of Earth is yellow and foods that particularly nourish this element are parsnip, squash, and carrot. These are generally sweet also (see below)
Taste – sweet	Each major organ has an associated taste. In this case excess sweet food can damage the Earth element. Conversely, small amounts of sweet taste nourish the Earth element
Season – sometimes described as late summer but more accurately is a centring between each of the 4 seasons	The energy of the centre is transformative. It moves in a circular direction. In cases of imbalance, it may result in the inability to move forward as with overthinking and excess analysis
Element – Earth	The Element correspondence reveals the connection of Chinese medical theory to nature. Each Element is connected to the others to provide, in health, a harmonious balance
Time – 9-11 a.m.	The 'time' of an organ is when its energy it at its maximum. It is best to eat a large breakfast when the energy of the digestion is strongest and not to eat late at night when it needs to rest. The time of the Stomach is 7-9 a.m.
Emotions – sympathy	An imbalance of the Earth element may manifest as oversympathy or lack of sympathy. Being oversympathetic may deplete Spleen energy. This is the difference between *mother* and *smother*. Mother also applies to the Earth element – Mother Nature
Mental aspect	Deals with the aspects of belief and faith, confidence and trust. Its paired organ, the Stomach, is to do with endurance, stamina and the ability to keep going. If there is Heat in the Stomach or its energy is scattered, there is no patience. If the energy of the Stomach is depleted, there is no endurance

Table 13.1: Holistic view of the digestion (Spleen function in Chinese medicine)

Tables 13.1 and 13.2 are descriptions of the gastrointestinal system according to holistic, energetic principles. These ideas are obtained from Chinese medicine but it may be that other practitioners such as homoeopaths see similarities with their system of medicine. It is our common experience that emotions and thoughts affect the digestive system. Homoeopathic remedies clearly show this connection in their remedy pictures. People know that certain emotional states are associated, for example, with diarrhoea or constipation. The ideas expressed in these Tables provide an explanation of these mechanisms. The organ which is considered in Chinese medicine to govern function of the digestive system is the Spleen.[1]

The gastrointestinal system and the lungs are the main organs after birth that provide the body with energy. It is clear, therefore, why there is so much debility and ill health in the West. Food and air are two items that are very much polluted.

Tremendous strains are put on the gastrointestinal system by eating food that is poor in quality. This may be a classical case of malnutrition when deprived of food. In the West, it is more likely to mean poor quality food due to farming methods and the use of pesticides and herbicides. It may be due to food processing techniques, e.g. canning, pre-cooking and freezing where old food is eaten. It may be due to cooking techniques such as microwaves.[2] Such treatment strips food of essential nutrients as well as its energy. This is dead food and cannot lead to health. When this is combined with rapid eating, irregular eating and eating when stressed, disturbances of the digestive system, together with general debility are easily explained. It is generally helpful to eat fresh food that has been grown or reared in healthier ways, either organically or by using the methods of biodynamic agriculture and permaculture.

Organ	Comments
Large Intestine	This organ is paired with the Lung. Its function depends largely upon the efficiency of the Lung. Mentally, it is to do with forgiveness and letting go. Its healthy functioning allows us to ease up and have a forgiving attitude. The role of the Kidney is important also as the Large Intestine is situated in the area controlled by Kidney function[3]
Small Intestine	This organ is paired with the Heart. Its function is to separate the pure from the impure. On a mental level, it is to do with awareness and sensitivity. It helps us with discernment, the ability to differentiate 'pure from impure'

Table 13.2: Information on energetic connections between organs of digestion and other organs

If one accepts that Spleen Qi drives the gastrointestinal system, then if we are to be healthy it is important to protect this Qi at all times. Qi is warm in nature. Therefore, Chinese medicine places great emphasis on eating warming foods,[4] particularly in cold climates. The advice regarding diet in cold northern climates is to eat mainly cooked foods such as porridge in the morning and to take soups, stews and casseroles. When cooking, the warming qualities of ginger and cinnamon also nurture Qi. It is helpful to avoid cold fruits, particularly of tropical origin, since these are more appropriate for hot climates. In the summer, when the weather is warmer, then it is more appropriate to eat occasional salads or fruit. The ingestion of large quantities of raw, cold food can only deplete Spleen energy and in the long run lead to general weakness. This is in contrast to common advice in the West that eating raw food will mean a greater intake of vitamins and minerals.

There are occasions when an intake of cold, raw food may be beneficial. This is when detoxification is appropriate. However, the use of such a technique without individualisation of the case may lead to serious consequences since there is a loss of body fluid and energy. The indiscriminate use of detoxification, particularly when linked with colonic irrigation or enemas, can deplete the body.

CLASSIFICATION OF GASTROINTESTINAL DISEASE

As can be seen from Table 13.3, the conventional classification is according to the site of the problem. The gastrointestinal system is studied in sequence from the mouth to the anus. Within each area, lists are made of the various problems that may occur. I have followed this pattern somewhat since there seems to be a fairly straightforward division between the upper and lower gastrointestinal tract. These produce symptoms in their respective areas.

Most disorders of the gastrointestinal system may be regarded as a disturbance of function. There may be some structural changes as with peptic ulceration or ulcerative colitis but these seem to me to be secondary to a functional disturbance. More serious disease such as diverticulitis and cancer are associated with marked physical changes and so are more difficult to treat. Table 13.4 lists diseases according to the site of symptoms rather than organ of origin. Mild disease is placed at the top of each section.

Disorders of the mouth
    stomatitis
Diseases of the tongue
    glossitis
    leukoplakia
    cancer
Diseases of the oesophagus
    reflux oesophagitis
    cancer
Diseases of the stomach and duodenum
    gastritis
    duodenitis
    peptic ulcer
    cancer of stomach
Diseases of the small intestine
    malabsorption
    Crohn's disease
Diseases of the large intestine
    ulcerative colitis
    irritable bowel syndrome
    diverticulitis
    cancer
Diseases of the anus
    haemorrhoids
    fissure
Diseases of the pancreas
    pancreatitis
    cancer
Diseases of the liver
    hepatitis
    cirrhosis
    cancer
Diseases of the gall bladder
    gallstones (cholelithiasis)
    inflammation (cholecystitis)

**Table 13.3: Conventional classification of gastrointestinal disease
(Those in italics are the most common)**

In terms of holistic medicine, most disorders in this system are relatively easy to treat. This is because the gastrointestinal system is, hierarchically speaking, a relatively superficial area of the body.

Upper abdominal symptoms (mild disease at the top)

Reflux oesophagitis
Hepatitis
Peptic ulcer
Gall stones (cholelithiasis)
Inflammation of gall bladder (cholecystitis)
Pancreatitis
Cirrhosis
Cancer of the stomach
Cancer of the pancreas
Cancer of the liver

Lower abdominal symptoms (mild disease at the top)

Anal fissure
Haemorrhoids
Irritable bowel syndrome
Diverticulitis
Inflammatory bowel disease
    Ulcerative colitis
    Crohn's disease
Cancer of the large intestine

Table 13.4: Holistic classification of gastrointestinal disease

ABDOMINAL PAIN

There are nine main questions to ask about pain wherever its site. These are reviewed here in relation to the gastrointestinal system.

Main site

Where is the pain? Ask for confirmation by pointing. Make sure that there is common understanding of whatever terms are used. Do not assume that the term 'stomach' or 'tummy' means the same thing to everyone. It can be useful to see the extent of the painful area and clues can be obtained by whether the person points with one finger or uses the whole hand to describe the site. At some stage see the area unclothed.

Figure 13.1 is a diagrammatic representation of the abdomen. It is divided into several areas, each with its own name. It is important to know these since they are a common method of describing sites of symptoms. References to them are made in homoeopathic repertories, for example.

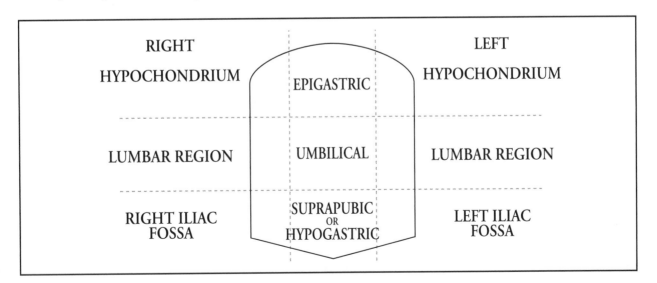

Figure 13.1: Division of the abdomen into named areas

In conventional medicine, the site of pain in the abdomen is seen as being related to the underlying anatomical structure. Problems with organs in the epigastrium lead to epigastric pain, problems with organs in the right iliac fossa lead to right iliac fossa pain, etc. A complete list is given in Table 13.5.

Area of abdomen	Organs in this area	Other organs which may produce pain in this area
Epigastrium	Oesophagus (lower end), stomach, duodenum, pancreas	Heart
Right hypochondrium	Liver, gall bladder	
Left hypochondrium	Spleen	
Umbilical	Small intestine	
Right lumbar region	Kidney, ureter	
Left lumbar region	Kidney, ureter	
Suprapubic (hypogastric)	Bladder (full), uterus (pregnant, fibroids)	Bladder,[5] uterus
Right iliac fossa	Appendix, ureter, caecum	Fallopian tube, ovary
Left iliac fossa	Sigmoid colon, ureter	Fallopian tube, ovary

Table 13.5: Organs contained within each area of the abdomen

Radiation
The pain may be felt in sites in addition to the primary area. Pancreatitis pain is felt in the epigastrium and radiates *through* to the back. Cholecystitis gives rise to pain in the right hypochondrium which radiates *round* to the back and the shoulder. The pain of renal colic is felt in the lumbar region and loin and can radiate to the groin or even the knee.

It is interesting that the occurrence of back pain may not be due solely to problems with the back. Organs are more likely to cause this symptom if they lie outside the peritoneal cavity. Examples would be pancreas, kidney and uterus.

Character
It can be difficult to describe the particular quality of pain but certain conditions are associated with characteristic qualities. Colic is a cramping pain, which comes in waves of worsening and relief, but the exact nature depends on the source organ. It is produced by hollow organs whose muscular walls are in a state of spasm such as small intestine, gall bladder, ureter, uterus and large intestine.

Colic of the gall bladder (biliary colic) or ureter (so-called renal colic) is typically severe and does not go away completely during remissions. However, the colic of small or large intestine origin does disappear before returning some time later. This is the type of colic seen in an acute enteritis, e.g. food poisoning.

Severity
Pain can be of any severity according to the cause or it can vary from person to person. As mentioned above biliary or renal colic is typically severe. Thresholds of pain are variable and different people will react to pain in greatly different ways. Usually, the more severe the disease is and the weaker the person, the more severe and intractable the pain will be.

Duration
Ask how long the pain has been present, not only this attack but also the whole process. Is this a recent event or have there been repeated attacks in the past? Appendicitis, for example, will have a short history of not more than 24 to 48 hours although some people do have recurrent subacute attacks – the so-called 'grumbling appendix'. Peptic ulcers on the other hand have a chronic course of many years with flare-ups, which last weeks or months.

Frequency
How often does the pain recur? With renal colic it will be every few minutes or so, with ulcer pain it will be every day or longer, perhaps every night (as in the case of a duodenal ulcer).

Time of occurrence
Conventional medicine sees a duodenal ulcer as being worse at night, bowel pain as being worse later in the day but otherwise the timing of an attack is seen to be of little significance. This is in contrast to holistic medicine where it is used as an excellent means of individual differentiation.

Changes of symptoms with the weather, seasons, temperature and times of day are of supreme importance in holistic medicine. They serve to help individualise the case.

Modalities

Does anything help the pain or make it worse? Ask the open question first and later suggest a list of holistics, if necessary, for selection. Peritoneal pain is worse for movement, peptic ulcer pain is better for vomiting, gastric ulcer is worse for eating, duodenal ulcer is better for eating, gall bladder disease is worse for eating fatty food and so forth.

Other modalities such as the effect of heat or cold, are often disregarded by conventional practitioners. Whereas, in holistic medicine the process of considering modalities is given much greater significance and is consequently more refined.

Associated phenomena

You should take note of any symptoms that also appear with the pain. For example, nausea with upper abdominal pain, diarrhoea with lower abdominal pain, vaginal discharge with gynaecological causes of lower abdominal pain.

From the questioning above, done in a careful and orderly way, most cases of abdominal pain can be diagnosed and examination of the abdomen would be a confirmation. Confusion can occur from the history, as with differentiating some cases of peptic ulcer from cholecystitis, but precise history taking will minimise this.

UPPER GASTROINTESTINAL DISTURBANCES

The gastrointestinal tract is essentially a hollow tube passing from the mouth to the anus. In any discussion, it is important to relate symptoms to a particular dysfunction. For example, disturbance of the passage of food through the gastrointestinal tract leads to constipation or diarrhoea. Reversal of the normal flow through the system leads to nausea and/or vomiting. Disturbance in flow at any particular site will lead to bloating, pain and discomfort.

The stomach is responsible for appetite and so disorders of the stomach may be associated with increased or decreased appetite. Any long lasting disturbance such as poor appetite or loss of fluid will lead to weight loss. Increased intake of food will usually lead to weight gain.

Upper gastrointestinal tract disturbances	Lower gastrointestinal tract disturbances
• Pain • Distension • Appetite changes • Nausea • Vomiting	• Pain • Distension • Constipation • Diarrhoea

Table 13.6: Summary of symptoms due to gastrointestinal tract disturbances

UPPER ABDOMINAL PAIN

General overview

This is a common symptom and may be due to many underlying disturbances. Most of these are not serious in the sense of being life-threatening but frequently interfere with people's life-style, habits and activity. Essentially, I am discussing here pain in the epigastrium and right hypochondrium. Pain in the left hypochondrium does occur but it is unusual.

OESOPHAGEAL DISEASE

The oesophagus is a hollow muscular tube, which transports food from the mouth the stomach. It has no digestive or absorptive function. Disturbances here lead to symptoms of dysphagia (difficulty swallowing), a sensation of something being stuck and pain.

Reflux oesophagitis

This is an inflammation of the oesophagus. This condition is more common in middle age or elderly women and in those who are overweight or in pregnancy. It is associated with passage of acid from the stomach into the oesophagus.

A common term that is often applied to this condition is hiatus hernia.[6] This is a technical label, which refers to the upper part of the stomach passing through the hiatus of the diaphragm.

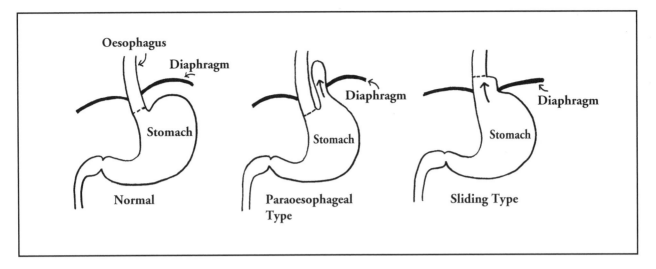

Figure 13.2: Different types of hiatus hernia

Hiatus Hernias

There are two types of hiatus hernia. There is the common 'sliding' hernia and the unusual 'paraoesophageal' or 'rolling' type. With a 'sliding' hernia, the oesophago-gastric junction slides up into the chest. It occurs in about 1 in 3 people at the age of 50 years. The 'paraoesophageal' or rolling hernia is where some of the upper part of the stomach passes alongside the oesophagus up into the chest. It may be associated with difficulty swallowing and a sensation of a blockage in the oesophagus as there may be obstruction to the passage of food.

Hiatus hernia does not produce symptoms. It is the *function* of the junction between the oesophagus and stomach that is the determining factor as to whether symptoms develop. If the oesophago-gastric junction is weakened, acid can pass back up into the oesophagus. The lining of the oesophagus is vulnerable to attack, as its mucus membrane is not designed to resist the effects of acid. Inflammation occurs and this leads to the classical symptoms of this condition. Such a hernia may or may not be associated with acid reflux. It can only be diagnosed by a barium meal X-ray.

The older treatment for hiatus hernia was by a surgical approach through the chest wall to fix the stomach firmly below the diaphragm. This was singularly unsuccessful and many people had exactly the same symptoms after the operation as they did before. The key is how something works, not what it looks like[7] – function is more important than structure.

Symptoms

The classical clinical feature of reflux oesophagitis is 'heartburn'. This is a burning sensation felt behind the sternum, which may begin at the upper part of the epigastrium and radiate upwards. It is precipitated and worsened by bending, stooping, lifting and straining. It is particularly troublesome at night when lying. There may be regurgitation of food on lying. The pain is better when the position is changed to sitting and is better after food or alkalis. Change of pain with change of posture is typical of this condition and is not really seen with any other cause of chest pain – see Page 104. Often there is blood loss from the inflamed area and iron deficiency, if not obvious anaemia, is common.

Complications

Complication	Symptoms to look for
Stricture (narrowing) due to scar formation	Difficulty swallowing developing over months and years, sensation of food sticking in chest
Anaemia	Pallor, tiredness, light-headedness, palpitations, anxiety
Haemorrhage	Vomiting blood

Table 13.7: Complications of reflux oesophagitis

Investigations

Gastroscopy will reveal the inflamed area and barium meal may show evidence of hiatus hernia. The complications of ulceration and stricture may be seen. Simple inflammation cannot be seen by X-ray procedures.

Treatment

Treatment (mildest to strongest)	Comments
General advice	Reduce alcohol consumption, stop smoking, raise the head of the bed, reduce excess weight. Stopping smoking is beneficial as nicotine leads to a rise in the secretion of gastric acid and is the most important single factor in avoiding further damage. All medication taken should be reviewed as many drugs lead to upper gastrointestinal problems especially aspirin, non-steroidal anti-inflammatory drugs and corticosteroids
Antacids	Antacids can neutralise gastric acid to some extent and will give immediate relief to inflammatory problems of the upper gastrointestinal tract. However, with continual usage they lead to the production of more acid because the body tries to maintain a certain level of acidity in the stomach. Problems are experienced when people try to come off them since the stomach is exposed to the full force of an increased acid secretion. Magnesium trisilicate (caused diarrhoea) aluminium[8] hydroxide (causes constipation) are the common ones
Alginate-containing antacids	These are taken as a liquid, which lies on top of the stomach contents like a foam. When acid passes into the oesophagus only the drug is in contact with the mucosa. Therefore, it protects the oesophagus from further contact with the gastric contents. It is of variable effectiveness
Histamine (H[2]) blockers	Described under peptic ulceration below
Proton pump inhibitors	Described under peptic ulceration below
Prokinetic agents	Described under peptic ulceration below
Helicobacter pylori eradication – 'triple therapy'	Some people with reflux oesophagitis have evidence of *Helicobacter pylori* infection. This treatment is described under peptic ulceration below
Surgery	This should be rarely considered because it is recognised that symptoms frequently continue

Table 13.8: Treatment of reflux oesophagitis

Holistic management

Treatment for this condition is very helpful when given along with appropriate dietary advice. Clearly smoking should stop. Most antacids can be taken when symptoms occur so the symptom picture can be more clearly seen.

Histamine (H[2]) blockers should be approached more circumspectly as stopping them can lead to a rebound of the original symptoms, whether pain or bleeding, and this can occur several years after starting them.

Gastritis

This is inflammation of the stomach and is common. There are acute and chronic types depending upon the presentation.

With acute gastritis, there may be simple inflammation, superficial ulcers (erosions) or ulcers. Common causes include aspirin, non-steroidal anti-inflammatory agents and alcohol. They are also seen in association with stressful situations, burns, injury, and kidney and liver disease.

Chronic gastritis is mainly of two types. There may be long-standing injury due to aspirin or non-steroidal anti-inflammatory agents or an autoimmune type, which is associated with pernicious anaemia. The latter condition may be associated with other autoimmune diseases such as hypothyroidism and Addison's disease and in severe cases may lead to cancer of the stomach.

Symptoms

Acute gastritis is characterised by strong symptoms of epigastric pain and vomiting. There may be vomiting of blood in cases of erosion or ulceration.

Chronic gastritis is considered in the conventional texts to be asymptomatic but in my experience leads to anorexia and nausea particularly in the morning. There may be vomiting of mucus. Intermittent epigastric discomfort will be experienced and there may be belching, upper abdominal distension and an unpleasant taste in the mouth.

Some people with stomach disorders develop symptoms in the mouth and gums. There may be ulceration or bleeding gums and there will be signs of inflammation (gingivitis).

Investigations
Gastroscopy will reveal inflammation. There may be ulceration in cases of acute gastritis. In chronic gastritis there is a reduced level of gastric acid and there may be evidence of anaemia with low levels of Vitamin B_{12}. A barium meal shows smoothness of the stomach lining in chronic gastritis.

Treatment
It is important to remove the cause of the gastritis if there is one. Pernicious anaemia will be treated with Vitamin B_{12} injections for life and regular monitoring of haemoglobin levels. Stopping Vitamin B_{12} treatment without effective holistic treatment and monitoring of serum levels is potentially hazardous.

Holistic management
The holistic management of gastritis is the same as for peptic ulcer below.

Peptic ulcer

This is a generic term, which is used to describe any ulcer occurring in the presence of acid. This may be the lower oesophagus, stomach, duodenum, jejunum after gastric surgery and in the ileum adjacent to a Meckel's diverticulum. The latter is present in 2 per cent of people and situated 2 ft from the terminal ileum and secretes acid.

Ulceration at the lower end of the oesophagus occurs in connection with reflux oesophagitis. I shall concentrate here on ulcers of the stomach and duodenum, as they are the common ones seen in clinical practice.

About 2 per cent of the adult US population have an active peptic ulcer and about 1 in 10 develop a peptic ulcer at some time in their life. There are 500,000 new cases of peptic ulcer each year in the US. Around one in seven of the population in the UK develop a duodenal ulcer at some time in their life. They are two or three times more common than gastric ulcers. Duodenal ulcers are four times more common in men whilst gastric ulcers are twice as common. There is a definite relationship between cigarette smoking and delayed healing due to an increase in gastric acid secretion.

There is often a family history of ulceration and so hereditary factors may be important. However, members of the same family tend to have similar dietary and emotional features, so it is not as simple as it seems.

Why some people develop ulcers is not well understood in conventional medicine. There are theories of excess acid production and of weakened mucosa. However, the main thrust of diagnosis and treatment is to consider acid production and see how to reduce it and its effects. This is in keeping with the philosophical viewpoint of an external factor causing disease. Conventional medicine does recognise that certain factors can damage the mucosa including drugs, e.g. aspirin and the non-steroidal anti-inflammatory agents, emotional upsets (although this is open to debate in conventional circles) and irregular eating habits. The most important recent development in the diagnosis and treatment of peptic ulcers is the discovery of an association with *Helicobacter pylori* – an organism found in some people with peptic ulcers.

In terms of individual ulcers, gastric ulcers are usually associated with low acid secretion unless they are around the pylorus in which case they have more in common with duodenal ulcers. It would seem, therefore, that gastric ulcers are associated with an abnormality of the stomach wall as ulceration occurs in the presence of decreased acid secretion and there is also an increased risk of stomach cancer in such people. Duodenal ulcers are associated with increased acid levels which then lead to erosion of the mucosa.

Symptoms
The distinction to be made between duodenal and gastric ulceration is not always an easy one. With a careful history however, it is possible to have an idea about the site of the problem.

The main symptom of any ulcer is chronic episodic pain over months or years. Some people present with the complications of the ulcer such as bleeding, perforation or obstruction of the gastric outlet due to scarring with little history of previous problems. A duodenal ulcer typically has a prolonged natural history of up to 20 years and although drugs may affect an acute situation this long natural history is unaffected. Gastric ulcers are seen as being less chronic in nature.

All ulcer pain is felt in the epigastrium directly in the middle or slightly to the right. It is localised and most people point with one finger. This is not seen with any other condition. The pain is often related to food but this can be variable. Classically, a duodenal ulcer leads to 'hunger pain', that is, pain between and before meals. It is relieved by eating and people often wake 2 to 3 hours after going to bed. Many people put on weight because they eat to relieve the pain. They keep a glass of milk and biscuits by the bed to eat in the night if there is pain. Gastric ulcer, on the other hand, leads to pain that is less regular. It comes on 1 hour or so after eating and rarely at night. People are afraid to eat because it causes pain and so they usually lose weight.

The pain of an ulcer is better with antacids and better with vomiting. This episodic pain continues for days and weeks and then usually disappears even with no treatment. It will recur in most cases some weeks or months later. There are commonly milder symptoms in the intervening period or some people may be very well between attacks.

Relapses of the ulcer and pain are commonly linked to alcohol intake, poor diet or emotional stress. In some cases the pain may only be felt as mild discomfort or as a distended feeling in the upper abdomen. Other symptoms include nausea, vomiting, constipation or diarrhoea, poor appetite or increased appetite, belching, abdominal distension, rumbling in the abdomen. Vomiting is not a major feature but when it does occur it relieves the pain. Severe vomiting may lead to weight loss and could indicate one of the complications of ulceration.

On examination, there is local tenderness with perhaps some upper abdominal distension.

Symptom	Gastric ulcer	Duodenal ulcer
Pain	Epigastrium, localised	Epigastrium, localised
Vomiting	Yes, relieves pain	Yes, relieves pain
Effect of eating	Worsens pain	Relieves pain
Time of pain	After meals	Before meals, at night
Appetite	Often poor because afraid to eat	Good

Table 13.9: Summary of differences between symptoms of gastric and duodenal ulcers

Investigations

Barium meal and gastroscopy are the standard investigations and will show most but not all ulcers. Gastric function tests on secretions collected via a tube passed into the stomach may reveal changes in the levels of gastric acid. Gastric ulcers may be associated with low gastric acid output and duodenal ulcers with raised levels.

Helicobacter pylori can be detected by several methods. A urea breath test is used as a quick screening method and to monitor the effectiveness of treatment. Levels of immunoglobulin antibodies may be measured for diagnosis or as a research tool. Endoscopy allows for three tests on the presence of *H. pylori*: the examination of gastric mucosa for the presence of *H. pylori*, culture of the organism and the rapid urease test.

Complications

Complication	Symptoms to look for
Pyloric stenosis[9]	Copious vomiting containing food eaten 12 or more hours before, projectile vomiting, upper abdominal distension with splashing sounds
Haemorrhage	Vomiting blood, black tarry stools (melaena[10])
Perforation	Severe abdominal pain, abdominal rigidity, immobility, shock – low blood pressure, rapid pulse
Penetration into pancreas	Severe epigastric pain radiating through to back, abdominal rigidity, immobility, shock, low blood pressure, rapid pulse

Table 13.10: Complications of peptic ulcer

Treatment

Treatment (from mildest to strongest)	Comments
General advice	No dietary advice is given as a rule other than avoiding the foods which may exacerbate symptoms. The conventional view is that diet has little, if any role, to play in the genesis and healing of ulcers. Stopping smoking is encouraged as nicotine leads to a rise in the secretion of gastric acid and is an important factor in allowing healing to take place. All medication taken should be reviewed as many drugs lead to upper gastrointestinal problems especially aspirin, non-steroidal anti-inflammatory drugs and corticosteroids. No-one with a history of ulceration or indigestion should take them. It is common now to see non-steroidal anti-inflammatory drugs combined, in the same tablet, with histamine (H_2) blockers. This strange practice is similar to prescribing antibiotics with corticosteroids or antidepressants with tranquillisers
Colloidal bismuth[11]	This is an older drug, which actually heals as well as the histamine blockers but with a longer symptomatic response. It also has an action against *Helicobacter pylori*
Histamine (H_2) blockers	Cimetidine and ranitidine decrease the amount of gastric acid secreted. They have to be given over a prolonged course to produce resolution of the inflammation. Relapses are common after stopping the drug no matter how long it has been taken. They are expensive and have some unpleasant side-effects including breast development in men. They produce a state of low gastric acid, which is consistently found in those with cancer of the stomach. There is some evidence to suggest, therefore, that these drugs may lead to the development of stomach cancer
Proton pump inhibitors	These lead to an almost total reduction in gastric acid secretion and are commonly used. They include omeprazole, pantoprazole and lansoprazole
Prokinetic agents	Metoclopramide causes the stomach to empty quickly and increases contraction of the cardiac sphincter. It is also used in the symptomatic treatment of nausea. It acts via the central nervous system and so its side-effects mainly appear there with symptoms similar to those of Parkinson's disease. Cisapride acts increases oesophageal peristalsis and may be given long-term
Helicobacter pylori eradication – 'triple therapy'	This is considered to lead to the healing of 90 per cent of peptic ulcers. Such a treatment fits neatly into the conventional view that an external event causes disease. The organism is increasingly resistant to some antibiotics particularly metronidazole. <ul><li>Proton pump inhibitor, omeprazole</li><li>Metronidazole</li><li>Antibiotic, e.g. clarithromycin or a penicillin such as amoxycillin</li></ul>
Surgery	This is rarely performed now and only in cases of perforation or severe intractable bleeding

Table 13.11: Treatment of peptic ulceration

Holistic management
The causes of epigastric pain in terms of Chinese medicine are many and varied. There is a general division in to conditions of excess and those of deficiency. The energetic diagnosis in each individual case will determine the specific symptom picture, modalities and associated symptoms. This is why the descriptions given above can only ever be rough approximations. Chinese medical syndromes that may give rise to epigastric pain are:

- Spleen Qi Deficiency
- Spleen Yang Deficiency
- Damp-heat injuring Spleen
- Stomach Yin Deficiency
- Stomach Cold
- Stomach Fire Blazing
- Stomach Phlegm-fire
- Stomach Damp-heat
- Food Stagnation in the Stomach
- Blood Stagnation in the Stomach
- Liver Qi invading Stomach.

Regarding the current emphasis of treating *Helicobacter pylori,* any organism appears secondarily and so the use of antibiotics can only lead to a worsening of the underlying imbalance. In terms of Chinese medicine, the use of antibiotics, which are Cold and Damp in nature, will relieve symptoms due to Stomach Fire or perhaps Yin Deficiency. However, they severely deplete Spleen Qi and cause Accumulation of Damp.

Case one

A man of 50 years came for treatment of his diarrhoea. He had suffered from epigastric pain for many years each Christmas. Each episode would last about 1 month and would settle with simple antacids. On one occasion, 5 years prior to his coming to see me he went to see his doctor. Because he was covered by a private health scheme, his doctor referred him to a surgeon who performed a vagotomy and pyloroplasty operation.[12] He developed diarrhoea immediately after the operation and this continued daily. Whenever he ate, he would have symptoms of light-headedness, dizziness and would have watery diarrhoea. There would occasionally be undigested food in the stools. He had lost about 21 lb in weight over the past year and for the last 6 months had felt quite ill. His appetite was poor and he quickly felt full when eating.

His diarrhoea would be at least three times daily despite the daily prescription of a codeine derivative – loperamide. Codeine is methylmorphine. They are derived from the opium poppy and classed as narcotics. They have a primarily heating effect on the Heart and Lungs leading to emotional and mental changes that bring feelings of detachment and invulnerability. The heat is passed down into the intestines and dries the stools producing the typical side-effect of constipation. This is the reason they are used to treat diarrhoea.

In terms of Chinese medicine, the diagnosis was Spleen Yang Deficiency. This means that the energy of the Spleen was very weak and unable to transport and transform food. The cause was the operation some 5 years previously. This clinical picture is commonly seen after upper abdominal surgery.

Interestingly, his tongue should have been pale, wet and swollen but at his first visit was red and thin. This was because of the heating and drying effects of the drugs.

Treatment was directed at strengthening the Spleen with acupuncture and herbs. I gave him advice to eat warming foods with the addition of ginger and cinnamon. Within 1 month, he had improved markedly with no watery stools and a reduced number of bowel movements each day. He was able to stop his drugs quite quickly. He was left with symptoms of excessive rumbling in the abdomen but this settled over the next few months of treatment.

This case reveals several points. Firstly, even when structural damage is present it is possible for people to improve. Secondly, the conventional treatment of peptic ulcer tends to make people worse. Thirdly, be careful before having conventional treatment which is private as this may tempt overzealous practitioners to try the more expensive yet more dangerous options.

Case two

A man of 64 years came for treatment of his stomach symptoms. He had trouble with his digestion for over 30 years, mainly an uncomfortable feeling in the epigastrium. A gastroscopy revealed inflammation and he was given 'triple therapy' to eradicate *Helicobacter pylori* infection. This had not helped his symptoms and he was now on omeprazole long-term.

His bowels were generally irregular and he would miss days completely. He had bloating in the abdomen with pain in the left iliac fossa which would improve after defaecation. He would feel weak and lethargic whenever his symptoms occurred. I made a diagnosis of Spleen Qi Deficiency and treated him with acupuncture and a herbal formula to strengthen his digestion. After some 6 months of treatment, he felt much better, his energy was good and his digestive symptoms were minimal. He would still have some discomfort if he ate poor quality food or when he was rushing.

This case reveals a common experience of holistic practitioners that digestive disorders are very amenable to treatment and most people do well. The previous use of 'triple therapy' is common and is not as widely effective as conventional practitioners would have us believe.

Case three

A girl of 13 years came for treatment. She was suffering from very sharp pain in the epigastrium. She described these as being 'like bubbles being popped with a knife'. It was accompanied by a blocked feeling near her chest, bloating and a desire to burp or vomit. Vomiting did not relieve the pain.

She also had headaches with knife-like pain. She had been the victim of an arson attack 2 years earlier and though she had escaped unhurt she still had nightmares about it and had a fear of fire. She hated the people responsible for the attack.

She was prescribed Hepar sulph 30c. Immediately after taking it she vomited three times and the epigastric pain disappeared, generally she was in a better mood and had the pain less frequently after that. She repeated the remedy as

237

needed and 10 months later all the symptoms were much improved. Two years later she is still well.

GALL BLADDER DISEASE

The gall bladder is a small hollow organ situated beneath the liver. Its function is to store bile secreted by the liver. Bile contains bile salts, cholesterol and the breakdown products of haemoglobin from red blood cells. It is also an important means of excreting substances from the liver. There are two main conditions of the gall bladder. These are gallstones, (cholelithiasis) and inflammation (cholecystitis). Although I consider these separately below for the purposes of description, in reality they commonly co-exist. Gallstones in the gall bladder may produce inflammation and inflammation is a common precondition for the development of gallstones.

Gallstones

Conventionally, gallstones are considered to be more in people who are over 40 years of age, overweight and female (especially if they have children).

There are three varieties of stone commonly found which are classified according to their composition. Cholesterol stones make up 20 per cent, 5 per cent are bile pigment stones and the remaining 75 per cent are mixed in nature. According to conventional medicine, the causes of gallstone formation are not well understood but seem to be related to several factors.

Cholesterol is an important constituent of bile. Disturbances in cholesterol metabolism or raised serum cholesterol levels may lead to the production of cholesterol stones and they are more commonly seen in women who take the oral contraceptive, in pregnancy and diabetes mellitus.

Pigment stones are more common in cases of anaemia due to red blood cell breakdown because excess bile pigment is excreted.

This does not explain the vast majority of gallstones that are present and it may be that there is some alteration in the concentration of bile constituents. Substances normally in bile exist in a supersaturated solution; i.e. they are present in concentrations far exceeding normal solutions. Any small change may result in the precipitation of substances from the solution.

Symptoms
These are variable and depend upon the site of the gallstones. In most people they cause no symptoms and merely lie in the gall bladder to be found at routine investigation, in the case of an operation for another reason or at post-mortem examination. Symptoms occur when the gallstone starts to move.

If they impact at the exit of the gall bladder or in the cystic duct, there may be biliary colic or cholecystitis. Biliary colic is the classic symptom picture that presents when a stone obstructs the exit to the gall bladder. Typically, pain comes on after a meal. It is severe in nature and lasts for several hours. It is felt in the right hypochondrium or epigastrium, often radiating to the right scapula. The person is restless, cannot get comfortable and there is associated vomiting and sweating. After an hour or so the pain subsides to be replaced by tenderness in the right hypochondrium. Attacks occur at irregular intervals.

If the gallstone passes into the common bile duct and blocks it, this prevents bile from entering the duodenum. The obstructed bile backs up into the liver and spills over into the blood. This causes a form of jaundice known as obstructive jaundice.

Rarely the stone may ulcerate through the gall bladder wall into the duodenum or colon. Acute cholecystitis is more common in the presence of gallstones and this is described below.

Cholecystitis

This is an inflammation of the gall bladder wall. It is frequently, though not always, associated with gallstones. Inflammation is not usually associated with organisms and is not infective in nature.

Symptoms
Pain is more persistent in contrast to biliary colic. There are additional signs of inflammation such as fever, toxaemia, and rapid pulse rate. There is also abdominal tenderness. Ninety-five per cent of cases are associated with gallstones. Chronic cholecystitis is typified by repeated attacks usually precipitated by food, particularly fatty food. Abdominal distension, flatulence and/or belching are common associated symptoms.

Investigations of gall bladder disease

About 10 per cent of gallstones are visible by plain X-ray examination since few contain calcium. The common investigation performed these days is ultrasound. Additional information may be gathered by oral cholecystogram, intravenous cholangiogram, barium meal and liver function tests.

Treatment

In the acute stage, cholecystitis is treated with antibiotics, despite the common absence of bacterial infection, and pethidine for the relief of pain. After the acute phase has subsided then the gall bladder is usually removed 2-3 months later.

The operation of cholecystectomy is common and is considered to be the treatment of choice. Other treatments are only considered if surgery is refused. The operation is increasingly perfored as a laparscopic procedure necessitating a shorter stay in hospital. The mortality rate of this surgery is less than 0.1 per cent with complications including wound infection, injury to the bile duct in 0.5 per cent and stones remaining in the bile duct. Cholecystectomy invariably leads to diarrhoea since there is an impaired ability to digest and absorb fats. Also, a number of people continue with the same symptoms and are subsequently diagnosed as having irritable bowel syndrome or a variant.

Cholesterol stones can be dissolved by chenodeoxycholic or ursodeoxycholic acid. This is long term treatment of up to 2 years and half of gallstones reappear when treatment is stopped. The treatment has side-effects of liver damage and diarrhoea. They may render oral contraception ineffective.

Holistic management

The main advantage of holistic medical treatment is that it rectifies the underlying imbalance. This will prevent, or at least minimise, the development of more gallstones. There are naturopathic treatments available such as the 'liver flush' to allow the body to pass gallstones. This is a pure diet or fast over several days followed by the drinking of a pint of olive oil with lemon juice. This causes the gall bladder to contract and the gallstones to expel. In my experience it is an effective means for removing gallstones without the need for surgery.

Homoeopathy and Chinese medicine are also effective for this condition. When I was training in acupuncture in China, we saw many people treated with acupuncture, particularly ear acupuncture. In terms of Chinese medicine, this condition usually corresponds with Damp-heat in the Liver and Gall Bladder.

Some people request surgery despite the holistic treatments available. The use of ultrasound to break up the stones is helpful since the gall bladder can be conserved. The subsequent use of holistic medical treatment can prevent the recurrence of more gallstones.

Case one

A woman of 54 years came for treatment with symptoms of upper abdominal discomfort, belching, nausea and poor appetite. Her bowels were normal and regular. She tended to feel tired easily. I made a diagnosis of Spleen Qi Deficiency and Damp-heat Accumulation in the Gall Bladder. She had had investigations at the local hospital which had shown the presence of gallstones.

I treated her with acupuncture and Chinese herbal medicine for some 3 months. She obtained a lot of relief although her symptoms did not disappear completely and she stopped coming for treatment. I saw her again about 1 year later. She had had a cholecystectomy but the symptoms had returned after the operation the same as before. The only difference now was that she had a tendency to loose stools. I resumed treating her as before with some relief. Her treatment continues but after four months she is generally well with increased levels of energy. Her abdominal symptoms are much improved although they tend to worsen if she eats poor quality food or irregularly.

This situation of abdominal symptoms that remain the same after gall bladder surgery is common. It shows the presence of gallstones is no guarantee that the symptoms are due to these and assumptions are made that lead to surgical interventions. My opinion would be that surgery should only be used for those people with intractable difficulties for which no other option has been of benefit.

PANCREATIC DISEASE

The pancreas is a combined exocrine and endocrine organ situated behind the peritoneal cavity at the level of the duodenum and lower stomach. In this section, I am dealing with the pancreas in its exocrine function. Endocrine disturbances of the pancreas are dealt with in Chapter 15 – Endocrine system.

The pancreas secretes enzymes, which have an important role in the digestion of proteins, fats and carbohydrates. It does so in response to food eaten.

Pancreatitis

This is an inflammation of the pancreas. It is unusual but severe in its symptoms. There are considered to be various causes in conventional medicine with excess alcohol intake and associated gall bladder disease being the commonest. It may occur as part of mumps[13] in post-pubertal people when it is mild and merely uncomfortable. The symptom picture described below is of the non-mumps type.

The underlying process is not completely understood in conventional medicine. There may be several factors such as the passage of bile (an irritant) up the pancreatic duct and digestion of the pancreas itself by pancreatic enzymes. Whatever the process, the accompanying inflammation is severe and widespread.

Symptoms
The severity of the attack may vary. There is epigastric pain radiating through to the back. It can vary in strength from mild discomfort to severe pain. There is associated nausea and vomiting. On examination, the epigastrium, and perhaps the whole abdomen, is tender and rigid with rebound tenderness.[14] These signs are typical of a severe attack. There may be rapid pulse rate, low blood pressure, pallor and sweating.

Some people have milder attacks denoting a more chronic picture. Attacks of pain are milder but more frequent. The pain is epigastric radiating through to the back. Alcohol intake is often the cause of an attack. Weight loss is common together with anorexia. In long-term disease, the absorption of fat is affected leading to diarrhoea with greasy and pale stools. Some people may develop diabetes mellitus if enough of the pancreas is damaged to enough affect insulin production.

Investigations
Most people with an acute attack will be admitted to hospital due to the pain and shock. Perforated peptic ulcer is the other condition that may give rise to similar symptoms. Serum amylase is the usual method of diagnosis since this is raised in pancreatitis. It needs to be five times the normal level as a rise also occurs in gall bladder disease and perforated peptic ulcer. This, together with the history and examination, is usually enough to allow a diagnosis to be made.

Other investigations performed include ultrasound to detect gallstones and pancreatic swelling, MRI scans and contrast-enhanced dynamic CT scanning which is very helpful in making a diagnosis. If there is any doubt it may be necessary to perform a laparotomy to exclude surgically correctable problems such as a perforated peptic ulcer.

Treatment
This is mainly supportive with pain relief and fluid replacement. There is no specific treatment for this condition. There is a significant mortality rate in acute episodes ranging from 1 per cent in mild cases to 50 per cent in severe ones.

Chronic cases are advised not to drink alcohol and may be given pancreatic enzyme supplements. A low fat diet is recommended. Surgery may be attempted in cases of severe intractable pain with variable results.

Cancer of the pancreas

This is the fifth most common cause of cancer death in the UK and US. Men are affected more than women and most people are over 60 years of age. Various reasons have been cited for the increasing incidence including smoking, alcohol and coffee.

Symptoms
The cancer may arise either in the head or the body and tail of the pancreas. The clinical picture varies slightly depending upon its site. Cancer of the head of the pancreas leads relatively early to obstruction of the common bile duct. Jaundice without pain is the typical first symptom. Later, there is usually the development of epigastric pain or discomfort with weight loss.

Cancer of the body or tail of the pancreas leads to epigastric pain, anorexia and weight loss. The pain is typically dull, constant and boring in nature, which radiates through to the back. It is often better for sitting forward or lying face down. On examination, a lump is felt in the epigastrium in about 20 per cent of people.

Investigations
Ultrasound or CAT scan usually makes the diagnosis. Needle biopsy confirms the nature of the disease.

Treatment
Only 2 per cent of people with cancer of the pancreas survive 5 years. This is because the pancreas is deep within the body

and comes to notice relatively late. Some surgeons perform total pancreatectomy but the operation has a mortality rate of 5 per cent. Inserting a plastic tube to bypass the obstruction can relieve jaundice. This is usually performed by endoscopy.

Holistic management

Please see Chapter 6 – Cancer. Recently, the US National Cancer Institute has funded a trial of holistic treatment of advanced pancreatic cancer. The so-called Gonzalez regimen is similar to many other such treatments of cancer comprising dietary changes, nutritional supplements and 'detoxification' through coffee enemas. Preliminary results show that people following such a regime survive 17 months more than those who had conventional treatments.[15]

PERITONITIS

This is the inflammatory reaction of the peritoneum to an irritant. There may be several underlying processes such as infection related to appendicitis or acid as part of a perforated gastric ulcer. Appendicitis is the common cause.

Symptoms

These are usually clear cut and unmistakable. There is the sudden onset of abdominal pain. This is typically severe in nature and is worse for movement. The person lies still. The abdominal muscles over the affected area are rigid in an attempt to protect the underlying inflamed tissues. The abdomen is still and motionless. There is tenderness to the touch and this is magnified when the examining hand is suddenly removed from the abdominal wall. This is called 'rebound tenderness'. There is associated shock with rapid pulse rate and a low blood pressure. If it is secondary to a condition such as appendicitis then the initial signs are of that particular complaint (see details of gastric ulcer above and appendicitis below).

Acute appendicitis

This is usually seen in young people. There has been a rapid increase since 1900 and is probably related to our diet and sedentary existence. It was unheard of in Africa when the first missionaries arrived there but once Western 'civilisation' arrived so did appendicitis.

Symptoms

The symptoms are slightly different to the classical appearance of peritonitis. The underlying process is more gradual than a perforated peptic ulcer. The pain of organ inflammation tends to be nondescript and central in location. The pain becomes more severe and localised once the inflammation spreads to the parietal peritoneum which lines the abdominal cavity.

There is a short history of vague central abdominal pain, which migrates to the right iliac fossa over several hours. It is eventually localised to McBurney's point.[16] There is also nausea, malaise and unpleasant breath. There may or may not be vomiting. The pulse is often raised and there may be a slight fever.

On examination, there is tenderness, rigidity and rebound tenderness in the right iliac fossa. More widespread rigidity occurs later. This typical appearance occurs in about 50 per cent of cases. In the remainder, it varies with the location of the appendix. The differential diagnosis of pain in the right iliac fossa is discussed in Chapter 18 – Women's Health.

Treatment

Conventionally, this is by surgery although acupuncture is definitely effective in the early stages. Another consideration is that a significant number of appendices removed at operation are normal, thus showing the diagnosis to have been incorrect.

Holistic management

In terms of Chinese medicine, this corresponds to Intestinal Abscess. It is associated with one of three syndromes – Stagnation of Blood, Accumulation of Damp-heat and Toxic Heat. Several factors including irregular eating and the intake of cold and raw foods cause it. There are treatments available and in mild cases it would be reasonable to use them. Hospitalisation is necessary in cases where toxicity is marked with fever, rapid pulse rate, and severe pain with guarding[17] and rigidity.

LOWER GASTROINTESTINAL DISEASE

The disorders here are located in the small and large intestines. They lead primarily to disturbances of bowel habit.

Inflammatory bowel disease

This is disease of the bowel where inflammation is the characteristic feature. Crohn's disease (also known as regional ileitis) and ulcerative colitis are extremely common and becoming more so.

An autoimmune process causes the inflammation. There is evidence of antibodies attacking the intestine. Although the two diseases are considered separately and always described differently in conventional medical textbooks, they seem to be two examples of the same process. They merely affect slightly different areas of the intestine to a differing degree.

Ulcerative colitis is commoner in 20-40 year olds whilst Crohn's disease is seen in a slightly younger age group (late teens to early twenties). Crohn's disease primarily affects the last part of the small intestine (ileum) although it can involve any part of the gastrointestinal tract from the mouth to the anus. It affects the colon in 15-20 per cent of the cases. Ulcerative colitis, as its name suggests, primarily affects the colon and in particular the rectum.

Symptoms

The symptoms of ulcerative colitis are commonly diarrhoea, mucus, blood, and tenesmus,[18] together with systemic symptoms of ill health, anorexia and tiredness. The condition frequently remits and relapses with exacerbations related to dietary indiscretions or emotional stress.

The symptoms of Crohn's disease are markedly similar. Abdominal pain is more frequent in the right iliac fossa whilst the systemic symptoms such as fever, anaemia and weight loss are more severe.

Symptoms of Crohn's disease are certainly more severe and this reflects the greater degree and depth of inflammation. In ulcerative colitis it is merely the mucus membrane that is affected whereas with Crohn's disease all three layers of the bowel wall are involved in the inflammation. Fistulae are well-recognised complications of Crohn's disease. They allow the passage of faeces from inside the intestines to other areas. These include other areas of the intestine, the abdominal wall, perineum, vagina and bladder.

Investigations

The diagnosis of inflammatory bowel disease is primarily made by the clinical history. However, there are typical appearances, which may be seen on barium X-ray examinations. A barium meal and follow-through[19] will reveal typical appearances in the case of Crohn's disease. A barium enema is performed in cases of ulcerative colitis where colonoscopy will reveal inflammation. Blood tests reveal evidence of anaemia. There may also be deficiency of iron and folic acid.

	Crohn's disease	Ulcerative colitis
Area mainly affected	Small intestine – terminal ileum	Large intestine – rectum
Tissue affected	All three layers of the bowel wall	Mucosa only
Age group	Late teens to early 20's	20-40 year olds
Diarrhoea	Yes	Yes
Mucus	Yes	Yes
Blood	Yes	Yes
Systemic symptoms	Yes – tend to be severe	Yes – tend to be mild
Fistulae	Yes	No
Diagnosis	Barium meal and follow-through	Barium enema, colonoscopy

Table 13.12: Comparison of ulcerative colitis and Crohn's disease

Complications

Complication	Symptoms to look for
Skin rashes	Dark discolouration over shins, nodular, tender (erythema nodosum)
Arthritis	11 per cent of those with Crohn's disease and 14 per cent with ulcerative colitis. Single joints affected with no long-term damage. Look for swelling, redness, heat and pain
Liver disease	Usually asymptomatic. Look for right hypochondriac pain, nausea, anorexia, and jaundice
Iritis	Pain, discomfort in the light, redness around the cornea, blurred vision
Deep venous thrombosis	Pain in calf of leg, swelling, and tenderness
Stomatitis	Sore mouth, redness
Toxicity	Fever, weight loss, severe diarrhoea
Perforation	Rare. Symptoms of peritonitis. Severe pain, rigidity of abdominal muscles, rebound tenderness, fever, shock
Kidney stones	Only in Crohn's disease. Loin pain of a colicky nature, vomiting, frequent urination, blood in urine
Cancer	Obstructive symptoms of distension and colicky abdominal pain. There is change in bowel habit, bleeding

Table 13.13: Complications of inflammatory bowel disease

Treatment

The conventional medical treatment of both conditions is similar. Antidiarrhoeal agents such as codeine and its derivatives may be used to control the symptoms of loose stools.

Corticosteroids are used in more severe disease. They are applied locally by enema to treat the rectum and orally where there is more systemic involvement. If corticosteroids cannot control the symptoms, immunosuppressive agents are given, e.g. azathioprine. Surgery is occasionally performed in acute emergencies only. It is well known that the removal of an affected part of the bowel in Crohn's disease leads to spread of the inflammatory process to uninvolved areas. In addition, the development of fistulae is common. Surgery should be reserved for cases of Crohn's disease with severe complications.

Treatment (from mildest to strongest)	Comments
Antidiarrhoeal agents	Symptomatic treatment for diarrhoea. Examples used are codeine and its derivatives, loperamide, lomotil
Sulphasalazine	Combination of aspirin and sulphonamide antibiotics. Also used in rheumatoid arthritis
Corticosteroid (enema)	Local application of corticosteroid to bowel wall
Corticosteroid (oral)	Systemic use
Immunosuppressants	Powerful drugs also used in cancer chemotherapy, e.g. azathioprine
Surgery	In ulcerative colitis – total colectomy with ileostomy Crohn's disease – small bowel resection

Table 13.14: Conventional treatment of inflammatory bowel disease

Holistic management

Inflammatory bowel disease is relatively commonly seen in the clinic. This is because conventional treatment is of variable effectiveness and people continue to have symptoms for many years. There may be relapses and remissions dependent upon dietary habits and emotional states. People may seek help at the time of a relapse or when symptoms are somewhat calmer in an attempt to prevent a flare-up.

In terms of Chinese medicine, these conditions often correspond to Damp-heat in the Large Intestine. Underlying Spleen and Kidney Yang Deficiency is common, as is some degree of Liver Qi Stagnation. The Intestines are a common site of emotional stagnation and they may manifest symptoms at times of emotional stress. It is interesting that the connection of the Small Intestine with the Heart explains how anxiety may lead to bowel disturbances. The connection between the Lung and the Large Intestine explains how feelings such as grief and loss may lead to bowel disturbances.

Case one

A woman of 30 years came for treatment with a 15-year history of ulcerative colitis. The course of her symptoms over that time was variable but had worsened over the recent months. It had flared up again with increased workload and some stressful situations at home. She was currently taking 20 mg prednisolone (corticosteroid) daily. She had previously been on sulphasalazine but had had to stop taking it because it damaged her blood.

When her symptoms were severe, she would have diarrhoea up to 20 times per day with urgency, blood, mucus and undigested food. At the time she came to see me it had settled to about twice daily with slight urgency. She would still have undigested food in the stools from time to time but no blood or mucus. She had increased in weight by over 20 lb since starting the corticosteroids. They also had increased her appetite and made her feel somewhat hyperactive and manic.

The diagnosis in terms of Chinese medicine was Spleen and Kidney Yang Deficiency, Heart Blood Deficiency and Liver Qi Stagnation. Treatment was aimed at strengthening her energy so that at some point she would be able to reduce her corticosteroids. It is important in such cases to take things slowly and you would expect to treat such people for several years. The conventional rate of reduction of prednisolone is by 1 mg per month and this is without flare-ups of the original condition along the way. It may sometimes to be possible to reduce slightly quicker with the support of holistic medicine but to get someone off 20 mg is slow work.

After some months of treatment, she was able to reduce her prednisolone. This was done gradually but the dose was increased when she had a flare-up after a colonoscopy. However, this lasted a shorter time than her previous flare-up after a colonoscopy and was controlled with a lower dose of prednisolone. She progressed very well until after 6 months she was down to 9 mg daily. Her stools were virtually normal. She had more energy and felt strong. Along the way, the hospital had suggested to her that she should stop her corticosteroids as they had terrible side-effects long-term and to go on azathioprine. An interesting suggestion in view of the fact that azathioprine is much more damaging to the immune system. It is an immunosuppressant and used in some cancer chemotherapy treatments.

She declined this offer of changing treatment. She subsequently had a great flare-up of her symptoms, which could not be controlled by my treatment. It did help to some extent but she had diarrhoea some eight times daily with blood and mucus. She eventually decided to increase her prednisolone to 30 mg eventually to control the symptoms and after 6 weeks she was able to begin reduction once more.

She had previously told me that her symptoms were always worse in the autumn but I had attached no especial importance to this. After some discussion of what was happening, it became clear that the cause of this episode was her son starting school. The sense of loss was marked. It is interesting that the Lung, in terms of Chinese medicine, is paired with the Large Intestine and affected by grief and loss. What was more important was that she came to recognise that there was a connection with her own past. Her family had broken up when she started school and this echo had led to her recent flare-up. The fact that this had now come to consciousness was clearly therapeutic and part of the general movement towards cure. She was able to continue her improvement by continuing treatment and addressing underlying emotional issues.

Case two

A man of 42 years came for treatment with a 9-year history of Crohn's disease. He had had several bowel operations in the past 7 years with removal of narrowed sections. His current symptoms were diarrhoea with urgency, which would contain blood and mucus when severe. He had lost some 7 lb in weight over the years. His energy levels were low and he had continual feelings of tiredness. His digestive problems actually dated back 20 years to an acute episode of diarrhoea with haemorrhoids in the Far East. This is a common story in people with Crohn's disease that symptoms develop after gastroenteritis, dysentery or related problem. When his bowels were particularly troublesome he would develop pustular spots over his lower back. His current medication was:

- azathioprine 250 mg three times daily
- prednisolone 10 mg daily
- codeine phosphate 30 mg three times daily.

His medication revealed the underlying severity of his condition and it was important to wait for his condition to improve before any attempt was made to alter their dosage.

The Chinese medical diagnosis was Spleen and Kidney Yang Deficiency, Blood Deficiency and Damp-heat Accumulation in the Intestines.

Treatment was directed at alleviating the underlying problem, namely the weakness of the Spleen and Kidney. He improved generally with herbs and acupuncture but it was not until after 6 months of treatment that we felt confident to begin reduction of the drugs. This was done slowly with the most powerful reduced first,[20] i.e. azathioprine.

Improvement continued over the ensuing months and it was possible to reduce and then stop his medication. Along the way, he addressed and resolved some long-standing emotional difficulties, which helped the healing process.

Diverticular disease

This is a condition that occurs in the colon and especially the descending and sigmoid areas. It is considered to be due to a weakening of the wall of the colon, perhaps associated with raised intra-colonic pressure. Small pouches (diverticuli) appear in the colon. It occurs in mid to late age with women more commonly affected than men. Symptoms are only present if there is associated inflammation and then the term used is diverticulitis.

Symptoms
As mentioned above, symptoms are only present if there is associated inflammation. There may be a history of constipation or other bowel disturbances in those with diets rich in fat and refined carbohydrates but lacking in dietary fibre.

Pain and tenderness are common particularly in the left iliac fossa. There is constipation and/or diarrhoea. Rectal bleeding can occur and although not common it may be severe.

An inflammatory mass may appear as the process continues. This may interfere with intestinal function to the extent that intestinal obstruction may develop. In such cases, it can be difficult to tell the difference between diverticulitis and cancer of the colon. Even after biopsy there may still be doubt about the diagnosis.

Treatment
This mainly consists of symptomatic and supportive measures, which include bed rest, and painkillers Antibiotics are invariably given for acute episodes. Surgery may be needed in cases of intestinal obstruction and this involves resection of the affected area. There is a definite correlation between the incidence of this disease and the low level of dietary fibre in the western world.

Irritable bowel syndrome

This is defined as 'abdominal pain with no organic cause'. It is also known as spastic colon. The cause is uncertain in conventional medicine but it is noted that anxiety is a common associated symptom. It is more common amongst women in the 20-40 age group. It is a disturbance of the function of the large intestine.

Symptoms
There is pain in the lower abdomen, which may be focused in the right or left iliac fossa. This is better for defaecation and worse for eating. Emotional upsets may also cause an exacerbation. Abdominal distension and flatulence are associated symptoms. The pain may vary from site to site. Attacks tend to be episodic and may be severe.

There may be evidence of mucus in the stools. Alternating constipation and diarrhoea is common. The stools may have the appearance of rabbit droppings or be thin and ribbon-like. Cancer of the large intestine may also present with alternating constipation and diarrhoea but it is of recent onset and tends to be progressive. Here it is intermittent and frequently related to mood.

Investigations
The diagnosis of irritable bowel syndrome is primarily made from the clinical picture. However, occasional investigations may be performed to exclude bowel obstruction. These will be colonoscopy and barium enema.

Investigations may also be done to exclude infection in the intestines. Occasionally, symptoms may appear after an acute bowel infection.

Treatment
This is of variable effectiveness in conventional medicine. There is no effective treatment, which will relieve the symptoms on a long-term basis so a symptomatic approach is taken. Antispasmodics such as mebeverine or anticholinergics such as dicyclomine are common prescriptions. Diarrhoea is treated symptomatically with codeine or one of its derivatives. Tranquillisers or antidepressants are common prescriptions, particularly in women.

Holistic management

This condition reveals the close association between the emotions and the intestines. In Chinese medicine, this usually corresponds to Liver Qi Stagnation invading the Spleen.

Case one

A woman of 31 years came for treatment of recurrent attacks of abdominal pain. She would experience a stitching pain in the right iliac fossa which would be worse for pressure. It started when she took the oral contraceptive after the birth of her last child. She had had many investigations, all of which were normal. She was most anxious about her symptoms and was worried about bowel cancer. This would always be relieved after a normal investigation but would then recur particularly if her symptoms were marked. Her bowels were always difficult and although daily, it would be difficult to pass a motion and the bowel would not feel properly emptied.

I made a diagnosis in Chinese medicine of Liver Qi attacking the Spleen with underlying Kidney Yang Deficiency. I treated her with acupuncture and Chinese herbs as well as discussing diet. This combination of physical and psychological symptoms is common in this condition and reflects the deeper pathology than if the symptoms were only physical in nature. I treated her for almost a year with good results. At the end of that time, she felt well and generally much better in herself. Physically the pain in the abdomen had subsided and she had fewer thoughts of cancer. She finished seeing me and continued to work on underlying psychological issues with the help of a counsellor.

Haemorrhoids

These are varicose veins in the wall of the rectum. They are subdivided, conventionally, according to the symptoms that they produce.

First degree haemorrhoids are located in the lower rectum and upper anal canal. They bleed but do not prolapse. Second degree haemorrhoids prolapse on defaecation then reduce spontaneously or manually. The third degree type remain prolapsed outside the anus. Their cause is usually unknown according to conventional medicine but they are associated with conditions that lead to congestion of the pelvic venous circulation. So, chronic constipation is considered to be responsible in many cases. Pregnancy, of course, is a common association as is compression by a pelvic tumour. Cardiac failure may also lead to haemorrhoids.

Symptoms

Rectal bleeding is almost universal. The blood is bright red and usually occurs at defaecation. This is the only symptom in mild cases but in more severe types there may be itching of the anal margin, a mucous discharge and occasionally pain. The symptoms are not usually, in themselves, serious but they can be unpleasant and you must bear in mind the possible associated diseases mentioned above.

Conventionally, local treatment is given unless the occurrence of bleeding or persistent prolapse necessitates surgical intervention.

I am reminded here of a woman I treated with rheumatoid arthritis. When she first presented for treatment, most of her joints were swollen, stiff and painful. Treatment with acupuncture resulted in a marked improvement and after about 6 months she remarked, 'I have not felt this well for 20 years.' She commented that she was having some problems with haemorrhoids and that she was due to go into hospital the next week for an operation. I discussed this with her, informed her of the concept of suppression and said that her haemorrhoids would, with time, improve also. She decided to have the surgery.

Within 2 weeks her joints flared-up to become hot, swollen and painful. Some 4 weeks later she developed a painful, swollen right leg, which I thought clinically was a deep venous thrombosis. Investigations at the hospital proved negative but for some weeks I was greatly concerned about her health. The effects of suppressive treatment are common but not always so dramatic. In conventional thought it is seen as a coincidental event or perhaps as a 'complication' occurring after surgery, drugs and other treatment. It is important to inform people of the possible consequences of conventional treatment, not in an attempt to frighten them but as part of a general education about health and healing.

Treatment

Any serious cause for the haemorrhoids such as pelvic tumour or cardiac failure is excluded first. General practitioners will often prescribe creams druing initial visits, particularly if the problem is not very severe. The creams usually contain an anaesthetic and many contain a weak hydrocortisone.

Injection therapy is given for first and second-degree cases. The veins are injected with a solution of phenol which is an irritant and the walls of the veins stick together. It is a similar treatment to that of varicose vein injection. The procedure is reputed to be painless and is usually done as an outpatient. It may be repeated two or three times.

The operation of haemorrhoidectomy is done for third degree cases. It is extremely painful immediately after the operation especially when any attempt is made to defaecate.

Holistic management

Haemorrhoids are an indication of a constitutional imbalance affecting the large intestine. They cannot be treated locally in a curative way. The case described above reveals the possible consequences of such suppressive treatment. In terms of Chinese medicine, the usual corresponding syndrome is Damp-heat Accumulation in the Large Intestine. Implicit in this diagnosis is usually some degree of Spleen Qi Deficiency, Kidney Yang Deficiency and Liver Qi Stagnation. The exact pattern will vary according to the individual.

Case one

A woman of 34 years came for treatment of her infertility. She had been trying to become pregnant for over 3 years. Conventional investigations were all normal. She had few symptoms apart from general tiredness and lethargy. Before her period she would have some soreness of her breasts and the first day or so of her period was painful. She had loose stools every day but particularly in the mornings. She had glomerulonephritis as a child and two episodes of kidney stones in the past. I made a diagnosis of Kidney Yang Deficiency. This is a common energetic problem in women with infertility. I discussed the issue of treatment for her partner at the same time, as it is useful to treat both.

I treated her by strengthening her Kidney Yang and after some months, she had more energy and felt better in herself. Her bowels became normal. It was after about 4 months of treatment that things began to change significantly. Long-suppressed emotions started to come to the surface and she began to think about the general direction of her life and particularly her career.

At the same time she started to develop pustular spots on her back and face with constipation. Haemorrhoids also developed which were uncomfortable and itchy. These symptoms of Damp-heat in the Large Intestine were now more obvious because her general energy had improved and the emphasis of the pathology had moved to the surface. An adjustment of treatment to relax her Liver Qi and alleviate the Dampness and Heat in the Large Intestine resulted not only in improvement of her physical symptoms, but also more emotional freedom.

After 10 months of treatment, she felt generally well, energetic and mainly symptom-free. Although she did not become pregnant, she was emotionally more balanced and calmer. There is a sense of non-attachment to pregnancy and this may help conception to take place.

The question of 'results' can be an issue when attempting to determine if holistic medicine is 'successful'. Her presenting complaint remained unchanged but many changes had taken place resulting in an improved quality of life. A planned career change was further evidence of her altered perception and was part of her movement towards health.

Anal fissure

This is a split at the anal margin, which is frequently related to constipation. There is pain on defaecation and perhaps local bleeding. It is of minor significance although can be very painful. The pain is due to associated muscle spasm in the anal sphincter.

Conventional treatment is to use local creams containing local anaesthetic and corticosteroid. If this is insufficient, an operation is performed to stretch the anal sphincter under general anaesthesia.

In terms of holistic medicine, this condition may be seen as related to haemorrhoids with Heat in the Large Intestine.

CANCER OF THE GASTROINTESTINAL SYSTEM

Cancers of the oesophagus, stomach, caecum, colon, and rectum can be described in general terms because of their symptoms. As the gastrointestinal system is a hollow tube, the symptoms appear because of obstruction. The main symptoms are constipation, abdominal distension, colicky abdominal pain and vomiting. The focus of the symptoms depends on the site of the cancer. If it is higher up the gastrointestinal system, then vomiting is an early symptom, distension is slight or not at all and constipation occurs later. Conversely, vomiting starts later, abdominal distension is more marked and constipation occurs earlier, the lower down the gastrointestinal system the cancer occurs. Bleeding may also be seen.

The key symptoms to remember for large intestine cancer are change in bowel habit of recent onset with rectal bleeding.

Site of cancer	Symptoms	Comments
Oesophagus	Dysphagia first – sensation of swallowed food becoming stuck Vomiting later as the obstruction develops and eventually an inability to take anything orally other than fluids	If the dysphagia is felt in the lower third of the oesophagus it is a reliable indicator of where the cancer is situated
Stomach	Vomiting of blood Lump felt in upper abdomen Upper abdominal distension Constipation develops late	There may have been a pre-existing ulcer and so there may be confusion between the symptoms of the ulcer and those of the cancer
Large bowel	Caecum: changes in bowel habit occur late as faeces are liquid Rectum: constipation occurs early Marked abdominal distension Vomiting occurs late Bleeding – seen on the surface of the stool with rectal and anal cancers, mixed with faeces for others. The blood is redder the lower down in the bowel is the cancer Lump felt in abdomen – tends to hard, fixed, irregular	With rectal cancer there is desire to defaecate but no stools produced because of the growing lump in the rectum. This is known as tenesmus

Table 13.15: Symptoms of cancer of the gastrointestinal system

Oesophageal cancer

This is not a common condition and usually is seen in the 60-70 year age group. It is slightly commoner in men than women. Half of cases develop in the middle third of the oesophagus and one quarter in the lower third. In the UK there are 5-10 cases per 100,000 of the population which account for 2.5 per cent of all cancers. There is a particularly high incidence in China and some areas of Africa and Iran.

Symptoms
The tumour ulcerates and bleeds and can extend either up or down to cause narrowing and thus difficulty in swallowing. Progressive dysphagia is the cardinal presenting symptom starting with solids and then softer foods and finally liquids. Anyone who has these symptoms over a period of several months should be suspected of this diagnosis until proved otherwise. There is often discomfort in the chest, usually well-localised where the tumour is present. The condition worsens over several months and weight loss is common. At diagnosis, half of people have evidence of spread to local lymph nodes. Weight loss and anorexia are invariably associated symptoms.

It is possible to develop dysphagia as a complication of simple reflux oesophagitis. In this case, it is not progressive and there is a past history of the typical pattern of heartburn.

Investigations
Barium meal will show the narrowing of the oesophagus but oesophagoscopy and biopsy offer the definitive diagnosis.

Treatment
Usually, by the time of diagnosis, there is direct invasion of surrounding structures or lymph node involvement so that surgery is impossible. Cure, in conventional terms of a 5-year survival rate, is seen in only 2 per cent of cases. Some people have treatment by means of radiotherapy and chemotherapy, which are only seen as being palliative. Operation by means of oesophagogastrectomy is only possible in a small proportion. Surgery has a high mortality and morbidity. Dilation of the obstructing cancer and the insertion of an indwelling tube may give short-term symptomatic relief.

Cancer of the stomach

This is a relatively common cancer and is the third commonest cause of cancer deaths in the UK. It is relatively low in incidence in the USA yet high in Japan. Men are more frequently affected than women. Cancer of the stomach is more likely to occur in those with low gastric acid levels. Cancer of the stomach spreads to liver, bone, brain and lung.

Symptoms
Epigastric pain is common and is identical to that of peptic ulcer. Constant pain and the appearance of other symptoms suggest the diagnosis of cancer. The pain may be severe. Associated symptoms include vomiting, anorexia, dysphagia (when cancer is near the entry of the oesophagus) and vomiting of blood.

Some people present with abdominal swelling and jaundice which are evidence of malignant spread to the abdominal cavity or liver. About half of those presenting will have a lump in the epigastrium with tenderness. Weight loss is common. An enlarged lymph node may be found in the supraclavicular fossa.

Investigations
Barium meal will reveal up to 90 per cent of cases. Gastroscopy with biopsy is used to confirm the diagnosis. In cases to be considered for surgery, ultrasound and CAT scans are performed to detect secondary spread.

Treatment
Surgery is associated with a 5-year survival rate of 10 per cent, which has remained the same for the past 25 years or so. Sixty-five per cent of cases are inoperable at the time of diagnosis. Chemotherapy is merely associated with a poorer quality of life.

Cancer of the large intestine

This is the second most common cancer in the UK yet it is rare in Africa and Asia. There are increased rates of this cancer when diets are high in meat and fat but low in fibre. Ulcerative colitis may predispose to the development of large intestine cancer.

Symptoms
The precise clinical picture depends upon the site of the cancer. In the left side there may be changes in bowel habit such as constipation, alternating constipation and diarrhoea or just diarrhoea. Blood may be seen mixed in with the faeces.

Cancer of the caecum or ascending colon may merely present as an anaemia of unknown origin as the stools are liquid and obstruction occurs late. A palpable lump may be found in some. If spread has occurred to the liver this organ may be enlarged.

Investigations
Full blood count is performed. Diagnosis is made by barium enema with confirmation by colonoscopy and biopsy. Abdominal and rectal ultrasound are performed prior to surgery.

Treatment
This is primarily surgical with removal of the affected part of bowel and joining of the cut ends. The overall 5-year survival rate is 50 per cent depending upon the stage at the time of diagnosis.

Cancer of the liver

Here, I shall discuss secondary cancer of the liver that has spread from other sites, which is the commonest liver cancer and is frequently the result of cancer of the gastrointestinal tract, breast and lung.

Symptoms
These are variable and there may be none in the early stages. Liver enlargement is seen later with perhaps jaundice and discomfort in the right hypochondrium.

Investigations
Diagnosis is made by means of CAT scan, magnetic resonance scan or ultrasound.

Treatment
This is frequently by means of chemotherapy but with poor results. The usual consequence of such treatment is merely a greatly diminished quality of life.

DISEASES OF THE LIVER

The liver is a large organ situated under the diaphragm in the right hypochondrium, extending partly into the epigastrium. It weighs about 3 lb in the average adult. The liver performs many functions, most of which are metabolic in nature. The liver has an important role in the metabolism of carbohydrate, fat and protein. It deals with the removal of drugs and hormones by a detoxification mechanism. Various drugs are excreted into bile and thereby removed from the body such as antibiotics, e.g. penicillin, amoxycillin, erythromycin and sulphonamides, steroid hormones and thyroxine.

The liver is important for the excretion of bile salts, storage of glycogen, vitamins A, B, D, E and K and minerals – particularly iron and copper. It has a function in removing red and white blood cells from the circulation and some bacteria. It can be seen from this list that the liver, physiologically, is a very important organ. It receives substances absorbed from the stomach and intestines since it receives blood draining from the gastrointestinal system. It is, therefore, the first organ that is exposed to potential toxins.

Jaundice

This is a yellowish discolouration seen in the skin, mucous membranes and conjunctivae. In conventional medicine, it indicates that the amount of bilirubin in the blood is more than 30-60 mmol/l. Bilirubin is one of the breakdown products of haemoglobin and is excreted in bile. The others, iron and globin, are recycled.

Levels of bilirubin in the blood may rise as a result of three mechanisms:

- increased breakdown of red blood cells leading to increased amounts of bilirubin – pre-hepatic jaundice
- liver disease leading to inadequate metabolism of bilirubin – hepatic jaundice
- obstruction to excretion of bile leading to a backup of bile and thence bilirubin in the body – post-hepatic jaundice.

The distinction between hepatic and post-hepatic causes is not always a clear one since liver disease and bile obstruction may be present at the same time. However, the causation and treatment are different in each case.

Pre-hepatic jaundice

An example of increased red blood cell breakdown is haemolytic anaemia. There will be jaundice together with symptoms of anaemia. The discolouration is typically pale yellow with normal urine and stools.

An unusual type is a congenital disorder of bilirubin metabolism. This is Gilbert's syndrome, which affects up to 5 per cent of the population. It is usually without symptoms but may be discovered on routine blood testing as a raised bilirubin level. There are no signs of liver disease but there may be a family history of jaundice.

Related disorders include Crigler-Najjar, Dubin-Johnson and Rotor syndromes. These are all rare.

Hepatic jaundice

This is the appearance of jaundice due to disturbances in liver function. It may be due to acute liver disease as in hepatitis or in more chronic conditions such as cirrhosis.

Post-hepatic jaundice

This is the appearance of jaundice due to an obstruction to bile flow. It may be called obstructive jaundice. Gall stones and cancer of the head of the pancreas are the two conditions to consider here.

Hepatitis

This means, literally, inflammation of the liver. In common parlance, it is associated with an infecting organism although strictly speaking it includes cirrhosis and other inflammatory liver diseases. Viral hepatitis can be of several types, A, B or C, D or E. Other viruses which may cause a hepatitis include cytomegalovirus, the virus of glandular fever (Epstein–Barr virus) and the yellow fever virus.

Type A

This is also known as 'infectious hepatitis'. It develops due to the contamination of food or water by faeces. It rarely may be spread by blood or body fluid contact. Various factors such as overcrowding and poor sanitation lead to greater risks as in underdeveloped countries and institutions. The incubation period is 1 month. People are infectious 2 weeks before the onset of symptoms and for 1 week after. There is no carrier[21] state.

Symptoms
These are chills and fever, malaise, and anorexia. There are gastrointestinal symptoms such as nausea, diarrhoea, vomiting and upper abdominal pain. Jaundice develops with dark urine, yellow sclerae and pale stools. The appetite gradually recovers and the nausea settles. People gradually improve in 3 to 6 weeks. Virtually everyone makes a full recovery. It is common to suffer debility for some 2 to 3 months after the infection.

Investigations

These are performed similarly in all types of hepatitis. Liver function tests are raised – serum AST and ALT. The serum bilirubin is raised. The serum aminotransferase may be raised for up to 6 months after an infection. Bilirubin is found in the urine.

Treatment

There is no specific treatment. The improvement of social hygiene helps to prevent attacks. Passive immunisation with human gammaglobulin is said to give 3 months protection. There is a vaccine available which stimulates antibody production in an attempt to produce active immunisation.

Hepatitis A vaccination is recommended for travel to countries where water supplies are at risk of contamination particularly with sewage. The vaccine is considered to be of variable effectiveness and people who travel to India report differing accounts of its worth. The vaccine itself produces symptoms of flu-like illness and tiredness commonly as well as headache and bowel disturbances.

Type B

This is known as 'serum hepatitis'. It is spread by the same methods as Type A but blood and body fluid transmission is much more common. The incubation period is 3 months. There is a carrier state where people continue to be infectious and contact with their blood or body fluids may lead to infection and the development of symptoms.

Symptoms

These are similar to those of Type A hepatitis except they are more severe. Around 25 per cent develop an urticarial or maculo-papular rash, joint pains and fever.

One in 20 people go on to develop chronic hepatitis. There are asymptomatic carriers of the disease which raises public health questions regarding donation of blood and sexual relationships, similar to those we see in the HIV and AIDS debate.

Investigations

These are the same as for Hepatitis A.

Treatment

Bed rest and an adequate diet are the most important measures taken. Corticosteroids are given if the vomiting is severe. No alcohol should be taken for 6 months after the infection. Oral contraceptives are considered to be safe when the liver function tests are normal.

There is no specific treatment currently available. A trial of an antiviral drug, fialuridine, was stopped in 1993 after two people died and a third required a liver transplant. Three further people may require liver transplants in the near future. There were 20 people on the trial.

Most people recover completely although some remain as carriers. Some people go on to develop chronic hepatitis whilst around 1 per cent develop a severe form and die.

Passive immunisation by means of human gammaglobulin is given to medical staff on exposure and to newborn babies of Hepatitis B positive mothers.

Active immunisation by vaccination is recommended to all healthcare personnel, members of emergency teams and rescue services, morticians and people with haemophilia.

Hepatitis B vaccination is recommended by some authorities for all babies which seems unnecessary considering babies are not at high-risk of contracting the disease (or indeed at any risk) as it is essentially a disease contracted either through sexual activity or exposure to contaminated blood products. In Italy the vaccine is compulsory.

The vaccine produced prior to the early 1990s was obtained from human blood – homosexual men who had contracted Hepatitis B. This older vaccine continued to be used even after the production of a genetically engineered vaccine was developed until all the old supplies had been used up. Whilst the process of producing the vaccine may have removed all risk of transmitting other blood-borne diseases, the genesis of AIDS, Hepatitis B, Hepatitis C and others is not completely understood.

The first country to attempt a mass vaccination campaign against Hepatitis B was New Zealand in 1988. It ended in failure due to the large number of reported side-effects and subsequent illnesses in babies who had been vaccinated. Almost 1 in 50 children developed such wide effects as 'lethargy, malaise, diarrhoea, asthma, arthritis, Guillain-Barré syndrome, faintness, pallor, loss of consciousness and drop in blood pressure.'[22]

Type C

This was recognised in 1988 and has been a great problem for the recipients of blood and blood products over the past 20 years or so. Up to 90 per cent of intravenous drug users are affected and around 80 per cent of people with haemophilia in the UK have been infected. It is believed that sexual transmission is unusual.

Symptoms
Most infections are unnoticed with no or mild symptoms. There may be an influenza-like illness with jaundice. The main difficulty with Hepatitis C is its long-term course.

Investigations
These are the same as for Hepatitis A.

Treatment
There is no specific treatment although interferon may be recommended. This has many and severe side-effects and unfortunately people are sometimes unduly pressurised to take it. At least half of people go on to develop chronic liver disease with cirrhosis in 20-30 per cent, and of these 15 per cent can develop liver cancer.

It is important to take precautions of screening transfusion blood against contamination as well as avoiding unnecessary contact with blood and body fluids. Currently, in Ireland, there is a legal tribunal uncovering the facts behind Hepatitis C infection in haemophiliacs and women who were given anti-D immunoglobulin in the 1980s. There have been some deaths and dealing with the effects of such infection is an everyday reality for a large number of people who received medical treatment in good faith with no mention of the possible health risks.

Type D

This is particularly seen in intravenous drug users but may affect any of the groups susceptible to Hepatitis B infection. Infection with Hepatitis B and D is more severe in its symptoms. Investigations are the same as for Hepatitis A.

Type E

This is transmitted through contaminated water and has similar symptoms to Hepatitis A. It is more common in developing countries. It causes death from hepatic failure in 1-2 per cent of people affected which rises to 20 per cent in pregnant women. It does not lead to chronic hepatitis and there is no carrier state.

Chronic hepatitis

This is defined as the continuation of hepatitis for longer than 6 months. The hepatitis may be one of the infective kinds mentioned above or may be autoimmune in nature or due to medication. Most people progress to cirrhosis although some pursue a more benign course with minimal changes in liver function and mild liver enlargement.

Treatment
The main treatment which will be recommended is with alpha-interferon for periods of up to 6 months. It can clear the infective agents from the blood but often at a large cost in terms of side-effects. There are many such effects including influenza-like illnesses, headaches, loose stools, depression, tiredness and feelings of ill-health and hair loss. The bone marrow is affected so that platelet counts may be low. There may also be more severe effects such as infections, severe depression and heart and kidney failure.

Holistic management of hepatitis
In terms of Chinese medicine, hepatitis usually corresponds to an Invasion of Dampness and Heat creating disharmony between the Spleen and Liver. The particular emphasis depends upon the precise symptoms. Treatment by holistic medicine is definitely effective for such conditions and hepatitis is one of the diseases curable by Chinese medicine as defined by the World Health Organisation. Early and continuing treatment is effective in minimising symptoms and slowing or reversing progression to more chronic forms of the disease.

Case one
A man of 35 years came for treatment after being infected with Hepatitis C with contaminated blood. He was diagnosed some 6 years previously. He had taken alpha-interferon for 9 months but had to stop because of the strong side-effects. He had been told by his hospital consultant that he had mild to moderate liver damage. His main symptoms were tiredness which was variable. His bowels were generally sluggish and he would be constipated from time to time. In terms of Chinese

medicine, he had Spleen Qi Deficiency and Liver Blood Deficiency. I treated him with acupuncture initially and added herbal formulae later. The main changes he noticed with the treatment were improvements in energy levels and his bowels settled to become more regular. He also paid attention to his diet by eating fresh, organic food and avoiding coffee, alcohol, greasy food and 'junk' food. His treatment continues.

Case two

A woman of 55 years came for treatment after she had been diagnosed with Hepatitis C some 5 years previously. She had received contaminated anti-D immunoglobulin some 20 years previously after the birth of her last child. Her main symptoms were bloating in the abdomen, discomfort in the right hypochondrium and flatulence. Her sleep was disturbed. She was attending the clinic at the local hospital regularly which she found quite an ordeal as they would concentrate on her abnormal liver function tests and the possibility of developing cirrhosis or liver cancer at some future date. Interestingly, she was taking hormone replacement therapy which has a recognised side-effect of affecting liver function tests.

I made a diagnosis of Spleen Qi Deficiency, Blood Deficiency and Liver Qi Stagnation. I treated her with acupuncture as she was too worried to take Chinese herbs. Her hospital consultant had told her that Chinese herbs cause liver damage. At one point, it was suggested that she also stop acupuncture as that might affect her liver adversely.

The main effects of treatment have been on a psychological level. She has become more confident, less afraid of the disease and what she was told about it and is generally taking more charge of her situation. She is exploring ways in which she can maximise her health. She stopped the hormone replacement therapy as such a prescription can only make the liver more diseased. Her bowel symptoms are more comfortable now, she has less bloating and her bowels are more regular. Her treatment continues.

Cirrhosis

This is chronic liver disease where there is death of liver cells associated with regeneration and fibrosis. The regeneration here occurs in a haphazard manner and contributes to the obstruction to hepatic blood flow that leads to the typical features. The commonest causes are alcohol ingestion and post-hepatitis B or C infection.

Symptoms

These are many and varied. There is enlargement of the liver at first with eventual shrinkage as scarring develops. An enlarged spleen is common. Spider naevi are found on the skin of the upper body. They are small, distended blood vessels of reddish appearance with small vessels radiating out from them. The palms of the hand become reddened. Finger clubbing is seen occasionally. Thickening of the tissues of the palm of the hand is typically seen in cirrhosis of alcoholic origin. Hormonal abnormalities lead to breast enlargement and testicular atrophy in men. There may be loss of libido and amenorrhoea.

Oedema is common and seen in the ankles. Fluid collection in the abdomen (ascites) leads to abdominal distension. There may be vomiting of blood and melaena. Itching is common. Mental symptoms include drowsiness and confusion.

Investigations

Liver function tests on the blood reveal raised serum alkaline phosphatase and serum aminotransferase. In severe cases, many blood tests are abnormal. Liver biopsy is frequently performed to determine the exact nature of the abnormality. Other investigations include ultrasound scan, barium meal and gastroscopy.

Treatment

This is primarily supportive to prevent further damage to the liver. In milder cases, there may be no advice given about diet or abstinence from alcohol (unless it is alcoholic cirrhosis). In cases of severe liver disease, treatment is directed at the complications which develop. These include oesophageal varices, ascites and eventual kidney failure.

REVIEW OF SYMPTOMS

Some are of great importance both in terms of their effect on the person and their value to us to help reach a diagnosis.

Pain

This is most important and with careful questioning a lot of information can be obtained. Subsequent examination will in most cases serve to confirm the information gathered during the history. There are questions to ask in every case of pain and a structured approach ensures that nothing is missed. This was discussed on Pages 103 and 229.

Heartburn

This is burning pain felt in the centre of the chest behind the sternum. It may start in the epigastrium and radiate up towards the throat. Any pain in the chest should be differentiated from the pain of a heart attack.

Loss of appetite

This is known as anorexia and conventionally it is seen as due to:

- psychological disorders such as depression, anorexia nervosa[23]
- stomach disease such as gastritis
- general disease such as acute fevers or severe chronic disease such as cancer.

Increased appetite

This may occur with disorders of the upper gastrointestinal system depending upon the precise energetic diagnosis. In conventional medicine, the conditions to consider are diabetes mellitus, hyperthyroidism and bulimia nervosa. The first two are characterised by increased appetite with weight loss, an unusual combination. Bulimia nervosa, as with its related condition anorexia nervosa, is accompanied by disturbed perception of body image.

Waterbrash

This is sudden filling of the mouth with saliva or tasteless watery secretions. It is seen in association with upper gastrointestinal tract disease such as a duodenal ulcer.

Taste in the mouth

In homoeopathy and Chinese medicine, this is an important indicator of an internal organ problem. Its connection with organs in terms of Chinese medicine is shown in Table 13.16.

Taste	Element	Organs
Sweet	Earth	Spleen/Stomach
Spicy (pungent)	Metal	Lung/Large Intestine
Sour	Wood	Liver/Gall Bladder
Salty	Water	Kidney/Urinary Bladder
Bitter	Fire	Heart/Small Intestine

Table 13.16: Tastes and their corresponding organs[24]

In conventional medicine, cases of 'halitosis' or bad breath are seen as due to gum disease, dental decay or infected lung lesions such as lung abscess. In the absence of these most people who complain of bad breath, unpleasant taste in the mouth or other tastes such as metallic are labelled as being imaginative or frankly neurotic.

Vomiting

This is a common symptom and is a more extreme form of nausea. In conventional medicine, it is seen as occurring in a wide range of differing conditions not always linked to gastrointestinal tract disease. Causes include:

- drugs – prescribed and social
- upper gastrointestinal disease
- appendicitis
- meningitis
- infections, e.g. pyelonephritis
- migraine
- pregnancy
- travel sickness
- heart attack.

The appearance of material which looks like 'coffee-grounds' in the vomit is characteristic of bleeding in the upper gastrointestinal tract. The blood has been altered by gastric acid and so takes on a brownish or black appearance. Iron medication can give a similar appearance. In children, vomiting may be the first indication of an infection. All children with fever and vomiting must be checked for otitis media, urinary tract infection and chest infection.

Vomiting with no preceding nausea occurs in brain tumour and is due to direct stimulation of the vomiting centre in the brain. Vomit with large amounts of food or containing food eaten a day or so ago indicates pyloric obstruction. Epigastric pain relieved by vomiting is characteristic of a peptic ulcer.

Regurgitation

This is the appearance of recently swallowed food in the mouth but not vomiting. It occurs after meals and there may be a bitter taste (bile) or acid (gastric juice) taste. It is not common in adults but babies can have frequent episodes.

Dysphagia

This means difficulty in swallowing but is also used to mean the discomfort felt when food becomes lodged in the oesophagus. It should be differentiated from *globus hystericus,* which is a sensation of a lump, felt in the midline above the suprasternal notch. This is associated with emotional symptoms and in Chinese medicine corresponds to the plum-stone throat in Stagnation of Liver Qi. It is not of structural significance although people are often concerned as to whether they have a malignant condition. Lumps felt to the side of the throat are of much more serious significance and may indicate carcinoma.

Dysphagia is seen in cancer of the oesophagus where there will be a progressive history over several months. First solid food sticks then softer food and in later, advanced cases, swallowing any liquid including saliva is impossible. The site of the sensation is an accurate representation, in the lower third of the oesophagus, of the actual site of the problem. Elsewhere the approximation is less exact. Dysphagia can also occur due to scarring of the oesophagus in cases of oesophagitis. This is not progressive as with cancer and there will usually be a history of heartburn.

Flatulence and belching

Symptoms of 'wind' or abdominal distension are pretty much disregarded by conventional medicine. They are considered to be due to air swallowing in anxious individuals or excessive intake of gas-forming substances, e.g. sodium bicarbonate, beans. For the purposes of easy learning, abdominal distension is seen as being due to:

- fat
- fluid
- faeces
- flatus
- foetus.

Other than these, little attention is paid. However, distension of the abdomen is very common particularly in women and is very much related to the function of the Liver, Spleen and Kidney. When I was in general practice I saw many women with this problem. They would wake up in the morning with a flat abdomen and by the evening looked as if they were more than 4, 5 or even 6 months pregnant. Conventionally this is puzzling and is seen as either a neurosis or an imaginative exaggeration.

Case

A woman of 25 years came for treatment with symptoms of abdominal distension after eating. She would develop pains in the hypochondria, flatulence and belching. Her bowels were often constipated. She had difficulty sleeping until about 1.30 am. The only medication she took was the oral contraceptive.

In terms of Chinese medicine, this is a classical case of Liver Qi Stagnation invading the Stomach and Spleen. The major contributing factor is the oral contraceptive, which stagnates Liver Qi. Treatment was aimed at relaxing the flow of Liver Qi and we discussed the role of the oral contraceptive in causing Liver Qi Stagnation.

In terms of conventional medicine, this would probably be labelled as irritable bowel syndrome. There is no understanding in conventional thought that the oral contraceptive can cause such symptoms.

Constipation and diarrhoea

The conventional texts state that 10 per cent of people have less than one bowel movement per day and 1 per cent have less than three per week. Constipation is usually defined in terms of the frequency of bowel action as above but what is also important is the consistency of the stool. Faeces that are dry, hard or difficult to pass are an indication of constipation. Another thing to consider is the length of time it takes for material to pass through the gastrointestinal tract. Normally this takes around 18 hours but for most people in the West it is a lot longer than this. Although we may pass faeces every day it may be from food taken in several days ago or longer. This is undoubtedly related to the higher incidence of gastrointestinal tract cancer in the West.

Diarrhoea is the passage of unformed stools several times each day. The term 'loose stools' may be reserved for the passage of unformed stools only once or twice per day. Always ask about the presence of blood and mucus in people with such symptoms.

Weight loss

This may not be a symptom to be considered in diagnosis if it is the result of a deliberate attempt to reduce weight by means of a regime of diet and/or exercise. As a symptom to be considered in the diagnosis, it will be part of a wider problem.

Anorexia, nausea and vomiting will lead to weight loss simply because there is a reduced intake of food. Malabsorption of nutrients as in small bowel disease, e.g. Crohn's disease or coeliac disease has the same effect. Ulcerative colitis, if severe, may lead to weight loss due to protein loss from the bowel. Many cancers lead to loss of weight but by no means all and wasting is particularly a feature of lung and intra-abdominal malignancy.

Weight gain

This may be a presenting symptom but is more usually part of the total case to be considered. In conventional thought it is usually seen as due to excess food intake. This is not the whole story as many people, particularly women, may be overweight and yet not overeat. The reason for this is related to the discussion at the beginning of this Chapter dealing with energetic concepts of the digestive system. If the digestive energy is depleted, *any* food taken may lead to increases in weight. This is more likely to occur in those who have had many years of cyclical diets, weight loss and excessive exercise. All of these practices lead to depletion in digestive energy and the inability to transform food. Weakness and tiredness are common as well as the collection of fluid.

Case one

A woman of 41 years complaining of being overweight for many years came for treatment. She had tried many different types of diet culminating in a stomach-stapling operation the year before. Her food intake was not particularly excessive. The only time she would lose weight would be with amphetamines or a drastic reduction in calorie intake to around 800 per day. This is a common situation with women where low calorie diets are necessary thereby inducing a state of malnutrition. The recurrent cycle of dieting leads to further weakening of digestive energy and therefore greater difficulty in maintaining normal weight. The only way out of this is to increase metabolic rate. Artificial methods of boosting metabolism include thyroid hormone, amphetamines and appetite suppressants.[25] The healthy method is by means of holistic medicine, which seeks to correct the underlying energetic problem.

Her other symptoms included low back pain, water retention and a desire for sweet food worse before her periods. In terms of Chinese medicine, her diagnosis was Spleen and Kidney Yang Deficiency. The main aim of treatment is to strengthen her Spleen and Kidney energy so that, eventually, her own energy will be able to control fluids. Her weight will then come under control. This process is slow and requires long-term treatment. Additionally, body weight, size and shape are very much the result of our innermost mental self-images. Some degree of emotional and mental symptoms may arise during the course of treatment. Counselling, psychotherapy or other psychological approaches are invaluable additional methods.

Bleeding from the gastrointestinal tract

Cause	Number per 100 cases
Duodenal ulcer	35
Gastric ulcer	20
Acute gastric erosion, gastritis	18
Oesophageal tear	10
Gastric cancer	6
Oesophageal varices – seen in cirrhosis	5
Others	6

Table 13.17: Causes of bleeding from the upper gastrointestinal tract

This is not a common symptom but it is important to know that some causes are of serious significance. It can manifest in several ways according to the organ involved. From the upper gastrointestinal tract blood will be seen in vomit. Coffee-grounds appearance is indicative of a small amount of blood loss from the stomach where the blood has become blackened by the action of stomach acid. Fresh red blood is seen when the loss of blood is greater and can occur with peptic ulceration or occasionally cancer. One third of people with gastrointestinal bleeding have taken aspirin in the past 24-48 hours. All the non-steroidal anti-inflammatory drugs are associated with bleeding even when taken as suppositories.

Bleeding from the lower part of the gastrointestinal tract can manifest as fresh red blood if from the lower parts and as brownish or blackish if from higher up the bowel. Blood on the surface of the faeces indicates a rectal or anal problem, e.g. haemorrhoids, rectal cancer or rectal polyps. Blood mixed up with the faeces indicates a problem further up the bowel.

HOW TO RECOGNISE A SERIOUS CONDITION OF THE GASTROINTESTINAL SYSTEM

Diseases of the gastrointestinal system are common in our society and the symptoms listed above are extremely common. It is important to know how to recognise if a symptom arises from a serious situation. You can use Table 13.18 (below) as a guide to refer to when faced with a person who has one or more of these symptoms. I do not mention disease labels in the column on the right as I would not expect you to be able to diagnose conventionally. Seriousness can be assessed merely by reference to symptom pictures. However, you will be able to recognise that there are clinical appearances that would be diagnosed as a particular disease. For example, if you look at diarrhoea and its seriousness, you will see that this describes diseases such as severe gastroenteritis, ulcerative colitis or Crohn's disease and cancer.

Symptom	Comments
Nausea	Severe
Vomiting	Severe, persistent, progressive, in the very young or old, with blood, with food eaten days before, projectile
Anorexia	Severe, progressive, with mental symptoms of distorted body image
Increased appetite	With weight loss, with mental symptoms of distorted body image
Bloating	Progressive
Belching	Not serious
Flatulence	Not serious
Diarrhoea	Severe, persistent, progressive, in the very young or old, with blood, with mucus, alternates with constipation
Constipation	Severe, progressive, with blood, alternates with diarrhoea
Abdominal pain	Severe, with abdominal rigidity, with guarding, with rebound tenderness
Weight loss	Progressive, unexplained
Jaundice	Always unless mild in new-born

Table 13.18: How to recognise a serious condition of the gastrointestinal system

SUMMARY

Gastrointestinal disorders are common, reflecting dietary habits and emotional states.

They tend to be superficial in terms of energetic hierarchies and so relatively easy to treat.

More severe disease produces symptoms that are more serious in nature (see Table 13.18) or suggestive of obstruction.

---

[1] At first sight, there may be confusion about the use of this word. It a consequence of translation where words are used which already have a meaning to us in the West. The Chinese word is *Pi* and its designated counterpart in the West was considered to be the spleen. This was done before our current level of knowledge of conventional anatomy and physiology. The Spleen, as this is understood in Chinese medicine, is functionally more related to the pancreas and duodenum. For these reasons, any organs which are capitalised, e.g. Spleen, refer to the Chinese medical view.

[2] There are two issues about the use of microwaves. One is concerning the effect of the microwave radiation on humans and particularly adverse effects on behaviour and the immune system. There was the well-documented case of microwave radiation directed at the US Embassy in Moscow in the 1960s and 1970s. This led to changes in white blood cell counts and ultimately increased rates of cancer. This and other aspects of electromagnetic radiation may be obtained from *Subtle Energy* by John Davidson (CW Daniel, 1987).

The second issue of domestic microwaves is the effect on the food itself. Microwaves cook by agitating molecules. This has the effect of depleting the Qi or energy of the food. It also tends to dry out the food as a result of this rapid stimulation. People who mainly eat microwave cooked tend to develop Spleen Qi deficiency. They may also develop Yin deficiency due to this drying action.

[3] Colonic irrigation may be useful in some people with severe heat syndromes affecting the Large Intestine. In others, particularly if the energy is depleted, it will lead to further weakness. This is because the large volume of fluid passed into the Large Intestine will damage the Qi of the Lung and the Kidney.

[4] The energetic qualities of food and how to apply these to individual cases is a complex subject. Two excellent books are *Prince Wen Hui's Cook – Chinese Dietary Therapy* by Flaws and Wolfe (Churchill Livingstone, 1993) and *Chinese System of Food Cures* by Henry Lu (Sterling, 1986). *Recipes for Self-Healing* by Daverick Leggatt (Meridian Press, 1999).

[5] Anatomically, the bladder, uterus, fallopian tubes and ovary are situated in the pelvis. However, they may give rise to pain in the lower part of the abdomen. They cannot be palpated via the abdomen except in the case of a bladder full of urine or a uterus enlarged by pregnancy or fibroids.

[6] A hernia describes the passage of part of the intestine outside the peritoneal cavity. This usually occurs in the groin where it is called an inguinal hernia. It may also be seen in the upper thigh (femoral hernia), around the umbilicus (umbilical hernia), at the site of an abdominal operation (incisional hernia) or protrude through the hiatus of the diaphragm (diaphragmatic or hiatus hernia).

[7] Similar observations can be made about the discovery of gallstones in people with upper abdominal pain and those with back pain who may have radiological evidence of intervertebral disc prolapse. Surgical correction of the physical abnormalities frequently does not lead to relief of symptoms. I would refer you to details of these disorders for a further discussion of these two situations.

[8] Ingestion of large amounts of metallic salts can lead to disturbances in electrolyte concentrations in the blood giving rise to deficiency of some substances or overload with others. Despite information of a strong connection between the ingestion of aluminium and dementia, the widespread prescribing of compounds containing aluminium continues. In view of the weight of evidence about aluminium and dementia, it would seem unwise to continually ingest these substances.

The main sources of aluminium are drinking water, medicines, inhaled air (small amount unless in an industrial environment) and food. It has been known for about 100 years that aluminium is toxic to the central nervous system-- Dollken A. *Arch Exp Pathol Pharmacol* 1897;40:98-120.

There have been discussions for some years that aluminium may also be implicated in the genesis of dementia and related syndromes. It may lead to nerve cell deformities similar to those found in Alzheimer's disease – Klatzo I *et al. J Neuropathol Exp Neurol* 1965;24:187-99.

It has been reported that aluminium is present in increased concentrations in the brains of people with Alzheimer's disease – Crapper DR *et al, Science* 1973;185:511-13. Others have confirmed these findings – Candy JM *et al, Regulation of transmitter function: basic and clinical aspects.* Edited by Vizi ES, Magyar K (Amsterdam: Elsevier 1984;301-6) and by Perry EK *et al, Trends Neurosci* 1985;8:301-3.

Aluminium has also been shown to cause an acute dementia in people undergoing dialysis for kidney failure when present in dialysis fluid in relatively high concentrations – Alfrey AC *et al*, *N Engl J Med* 1976;294:184-8 and Rozas *et al*, *J Dialysis* 1978;2:459-70.

The main source of exposure is usually dietary especially tea or foods which have had aluminium added, e.g. raising agents, emulsifying agents, or canned goods. The amount in drinking water provides only a small proportion of the total dietary content but such aluminium tends to be more easily absorbed and therefore a greater source of pollution. Various studies have been performed which relate aluminium in drinking water to increased rates of dementia. Of the 10 studies available, seven have shown a connection – these include Martyn CN *et al*, *Lancet* 1989;i:59-62, Michel P *et al*, *Alzheimer's disease basic mechanisms, diagnosis and therapeutic strategies*. Edited by Iqbal K, McLachlan DRC, Winblad B, Wisniewski HM (Chichester: J. Wiley & Sons, 1991;387-9), Frecker MF. *J Epidemiol Community, Health* 1991;45:307-11, Forbes WF *et al*, *Lancet* 1991;338:1592-3, Flaten TP. *Environ Geochem Health* 1990;12:152-67.

A major source of exposure is the use of medicines which contain aluminium, of which the most important are the aluminium antacids – there is some evidence that they are related to demented states – Leventhal GH. Dissertation presented for the Doctor of Philosophy Degree, University of Tennessee, Knoxville, 1987. These are potentially a much greater risk as the dose is much higher than that of food and drinking water. Certainly, blood levels of aluminium are raised in those who take such drugs regularly – House RA. *J Occup Med* 1992;34:1013-17.

Other medicines that contain aluminium include enteric-coated aspirin and some antiperspirants and deodorants that are sprayed on the skin (some of which may be absorbed). A positive association with the use of antiperspirants and dementia – Graves *et al. J Clin Epidemiol* 1990;43:35-44.

Other sources of medical contamination include the inhalation of aluminium powder in the belief that it would protect miners from pneumoconiosis. This was used in Ontario, Canada in the 1950's. Examination shows that such exposure is related to central nervous system damage – Rifat SL *et al*, *Lancet* 1990;ii:1162-5.

[9] This is narrowing of the pylorus – the exit of the stomach. It is due to scar tissue secondary to ulceration. A rare, unrelated situation occurs in male babies causing projectile vomiting at around 3 months of age.

[10] If a peptic ulcer bleeds heavily there may be no vomiting to reveal its presence. It can pass through the intestines where the motions take on a black tarry appearance and is known as melaena. It can be confused with the stools seen with iron medication.

[11] Interestingly, this is another example of conventional medicine stumbling across a commonly appropriate energetic remedy. The homoeopathic potency of bismuth has symptoms in its provings similar to those of peptic ulceration.

[12] Surgical procedures on the stomach and duodenum as well as the use of histamine (H_2) blockers leads to depletion of Spleen Yang. This operation, which is not performed nowadays, was done to reduce acid secretion by the stomach. Cutting the vagus nerve supplying the stomach together with opening up the pylorus to aid flow of food into the duodenum had the effect of speeding up the passage of food into the lower gastrointestinal. This man exhibited the classic symptoms of what is called 'dumping syndrome'.

[13] Homoeopaths may use the mumps nosode (a remedy made from disease products of a case of mumps) to treat pancreatic disease.

[14] These are the classical signs of inflammation of the peritoneum - peritonitis. Such appearances are classed as a surgical emergency. The differential diagnosis of acute abdominal pain is discussed later in this Chapter.

[15] *BMJ* 2000;320:1690.

[16] This a point on the abdomen which overlies the usual anatomical site of the appendix. It is located one-third of the way along a line connecting the anterior superior iliac spine and the umbilicus.

[17] The abdominal muscles go into spasm to protect the underlying tissues and organs. On palpation, this is felt as a tenseness in the muscles.

[18] This is the desire to defaecate with no or little faeces passed. It occurs in association with inflammation of the rectum (proctitis) as here, tumour of the rectum and irritable bowel syndrome.

[19] This is a variation of the usual barium meal. Here, the passage of barium is 'followed through' to the small intestine and X-rays taken to visualise this area.

[20] Details of how to reduce combinations of drugs and in which order are given in, *The Prescribed Drug Guide – A Holistic Perspective* by Dr S Gascoigne (Jigme Press, 2001).

[21] A carrier is someone who remains infectious after the symptoms have subsided. This may be a permanent state. A small proportion of people may be carriers having had no symptoms or only a mild illness which passes unrecognised.

[22] *The Vaccination Bible*, edited by Lynne McTaggart (What Doctors Don't Tell You, 2000).

[23] The term 'anorexia' is sometimes used as shorthand for the disease anorexia nervosa which is characterised by disturbed perception of body image.

[24] The organs listed indicate their energetic nature as described in their relevant chapters and not the narrow physical sense of conventional medicine.

[25] The prescription of appetite suppressants is a potentially dangerous practice. They are stimulant in nature and rapidly lead to addiction. There are well described withdrawal syndromes. Some 400,000 people are prescribed such drugs in the UK. It costs the NHS about £1m per year. Drugs used include amphetamines, fenfluramine and dexfenfluramine.

14 CENTRAL NERVOUS SYSTEM

INTRODUCTION

The central nervous system can be a difficult system to understand because of its complex anatomy and it may also be taught in minute detail. Many students leave with the idea that it is totally incomprehensible and that they will never go near it again. I know from my own training that it took about three or so years of medical school before some of it started to mean anything at all.

For this reason, I spend some time giving an introduction to the central nervous system with a short, yet hopefully, clear description of its structure and function. I have divided the system into easily manageable portions although they actually function as a complete whole. However, this should make it more accessible. I have also resisted using many of the long and difficult names that abound in this area of the body.

OVERVIEW OF CENTRAL NERVOUS SYSTEM

Motor system

This, as its name suggests, deals with movement. Nerves of the motor system supply muscles that contract when activated. Such muscle contraction may be under voluntary control as in the case of arm or leg movements, or involuntary in the case of heart muscles. As the motor nerves pass through the lower part of the brain, this area may also be labelled the pyramidal system. As an analogy, the motor system can be likened to the engine, which moves a car. It is merely responsible for movement.

The distinction between voluntary and involuntary control is not absolute. Even so-called involuntary muscular movements are under some degree of voluntary control as we can alter our breathing within certain limits. The interest in Oriental philosophies and religions has revealed more about our ability to control these.[1] Involuntary muscle movements are influenced by the autonomic nervous system.

Movements are the result of the balanced contraction and relaxation of different muscle groups. A seemingly simple voluntary action, such as drinking a cup of tea involves a complex series of co-ordinated actions. As some muscles contract to move a joint in a certain direction, another muscle group has to relax. Yet another set of muscles will fix the joint around which the movement takes place. This co-ordination function is carried out by other parts of the nervous system.

There are two groups of nerve cells (neurones) that comprise the motor system – upper motor neurones and lower motor neurones. The upper motor neurone comprises cells in the motor area of the cortex of the brain. Nerve fibres from these pass down into the spinal cord to connect with nerve cells. They cross over to the other side as they do so. The exact level at which this occurs is not particularly important for our purposes but this means that upper motor neurones in a particular area of the motor cortex control muscle movements on the opposite side of the body.

The lower motor neurone is the nerve cell in the spinal cord from which nerve fibres leave to supply particular muscle groups of that region. At the same time, sensory nerves from the muscles pass back to the spinal cord to interconnect with the lower motor neurone. This interconnection is known as a reflex arc and is continually in operation to maintain tone in the muscle. It monitors the degree of tension or relaxation in a muscle and ensures, via this feedback mechanism, that a certain degree of tone is maintained.

The reflex arc is also the mechanism that results in tendon reflexes. These are the contraction of muscles that occur when its own tendons are tapped. The knee jerk (reflex) is commonly known and describes how the quadriceps muscle contracts as the patellar ligament is tapped. There are also tendon reflexes at the ankle, biceps, triceps and the supinator muscles.

Clearly, a disorder of the lower motor neurone will lead to different symptoms from the upper motor neurone. This is mainly because of the presence of the reflex arc. The exact clinical picture will depend upon whether the lower motor neurone is partially or completely non-functional. If the lower motor neurone is non-functioning the result is no movement (paralysis), absent tendon reflexes at that level and little tone in the muscle (flaccidity). Partial interruption to the nerve supply leads to weakness (paresis), reduced tendon reflexes at that level and reduced muscle tone.

If the upper motor neurone is the site of the problem then the reflex arc is still operating. A feature of the reflex arc is that it is very powerful. The normal influence of the upper motor neurone is one of sedation. The reflex arc becomes stronger when this influence is removed.[2] This is evidenced by paralysis (as the upper motor neurone is not functioning), increased tone (spasticity) and increased tendon reflexes. Wasting is minimal as the tone maintained by the reflex arc prevents this. These differences are summarised in Table 14.1.

Upper motor neurone	Lower motor neurone
Weakness or paralysis	Weakness or paralysis
Increased tone: spasticity	Decreased tone: flaccidity
Increased tendon reflexes	Reduced or absent reflexes in area affected
Plantar reflex – upgoing	Plantar reflex – unchanged
No muscle atrophy	Wasting of muscles
Contractures	No contractures

Table 14.1: Comparison of appearances of upper and lower motor neurone disorders

The clinical appearances listed in Table 14.1 will allow you to recognise some disorders of the motor system. These can be seen in Table 14.2.

Upper motor neurone disorders	Lower motor neurone disorders
Stroke	Polio
Brain tumour	Motor neurone disease
Motor neurone disease	Multiple sclerosis
Multiple sclerosis	Cervical and lumbar disc disease Peripheral nerve compression

Table 14.2: Examples of upper and motor neurone disorders

Symptoms of motor system disturbance include:

- Paralysis
- Weakness (paresis)
- Wasting
- Increased muscle tone (spasticity)
- Decreased muscle tone (flaccidity)
- Exaggerated tendon reflexes
- Reduced tendon reflexes
- Absent tendon reflexes
- Upgoing plantar reflex.

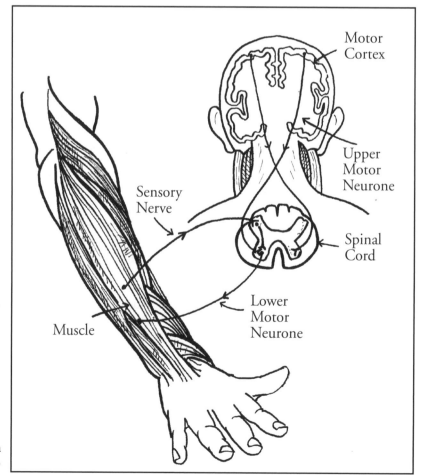

Figure 14.1 Motor System (Pyramidal System)

Extrapyramidal system

This is the part of the nervous system that modifies voluntary motor activity. There are several parts of the brain that do this including the basal ganglia. Disorders in this area lead to disturbance in voluntary movement control. There is a classical triad of symptoms that develop. There are disturbances in voluntary movement such as slowness, disturbances in tone such as increased tone or rigidity and the development of involuntary movements such as tremor. We see these in an illness such as Parkinson's disease, which is a disorder of the basal ganglia. Other, more unusual, disorders of the extrapyramidal system include Huntington's chorea.

To continue the analogy with a car, the extrapyramidal system can be compared with the clutch. This is responsible for the smooth control of movement. When we are learning to drive, we do so jerkily, slowly and tensely.

Symptoms of extrapyramidal system disorders include:

- Involuntary movements, e.g. tremor, hemiballismus
- Slow movement
- Increased tone.

Cerebellum

This is responsible for the co-ordination of movement. It is important in the maintenance of posture. This may be seen as being passive but information is being continually relayed to and from the brain and peripheries, telling central areas about the state of tension in the body, its position in space and in relation to other parts of the body. It is the cerebellum which co-ordinates this information and acts to control posture.

Toxic substances including lead, alcohol and anticonvulsants may damage the cerebellum. A variety of symptoms are seen including problems with posture, disturbances of walking (ataxia), head tremor, nystagmus, jerky speech, reduced tone and an intention tremor.[3]

Symptoms of cerebellar system disturbance include:

- Intention tremor
- Lack of balance
- Ataxia
- Nystagmus
- Reduced tone
- Jerky movements and speech
- Difficulties with co-ordination.

Sensory system

This is the area that is involved with sensation. It is the way in which we detect our external environment and inform central areas about it. There are several types of sense organ all dealing with different qualities of sensation. In the skin, there is superficial sensation such as touch, pain, warmth, and cold. At deeper levels there is sensation of deep pain, pressure and position. Vibration is recognised by a combination of deep and superficial sensors.

Some impulses in sensory nerve fibres do not reach consciousness and these deal with reflex functions and connections with the cerebellum as in co-ordination control. The impulses in the sensory nerves pass to the spinal cord and through the thalamus in the brain to the sensory cortex.

Sensory disturbances lead to different symptoms depending on which area is affected. In the case of a peripheral nerve, complete loss of function causes numbness. This is fairly obvious. However, nerves overlap in their distribution[4] so there may be a limited area with no sensation at all.

Partial loss of function may lead, at first, to symptoms such as pain, tingling and pins and needles. The term 'neuralgia' may be applied to such symptoms. Conditions that may interfere with function in such a way are frequently those that cause pressure on nerves. These include nerve entrapments, spinal tumour and prolapsed intervertebral disc. There may also be feelings of pain in deep structures such as muscles and ligaments supplied by the particular nerve. In severe cases, the motor part of the nerve may be affected leading to the symptoms of a lower motor neurone disorder described above.

In a neuropathy[5] there are particular nerves affected. The longest are most susceptible so the fingers and toes are the usual areas affected. Posterior root disorders lead to loss of some types of sensation but not others. This is because some nerves cross over to the other side and others do not. However, this is beyond the scope of this book as it represents complex neurological disease.

Disorders of central areas such as the thalamus produce pain on the opposite side of the body. It is typically unpleasant, severe and of a burning quality. People may develop this condition after a stroke and many such people attend pain clinics, which specialise in treating severe and intractable pain such as:

- tingling
- pins and needles
- shooting, stabbing or burning pains
- numbness
- loss of perception of touch, vibration, position, pressure, heat and cold.

Reflexes

A reflex is a nervous system connection between a sensor and an effector organ (e.g. a muscle or gland). There are two main points when considering the reflexes involving muscles. Firstly, there is a postural function. An example would be the reflex in a cat that always makes sure that it lands on its feet even if dropped upside down from a height. The second aim is to be protective and is evoked by stimuli to pain receptors. An example would be what happens when we touch something very hot. I need not describe the result with which we are all familiar. Rapid withdrawal that is not conscious, it is at a spinal level. It only comes to consciousness later.

Tendon reflexes

These are postural reflexes, which depend on the stimulation of sensory organs within the muscle when it is stretched. The most commonly known one is the knee reflex (or jerk). When the quadriceps is stretched and the tendon of the muscle tapped, the muscle will go into reflex contraction. It is a way of measuring the function of the reflex arc at a particular level in the spinal cord. Each reflex has a different level as shown in Table 14.3.

Reflex	Level
Biceps	Cervical 5 and 6
Triceps	Cervical 7
Supinator	Cervical 5 and 6
Knee	Lumbar 3 and 4
Ankle	Sacral 1

Table 14.3: Tendon reflexes and their spinal levels

If the tendon reflex is absent, it can be assumed that there is a problem with the lower motor neurone at or above that level. If the tendon reflex is increased, there is likely to be a problem with the upper motor neurone.

Superficial reflexes are to do with the skin and usually involve many levels. The response is a co-ordinated movement. There are many of them and a few have clinical significance. The plantar reflex is produced at the sole of the foot. Scraping along the outer edge of the sole and across to the base of the little toe elicits it. At the age of one year it is normally extensor. It then becomes flexor unless an upper motor neurone lesion is present. In which case it is extensor in type.

The corneal reflex provokes blinking of the eyelids and has two components. Therefore, it is only present if both parts are functioning correctly. The sensory portion is via the first (ophthalmic) division of the fifth cranial nerve and the motor portion is through the seventh cranial nerve.

Specific organs and pathways

Dysfunction in a nerve supply to organs such as the rectum and bladder may herald spinal cord compression, e.g. prolapsed intervertebral disc or spinal tumour. The bladder has a complex nervous control as it has voluntary and involuntary (reflex) mechanisms. There is a sympathetic nervous supply from the 1st and 2nd lumbar areas and this serves to relax the bladder and contract the sphincters. The parasympathetic supply is through an outflow at the second to fourth sacral levels, which serves to contract the bladder and relax the internal sphincter. The external sphincter is under voluntary control via the 2nd to 4th sacral areas.

The rectum similarly has this control. The sympathetic is inhibitory, that is it tends to stop bowel emptying ('holding on') and the parasympathetic is facilitatory ('letting go').

Autonomic nervous system

Unfortunately, the word 'autonomic' conjures up a similar meaning as 'automatic' although they originate from different words in the original Greek. Autonomic implies a self-governing (i.e. autonomous) or regulating function. Thoughts and emotions can affect it, in either a positive or a negative manner. A well-known example of how our minds can affect this system is the effect of meditation practices. They can lead to decrease in oxygen consumption, reduction in metabolic rate and blood pressure, reduction in heart rate and changes to brain waves characteristic of a relaxed state of mind.

There are two aspects to the autonomic nervous system, which have opposite functions. They are balanced in health. As with the endocrine system, it is one of the few areas, conventionally where the principles of Yin and Yang as understood by Chinese medicine may be recognised.

The parasympathetic aspect deals with relaxation and mainly involves the release of the neurotransmitter substance, acetylcholine. Anticholinergic drugs block this area. The nerve tracts that are part of this system include parts of the cranial nerves III, VII, IX and X, and parts of the outflow from the second to fourth sacral nerves.

The sympathetic aspect is stimulatory. It mainly involves the release of noradrenaline, a neurotransmitter. Betablockers inhibit its function. The adrenal medulla is an integral part of this system as it releases adrenaline and noradrenaline and is directly stimulated by sympathetic nerves. Nerve tracts in this system arise from all the thoracic and the first two lumbar nerve roots to form the sympathetic chain. The sympathetic division plays an important role in flight-or-fight responses.

Summary

From the foregoing discussion, the central nervous system is clearly a complex organ. It is not easy to accurately identify the site of any problem without an understanding of the anatomical connections of each nerve tract. This is not necessary for the holistic practitioner, as a holistic approach would not involve treating a localised area. However, it is useful to gain a general idea about the underlying process and site. This may help you in deciding whether to refer or not.

There are several key questions to consider when faced with a person with neurological symptoms. Firstly, do the symptoms suggest a peripheral or central location? Secondly, are the symptoms motor or sensory in type? For example, symptoms only present in the hand can be either a central problem or a local problem in the arm or neck. Symptoms present concurrently in a hand, leg and head must be due to a central problem. A knowledge of anatomy is helpful here.

Symptoms, which are only motor in type, may indicate a disorder such as motor neurone disease or polio, which only ever affect motor nerves. Symptoms, which are only sensory in type, may indicate a neuropathy that is sensory in nature such as that seen with diabetes mellitus or a mild compression, e.g. cervical spondylosis, prolapsed intervertebral disc. Symptoms, which are mixed in nature, may indicate a disease that affects several nerves at once, e.g. brain tumour, multiple sclerosis, more severe compression of a nerve.

The way in which symptoms appear may also give useful clues about the underlying process. Some diseases, by their nature, are rapid in onset over minutes or an hour or so. This would indicate either a disturbance in blood supply (as in stroke) or an infection (e.g. meningitis and encephalitis). A slower process over days or weeks, which is progressive, would indicate a tumour. A malignant tumour would clearly develop symptoms more quickly than a benign one. A more gradual onset over months would indicate a degenerative process such as Parkinson's disease. Some diseases have a typical history of relapses and remissions over months and years. Multiple sclerosis is an example of these.

Using these ideas, it is possible to formulate an opinion about the possible process. It may be necessary to seek referral in those cases that are rapidly changing.

In summary, you may consider the following to be of importance:

- do symptoms suggest peripheral or central location?
- are symptoms motor or sensory?
- is the onset rapid, slow or progressive?
- is there a history of relapses and remissions?

HOLISTIC VIEW OF THE CENTRAL NERVOUS SYSTEM

In this section, I shall discuss the ideas in Chinese medicine that generally correspond to the central nervous system. It is difficult for Westerners to consider that there may be different explanations for a group of functions and symptoms. This is particularly true in the case of the central nervous system and the endocrine system. In Chinese medicine, there is no precise system of organs and structures that can be identified as being identical with the nervous system. This is mainly because Oriental systems of philosophy are more concerned with function than structure.

Nevertheless, there are organ systems in Chinese medicine, which have a similar *function* to the nervous system. This is clearly the case since disorders of the nervous system are usually amenable to treatment by Chinese medicine. This is in direct contradistinction to conventional medicine, which is usually at a loss to know how to address such problems.

The most important organ system of Chinese medicine to consider here is the Liver. There are several associations with this organ, which I describe in Table 14.4.

Imbalances of Liver functions may manifest in many different parts of the body. This is partly related to the role of the Liver in maintaining the free flow of Qi and also to the course of the Liver channel. This starts in the big toe, passes up the inside of the leg through the genital area. It then passes up to the breast area and connections are made eventually with the eyes and the vertex of the head.

Symptoms such as abdominal bloating, constipation, breast pain, pains around the eyes and vertex may all be related to Liver imbalances. Disease labels in conventional medicine that may be the counterpart include hernias, irritable bowel syndrome, pain in the hypochondria, pre-menstrual tension and migraine.

Disturbances in the Liver's function of allowing the free flow of qi may lead to symptoms such as stiffness, tremor, tics, convulsions and so forth. Disease labels in conventional medicine, which may correspond, tend to be classified as central nervous system problems.

Association	Comments
Stores Blood	When the person is at rest and particularly when lying down, the Blood returns to the Liver. This is released during exercise and menstruation. Lack of Blood in the Liver may lead to gynaecological symptoms
Maintains free flow of Qi	This ensures the smooth and harmonious flow of energy throughout the body and its organs
Dominates tendons and movements	This ensures the smooth movement of joints. Disturbed function leads to stiff movements, cramps, and tremors
Manifests in the nails	Nails are seen in Chinese medicine as a 'by-product' of the sinews[6]
Opens into the eye	Each organ is connected to a sense organ. The function of the eye is very much related to Liver function
Paired organ is Gall Bladder	This is comparable with the conventional view that the liver and gall bladder are closely related
Colour – green	This is the colour of spring and the Wood element. In Chinese medicine, the colour is more accurately blue/green or cyan
Taste – sour	Each major organ has an associated taste. In this case excess sour taste can damage the Wood element
Season – spring	The energy of spring moves upward and outward as the branches of a tree (Wood element). This can be related to the function of the Liver in maintaining the free flow of Qi
Element – Wood	The Element correspondence reveals the connection of Chinese medical theory to nature. Each Element is connected to the others to provide, in health, a harmonious balance
Time – 1-3 a.m.	The 'time' of an organ is when its energy it at its maximum. Liver imbalances may make it difficult to sleep when going to bed
Emotions – anger	In health, this is assertiveness as befits the function of the Liver in allowing the free flow of Qi. Unbalanced, this may manifest as aggression, guilt, resentment or jealousy ('green with envy')
Mental aspect	The Liver is to do with a giving attitude. It is responsible for a kindly attitude and sharing. Its paired organ, the Gall Bladder, is responsible for decision-making

Table 14.4: Holistic energetic view of the Liver

INVESTIGATIONS

Any person who has a suspected condition of the central nervous system of a serious nature will have investigations performed. There are several reasons why they are done including the desire to:

- identify the exact nature of the disease
- classify how to treat the condition
- come to a conclusion regarding prognosis.

The common investigations applied are listed in Chapter 4 – Investigations. I shall discuss individual situations in relation to each disease.

CEREBROVASCULAR DISEASE

This is disease of the brain due to an interference with its blood supply. The usual problem is disruption to arterial blood supply by either haemorrhage or ischaemia (either as a result of thrombosis or embolism). The counterpart in the cardiovascular system is ischaemic heart disease leading to the clinical pictures of angina pectoris and heart attack. The comments I made in Chapter 7 – Cardiovascular system – in relation to the pathological processes of atheroma, thrombosis and embolism are relevant here.

The additional process that is of importance is bleeding (haemorrhage). In the brain, this is due to a rupture of a blood vessel usually associated with high blood pressure and atherosclerosis. Primary cerebral haemorrhage is the term used to describe the process that occurs with hypertensive people where there is bleeding into the substance of the brain. This is the 'burst blood vessel', the apopleptic attack. It is of abrupt onset and can occur with exercise. It may also occur after a particularly stressful incident. There is usually a severe headache with this condition and more than 50 per cent of people lose consciousness. The haemorrhage is often large and loss of consciousness is a sign that the condition is severe. Half of such people die within a few days.

Atherosclerosis is an extensive disease and does not affect one organ only. Each person will present their own symptom picture and the emphasis of the pathology will depend on the individual. If someone has had a stroke there may be evidence of heart disease. Conversely, if you see a person with coronary atherosclerosis there may also be evidence of damage to the central nervous system.

The common clinical condition associated with cerebrovascular disease is stroke. The precise clinical picture depends on the site and size or any damage and whether there are any unaffected blood vessels left supplying the same area of brain.

Stroke

This is rare before the age of 40 years and uncommon before the age of 50 years. It is found in 1 per cent of people over 60 years old and becomes more common with increasing age. It causes much ill health and leads to difficulty with mobility, dependence and rehabilitation. It occurs in 2 people per 1000 of the population each year and of these 1 will die as a result of this event.

Symptoms
The clinical picture usually evolves over a period of one to two hours. There is a loss of consciousness in a minority although drowsiness is common. Severe headache is unusual. The exact nature of the stroke depends on the site of the damage in the brain.

The commonest symptom is paralysis of one side of the body (hemiplegia). The face, arm and leg are affected in most cases. The side affected is opposite to the side of the problem in the brain. As I mentioned above in relation to upper motor neurone lesions, there is spasticity and increased reflexes. These features are not seen immediately but take a few days to develop as the spinal cord recovers from the 'shock' of the removal of cerebral influences.

There will be dysphasia (difficult speech) if the dominant hemisphere of the brain is affected. This is the left side in right-handed people and often also the left side in most left-handed people. Therefore, a right-sided stroke (of the body) will be accompanied by dysphasia in all right-handed people and in most left-handed people.

A milder symptom picture may present with temporary symptoms. This is named a transient ischaemic attack (TIA). There is also sudden loss of function in the central nervous system. It is followed within the hour by complete recovery. Most attacks only last a few minutes. They should be regarded as a warning of a possible stroke in the future.[7]

The symptoms depend on the site of the problem within the brain. They include loss of consciousness (rare), aphasia, sensory loss and weakness (rather than paralysis) on one side of the body, difficulty swallowing, double vision and vomiting. Vertigo is common and there may be ataxia.

Visual loss is common and the typical symptom is a transient blindness, which is said to be like a black curtain descending down the field of vision. It is called amaurosis fugax. Recovery is the reverse of this process. The frequency of attacks is variable and they may be due to small emboli of atheroma and clot breaking off the affected arterial walls.

Prognosis

There is a high mortality rate with stroke. Between a third and a half of sufferers die within the month after an attack, usually in the first few days. This is more common with haemorrhage (75 per cent die) than with embolism or haemorrhage (under 25 per cent). A poor outcome is more likely if there is coma, squint or a severe hemiplegia. Some 10 per cent of people have recurrent attacks of stroke. Around 30-40 per cent of *survivors* are alive after 3 years, which illustrates the severity of this condition. Common long-term problems include muscle weakness and speech difficulties.

Treatment

This tends to be supportive immediately after the event and then concentrates on rehabilitation in the long-term. Any underlying disease, such as diabetes mellitus or hypertension, is treated. The main aim is to minimise any disability and to try and improve function. Physiotherapy plays a large part in this. It is helpful in supporting, encouraging and aiding the person gain as much mobility as possible. Massage would also be useful here. Speech therapy and psychological support are important additions.

Transient ischaemic attacks are usually treated by anticoagulants. Aspirin inhibits platelet aggregation and can be used in conditions where there is a tendency to clot formation. It is frequently used in this disease. Other drugs used include dipyridamole, which has a similar function.

Holistic management

In terms of Chinese medicine, this condition is denoted Wind-stroke. There are three main features of such a condition and there are similarities with many other conditions that are labelled as of central nervous system origin by conventional medicine. Essentially, there is Heat, which causes the stirring of Wind. This carries Phlegm up to the orifices to cause loss of consciousness and to the channels, causing paralysis and numbness. The generation of Heat may arise from Deficiency of Kidney or Liver Yin leading to rising of Liver Yang. This is the correlation of hypertension with stroke (see Page 163). Alternatively, the Heat may arise from the excessive consumption of greasy and sweet food. Occasionally, the Wind may be of external origin in those people who are weak and deficient.

Specifically, therapies such as acupuncture can help the paralysis and the sensory problems that people have after a stroke. Techniques such as relaxation, Tai Chi or other exercises are also beneficial.

The problems posed by this condition are frequently long-term. There is a lot of money, time and energy spent on treatment. You will see people in your clinic who have problems remaining after a stroke and holistic medicine has a lot to offer such cases. If the person has had a paralysis or a sensory problem for many years then the chances of improving the situation may seem slim. However, I have seen and heard of cases where marked improvement has occurred several years after the stroke and so the recuperative powers in the central nervous system can be strong indeed.

OTHER DISEASES LEADING TO STROKE

The clinical appearance of stroke may also be the result of other pathological processes. For example, brain tumour may lead to the death of nerve cells either due to direct pressure or to obstruction of the blood supply. Brain tumour is described on Page 275.

Subarachnoid haemorrhage

This is an uncommon condition but one which you may come across. It is haemorrhage under the subarachnoid layer around the outside of the brain. The usual source is from a ruptured aneurysm. An aneurysm is a dilatation on an arterial wall and tends to be weaker than the rest of the blood vessel. The conventional belief is that they are congenital in nature and spontaneously burst to produce the typical symptoms.

Symptoms

There is a severe and sudden headache, which is usually occipital in site. It can come on so suddenly that the person may turn round because they think that they have been struck. There are signs of meningeal irritation. These are photophobia, neck stiffness and occipital headache. There will not be a fever, as you would expect with meningitis or encephalitis. There may be loss of consciousness for hours or days. Vomiting is common. Impaired function of the central nervous system does not always happen, but if it does the condition is clearly more serious. The danger is of a further rupture of another aneurysm.

This condition is fatal in many cases. Around 50 per cent of people are dead or almost so by the time of arrival at hospital – a further 10-20 per cent die in the next few days. The prognosis is more serious if paralysis is present or if another bleed occurs within the next few days.

Treatment

The conventional response is dependent upon the person's age. Computerised axial tomography scans are performed under the age of 60 years and angiography in that age group if the blood pressure is normal. Less than 5 per cent of people have a detectable abnormality.

Essentially, the management is to wait until the person's condition has stabilised. Rest and supportive treatment are important in the early stages. If an aneurysm is discovered by angiography, it will be clipped surgically.

EPILEPSY

Epilepsy is defined as the occurrence of recurrent convulsions or 'abnormal events'. It may be classified as 'seizure disorder', for which there are over 20 different types. About 3 per cent of the population have two or more such attacks in their lives. Some 250,000 people in the UK take anticonvulsant drugs. In the US, around 125,000 new cases of epilepsy are diagnosed each year.

It is classified by conventional medicine according to the appearances of the attack. The symptoms are of an epileptic convulsion and the particular form varies with each type. The diagnosis is necessarily confirmed and categorised with the aid of an electroencephalogram (EEG). It is considered to be a brief disorder of cerebral function associated with disturbance of consciousness accompanied by sudden, excessive discharge of cerebral neurones. The classification is as follows:

- Generalised
- Grand mal
- Petit mal
- Focal
- Temporal lobe
- Jacksonian.

The causes are usually unknown conventionally. There may be a family history and it is more likely to develop if one or both parents have epilepsy. It can develop secondarily to cerebral disease. The most common conditions here are brain tumours, a head injury and cerebrovascular disease. Other situations may lead to epileptic fits and these reflect the fact that it is possible for anyone to have an attack, if the conditions are right. These include hyperglycaemia, hypoglycaemia and withdrawal of drugs such as heroin, opiates and alcohol. One in 20 people with epilepsy are photosensitive and flashing lights, a flickering television or VDU can set off a fit.

Symptoms

I shall describe each type of epilepsy separately although you often see people who have what seems to be a mixture of types. This is difficult to explain conventionally. I treated a boy of 8 years once who had what was clinically petit mal and grand mal attacks but the diagnosis of the neurologist was of temporal lobe epilepsy (based mainly on the EEG finding). He was given carbamazepine, the main drug for temporal lobe epilepsy. The attacks changed in appearance only because this drug does not control this type of convulsion.

Grand mal or major attack

There is a prodromal stage, which can last for hours or days and is usually characterised by a change of mood. Then there may be an 'aura' which is uncommon in this type of epilepsy and is brief. If the person does go through this stage, it may merely be an awareness that a fit is about to happen. If so, they can lie down and prepare themselves to avoid injury.

If an aura is not experienced, the person goes suddenly into a *tonic* stage. There is generalised contraction of all the muscles in the body. The person may give a 'cry' as the air is forced from the lungs and falls to the ground. There is loss of consciousness and the contraction of all the musculature is sustained for about 20-30 seconds. There is no respiration and so cyanosis develops.

This is followed by the *clonic* stage, which involves spasmodic contractions of the muscles. There are typical jerking movements of the face, body and limbs. It lasts for about 30 seconds and there may or may not be incontinence of urine (usually) or faeces (rarely). The person may bite their tongue either in this, or the previous, stage.

Finally, the attack ends in a stage of relaxation. This is a flaccid, comatose state, which lapses into normal sleep. This lasts for a few minutes or half an hour. When consciousness is regained there is often a period of drowsiness and some confusion with a headache. A person should not be allowed to go home unaccompanied after an attack.

Petit mal or minor attack

This has a characteristic EEG pattern. Petit mal cannot be diagnosed medically without this. There is a transient loss of consciousness, which lasts for 10 to 15 seconds. The person stares blankly. In mild cases and at the onset they may pass unnoticed. They are accurately described as 'absences'. In children this condition may be mistaken for inattention, learning difficulties, deafness and so forth.

Temporal lobe epilepsy

This is the commonest type of focal epilepsy. There are strange symptoms of sensory hallucinations (of smell, taste, hearing or sight). They are frequently unpleasant such as smelling something offensive or hearing obscene words. People may think that others are swearing at them. There are often 'déjà vu' phenomena.[8] Déjà vu is also seen in schizophrenia and is certainly linked to altered states of consciousness although it is common in people with neither of these conditions.

Emotional changes are common. Consciousness is disturbed but not lost. There may be a situation known as automatism. This is behaviour that is not attended by conscious thought or awareness and, for this reason, has medico-legal implications.

Jacksonian epilepsy

Here, there is involuntary twitching of one limb or part of a limb. It may or may not spread further. There may be loss of consciousness although it is unusual. A single part of the body, such as the thumb, is usually the first place affected. The shaking spreads to involve the whole limb and, rarely, the whole body. Each episode lasts for several minutes. A temporary weakness or paralysis may follow the attack.

The significance of this type of epilepsy is that it usually develops in later life and may be caused by a structural abnormality such as a brain tumour.

Investigations

The definitive diagnosis is made with an EEG and conventional treatment cannot start until the exact type is known. Drug treatment for epilepsy suppresses the changes detectable by EEG.

Some types of epilepsy are secondary to structural problems of the brain such as tumours. Investigation will be undertaken if this is suspected. This will include brain scan – computerised axial tomography, magnetic resonance imaging (MRI) or a radioactive isotope scan.

Treatment

There is a social stigma associated with this disease and, in general, society is not very understanding. I remember that there was a boy in my class at school who had grand mal attacks fairly regularly and he was treated miserably by the rest of us. There was little attempt to understand the condition and this seemed to be the general attitude throughout the school.

The occupation opportunities of a person may be affected, as certain jobs are not considered suitable. Any job where loss of consciousness may be dangerous for the person or others is precluded. This covers such work as airline pilots, professional driving, steeplejacks, divers and anyone working with high voltage equipment.

The regulations concerning a driving licence differs slightly in different countries but essentially it is illegal to drive for 1 year after an epileptic fit or unexplained loss of consciousness. In the UK, someone can drive if there has not been a fit whilst awake in the previous year. When fits occur during sleep, the convulsions must have occurred only whilst asleep for the previous 3 years. The rules for truck drivers and public service vehicle drivers are far stricter.

There are certain precipitating factors. Common ones are lack of sleep (tiredness), fevers and television or flashing lights in those who are sensitive.

The first-aid treatment of an epileptic attack is to remove the person from potential sources of injury (such as furniture) and to loosen clothing. Wait until the attack has subsided and then place the person in the recovery position until consciousness is regained. The old advice about placing an object between the teeth to protect the tongue is no longer given, as the tongue will have been bitten early in the attack. If you attempt such a practice you may damage teeth or risk losing fingers!

Drugs remain the mainstay of conventional treatment. Different agents are used for different types of epilepsy.

Type of epilepsy	Drug used	Comments[9]
Grand mal	Phenytoin Phenobarbitone Carbamazepine Sodium valproate	Affects the liver. Commonly used. Heavily suppresses respiration Also used to treat neuralgias Commonly used. Affects the liver
Petit mal	Ethosuximide Sodium valproate	Main side-effects in the blood See above
Temporal lobe	Carbamazepine	See above

Table 14.5: Conventional treatment of epilepsy

Holistic management

In previous times and in other cultures, epileptics and people who could enter trance states were seen as being in touch with something powerful and perhaps useful. This potentially positive connotation is denied by Western society. We shy away from such things and prefer them to be hidden from us. This is also true of some mental and emotional disturbances. It is part of the holistic process of treatment to encourage people to reconnect aspects of themselves that have been suppressed.

The precise manifestation of an imbalance will vary from person to person. If blockages exist in the mental and emotional levels there may be the appearance of psychological disturbances and disorders such as epilepsy, which has physical symptoms. Cure involves an awareness of these levels and how they interact and seeks to transform these blockages. Curative treatment, in the case of epilepsy, may well release emotions that have been long suppressed. Coming to terms with these and learning how to handle them in a healthy way are the challenges of treatment.

In terms of Chinese medicine, epilepsy is considered to be in the same group of disturbances as mania and hysteria. There are common connections with these as they are all associated with the substances of Wind, Heat and Phlegm. They manifest in different ways according to the person. They may also be seen in relation to the three levels of mental, emotional and physical. Mania is a disturbance of the mental level and is described (see Chapter 16 – Psychological Disorders). In Chinese medicine, this term is used broadly to include the conventional labels of schizophrenia and mania. Hysteria is a disturbance of the emotional level and is described (see Chapter 16 – Psychological Disorders). Epilepsy is a disturbance of the physical level.

The treatment of these three disorders by conventional medicine may also be understood from an energetic viewpoint. Mania is treated by lithium and 'major' tranquillisers such as the phenothiazines. Hysteria is treated by 'minor' tranquillisers such as the benzodiazepines. Epilepsy is treated by anticonvulsants (of which the benzodiazepines are one example). These interrelationships are shown in Table 14.6.

Disorder	Conventional treatment	Comments
Mania	Lithium, antipsychotics such as 'major' tranquillisers	Sedative to the mental level. Side-effects damage the central nervous system causing tardive dyskinesia similar in its manifestation to Parkinson's disease
Hysteria	'Minor' tranquillisers	Sedative to the emotional level. Withdrawal may lead to mania (mental level), anxiety (emotional level) or convulsions (physical level)
Epilepsy	Anticonvulsants	Sedative mainly to physical level. Side-effects include damage to the central nervous system

Table 14.6: Conventional treatment of mania, hysteria and epilepsy

Treatment by holistic medicine is effective for epilepsy but it will almost always be complicated by the administration of anticonvulsants. Sudden withdrawal of these is dangerous and must not be attempted. Some 40 per cent of people with epilepsy can withdraw their drugs and have no problems, presumably because the original exciting cause has gone. The difficulty we have with each person is that we do not know if they are one of those 40 per cent.

Treatment must be accompanied by an awareness that hidden issues on a psychological level may arise. These can be dealt with as they appear but a general atmosphere of support and openness is helpful. It is beneficial to avoid as much stimulation as possible particularly drugs including coffee. This together with regular relaxation and a healthy diet (especially avoiding greasy, sweet and spicy food) will enhance recovery. It is certainly possible to gradually reduce medication after people's health begins to improve. How far you can go will vary from case to case.

Case one

A child of two came for treatment of fits, that began after the MMR vaccination at around 1 year old. Prior to this he had a history of chest infections and had been diagnosed as asthmatic. More recently he had ear and throat infections. The fits occurred daily and always came on when he was excited, cross or tired. It was as if he missed a breath, passed out and then stayed out as if he was asleep. This could last between 2 minutes and 2 hours and he would be tired on coming around. The longer he was 'out' the more tired he would be. His mother was waiting for a CT scan.

Despite his age, he had had many antibiotics and was on a bronchodilator inhaler three times daily as well as bronchodilator syrup. He had a very chesty cough and X-rays showed a shadow on his lungs. He tended to throw himself to the ground during tantrums. His sleep was restless and disturbed. There had been a premature death in the family due to TB many years ago.

The pattern of the fits, the shadow on the lung and the family history led to a prescription of Tuberculinum 30c. Four weeks later he was free of both inhalers and antibiotics and had no more fits. He no longer had tantrums and was sleeping much better. He had just caught chicken pox, but was managing well with them. His mother was provided with Rhus tox. to be given only if needed once the spots had emerged.

Case two

A man of 41 years, who was born deaf, came to be treated for headaches accompanied by nausea and a troublesome burning sensation at the pit of the stomach. The headaches had started more than 20 years before, more or less when he began his work as a dental technician. They became worse and worse until the pain was intolerable with daily fits.

Sometimes a throbbing head pain was the first symptom followed by nausea, but at other times the nausea, rising from the stomach, could appear first and then turn into a heavy throbbing sensation in the head. The symptoms used to last all day long if he didn't take painkillers, and left him stunned. He was an assertive man with a very strong personality. He made it very clear that he wanted to take something as effective, or even more effective, than the strong painkillers he was used to. He couldn't take time off work. Work was his religion and he had no time for anything else.

The remedy prescribed was Arsenicum Sulphuratum Flavus 30c also called Orpiment Dosage: 1 pellet as soon as symptoms appeared.

Other important and fundamental keynotes that led to the prescription included:

- restless
- sleeplessness (sleeping only 4/5 hours per night)
- fastidious – a perfectionist (others aren't normally up to his standard)
- gets angry when contradicted
- he generates heat
- worried about being on time and gets angry if others aren't
- always on the move
- always doing something
- cannot stop
- anxiety or fear of being a failure
- longing for confidence about the future
- a craving for chocolate that was so strong he said: 'When I eat it I'm as happy as if I've made love'.

The remedy worked well from the beginning and that's the only reason the patient managed to stay with the homoeopath. He wouldn't have allowed any 'second try'. Threatened fits became rare and symptoms responded to an acute administration of the remedy.

MULTIPLE SCLEROSIS (disseminated sclerosis)

This is the main example of a group of diseases that are associated with loss of the myelin sheath (demyelinisation) around the nerve fibre. This sheath of fatty material is essential for normal nerve function. The loss of myelin leads to abnormal function of whichever nerve or nerves are affected.

It occurs in 1 in 2000 people and the cause is unknown. There are about 250,000 people with multiple sclerosis in the US.

It occurs in geographical clusters and is commoner in the North and West of Europe, UK, northern United States, Canada, Iceland, Tasmania and southern New Zealand. This may be an association with damp and cold conditions. It is more common in those areas where people have a high intake of animal fats and certain dietary changes may lead to improvement.

Conventionally, there are considered to be genetic or autoimmune mechanisms involved. There is evidence from the study of disease incidence and antibody levels to suggest that multiple sclerosis may be linked to latent viral infections in the body. These, in susceptible people, disrupt the immune system so that it attacks the nervous system. Many viruses have been implicated but especially the measles virus.[10] This has implications for vaccination procedures, since these deliberately introduce such material into the body. Recent evidence indicates that 30-60 per cent of new attacks of multiple sclerosis occur soon after a common cold, influenza or other viral illness.

Symptoms

Initially there is an episode of symptoms reflecting a neurological disorder. The exact nature depends on the nerves involved as any nerve in the body can be affected. Typically, this includes an acute weakness of one or more limbs, the appearance of pins and needles or numbness, blurred or double vision (common), vertigo, loss of balance. Most people recover within 1 to 3 months of the onset of symptoms. There is a recurrence after a variable period of time and this is usually within 2 years.

In some people, the disease enters a stage of gradual increase in disability without remission. Most people recover to almost normal function but after each relapse there is a further degeneration in function and so the result is a step-by-step deterioration. Half of affected people enter a chronically progressive stage.

The motor dysfunction is of an upper motor neurone type. It is typically worse after a hot bath. There is often loss of balance and an intention tremor.[11] Sensory affections are common and include tingling, electric shock-like sensations and numbness. Mental changes also take place and the common one is depression. It is said in conventional texts that euphoria can also occur. However, as this is a side-effect of corticosteroid therapy, I think that it is much more likely to be as a result of such treatment than of the disease itself.

It is considered to be a progressive and chronic disease and 5 per cent die within 5 years. In the rest there is a variable course. A significant proportion (up to one third) has only the first attack. These cases are unlikely to seek a medical follow-up so the conventionally held view of almost certain deterioration is not valid.

Investigations

There is no single investigation that can lead to a definite diagnosis of multiple sclerosis. The diagnosis is made from the clinical history and an exclusion of diseases causing similar symptoms, such as brain tumour.

The investigations that are performed provide circumstantial evidence but must be considered in the light of the total picture. They include lumbar puncture and examination of cerebrospinal fluid, tests of visual evoked potential and scanning of the nervous system. This latter is by means of magnetic resonance imaging (MRI) or computed axial tomographic (CAT) scanning.

The MRI scan, in particular, is seen as a more sensitive indicator of the presence of areas of demyelinisation. However, it is not necessarilty infallible, as many things may give rise to the same appearances.

Treatment

In conventional terms, there is nothing that is considered to be curative. Corticosteroids are frequently given, as it is believed to lead to a more rapid and complete recovery of a relapse. This is a matter for debate even in conventional circles. There is certainly no documented evidence of benefit from long-term corticosteroid use. It tends, instead, to lead to serious side-effects such as osteoporosis, fluid retention, hypertension and cataracts.

One consideration is to attempt the relief of spasticity through drugs. These are of variable effectiveness. Urinary incontinence is common and an in-dwelling catheter may be necessary. Kidney infections are common as a result of the underlying urinary problem and the presence of the catheter.

An important aspect is support for the relatives as this disease is tremendously tiring for the carers.

Holistic management

You will definitely see people with this condition as they look for alternatives to the approach of conventional medicine. One issue to be considered is the effect upon the person of the label itself. As described above there is a wide range of variable courses of the disease. However, when a doctor in a white coat in a hospital tells you that you have multiple sclerosis, that will engender a sense of hopelessness and despair. There used to be an advertisement in the UK for an organisation that purports to help people with multiple sclerosis. It shows a woman's back with a tear in the photograph down the length of the spinal column and a (literally) spine chilling message about the effects of the disease. The phenomenon of the self-fulfilling prophesy is such that even if there were nothing wrong originally, many people would end up crippled after such pronouncements.

This is a difficult disease to treat as far as the holistic practitioner is concerned. This is particularly so since many people seek treatment when the disease is well established. It is important to have several approaches. Diet seems to be a major factor and especially the avoidance of animal fat.[12] This would fit in with the observation that multiple sclerosis occurs more commonly in damp[13] areas such as the UK and the North and West of Europe. Some people also benefit from removing gluten from the diet. I have known people who started to improve with treatment and then relapse after eating dairy products or meat. These foods tend to produce Dampness within the body, in terms of Chinese medicine. It is such observations that lead people to take oils such as linoleic oil and evening primrose oil for this condition.[14]

My approach to a person with multiple sclerosis is similar to someone with cancer. There are frequently psychological factors that play an important part in the genesis and the continuation of the disease. Looking at these emotional and mental factors may be of importance. Relaxation is also very beneficial.

In terms of Chinese medicine, this condition is usually seen as Wind in the Channels, which may be due to several causes. There may be Wind-damp directly invading the Channels and Organs. Otherwise, there is Deficiency of Kidney, Spleen or Liver leading to Wind because of Qi and Blood Deficiency. Phlegm and Dampness gather in the tissues giving rise to stiffness and numbness. Long-term the tendons and ligaments are damaged. Sometimes, the milder the symptoms, the harder it is to treat. People with Heat symptoms tend to do better because there is more energy in the system.

It is definitely possible for people to improve and I know of people who are leading a full and active life after a diagnosis of multiple sclerosis. When the disease has progressed and there is paralysis and other neurological symptoms, there is still much to offer. Treatment can help alleviate the worst of the pain or tingling. It can help the weakness. It can help the urinary and bowel problems of incontinence or impaction. You would expect the person to continue with symptoms but with an improved quality of life and comfort.

PARKINSON'S DISEASE

This is one of a group of diseases where there is a disturbance in the function of the extrapyramidal system. This system is like the clutch on the car and serves to act as a control of movement. Abnormalities here lead to three typical groups of symptoms. There is disturbance of voluntary movement, the appearance of involuntary movements and an alteration in the muscle tone. Another disease of the same part of the brain is Huntington's chorea.

In Parkinsonism, there is impairment of voluntary movement, rigidity and tremor. If these three symptoms co-exist in an elderly person then the diagnosis is usually made. The incidence is around 1 in 1000 of the population and this rises to 1 per cent in those over 60 years old. The pathological lesion is in the basal ganglia and involves a relative lack of the transmitter substances of that part of the nervous system. There are several causes in conventional terms:

- unknown in 75 per cent
- post-encephalitis especially encephalitis lethargica
- prescribed drugs, such as the phenothiazines used in schizophrenia, Alzheimer's disease and senile dementia
- head injury.

Symptoms

There is the gradual development of a tremor in the fingers and the forearms. It is slow in nature and is described as 'pill rolling', because it looks as though the person is rolling a pill between the thumb and index finger. Tremor of the head is rare. It is worse at rest and improves with purposeful movements such as attempting to pick something up. This is in contrast to the tremor of cerebellar disease, which gets worse the closer the hand moves to an object (intention tremor). The tremor of Parkinson's disease is typically worse with stress and with embarrassment.

The rigidity in the muscles is due to increased muscle tone. It is of a 'cog-wheel' type where passive movement of the arm, for example, reveals the intermittent nature of the rigidity. There are often fixed abnormalities of posture and the body appears to be in a permanent state of flexion. Movement is slow and there is a delay in the initiation of movements. It is difficult for a person to start to walk from standing or to stand from the sitting position. It is as if the person is moving in slow motion. Conversely, it is not possible to control the speed of walking and people may gather speed when walking downhill. There is a typical gait, which is short and shuffling because the legs cannot be picked up very well. The voice is quiet.

This is a severe, degenerative disease of the central nervous system. One in five people cannot cope independently with normal living and have to be supported in some way by family, friends or the health services.

Treatment

This is aimed at the cause, but this is only known in the minority of cases. The main aim of treatment is to minimise the worst symptoms of the disease. This is primarily with drugs designed to correct the chemical abnormalities in the affected area of the brain. Treatment is generally unsatisfactory as the disease continues to progress and side-effects increase despite changing dosages or medication. After 5 years of treatment about half of patients have some degree of side-effects which can be severe.

Treatment (mildest to strongest)	Comments
Anticholinergic, e.g. benzhexol, orphenadrine and amantadine	They are rarely used since the advent of L-dopa. Lead to dry mouth, blurred vision, retention of urine and confusion
L-dopa – in combination with a decarboxylase inhibitor[15] such as benserazide or carbidopa	Early use is associated with worsening of the symptoms in the long-term. There is an 'on-off' phenomenon where either the drugs do not work or they have strong side-effects. This can occur with no warning and despite a constant drug dosage. Originally L-dopa seemed to revolutionise the treatment of Parkinson's disease. People who had been almost seized up for years started to walk and move. Side-effects include nausea, vomiting, confusion, and visual hallucinations
Type B monoamine oxidase inhibitor	Selegiline may be given with L-dopa when this has ceased to work effectively as described above. Cardiovascular disease tends to worsen with this drug as would be expected as it is related to the antidepressants which are cardiotoxic
Dopaminergic agents, e.g. bromocryptine, lysuride, pergolide	Used when L-dopa is ineffective. The dosage is restricted by the appearance of side-effects, which include nausea, vomiting, dizziness, fainting, cold hands and feet and constipation
Surgery	This is the implantation of brain cells obtained from aborted foetuses. This has ethical implications. It is still at an experimental stage

Table 14.7: Conventional treatment of Parkinson's disease

Holistic management

In terms of Chinese medicine, this condition usually corresponds to Liver Blood Deficiency with Wind. Phlegm accumulates in the channels and muscles leading to stiffness and slow movement. The conventional drugs have a heating effect and mainly affect the Liver and Heart. The heating effect of the drugs is to dry the Phlegm and to help movement but leads to side-effects of restlessness and sometimes worsening of the tremor. Long-term, of course, they cause Liver Blood Deficiency and so can only worsen the disease.

CEREBRAL TUMOUR

This causes 2 per cent of deaths at all ages so is not that uncommon. The tumour is frequently a secondary development from a cancer elsewhere in the body but it can be a primary growth.

Benign tumours may develop in the brain and these will present with similar symptoms to those of malignant tumours. However, malignant tumours grow more quickly and symptoms develop more rapidly with clear progression. The treatment of both types may be the same. The main restriction for surgery is the site of the tumour. Some are not amenable to removal, as the operation would cause too much damage. Consequently, radiotherapy and chemotherapy may be given.

An exception to the above is the meningioma. This is a slow growing benign tumour on the meninges, the membrane that surrounds the brain. This can be removed surgically without damaging internal structures.

Symptoms

These are considered to be due to two factors. Firstly, there is the local effect on neighbouring tissues. Secondly, there is increased pressure as the tumour grows inside the rigid bony skull.

Local effects are due to pressure on adjacent brain tissue. There are symptoms dependent upon the particular nerve tract that is affected. There could be problems with motor nerves, sensory nerves, cerebellum and other areas. Symptoms here include weakness or paralysis, numbness, tingling, pins and needles, difficulties with balance and fits. The clinical syndromes that are seen include stroke and epilepsy.

The pressure inside the skull increases because there is no outlet for the cerebrospinal fluid. As the tumour expands in size the pressure rises. This leads to a headache, which is described as diffuse. It is worse for activities such as bending, coughing or straining. It is worse on waking and when lying flat. There is often clouding of consciousness, which varies from a mild degree of listlessness and drowsiness to deep coma. There may be the development of generalised epileptic attacks. Also, there is often dizziness and, typically, vomiting (with no preceding nausea) due to direct stimulation of the vomiting centre in the midbrain.

Investigations

The approach to this condition will depend on whether it is a primary or a secondary tumour. The presence of a secondary cancer means that the only treatment in conventional medicine can be palliative. There will be no attempt to cure (in the conventional meaning of the word). Therefore, the number of investigations will be limited, as surgery will not be an option.

If the cancer is primary, or suspected to be so, investigations will be carried out with several aims in mind. In conventional medicine, it is important to locate the exact anatomical site and to determine the histological appearances. This information defines the type of tumour and this will enable a decision to be made about whether surgery is a viable proposition.

Treatment

It is generally considered that surgery with or without radiotherapy offers the only hope for people with cerebral tumours. A year after diagnosis less than 50 per cent of people with malignant tumours are still alive.

Dexamethasone, a corticosteroid, is frequently used to shrink the tumour and any surrounding oedema. This may lead to short-term relief of symptoms only, as the underlying progress is not affected. It can be helpful for people to improve their level of consciousness in order to settle their affairs and connect with family relationships.

ENCEPHALITIS AND MENINGITIS

This is inflammation of the substance of the brain and the lining around the brain, respectively. They are considered together as they lead to similar symptoms. In conventional medicine, there are considered to be several causes of meningitis including:

- infection by bacteria, virus or fungus – encephalitis is almost always associated with viruses
- drugs
- dyes used in radiology
- blood – see subarachnoid haemorrhage

Symptoms

Both meningitis and encephalitis produce similar symptoms with meningitis having the more severe clinical picture. There is fever, severe occipital headache, photophobia and vomiting. Irritability and desire for quiet are common. The presence of a rash should be looked for and indicates severe disease.

Neck stiffness is found on examination, which progresses to opisthotonos and eventually convulsions. These symptoms are obvious when the disease has progressed. Recognition at an early stage is essential if complications are to be avoided. The symptoms frequently follow an upper respiratory tract but may occur directly. If there is any suspicion of meningitis, appropriate measures must be taken immediately. The death rate in treated cases is 15 per cent.

Encephalitis and viral meningitis have similar symptoms but milder. The exception is encephalitis caused by the herpes simplex virus. This is severe and has a death rate of at least 20 per cent.

Complications

Headaches are common after meningitis and encephalitis. In severe cases, there may be intellectual impairment.

Complication	Symptoms to look for
Venous sinus thrombosis or cerebral oedema	Drowsiness, squint
Septicaemia	Low blood pressure, rapid pulse, pale, ill and sweaty
Convulsions	Loss of consciousness, epileptiform attacks

Table 14.8: Complications of meningitis and encephalitis

Treatment

This is invariably with antibiotics after examination of cerebrospinal fluid obtained by lumbar puncture. They must be given early in the course of bacterial meningitis to prevent or minimise the occurrence of complications. Herpes simplex encephalitis is treated with intravenous acyclovir.

Holistic management

The main differentiation to be made is with meningism. This is the appearance of vague symptoms of neck stiffness, photophobia and headache with a fever. It is not serious and does not progress. If there is any suspicion of meningitis, antibiotic treatment and hospitalisation are necessary.

The occurrence of meningitis is due to general weakness of the immune system. Prevention depends on providing optimum situations for healthy childhood – see Chapter 19 – Children's Health.

In terms of Chinese medicine, this condition corresponds to Extreme Heat generating Wind. It is a consequence of pathogenic influences passing directly into deep levels of the body.

SPINAL CORD DISORDERS

Cervical spondylosis

This is a condition of chronic cervical disc degeneration. The term is applied to a particular appearance of the X-ray. It becomes more common with age. Many cervical spine X-rays in people over the age of 35 or 40 years will show some evidence of degeneration. Again we have a situation where many people have abnormal investigations but only a few will have symptoms.

It is not generally the degenerative changes themselves that give rise to pain but associated muscle spasm. There are many causes of muscle pains especially in the neck and so it may be inappropriate to assume that it is cervical spondylosis on the basis of an X-ray. This is why treatments by acupuncture, osteopathy, massage, aromatherapy and the like can frequently be beneficial.

Symptoms

The overriding feature is of a pain in the neck that is felt under the occiput and may radiate over the head into the forehead. It may, in severe cases, radiate to the area of supply of the nerve associated with the affected disc degeneration. These are usually the 5th, 6th, 7th and 8th cervical nerve roots. The pain in the neck is felt under the occiput and may radiate over the head into the forehead. There is often pain across the shoulders into the joint itself and in severe cases will radiate down the arm. There may be decreased tendon reflexes as this is a lower motor neurone problem.

On examination, the neck is stiff and there are reduced movements in the cervical spine. It may be worse in one particular direction than the others. There will also be tenderness under the base of the skull and in the trapezii muscles. The pain is worse for movement and especially those movements that involve use of the arms or neck. Window cleaning, carrying bags or weights, knitting, hanging curtains or washing and so on may lead to more pain.

Investigations

An X-ray of the cervical spine may reveal degenerative changes in people with neck pain.

Treatment

The main treatment is with drugs and physiotherapy. A collar is often used to restrict the movements in the cervical spine but only serves to help prevent the actions that cause pain. It will weaken the muscles in the neck and so, as with corsets for lumbago and sciatica, I usually tell people to only use them for specific situations.

Physiotherapy, in my experience, may make the problem worse and must be applied with care. Traction may be used in this condition and will do nothing for the spasm of the muscles of the neck but will lead to problems in the thoracic musculature. Also, treatment with heat or cold can be unhelpful as there is no attempt to individualise the case and ensure such treatment is appropriate.

The main drugs used are the group of non-steroidal anti-inflammatory agents, which are described in detail in Chapter 10 – Musculoskeletal system. Therefore, little benefit will be obtained and there is the risk of very serious side-effects from these drugs.

On occasion, people may be prescribed 'muscle relaxants'. These are invariably benzodiazepine tranquillisers such as diazepam. They are rapidly addictive and when prescribed for pain can only lead to depression.

Holistic management

In terms of Chinese medicine, this condition is due to Stagnation of Qi and Blood in the Channels. There may be several causes of this and underlying conditions. In an acute situation, particularly in those with strong energy, there may be an Invasion of Cold, Wind or Dampness. Injury may also play a part in some.

When the condition is more long-term, there may be underlying syndromes of Blood Deficiency. There may be associated tingling and numbness in the arms and hands. There are similarities here with carpal tunnel syndrome and repetitive strain injury. Tension and worry can generate neck pain and there may be connection with Stagnation of Liver Qi. The Gall Bladder channel passes over the shoulders and up into the back of the head and Stagnation here can give rise to pain due to a problem in its paired organ, the Liver. Remember that the acupuncture point, Gall Bladder 21 in the trapezius muscle is connected with the uterus. Women may exhibit pain here due to a uterine imbalance.

Case one

A man of 50 years came for treatment of his neck and shoulder pain after a road traffic accident some 16 years previously. He had severe pain in the right side of his neck and his right shoulder. He would have 'electric tingling sensations' in his right hand so that he would drop objects. He had pain in his right elbow, right side of his face and the outside of his right foot would feel cold. He was generally tired with a poor appetite and his sleep would be disturbed every night by pain. He was taking two types of analgesics daily with little relief. Such a pattern of symptoms after a neck injury is very common as it is not just the neck itself that is affected but the flow of energy up and down the spine is also obstructed. Headaches as well as tingling, numbness and pain in the limbs are common. I made a diagnosis of Liver Blood Deficiency and Kidney Yang Deficiency. I treated him with acupuncture only.

He made a slow recovery with each visit for treatment resulting in decreased levels of pain, increased energy levels and the sensations in his hand and foot returning to normal. He made many changes in his work schedule that also helped and after 4 months of treatment he has much less pain in his neck and shoulder. He will need to continue treatment for some time yet to consolidate this improvement and hopefully gain more relief.

Lumbago-sciatica

Lumbago is low back pain and is usually felt in the lumbar region. Sciatica is pain in the distribution of sciatic nerve and is felt in the buttock and down the leg. It may pass into the calf and foot in severe cases. The exact distribution of the pain depends on the particular nerve root affected but essentially it is either down the back or the side of the leg.

I have seen people develop pain in the back of this type with minimal trauma such as opening the boot of a car or washing the windscreen of a car. The onset may be sudden as in, 'my back has gone, doctor' or it may be gradual, over a period of days or even weeks. The lumbago may precede the development of sciatica by months or years.

The cause of lumbago and sciatica is often a source of much discussion. There are generally considered to be several scenarios. The most common source of pain is a strained muscle or ligament. Either can result from exercising whilst being out of condition (e.g. gardening when unused to physical exercise), overexertion (e.g. a lot of heavy lifting) or placing your back into a position it's not used to (e.g. twisting to reach something or doing a lot of sitting or standing still). These situations are more likely to lead to problems if there are other factors involved. These factors include poor posture, a weak back, in pregnancy, being overweight and wearing high-heeled shoes.

Rarely, back pain occurs when an intervertebral disc 'slips' or prolapses and presses on a nerve. Recent studies show that prolapsed discs are relatively common but rarely cause pain.

Back pain can originate from bones if the spinal joints are inflamed. Disease such as rheumatoid arthritis, ankylosing spondylitis and other autoimmune disorders can cause back pain. Osteoporosis may cause bone to weaken and if vertebrae fracture or compress, they can cause back pain and sciatic pain.

Psychological stress is associated with back pain and in some it may be considered to be the cause. Certainly, some patients with chronic back pain may be offered tranquillisers or antidepressants as a form of treatment.

Symptoms

In the case of lumbago, there is low back pain, which is brought on by bending. It may be better for heat or warmth. There is often tenderness over the lumbar musculature. Sciatic pain radiates down the leg in the distribution of the affected nerve root. It usually starts in the buttock and is felt down the back or side of the leg. It is typically worse for coughing, sneezing and movement. It may be difficult to move the leg and some people have excruciating pain and cannot move at all. Some people have sensory symptoms of 'pins and needles' or numbness.

In severe cases there will be evidence of motor involvement of a lower motor neurone type. There is weakness of the muscles of the affected nerve root. There are weak calf muscles and foot drop, i.e. inability to dorsiflex the foot in the case of 5th lumbar affection. There are weak quadriceps muscles and no knee tendon reflex in the case of 4th lumbar affection.

These more severe symptoms may indicate nerve compression of which two causes are considered important. Prolapsed ('slipped') intervertebral disc is when the disc is considered to herniate outwards and press onto the nerve. This can be due to trauma such as twisting the spine while flexed (e.g. lifting a heavy object incorrectly) or during childbirth. It is characterised by severe back pain frequently with radiation down the leg.

In the case of spinal cord compression from a spinal tumour the symptoms will be more severe, there will be a combination of motor and sensory nerve loss and the symptoms will be progressive. There will be little, if any, improvement with treatment.

Investigations
The main investigation will be an MRI scan. It will reveal if there is any compression of the nerve root and, if so, where this is present. Plain X-ray may reveal degenerative changes in the lumbar spine but these are so common that they cannot be relied upon to be the 'cause' of the problem. Similar comments were made in relation to cervical spondylosis.

Treatment
People are told to take complete rest, at first, when the pain is severe or with sciatica. Rest in bed is advised as the best way of attaining this. This may be continued for 2 to 4 weeks followed by back strengthening exercises for the next 10 to 14 days. A spinal support or surgical corset may be given.

If there is no improvement surgery is considered in order to remove what may be considered to be a compression of the disc on the nerve root. Laminectomy[16] relieves the pressure on the nerve. The same will also be considered if the condition is recurrent. A further surgical option in resistant cases may be spinal fusion.

Holistic management
In terms of Chinese medicine, there are two main syndromes that are seen. In people with strong energy, these symptoms are due to Stagnation of Qi and Blood in the Channels due to an Invasion of Wind or Damp or Cold. This is the type of situation where people develop acute lower back pain and find it difficult and painful to move. Treatment can lead to immediate relief. It is the situation where acupuncture and osteopathy have a well-known reputation for almost miraculous improvement.

There are far more indications, of course, for the use of osteopathy than merely backache. There are many conditions that benefit from manipulation and it is outside the scope of this book to list them all. Nevertheless, osteopathy provides an effective treatment for musculoskeletal conditions of many types. Cranial osteopathy is particularly helpful in chronic back conditions. It is extremely gentle and is more energetic in its diagnosis and treatment. I find a combination of acupuncture and cranial osteopathic treatment for chronic back pain to be extremely efficacious.

In terms of back pain, the Alexander technique is extremely helpful for remedying long-term postural problems. This may necessarily be on-going in order to correct spinal deformities. It works on very subtle levels and can be almost meditative in its methodology.

In weaker people, and this is the common situation in the West, there is usually an underlying syndrome of Kidney Deficiency. This is because the Kidney is responsible for the functioning of the lower back and knees. Treatment, in most cases, therefore, needs to be directed at underlying issues of Kidney function as outlined in Chapter 9 – Urinary system. Strong treatments of this condition may lead to worsening of symptoms, as the energy is not strong enough to cope. Gentle strengthening treatments are more appropriate and need to be applied long-term. In the short-term, the back pain may not change much but you will be looking for improvement on inner levels first.

All surgical procedures tend to further weaken the back and holistic practitioners may find treatment subsequent to these interventions have a less favourable outcome.

Case one
A man of 45 years came for treatment of his acute back pain. He had injured his back whilst lifting a heavy object and he was in marked discomfort when I saw him in the clinic. He had severe low back pain, with reduced movements of his lumbar spine and he held himself stiff as movement exacerbated the pain. His diagnosis in terms of Chinese medicine was Stagnation of Qi and Blood in the Urinary Bladder channel. I treated him using two points on the back of his hand for acute low back pain, Yaotong. I asked him to move his back as I manipulated the needles and within 10 minutes his back was feeling much looser and less painful. I followed this up with local points in his back and local heat. After a 30-minute

treatment his back was feeling sore but more mobile and not painful. The next day he was fine, he felt pain-free and his back was moving normally. Treating acute back pain in someone who is healthy and fit is very satisfying as improvement is almost immediate. Whilst I was in general practice, I used to treat acute back pain with ear acupuncture and people were amazed that they could feel better so quickly.

Case two

A woman of 38 years came for treatment of her back pain. It had started some 6 months previously with a 'crick' in her neck that had gradually worsened. When I saw her, she had pain in her neck radiating down to the thoracic area that then continued to the lower back and her right leg. She would develop pins and needles in her right leg on walking. Her pain was so severe at times that she could hardly walk and the painkillers she had to take made her feel ill with nausea, headaches and migraine. Her energy was low and she felt constantly tired. She had a tendency to loose bowels with rich food. I made a diagnosis of Spleen Qi Deficiency, Kidney Yang Deficiency, Liver Blood Deficiency and Stagnation of Qi and Blood in the Urinary Bladder channels of her lower and upper back. In such a case, gentle strengthening and tonifying treatments are of great importance and treatment tends to be prolonged. She had already been seeing a cranial osteopath for several months with some improvement in her symptoms. I find that a combination of Chinese medical treatment and cranial work to be extremely efficacious in such cases.

I treated her with acupuncture and Chinese herbal medicine. After the first treatment she had a slight improvement in her back pain, however, it did not last long. It was after the second treatment that she reported improved energy levels and said that her back and neck were much better with less pain. I did not expect her to improve so quickly and the fact that she had done so was an indication that her constitution was generally good and that after some further treatments she could expect to feel much better. She has now been having treatment for 7 months and her back is generally good. She has some discomfort if she sits or stands for long periods but otherwise her activity is not limited and she has little pain. Her energy is good and her life is much more comfortable. Her treatment continues but I am extremely optimistic that she will be pain-free and without symptoms.

Case three

A boy of 10 years came for treatment. He had suffered severe pains in his right lumbar area, which felt like needles or swords, since the age of 5. These pains went from his back through to his abdomen. The pains were better for bending over and also for pinching his back. At 8 years the pains returned and it was suspected that it might be due to a longer rib. Recently the pains had worsened and despite many investigations nothing could be detected.

Strangely the child had been born with a fractured skull and then at 18 months he had a very bad fall in which he hit his head and broke his front teeth. There was talk of having to open the skull to release the pressure caused by the injury, but the swelling went down of its own accord.

The boy had very strong opinions about most things and used the word 'hate' all the time. He hated untidiness. He hated people who moved his things. He hated reading and spelling (but liked maths). He hated being away from home even for a short time. He hated heat. He loved poached eggs and they had to be cooked to perfection – he did this himself. He said if he could he would eat three or four a day. He could be constipated for up to a week and it didn't really bother him. He had pain in the base of his right little finger and in both ankles.

This was a textbook case of Calc. Carb. (a remedy made from the inside of the oyster shell). Early on his protective covering (skull) was damaged twice, leaving him feeling vulnerable and in need of order and structure in his life. This was why he hated spelling, because of the lack of logic and order, but enjoyed maths where 2+2 is always 4.

I gave him Calc. Carb. 1M and after one hour all his symptoms including the severe back and abdominal pain got much better and this lasted for 3 weeks. He lost his desire for eggs. His reading improved. He didn't feel the need to be at home so much and was in better form. He told me he was happy he had come for treatment. The remedy was repeated as needed.

DISEASES OF THE PERIPHERAL NERVES

Mononeuropathy

This is disease of a single nerve. It is usually due to injury or compression. A typical example of this is carpal tunnel syndrome – Page 185. Another common situation is injury of the ulnar nerve at the elbow, the radial nerve in the axilla[17] or the peroneal nerve at the knee. The clinical picture is of a lower motor neurone weakness with sensory loss. They may take up to 4 to 6 weeks to recover.

A multiple form is seen in systemic diseases. These include:

- diabetes mellitus
- autoimmune disease, e.g. systemic lupus erythematosus, polyarteritis nodosa, temporal arteritis, rheumatoid arthritis
- sarcoidosis
- AIDS.

DISORDERS OF THE HEAD AND FACE

Trigeminal neuralgia

This condition occurs mainly in the elderly and is of unknown cause in conventional medicine. It is also known as 'tic douloureux'.

Symptoms
There is pain in the face in the distribution of the fifth (trigeminal) cranial nerve. Maxillary and/or mandibular divisions are usually affected. It is rarely felt around the temple or eye and most people have pain over the upper and lower jaws. Particular areas, which are troublesome, are the gums, the edge of the nostril and in front of the ear. The pain is characteristically severe and sharp or stabbing. It occurs in episodes where there will be pain every day and probably all day for several days, weeks or months. It is sharp in nature and can be excruciating. There are often trigger areas where contact such as washing, brushing the teeth or eating will set off attacks of pain. There are remissions when the pain goes but these become shorter and shorter as time passes.

Treatment
This is usually with carbamazepine, an anticonvulsant. It is frequently used for any neuralgic condition. It works to a variable extent and there are side-effects on other parts of the central nervous system. I treated a woman with this condition who, whenever she took this drug, would develop weakness in her legs and would have to use a wheelchair.

Some people may be given benzodiazepines or phenytoin. The aim of all the drug treatments is to sedate the central nervous system and damp down its activity.

Surgical destruction or injection with alcohol may be used in intransigent cases to destroy the nerve function. This leads to numbness in the face.

Holistic management
In terms of Chinese medicine, the usual syndromes that correspond are Wind-heat Invasion, Fire in the Liver and Stomach or Yin Deficiency with Yang excess. It frequently comes on after a shock – emotional or physical and, in my experience, treatment with acupuncture is very effective.

Facial paralysis (Bell's palsy)

This is a disorder of the seventh cranial nerve of unknown cause. It is considered to be associated with oedema of the facial nerve as it passes through the facial canal in the base of the skull and this may be associated with a viral infection. Men are just as likely as women to suffer from it and it can come on at any age.

Symptoms
There is a one-sided facial paralysis where the person cannot close the affected eye. The mouth is drawn over to the opposite side and saliva and fluids may escape from the corner of the mouth. There is paralysis of the upper and lower parts of the affected side of face. The taste may be affected over the front two-thirds of the tongue. It typically lasts for several weeks and then subsides. Some people (15 per cent) are left with a chronic weakness where wasting will be evident. There is considered to be recovery in 85 per cent of cases after 2 to 3 weeks, which is usually complete after 2 to 3 months. Recovery may take many months.

This is an example of a lower motor neurone type of paralysis. If the forehead muscles are normal on both sides then the facial paralysis is of the upper motor neurone type as will occur in a stroke and the approach to this will be completely different. It is important to make this differentiation.

Treatment
There is little which is effective since the cause is not known. Corticosteroids are often given in a short reducing course. Around 60 mg daily are given at first, reducing to zero over a week or 10 days. In some cases, adrenocorticotrophic hormone

(ACTH) may be injected to stimulate the person's own corticosteroid levels. Care is taken to reduce or prevent problems of corneal damage, as the eyelid cannot close on the affected side.

Persistent cases are treated by cosmetic surgery perhaps with an attempt to reactivate the nerve by joining it to a normal nerve.

Holistic management

In China, it occurs in large numbers in the spring and is due to the winds that appear at that time of year. Certainly people often report that it came on after they were in a draught. In terms of Chinese medicine, this is a case of Wind-cold Invasion affecting the channels of the face. In the West, there is almost always an underlying deficient condition, which allows for this invasion.

Headache and migraine

This is a pain in the head. It is very common and probably there isn't anyone who does not suffer from this at some time in their lives. Many people have recurrent problems. An occasional one is probably a 'normal' reaction to many influences either physical or emotional. However, if they become severe or frequent, they indicate a chronic imbalance.

There are many different associations with the symptom of headache. In conventional medicine, the search is for an underlying physical cause, which can then be treated – usually in the head or neck. The vast majority of causes are seen in Western medicine as being non-serious. The exceptions to this are cerebral tumour, meningitis and cerebral vascular problems.

Cranial arteritis is seen in the elderly. Such headaches tend to be severe and diffuse. Temporal tenderness is only one manifestation. They are usually severe enough to be troublesome at night and interfere with sleep.

Pain can be referred from eye diseases such as glaucoma and iritis. They are frontal in site and there are the signs of the underlying disease. 'Eye strain' is conventionally considered to be an uncommon situation and certainly rarely regarded as a cause of headaches. However, some people who overuse their eyes, especially in conditions of poor lighting and when tired will develop headaches.

Nasal or sinus disease can produce pains in the head and these can be severe. The most usual sinus to be involved is the maxillary. Pain is felt in the face with tenderness over the sinuses. There will also be the other symptoms of sinusitis.

Dental conditions can cause headaches, usually frontal, or in the face. Tapping on the suspected tooth will produce pain. Such causes of pain are notoriously difficult to pin down on occasion and I have known people to have recurrent dental surgery in an attempt to track down the source of the pain.

Aural conditions lead to headaches as in cases of otitis media or mastoiditis.

Cervical spondylosis is commonly associated with headaches. They are usually occipital in site. The pain is felt at the back of the neck, up into the head and can on occasions radiate into the frontal area. It can be severe with limitation of movement of the neck and perhaps creaking and cracking.

A cold stimulus on the soft palate leads to a frontal headache in the so-called 'ice-cream headache'.

Neuralgias in the head and face typically cause severe pains. Trigeminal neuralgia is usually in the face although if the ophthalmic division of the nerve is affected then it will be felt further up the head. It is classically episodic and sharp. It occurs in paroxysms and is intractable. The pain of post-herpetic neuralgia however is continuous and burning in quality. It follows on from herpes zoster of the face and here it is usually severe.

Meningeal irritation is a situation that indicates a serious and possibly life-threatening situation. The three diseases to bear in mind are encephalitis, meningitis and subarachnoid haemorrhage. The pain is generalised but is worse occipitally. It is continuous, of an aching or boring quality and there are signs of 'meningism'.[18] This is evidence of meningeal irritation, which exhibits itself as photophobia and neck stiffness. The neck stiffness can be elicited by raising the neck and trying to put the person's chin on their chest. This will produce marked pain in the occiput and will reveal a lot of neck stiffness. A fever is often in evidence with the first two conditions.

Investigations

This depends on the history. Conventional medicine considers about two or three conditions particularly serious and the person will be investigated if these are suspected. Otherwise, treatment is instituted with no further action being taken.

Migraine

These are periodic headaches, which are typically one sided in site. The term migraine is derived from 'hemicrania' – one side of head. In conventional medicine, migraine is considered to be due to a disturbance in blood flow to the brain. There is firstly constriction of blood vessels followed by vasodilatation. It is constriction in the blood vessels, which is associated with the visual symptoms and dilatation that leads to the classical headache. This explanation explains the emphasis in conventional treatment of using drugs that affect blood flow. Three-quarters of people with migraine have a family history of this condition.

Symptoms

Visual disturbances such as flashing or coloured lights are a common association. There may be vomiting during an attack. There are several precipitating factors where the headaches are more likely to occur. They are more likely around times of emotional stress or anxiety and around menstruation. They may also be triggered by flashing lights, or certain foods. They usually occur between puberty to middle life and come in paroxysms.

An attack is different for each person but typically it starts with visual symptoms as described above. In severe cases there may even be pins and needles or weakness of one part or half of the body. This can last for up to half an hour. Then the pain starts, usually in one spot around the temple and spreads to the whole of one side of the head. It is severe, throbbing and there may or may not be vomiting. There is usually a degree of photophobia. There is often pallor, sweating and an attack may be so severe that the person may be prostrated. Many people end up in bed and have to lie in a darkened room. Tiredness is a common association and some people may feel weakened for a day or so after an attack. They typically occur at periods of relaxation and so weekends and the first few days of a holiday are common times for migraine.

Treatment

It is helpful for some people to avoid triggers especially if it is something specific such as red wine or prawns. Drugs are frequently used conventionally. They may either be those that are designed to prevent attacks or those to be given during an attack.

Treatment	Comments
Diuretic	Aims to reduce fluid retention. Variable effectiveness. Described in detail on Page 107
Paracetamol with buclizine	Simple analgesic with antihistamine
Ergotamine	Powerful drug that constricts arteries. When used in excess it may cause gangrene
Tranquilliser	Used on the assumption that there is an emotional basis. Rapidly addictive and causes depression when used for pain
Clonidine	Also used in high blood pressure and flushing attacks. Dangerous to stop suddenly
Betablocker	Described in detail in Chapter 7 – Cardiovascular system. Weakens the digestion, heart and kidneys
Sumatriptan	New, powerful drug. When used frequently it tends to lead to more migraine attacks presumably due to a depleting effect
Methysergide	Powerful drug related to lysergic acid diethylamide (LSD). Causes fibrosis in the abdomen with horrific consequences. Must not be given for more than 6 months continuously. Must be withdrawn slowly

Table 14.9: Conventional treatment of migraine

Holistic management

The conventional label of migraine is a loose collection of different energetic entities. In terms of Chinese Medicine there are common associations with Stagnant Liver Qi, Stomach Heat or Liver Blood Deficiency. With imbalances of the Liver there may be a particular association with emotional disturbances or the menses. In the case of Stomach Heat, the headaches will be worse with dietary factors such as red wine, chocolate and shellfish – all of which are heating energetically. Liver Blood Deficient headaches tend to be worse with standing, overwork and during or after menstruation.

The typical site of the headache will tend to be temporal with Liver pathologies whereas they are frontal with a Stomach imbalance. Associated symptoms include irritability and visual disturbances with Liver imbalances. This type of headache will be precipitated or exacerbated by the oral contraceptive which Stagnates Liver Qi.

Vomiting is common if the Stomach is primarily involved. Clearly the Stomach and Liver functions are closely interwoven as combinations of these symptoms may occur.

Case one

A woman of 32 years came for treatment of her migraine headaches. These had begun at the age of 15 years but had been worse for the past 9 years. They took the form of right-sided headaches mainly around the right eye. Occasionally, the pain would pass back to the right side of the occiput. Nausea and sometimes vomiting always occurred with the headache. She had attacks twice each month but also had what she described as ordinary headaches more often. These would affect the temples and forehead for several days each week.

Her general energy was low and particularly so in the afternoon. She had low back pain regularly and a tendency to loose motions. Her periods tended to be heavy at the beginning with some cramping pains. The diagnosis, in terms of Chinese medicine, was Spleen Qi Deficiency with Damp Accumulation and Liver Qi Stagnation.

I treated her with acupuncture and herbs together with general advice about diet to strengthen the digestive energy and relaxation. She worked long hours in the city with much travelling each day. Gradually, after a couple of month's treatment she began to feel better with more energy and less headaches. Her migraines declined in number to once per month (before menstruation) and then stopped completely. After 6 months of treatment she felt well with only occasional headaches when she was overtired or particularly stressed.

Case two

A woman of 35 years came for treatment of her migraine headaches. She had them on and off since she was 13 years old. They resumed whenever she felt particularly stressed. Her energy was slightly low. The migraines took the form of pain in the occipital region, which passed over the head to above the left eye. She would have associated nausea and dizziness. Her other symptoms included abdominal bloating and slight oedema before her periods.

In terms of Chinese medicine, this is Liver Qi Stagnation with Spleen Qi Deficiency. Her energy was not so low as in the case described above. This was reflected in treatment as she responded very quickly. Her headaches disappeared after three treatments and she had a few more treatments to consolidate her progress. She had also had other holistic medical treatments in the past because she was keen on avoiding suppressive, chemical forms of treatment. She also had a strong interest in the philosophical views of holistic medicine. Such people respond much more quickly and effectively to treatment.

Case three

A boy aged 12 years came for treatment of his migraine attacks. These were very severe and during them he was tempted to jump out of the window. For this reason he wanted his mother to stay with him. He would bite both his own hand and his mother's during the height of the pain. This was throbbing, left-sided and began over the eye. It was worse for any light and was accompanied by stomach cramps and vomiting. The migraines often came on after over-excitement. He also suffered from asthma and this too became worse after excitement or exertion.

He was prescribed Glonoine 30c not only because it is a classic migraine remedy, but also because one of the symptoms it can produce is the desire to jump out of the window. Let like be cured with like...

The migraines became much less frequent, at one point he went over 18 months without one. If he did get one it could be nipped in the bud with Glonoine. However the asthma did not respond much to the remedy and after reviewing the case, the prescription has now been changed to Veratrum.

HOW TO RECOGNISE A SERIOUS CONDITION OF THE NERVOUS SYSTEM

Diseases of the central nervous system are common in our society and the symptoms listed below are extremely common. It is important to know how to recognise if a symptom arises from a serious situation. You can use Table 14.10 as a guide to refer to when faced with a person who has one or more of these symptoms. I do not mention disease labels in the column on the right, as I would not expect you to be able to diagnose conventionally. Seriousness can be assessed merely by reference to symptom pictures. However, you will be able to recognise that there are clinical appearances that would be diagnosed as a particular disease. For example, if you look at the comments about headache (in the following Table), you will see that this is the appearance of a brain tumour.

Symptom	Comments
Headache	Progressive, severe with short history, with other central nervous system symptoms
Tremor	Severe, progressive
Numbness	Severe, progressive
Paralysis	Always
Tingling	Severe, progressive
Dizziness	Severe, progressive
Convulsions	Always
Loss of consciousness	Not if short duration with specific trigger (see Page 94)
Stiffness	Severe
Pain	Severe

Table 14.10: How to recognise a serious condition of the central nervous system

SUMMARY

Conventional anatomy and physiology of the central nervous system is complex.

The essence of physiology is the important aspect and this knowledge of function can provide most of what a holistic practitioner needs to know.

Symptoms of central nervous system dysfunction are similar in many varied disorders. It is their development and timing that are the important factors in determining the underlying process.

Conventional medicine is not particularly effective at treating such disorders.

Holistic medicine can offer people real benefits, sometimes to a surprising degree, in central nervous system disease.

You must know the presenting symptoms of the life-threatening conditions, i.e. meningitis, brain tumour.

---

[1] *Rainbow of Liberated Energy* by Ngakpa Chögyam (Element, 1986) contains, in the Introduction, an account of the effect of meditative practices on the EEG.

[2] Evidence of this can be seen when the influence of 'higher centres' is removed. People who are insane or emotionally charged are very strong and may require several others to control them. Experts in various forms of martial arts can be solidly planted on the ground to the extent that several people cannot knock them over. There are cases of mothers who have seen their children run over by cars. They have been able to lift vehicles off their children.

[3] This is a tremor which gets worse on movement.

[4] The area of skin supplied by a specific nerve is called a dermatome. Maps of such areas and the nerves supplying them can be found in anatomy books.

[5] This is disease of a peripheral nerve. There are many causes and some are discussed later.

[6] *The Foundations of Chinese Medicine* by Giovanni Maciocia (Churchill Livingstone, 1989).

[7] Five years later, 1 in 4 are dead due to heart attack or stroke and 1 in 6 have had a stroke.

[8] A feeling of being in a familiar place or having done the same thing previously.

[9] All anticonvulsants may damage the blood but particularly ethosuximide and phenytoin. The latter can actually lead to lymphoma – cancer of the lymphatic system.

[10] Kinnunen, Esko *et al. Archives of Neurology,* 1990;47(7):743(4).

[11] This is a tremor which increases with movement as the object is approached. It is typical of a co-ordination difficulty due to cerebellar involvement.

[12] A survey of 134 people with multiple sclerosis over a course of 34 years showed that a low-fat diet leads to significantly less deterioration and lower death rates from the disease. It works best at an early stage of the disease. Swank, R.L., *et al. Lancet,* 1990;336(8706):37(3). Also, Swank, R.L. *Am J Med Sci* 1950;220:421-30. Also, Swank R.L. *Nutrition* 1991;7:368-76.

[13] Here I am relating the intake of foods which generate mucus in the body with the climatic factor of dampness.

[14] This has been confirmed by studies such as Millar JHD, *et al. Br Med J* 1973; 1:765-8 and Bates D, *et al. Br Med J* 1978;2:1390-1.

[15] This allows a lower dose of L-dopa to be taken thus reducing side-effects of nausea which otherwise may prevent its use.

[16] In my experience, many people who undergo laminectomy gain little relief. Relapses are common in the months after surgery. A study of workers who had undergone laminectomy showed that they were six times more likely to develop back injuries. James R, *et al. Journal of Occupational Medicine,* 1990;32(5):468(5).

[17] This is known as 'drunkard's' palsy as it occurs after falling asleep with the arm over the back of a chair.

[18] A difficulty arises in diagnosis because meningism of a lesser degree may be seen in children with upper respiratory infections and fever. The symptoms are mild and do not progress. This situation and early meningitis can be confused in the unwary.

15 ENDOCRINE SYSTEM

INTRODUCTION

The endocrine system is where conventional medicine recognises the concept of balance. There are control mechanisms that maintain hormone levels within narrow limits. In addition, hormones from the same or different organs may have effects that are opposite to each other. These need to be in balance for the body to function efficiently. For example, in the case of blood sugar control, insulin and its opposite hormone, glucagon, are partially responsible for maintaining sugar levels in the blood within closely determined limits. Other hormones such as corticosteroids, adrenaline and noradrenaline also have a part to play in this.

In endocrine disturbances, there may be overactivity or underactivity. Each of these presents a particular symptom picture that has a close relationship with conditions recognised by Chinese medicine. Homoeopaths may also recognise remedy pictures in the descriptions given later. In terms of Chinese medicine, the duality of Yin/Yang philosophy can be recognised in the extreme states of imbalance seen in endocrine disorders. For example, overactivity of the adrenal gland can be recognised as an excess of Yang energy and underactivity of the adrenal gland as a lack of Yang energy, i.e. a Yin state. These comments are amplified when discussing each disease in turn.

There has been rapid progress recently in the conventional investigation of endocrine disease. It is now possible to determine blood levels of many hormones and so gross dysfunction can be diagnosed more accurately. Disorders that are the result of too little of the respective hormone being released into the circulation are treated by replacement. Other endocrine disorders are due to overactivity and treatment, conventionally, comprises either partial removal (or destruction) of the gland, or the use of a chemical which blocks the action of the hormone released by it.

When treating people people who either have severe disease or who take replacement hormones, holistic practitioners need to be aware that the situation may be life-threatening. Care must be taken with such cases. If hormone replacements are stopped or reduced without adequate checks on blood levels there may be serious problems. For example, it is manifestly dangerous for a person with diabetes mellitus taking daily insulin injections to reduce or stop insulin without effective treatment of the underlying condition. This is true for all endocrine abnormalities.

An additional factor to consider is the general effect of holistic medical treatment on a person's hormone balance. Holistic treatments do not treat one specific area. It is necessary to bear in mind the effect on endocrine hormones whatever the presenting symptom. There are significant numbers of people taking regular hormone replacements[1] who will come for treatment of what they consider to be an unrelated problem. Careful case taking will involve asking for details of any medication they are currently taking. Since holistic medicine may improve endocrine function as the person recovers, reduction of prescribed replacement hormones will be necessary to avoid overdosage. Monitoring is of prime importance to ensure that such situations are handled safely and appropriately.

ANATOMY AND PHYSIOLOGY

I want to spend some time describing the essential features of the endocrine system. In addition, I shall introduce some information that may be new to you but will hopefully serve to make some connections with holistic medical views. Before studying disease of the endocrine system you will need to familiarise yourself with its anatomy and physiology. Check that you are able to:

- list the organs contained in the endocrine system
- state the hormones secreted by each organ
- describe the function of these hormones
- explain the homeostatic mechanisms and feedback systems of the endocrine system.

The endocrine system is composed of the hypothalamus, pituitary and various end organs,[2] the most important of which, for clinical purposes, are the thyroid, ovaries, testes and adrenal glands. All these organs are interconnected and are influenced by feedback mechanisms of control – Table 15.1.

```
Hypothalamus
Pituitary
Pineal
Thyroid
Parathyroid
Pancreas
Adrenal
Ovary
Testis
```

Table 15.1: Endocrine organs

The hypothalamus can be considered as the centre. It releases hormones, which influence the pituitary. This, in turn, secretes hormones to stimulate a relevant end organ. For example, thyrotrophic-releasing hormone (TRH) is released by the hypothalamus and stimulates the production by the pituitary of thyroid stimulating hormone (TSH). This, in turn, stimulates the thyroid gland, which releases thyroxine (T_4) and tri-iodothyronine (T_3). These circulating levels of T_3 and T_4 influence hypothalamic function.

If the circulating levels of T_3 and T_4 are low, the hypothalamus increases its production of TRH. If circulating levels of T_3 and T_4 are high, the hypothalamus reduces the secretion of TRH. In this way, levels of T_3 and T_4 are kept within normal limits. There are similar *negative feedback* mechanisms for the adrenal gland, testes and ovaries. The parathyroid and pancreas have a different mechanism as they produce hormones in response to blood levels of the substances they control. Specifically, the parathyroid responds to blood calcium levels and the pancreas to blood sugar levels.

The secretion of hypothalamic hormones is dependent upon a wide variety of stimuli – nervous, metabolic, physical and hormonal. The hypothalamus is the interface between the endocrine system and the central nervous system. It is the means by which external events influence the endocrine system. It responds to changes in temperature, to the amount of light in the environment and to psychological factors. This validates the Chinese view that natural life cycles and the environment have important roles to play in human health.[3] Awareness of the workings of the hypothalamus represents the beginning of an understanding in conventional thought that human beings do not exist in splendid isolation. Sadly, such ideas are not reflected in available treatments.

The endocrine glands may also be considered from the viewpoint of the chakras. The testes and ovary relate to the base chakra, the adrenals to the chakra around the kidney area, the pancreas to the solar plexus, the thymus to the heart chakra, and the thyroid to the throat chakra, the pituitary to the brow and the pineal to the crown chakra.

CLASSIFICATION OF ENDOCRINE SYSTEM DISEASE

The most important organs to consider, in terms of clinical significance, are the thyroid, ovary, testis and adrenal. Conventionally, the classification centres on the physical organ that is responsible for the imbalance – Table 15.2.

It can be seen that there is no mention of hypothalamic disorders as they are extremely difficult to diagnose. Therefore, the interconnections between the hypothalamus and the external environment and psychological state are completely missed by most conventional practitioners. The main treatments (applied to the diseases listed) focus on the end organ, for example, thyroid or adrenal. This is a classical case of suppression, in any terms, since the root is not treated. The administration of hormones only serves to suppress endocrine system function.

Hyperthyroidism (overactivity of the thyroid gland), for example, is frequently the result of a psychological disturbance. Removing part of the gland surgically or destroying the gland by radioactivity does nothing to resolve the underlying imbalance.

```
Pituitary gland
        Tumours of the pituitary
        Pituitary overactivity
        Pituitary underactivity
                Diabetes insipidus

Thyroid gland
        Goitre
        Hyperthyroidism
        Hypothyroidism
        Hashimoto's thyroiditis
        Subacute thyroiditis
        Tumours of the thyroid gland
                Benign tumours
                Carcinoma

Pancreas
        Diabetes mellitus

Adrenal gland
        Adrenal Cortex
                Overactivity
                        Cushing's syndrome
                        Hyperaldosteronism
                Underactivity
                        Addison's disease
        Adrenal Medulla
                Phaeochromocytoma
```

Table 15.2: Conventional classification of endocrine disease (italics indicate those of most clinical importance)

A more practical classification, from the point of view of a holistic practitioner, is to consider the severity of the disorder and the pace of change. Thus, a disease such as diabetes mellitus, which may produce rapid deterioration in health, would be more severe than hypothyroidism, which presents with a much slower clinical progress – Table 15.3.

```
        Mild disease

        Hyperthyroidism
        Hypothyroidism
        Cushing's syndrome
        Diabetes mellitus
        Diabetes insipidus
        Addison's disease

        Severe disease
```

Table 15.3: Energetic classification of disease of the endocrine system

DIABETES INSIPIDUS

This is an uncommon disease that may be confused with diabetes mellitus. The word 'diabetes' refers to the passage of large volumes of urine and before urine testing was available tasting the urine made the distinction between these two diseases. People with diabetes insipidus pass large quantities of urine that is bland to the taste whilst those with diabetes mellitus pass large quantities of urine that is sweet.

In conventional medicine, there are two types of diabetes insipidus. A cranial form is associated with an inadequate production of antidiuretic hormone (vasopressin) by the pituitary gland. A renal type is when the kidney is unresponsive to the effects of vasopressin.

All types of diabetes insipidus are rare. The cranial type may either occur after meningitis or head injury or be the result of a pituitary tumour. Diabetes insipidus due to kidney unresponsiveness may be genetic, due to the effects of heavy metal poisoning or treatment with lithium.[4]

Symptoms

There are the characteristic symptoms of frequent urination, the persistent passage of large quantities of pale urine and constant thirst. The person may pass up to 20 or more litres of urine in 24 hours. The urine is clear in appearance. As dehydration develops there will be confusion and eventually fits and unconsciousness.

Investigations

The usual method of diagnosing cranial diabetes insipidus is to withhold water and measure the specific gravity of urine, which does not rise in this disease. It will do so if vasopressin is given. The main distinction to be made is between this condition and diabetes mellitus.

Treatment

This is usually with the long-acting type of vasopressin, desmopressin (DDAVP). It is given intranasally or intramuscularly. The dosage in each case is individually assessed depending upon how much urine is produced. Other drugs that may be used include thiazide diuretics, carbamazepine or chlorpropamide. Thiazide diuretics remain the only effective drug therapy for renal diabetes insipidus and reduce urine volume in this condition by about 50 per cent.

THYROID GLAND

The thyroid gland produces two hormones, thyroxine (T_4) and tri-iodothyronine (T_3), which control the rate of the metabolism. Production of these hormones is influenced by thyroid stimulating hormone (TSH) from the pituitary gland. The gland itself is situated over the thyroid cartilage in the neck and upper end of the trachea. It may be palpable in women with no other indications of thyroid imbalance. Embryologically, the thyroid gland originates in the pharynx between anterior and posterior sections of the tongue. It migrates downwards to its eventual position in the throat along the thyroglossal duct. If this duct persists beyond foetal life, cysts may occasionally develop in children. This connection between the thyroid gland and the tongue, throat and larynx is explored later – Page 293.

The two main clinical syndromes of the thyroid gland are overactivity and underactivity. They provide excellent examples of the need for balance within the body to prevent the appearance of the extremes that result from the over or under production of hormones. Both syndromes are primarily autoimmune in nature as the body produces antibodies against the thyroid gland. In overactivity of the thyroid gland, hyperthyroidism, these antibodies serve to stimulate the thyroid gland. In underactivity of the thyroid gland, hypothyroidism, these antibodies are destructive in nature. The natural history of thyroid disease is firstly to respond to the autoimmune disturbance by stimulation and then by exhaustion. This is a common feature of all organs in that the first stage of disease is characterised by overactivity that is eventually replaced by non-reaction.

Hyperthyroidism[5]

This is overproduction of the thyroid hormones, thyroxine (T_4) and/or tri-iodothyronine (T_3). Frequently, there are associated autoimmune disorders such as diabetes mellitus and pernicious anaemia.

Hyperthyroidism is common. It affects about 1 in 20 women at some time in their lives, most commonly between 15 and 20 years of age. Men are rarely affected with nine times more cases seen in women. There are increased levels of thyroid hormone in the blood so levels of thyroid stimulating hormone are reduced sometimes to extremely low levels. This is an attempt by the pituitary to reduce the amount of stimulation to the thyroid gland. There is invariably an associated goitre.[6]

In most people with hyperthyroidism, the thyroid gland is either generally overactive or there are several nodules which are overproductive of thyroid hormones. The general overactive type with diffuse goitre is seen in young people. The cases involving nodules (toxic nodular goitres) tend to occur in older people.

Symptoms

The symptoms of hyperthyroidism are conventionally explained as due to an overproduction of thyroid hormones. These are responsible for controlling the metabolic rate, i.e. the amount of energy consumed by the body. A by-product of energy usage is heat and so many of the symptoms are related to this:
- feelings of (internal) heat with intolerance to (external) heat
- sweating
- increased appetite yet weight loss
- raised heart rate
- palpitations
- diarrhoea
- tiredness
- anxiety
- tremor of the fingers
- thyroid gland enlargement (goitre) – this is common and is usually a soft, diffuse swelling of both lobes.

Other features are difficult to explain conventionally:

- exophthalmos
- pretibial myxoedema[7]
- finger clubbing[8]
- reduced fertility
- menstrual irregularities
- muscle weakness.

Exophthalmos is a protrusion of one or both eyes. It can be detected in most cases because it is possible to see the white sclera above and below the iris. Exposure of the cornea may result from eyelids failing to close properly leading to keratitis. There is grittiness in the eye and excessive watering. The conjunctivae can become red and swollen. Double vision can be present because of the weakness of extraocular muscles. It is first detected when the person is asked to look upwards and outwards.

In some, exophthalmos may precede the development of the symptoms of hyperthyroidism by some months or years. The conventional treatment of hyperthyroidism has no effect on exophthalmos which would again confirm that the underlying process is unaffected by such treatment.

The natural history of hyperthyroidism is variable. Some people recover within a few months or a year whilst others have more persistent problems. A few develop a 'thyrotoxic crisis', which is uncommon as drug therapy is given to all. This is a state of severe mental and physical exhaustion with delirium, delusions or mania, dehydration, palpitations, oedema and fever. The person literally 'burns up'.

Complications

Complication	Symptoms to look for
Cardiac failure	Oedema, breathlessness
Thyroid (thyrotoxic) crisis	Extremely rapid heart rate, high fever, severe agitation

Table 15.4: Complications of hyperthyroidism

Investigations

There are raised levels of thyroxine (T_4) and tri-iodothyronine (T_3) with reduced or virtually absent levels of thyroid stimulating hormone. There are a wide range of normal results and errors occur so several estimates are the ideal. The presence of minor symptoms with blood levels near normality may not need immediate conventional treatment. It is the complete picture that is more important and as with all investigations, single estimations should be viewed as only one aspect of the case. A radionuclide scan of the thyroid may be used to assess the appearance of the thyroid gland.

Treatment

The aim of conventional treatment is to achieve normal blood levels of thyroid hormones. There are three methods of doing this.

Antithyroid drugs

Antithyroid drugs block the function of the thyroid gland and thereby reduce the amount of thyroid hormone produced. A commonly used example is carbimazole in the UK and its relative, methimazole, in the US. Propylthiouracil is occasionally used in the event of allergy to carbimazole.

Antithyroid drugs are given initially for 3 to 4 weeks, according to the severity of the condition and the size of the goitre. Thereafter, the dose is reduced according to symptoms. The aim is to maintain a normal thyroid state with as little medication as possible. The normal dosage of carbimazole is between 5 and 30 mg daily.

Overtreatment with antithyroid drugs will result in increased thyroid stimulating hormone production by the pituitary and an increase in thyroid size. Carbimazole may be given as sole treatment or as a preparation for surgery. If used alone, these drugs are given for at least 1 year and restricted to people who do not have a large goitre.

Just under half of people treated in this way recover and do not require further treatment. The probability of relapse after 6-12 months treatment with antithyroid drugs is more likely in the presence of autoimmune disease.

Antithyroid drugs may produce toxic effects. The most common is a rash and the most serious are blood disorders, agranulocytosis being the most frequent. Routine white cell counts are of little value in its early detection as it occurs with dramatic suddenness. People taking these drugs must be told to report a sore throat and to stop the drug immediately until it is clear whether agranulocytosis has occurred or not.

Betablockers are commonly given in addition to specific antithyroid drugs to reduce symptoms of palpitations, increased heart rate, anxiety, tremors, sweating and so forth. These are merely symptomatic in their action and have no influence on the thyroid gland itself.

Surgical treatment
This is usually applied if the person is too young for radioactive iodine or antithyroid drugs have failed. People with large goitres may be offered surgery no matter what their age. Men are considered to relapse more often after antithyroid drug treatment and so may be considered for surgery earlier rather than later.

The amount of thyroid gland that is removed at operation is based upon an assessment made by the surgeon. Clearly the function of the thyroid gland is reduced after partial removal and about 4 out of 5 people who have a partial thyroidectomy have no problems for around 3-5 years. In 15 per cent there will either be a recurrence of the hyperthyroidism or hypothyroidism will develop after the operation. This latter situation requires the administration of thyroxine supplements.

Local effects of surgery to the thyroid may include damage to the recurrent laryngeal nerve, which occurs in a small percentage of people and will produce temporary hoarseness. The normal function of both vocal cords should be confirmed before surgery and checked after surgery. The parathyroid glands, which are usually situated in the substance of the thyroid gland, may be temporarily damaged by the surgery or occasionally removed leading to disturbances of calcium metabolism. Damage to the parathyroid glands may lead to persistent low calcium levels in the blood and so long-term follow-ups should include checks for cataracts and any mental disturbance. Second operations on the thyroid gland often damage the recurrent laryngeal nerve and the parathyroid glands and so are rarely done. The appearance of hyperthyroidism after surgery is always treated with radioactive iodine.

Radioactive iodine
Using radioactive iodine destroys a proportion of the gland. Iodine is concentrated in the thyroid gland as it is an integral part of the thyroid hormone molecule. Administration of radioactive iodine concentrates radioactivity in the thyroid gland and this destroys the thyroid cells. It is mainly used for people over the age of 40 years and certainly when having children is no longer a likelihood. It may also be given to young people who have been sterilised or if they have an associated condition which shortens life expectancy. The actual dose to be administered is difficult to calculate accurately for various technical reasons. Regular review is essential until such time as the person has become hypothyroid and is on a suitable life-long replacement dose of thyroxine. As with surgical treatment, there is no attempt to affect the underlying process. Hypothyroidism affects most people within 20 years following treatment with radioactive iodine.

Hypothyroidism

This is underactivity of thyroid gland function. It is occasionally due to pituitary disease but the common situation in clinical practice is autoimmune disease where there may be a history of hyperthyroidism. There may be a history of conventional treatment of hyperthyroidism, i.e. drugs, surgery or radioactive iodine. Some cases develop spontaneously with no previous history of overactive thyroid function.

Hypothyroidism is primarily seen in women and there is almost always an associated goitre. Inflammation may be an important feature where thyroiditis may be diagnosed.

An uncommon cause of hypothyroidism nowadays is iodine deficiency. This is more common in areas a long way from the sea. Iodine, essential for the normal functioning of the thyroid gland, is found in abundance in seafood, seaweed[9] and the like. The connection between such a clinical appearance and mountainous areas was noted by the Chinese during the Sui dynasty in the 6th century AD. 'Derbyshire neck' is the term used in the UK and reflects the distance of this English county from the sea. Such a development is unusual now due to the addition of iodine to table salt. The first response of the body to reduced iodine intake is goitre and eventually symptoms appear due to thyroid underactivity.

Symptoms
The commonest situation is in adult life where there is a decreased metabolic rate. The consequence of this is a general slowing of physical and mental functions. There is a feeling of coldness and sensitivity to cold. Associated features include dry skin, coarse, dry hair, constipation, gain in weight, tiredness and vague generalised pains. The outer third of the eyebrows becomes thin and sparse.

Menstrual disturbances are common and mental symptoms, such as forgetfulness, lack of concentration and eventually confusion are common. There may be tingling of the fingers and there is a general appearance of pallor. In severe cases, the face and eyelids become swollen, sweating is absent and the voice is husky. The pulse is slow and tendon reflexes delayed. In some, there is the appearance of psychotic symptoms such as hallucinations and delusions. The end stage of the mental symptoms is coma. Body temperature is low. In the early stages of hypothyroidism, the symptoms may be attributed to ageing. A careful history and examination will reveal the true diagnosis.

In children and especially infants it may be difficult to recognise. There may be poor performance at school and a lack of interest in games. In infants there may be constipation and poor feeding, a general 'failure to thrive' and a failure to attain the usual developmental milestones at the appropriate age. The development of the brain is dependent on thyroid hormones and so a delay in diagnosis at this stage may lead to permanent mental impairment.

Investigations
There are reduced levels of thyroid hormones in the blood and a raised level of thyroid stimulating hormone. There may be thyroid antibodies in the blood.

Treatment
This is with thyroxine supplementation, which initially is given at a low dose and increased gradually over several weeks. The normal maintenance dose is 0.15 to 0.2 mg per day.[10] Annual checks of thyroxine levels are necessary to ensure that supplementation is adequate as the underlying disease process may be progressive.

There are a number of people who present to medical practitioners with non-specific symptoms of tiredness, gaining weight, coldness, depression and the like and they may be subjected to evaluation of thyroid hormone levels. Thyroxine may be given to such patients, even if the thyroxine level in the blood is at the low end of normal. In addition, you may still see some people who are given thyroid hormone on the basis of being overweight. That is clearly an inappropriate way in which to treat such problems. The administration of thyroid hormones leads to a reduction in the person's own thyroid gland function. Over the course of the next year to 18 months, the dosage of thyroxine will be increased, as the person's own production declines. They may not have had a thyroid deficiency to begin with but they certainly end up with one.

Holistic management
If overactivity and underactivity of the thyroid gland are considered together, clearly there is a gradual process of disease with these two being merely extremes. The natural history of thyroid gland disease is for hyperthyroidism to wane as time goes by, to be replaced at some later date by hypothyroidism. Since the conventional treatment of hyperthyroidism involves removal or destruction of part of the gland, hypothyroidism becomes more likely. Whilst the majority of people who become hypothyroid after surgery do so within the first 6 months or 1 year, there is a low but steady further incidence with each year after surgery. Because of this, all people who have received conventional treatment for hyperthyroidism must have annual checks of circulating thyroid hormones.

In terms of Chinese medicine, hyperthyroidism results from emotional distress or frustration. These feelings prevent the energy of the Liver and Spleen from flowing through the channels and Fire is generated which depletes the Yin of the Heart. This causes Phlegm to accumulate which gradually obstructs the channels of the neck, thereby leading to goitre. Enlargement of the thyroid gland (goitre) and disturbances of thyroid function are common some 6 to 12 months after an emotional shock.

The throat area is associated with communication – also see Page 290. I would also suggest that this is why thyroid diseases are much more common in women than men. Women may be aware of their feelings but may also experience difficulty expressing them, since society generally teaches them not to do so. This energy then becomes blocked and causes pathology in the neck and throat area.

It is certainly valid to treat people who have hyperthyroidism by means of holistic medicine but you should be aware of the complications of hyperthyroidism and their symptoms. Severe cases need to be treated with more care and monitored more closely.

When treating people with hypothyroidism it is helpful to remember that holistic treatment may improve thyroid gland function. Their requirements for thyroxine supplementation may decline and so it is wise to monitor thyroxine perhaps every 6 months instead of the usual 12 whilst undergoing treatment.

Case one
A woman of 31 years came for treatment of her hyperthyroidism. She had had an episode of illness 4 years previously after a bereavement when she felt very tired with no energy. She had several attacks of sore throat over a period of some months for which she received antibiotics. She had subsequently been diagnosed as suffering from hyperthyroidism and had been given

carbimazole. After 10 months of treatment her thyroid gland was still overactive and her hair was now falling out. Her white cell count was reduced which is a relatively common side-effect of this medication. She had stopped her carbimazole some 6 months before seeking treatment at my clinic. Her main symptoms were pins and needles in her arms and legs, great intolerance to heat, tiredness, metallic taste in the mouth, a constant feeling of agitation, sweating, sore and swollen tonsils which would often have yellow discharge from them, palpitations which would be worse premenstrually and thirst. Her thyroxine level at her first visit was 69.8 nmol/l (normal 9.1 – 23.8 nmol/l). Her TSH levels were unrecordable at less than 0.05 (normal 0.6 – 4.3).

I made a diagnosis of Blood Deficiency particularly of the Heart leading to Heart Yin Deficiency secondary to Liver Qi Stagnation. There was also some Heat in the Lung. I treated her with acupuncture and Chinese herbs. After 2 months of treatment she felt somewhat better with few attacks of palpitations and no pins and needles. The course of her treatment subsequently was slow but she made progress both with her symptoms and her thyroid function. Her thyroid hormones were unchanged for the first 12 months of treatment although, by that time, many of the symptoms of heat had abated, she had much more energy and she felt generally well. Her thirst and metallic taste also eased as did the throat symptoms. After 18 months of treatment her thyroid hormone estimations were normal. She continues to receive treatment occasionally now for her underlying Heart Blood Deficiency.

Case two

A woman of 37 years came for treatment after a diagnosis of hypothyroidism. She had a baby of 6 months and had been well during the pregnancy except for excessive weight gain. After the birth, which was uneventful, she developed tiredness and lethargy. She had not lost weight since the delivery. Her appetite was generally poor and she tended to suffer from constipation. Her Chinese medical diagnosis was Spleen Qi Deficiency, Kidney Yang Deficiency and Blood Deficiency.

Pregnancy is a drain on Blood and Qi that in some women can lead to symptoms. It is helpful, if possible, to treat women before conception but certainly during pregnancy and after delivery.

The thyroxine level was 35 nmol/l 4 months before treatment and 21 nmol/l 2 months before. She was advised to take thyroxine but sought holistic medical help in an attempt to deal with the problem. I gave her herbs and acupuncture and she felt generally better with more energy. We decided not to repeat the blood test as this would not have changed the management of the case and because she was symptomatically improved. The thyroxine level was checked 10 months after treatment had begun and was normal.

Goitre

This is any enlargement of the thyroid gland. It is more common in women. When seeing a person with such a condition, it is important to consider certain factors:

- size
- shape
- consistency – soft or hard
- symmetry
- generalised or local
- presence or absence of pain
- irregularity of surface
- mobility of the thyroid – the thyroid normally moves on swallowing
- presence or absence of enlarged lymph glands in the neck
- are there symptoms of underactivity or overactivity of thyroid function?*

(* Blood tests may help in this regard but use them as a guide not as an absolute statement.)

Thyroid enlargement is usually noticed due to its appearance since symptoms are absent or minor in most cases. In some, where the enlargement is marked, there can be difficulty in swallowing or breathing because of pressure on the oesophagus or trachea.

There are various causes of goitre in conventional medicine – Table 15.5.

Cause of goitre	Comments
Puberty	Diffuse enlargement. No associated symptoms
Pregnancy	Diffuse enlargement. No associated symptoms
Hyperthyroidism	Diffuse enlargement, firm. Symptoms of hyperthyroidism
Hypothyroidism	Diffuse enlargement, firm, rubbery. May be soft or hard. Symptoms of hypothyroidism
Thyroiditis	Diffuse enlargement that is painful. Fever and malaise
Drugs	Female sex hormones,[11] sulphonylureas
Iodine deficiency	Smooth, soft enlargement
Cancer	A single lump, painful, short history, enlarged lymph glands in the neck
Cysts/benign tumours	Lumps in the thyroid – one or several. If several then unlikely to be cancer

Table 15.5: Causes of goitre

Investigations

These will include thyroid function tests, mainly estimations of thyroxine (T_4), tri-iodothyronine (T_3) and thyroid stimulating hormone. Radioactive scans of the thyroid are done in many cases since the thyroid will concentrate the radioactive substance in an active area. Ultrasound scans can also give information about whether an enlarged area within the thyroid is solid or cystic. Cystic areas are rarely malignant. Biopsy of the thyroid gland using a needle is an increasingly used technique.

Treatment

This depends upon the cause.

Hashimoto's thyroiditis

This is a firm, diffuse enlargement of the thyroid gland, which may or may not be associated with underactivity of the thyroid gland.

Symptoms

There may be aching in the gland and mild dysphagia depending upon the extent of the enlargement. It is most common in middle-aged women and is autoimmune in nature. Virtually all people with this condition have antibodies to thyroid tissue in their blood.

Treatment

This is by means of thyroxine (0.2-0.3 mg daily) to reduce the functioning of the gland and so lead to a reduction in size. Corticosteroids are given in addition to treat the autoimmune aspect.

Subacute (De Quervain's) thyroiditis

This is a painful condition of the thyroid usually associated with enlargement. It is considered to be associated with a viral infection. Thyroid function is reduced and may recover spontaneously or persist.

Treatment

This is treated in the same way as Hashimoto's thyroiditis.

Holistic management of goitre

The symptom of goitre is only one part of the whole case. The exact management will depend upon the individual. In terms of Chinese medicine, goitre is associated with living in the mountains and a long distance from the sea. This observation was noted in the 6th century AD and corresponds with the modern view of low iodine levels.

In Chinese medicine, there is also a belief that goitre is related to emotional causes where emotional distress interferes with the flow of Qi, allowing Dampness and Phlegm to coagulate and obstruct the channels. In this situation it would be important to transform the Phlegm rather than to disperse it (break it up) since the Phlegm Accumulation represents a gathering of the emotions. The use of local treatments, e.g. with acupuncture, may disperse the swelling and stronger treatments can break up the stagnation. This can, however, lead to the sudden release of strong emotional states that overwhelm the person.

It is reasonable to treat goitre by means of holistic medicine but expect progress to be slow, particularly in terms of the actual size of the gland. In my and other practitioner's experience, results tend to be very good. You will have to be more circumspect in underactivity or overactivity of thyroid function and if cancer is a possibility.

Tumours of the thyroid gland

Benign tumours may produce thyroxine and so produce a syndrome identical to hyperthyroidism described previously. They are removed surgically.

Cancer of the thyroid gland is uncommon. It accounts for 1 per cent of all cases of cancer in the UK and about 400 deaths per year. In advanced cases, it can be recognised by its hardness, irregularity and adhesion to surrounding tissues. There may be associated glandular enlargement. In early cases it may present as a single nodule that is seen as being non-functional (a 'cold' area) on radioisotope scan.

Treatment

This is by means of total thyroidectomy together with thyroxine replacement. Local radiotherapy is also used if there is secondary spread. The majority of thyroid tumours spread locally and then metastasise to the lung or bone. Prognosis is variable depending on the exact type.

Holistic management

Issues for holistic practitioners in relation to cancer are discussed in Chapter 6. Note that thyroxine supplementation cannot be altered whenever there has been total thyroidectomy.

DIABETES MELLITUS

In conventional textbooks, diabetes mellitus is usually placed with disorders of metabolism. The term 'diabetes' means excessive urination and 'mellitus' is derived from the Latin for honey. Colloquially, it may be known as 'sugar diabetes' to serve as a distinction from the rarer diabetes insipidus.

The primary feature of diabetes mellitus is raised blood sugar levels due to an inadequate production of insulin by the pancreas. The key to understanding this disease is to appreciate the ways in which the body balances blood sugar levels.

Simply stated, carbohydrates can only be absorbed as simple sugars.[12] More complex carbohydrate sources such as starches and complex sugars have to be broken down into simple sugars before absorption can occur. These enter the blood and may be used as an energy source immediately or stored as glycogen in the body for use at some later date. The body attempts to maintain blood sugar levels within fairly narrow limits (3.5 to 6.0 mmol/l).

The pancreas secretes insulin in response to circulating levels of blood sugar. Insulin allows glucose to enter the cells more readily and facilitates the storage of glucose as glycogen, i.e. reduce blood sugar levels. Conversely, low levels of insulin lead to the breakdown of glycogen stores into glucose and a reduced ability of the cell to absorb sugar. The net result is an increase in blood sugar levels.

Other hormones play a role in regulating blood sugar levels. Glucagon (from the pancreas) together with adrenaline and corticosteroids (from the adrenal glands) raise blood sugar levels. Adrenaline and corticosteroids are released in response to stressful situations and so blood sugar will rise as a result. Similarly, if the blood sugar is low, these hormones are released and so people feel anxious, sweaty and irritable with a rapid pulse.

In the West, many diets include a high intake of carbohydrates especially of the refined type. In addition, we may have irregular eating habits and use stimulants such as alcohol, nicotine and caffeine.

Such habits cause large swings in blood sugar. The blood sugar rises quickly because a diet rich in refined carbohydrate leads to rapid absorption of sugars. Large amounts of insulin have to be produced in response. A rapid fall in blood sugar follows, as there are no complex carbohydrates to be broken down more slowly and to allow gradual absorption of sugar.

The low points of blood sugar levels are known as hypoglycaemic episodes. They are associated with feelings of hunger, sweating, anxiety, irritability and agitation as stress hormones such as adrenaline and corticosteroids are released in an attempt to normalise blood sugar levels. Commonly, a between meal snack or sugar food will be taken to relieve such symptoms. This causes another peak in blood sugar level with a consequent release of insulin. On a daily basis, the pancreas produces large amounts of insulin and the adrenal gland secretes large amounts of adrenaline and corticosteroids. All these factors lead to great fluctuation in blood sugar levels. Exhaustion of the pancreas and adrenal glands occur if this continues for a long period of time. As the pancreas fails, the production of insulin declines leading to permanently raised blood sugar levels, i.e. diabetes mellitus.

The way to remedy and prevent this situation is by smoothing out the extremes of blood sugar levels. It is helpful to avoid refined carbohydrates, overuse of stimulant drugs and to live a relaxing life-style in order to reduce circulating levels of stress hormones. In this way, the peaks and troughs of blood sugar swings will be minimised. This, in itself, can radically affect health as people feel more energetic, less stressed and specific symptoms of a wide variety may be alleviated.[13]

Factors decreasing blood sugar	Factors increasing blood sugar
Exercise Relaxation (because less stress hormones released) Insulin Diet (reducing intake of carbohydrate but especially those of the refined type)	Food (particularly carbohydrates but especially those of the refined type including alcohol) Lack of exercise Stressful situations (due to adrenaline and corticosteroid release) Stimulant drugs, e.g. nicotine, caffeine Glucagon

Table 15.6: Factors affecting blood sugar levels

The disease of diabetes mellitus is when there are inadequate levels of insulin for the requirements of the body. Consequently, blood sugar levels start to rise. Conventionally, there are two types of diabetes mellitus. Insulin dependent diabetes mellitus (also known as IDDM or Type 1 diabetes) is due to an almost total absence of insulin production by the pancreas. It requires the administration of insulin by injection to control sugar levels. The second type is non-insulin dependent diabetes mellitus (also known as NIDDM or Type 2 diabetes) and is due to a relative lack of insulin production. That is, there is insufficient production of insulin for the needs of the body. It is usually treated by diet with or without prescribed medication taken orally. The medication stimulates the pancreas to produce more insulin.

As with most diseases, there are combinations of constitutional and environmental factors. In insulin dependent diabetes, constitutional factors are more important. The presentation tends to be acute and occurs in childhood, particularly around 10 to 13 years. The incidence is currently rising in the West.

In non-insulin dependent diabetes, environmental factors are more important. The person may be overweight and have a long history of poor diet with excess intake of refined carbohydrate.

Whatever the type of diabetes, it frequently develops in the weeks and months after a shock or injury. This may be physical (as in cases of road traffic accident) or emotional (as with bereavement, separation, loss or some other kind of psychological stress). There is evidence to show that diabetes of both kinds is related to autoimmune factors. The suddenness of the onset is an indication of the rapidity of action of insulin. There may have been damage to pancreatic function by the immune system for some time prior to the appearance of symptoms.

The two types of diabetes mellitus are variations of the same disease process. I shall describe diabetes mellitus as a whole and where relevant point out distinctions between them.

Symptoms

Diabetes mellitus may present in several ways. In mild cases, where symptoms may be absent or unnoticed, routine examination of the urine may reveal sugar (glucose). This, in most cases,[14] indicates diabetes. The two main presentations of diabetes reflect the insulin dependent and non-insulin dependent varieties discussed previously.

Insulin dependent diabetes occurs mainly in adolescents and children hence its other name of juvenile-onset diabetes. It is acute in onset and a high blood sugar level causes the main symptoms. As sugar levels in the blood rise, the sugar spills over into the urine. Extra water is excreted and so excess urination, dehydration and thirst are primary symptoms. Eventually there will be weight loss and toxic symptoms of vomiting and breathlessness. Over the course of a few days the child becomes rapidly and progressively ill. Coma and death follow unless treatment with insulin is instituted. Before the use of insulin in the 1920s, all such cases ended in death.

One of the main difficulties is the presence of ketones. Energy is normally obtained from sugar. If this is not possible fat is broken down as an energy source. By-products of fat breakdown are ketones. These are toxic, acidic and have the odour of pear drops. Acetone is a related substance. Ketones are dangerous and are common in acute situations of hyperglycaemia. Other situations leading to ketone production are fasting and malnutrition. This is one of the dangers of very low carbohydrate diets that are proclaimed as helpful in weight loss. I remember when I worked in hospital practice that a woman was admitted for weight loss. She was put on a low carbohydrate diet (around 200 calories per day). She started to lose weight but after 2 weeks had a heart attack and died. Whilst this may not entirely have been due to ketosis, such diets are potentially hazardous.

Non-insulin dependent diabetes is usually much slower in its onset. It occurs in older people (hence its other name is maturity-onset diabetes). Being overweight is a common precursor. There may be a relatively long history of raised blood sugar levels leading to tiredness and lethargy. Depending upon the height of blood sugar there may be thirst and excessive urination. These symptoms will be much milder than those of the insulin dependent type. Weight loss develops as the disease progresses. The development of ketones is unusual. A common feature of the developing diabetic is a complaint of epigastric pain.

Complications

These are many and varied. Firstly, there are the complications of the acute situation and these are commoner in insulin dependent diabetes at first presentation.

Secondly, there are long-term consequences of diabetes mellitus. These arise because of the disruption in carbohydrate metabolism. Even with treatment, such metabolism does not return to normal. Most diabetics, therefore, have long-term problems with fat metabolism, as the body cannot completely handle these basic energy sources normally. The long-term complications are occasionally the first things to present. This is the situation in some cases of the non-insulin dependent type where the symptoms of high blood sugar may be mild or unnoticed.

Complication	Symptoms to look for
Short-term	
Hyperglycaemia	Tiredness, thirst, excess urination, dryness
Hyperglycaemic coma	Unconsciousness
Ketosis	Rapid respiration, pear-drop smell on breath or urine, nausea or vomiting, feels ill
Long-term	
Atherosclerosis	Cold limbs, pain in calves on walking, absent peripheral pulses
Diabetic neuropathy	Tingling and numbness especially in extremities. Feet more than hands
Retinal damage	Impaired vision
Glomerulonephritis	Oedema, loin pain, haematuria

Table 15.7: Complications of diabetes mellitus

Diagnosis

This may be made clinically according to the precise symptom picture given above. Confirmation is by means of blood testing. Two fasting blood sugar levels above 6.7 mmol/l or random samples over 10 mmol/l are sufficient to diagnose diabetes mellitus. A glucose tolerance test[15] is only considered to be necessary in borderline cases.

Sugar in the urine is not, in itself, adequate proof of diabetes mellitus and blood tests must be performed in such cases.

Other routine tests performed once the diagnosis has been established include urinalysis for protein, full blood count, urea and electrolytes and a fasting blood sample for cholesterol and triglycerides. This last test is only valid once blood sugar levels have been controlled.

Treatment

The main aim of conventional treatment is to maintain relatively normal levels of blood sugar throughout the day. Dietary restrictions are placed on carbohydrate intake, particularly sugars.

In addition, agents that reduce blood sugar may be required. These are of two types. Insulin itself may be administered in severe cases where other methods of blood sugar control would fail. This is given to those of young age with insulin dependent diabetes and some older people whose symptoms are too severe for control by other means. Oral hypoglycaemic drugs, which stimulate pancreatic function, are given to those older people where dietary restriction alone is inadequate but the case is not so severe that insulin is necessary.

Hypoglycaemic agents may reduce the level of blood sugar too much and lead to low blood sugar or hypoglycaemia. This is not the hypoglycaemia that we may all sometimes feel if we miss meals or are very tired. In treated diabetes mellitus, the blood sugar may fall so low as to be life threatening. There are similar symptoms of hunger, sweating, agitation and so forth. As the blood sugar level continues to fall there is the appearance of confusion. Eventually coma and death will occur. Some people think that such hypoglycaemia develops as part of the disease. In fact, it is a result of the *treatment* of diabetes mellitus.

The optimal treatment of diabetes mellitus, therefore, is to tread a line between the extremes of hyperglycaemia and hypoglycaemia. The essence of good management is a restriction of diet, a regulated life-style in terms of exercise and stress levels and to monitor blood or urine sugar regularly. Nowadays, most diabetics use blood checks. A level of between 6 and 8 mmol/l is about right. Tests performed before meals will give a good idea of what is happening to blood sugar levels throughout the day.

Urine testing is less commonly performed nowadays. Ketones may be tested by dipstick at the same time. Dipstick tests are used rather than the older tablet method. There are drawbacks to urine testing. These include:

- urine sugar is a reflection of the situation in the blood some time previously
- the level of sugar in the urine is a reflection not only of blood sugar but also of kidney function
- negative urine tests give no indication of blood sugar levels.

The diet of a person with diabetes mellitus is similar in many respects to that which is considered generally healthy. Carbohydrate intake needs to be based on unrefined, complex substances rather than simple sugars. Fat intake needs to be limited, particularly in diabetics who have a tendency to premature atherosclerosis. In terms of calories, 15 per cent should be obtained from protein, 35 per cent from fats and 50 per cent from carbohydrate. For those who take insulin, regular snacks between meals are required to prevent low blood sugar levels at those times.

It is notoriously difficult for most of us to change our habits and particularly our eating habits. People with diabetes need information about their condition and how diet may affect it together with support to put necessary changes into action. In this way, rather than being something imposed from the outside, the control of diabetes is managed by the individual themselves.

Commonly used methods of reducing blood sugar levels are insulin by injection and oral hypoglycaemic agents. In the case of insulin, there are several routines used. Frequently, long-acting insulin is administered in the evening and three doses of short-acting insulin before each meal during the day. In this way a relatively smooth degree of control is attained in most people. The blood is tested before each meal and the amount of insulin given is dependent upon the result.

Insulin, formerly, used to be obtained from the pancreases of pigs or cattle. Such pork and beef insulin have, to a large degree, been replaced by human insulin produced synthetically. The changeover to human insulin has led to problems with sudden attacks of hypoglycaemia but no warning symptoms. This has resulted in some deaths since human insulin was introduced.

The injection of insulin is clearly not physiological and so control of blood sugar levels is not perfect. The absorption of injected insulin is variable, it enters the systemic rather than the digestive circulation, delaying absorption and there are individual variations of response.

The second type of control is by means of oral hypoglycaemic agents. Essentially, these stimulate the pancreas to produce more insulin. They are only appropriate for those with milder diabetes mellitus. Certainly, almost all diabetics who develop the disease at a young age will require insulin. There are two main groups of drugs available. The sulphonylureas, such as tolbutamide and chlorpropamide, are commonly used. They are contraindicated in pregnancy and may damage the liver. Hypoglycaemia may be produced which can be severe and long lasting.

Biguanides are the other group available. Metformin is the usual example and is reserved for those in middle and old age. It may induce anorexia, indigestion and diarrhoea. Some people develop an acidotic reaction, which is potentially life threatening. It is not licensed for use in the US.

Holistic management

In terms of Chinese medicine, diabetes mellitus usually corresponds to 'thirsting and wasting disease'. It is the generation of Internal Heat due to the excessive intake of sweet and greasy food or emotional stagnation. The Heat damages the Yin leading to the classical symptoms. The condition is further divided into upper, middle and lower types depending upon the presence of thirst, hunger and frequent urination respectively. In clinical practice, there is usually a mixture of the three types seen.

Insulin, therefore, has an effect of cooling the Heat and moistening the Yin. This is why heat signs are not commonly seen in treated diabetics. However, the cooling effect will also damage the Spleen Qi further and lead to digestive symptoms, desire for sweet food, oedema and Damp-phlegm Accumulation.[16]

Case one

A man of 25 years came for treatment of his diabetes mellitus. He had first developed this at the age of 8 years when his grandmother died. He had been very close to her as she had mainly been responsible for his upbringing.

He generally felt exhausted. He had loose stools at least five times each day. His current insulin dosages were 26 units of long acting at night and variable amounts of short-acting three times daily (usually around 8, 10 and 8 units). His blood sugar estimations were unstable.

- Fasting – 20 mmol/l or more
- Midday – 15 mmol/l
- Tea time – 15 mmol/l
- Evening – 15 mmol/l.

These blood levels were an indication of his life-style, which was quite irregular. He had a large intake of cigarettes, coffee and recreational drugs with late nights and a stressful job. It is important to be careful with such cases at these blood levels of sugar. It is more worrying if there are ketones in the urine or strong symptoms of thirst and frequent urination.

In terms of Chinese medicine, his diagnosis was Spleen Yang Deficiency, Kidney Yang Deficiency, Liver Qi Stagnation and Heat in the Stomach. I decided to begin with improving his digestive energy and we discussed the effect of treatment on his blood sugars.

Some two days after treatment, he noticed that his blood sugars were more moderate and when he returned one week later they were much more stable.

- Fasting – usually 10 but on one occasion 5 mmol/l
- Midday – 5 mmol/l
- Tea time – 5 mmol/l
- Evening – 5 mmol/l.

Over the course of the next few weeks, his blood sugars continued to regularise. He began to change his dietary and drug habits as he felt better and his energy returned. It is a common finding that people can change their lives when they have the energy to do so. It is rarely, if ever, beneficial to lecture people about their 'bad habits' in the hope that they will change. Such change only comes from within, certainly if it is to be long lasting and effective.

In the next few months, he progressed to reducing his insulin dosage until he was taking 20 units of long acting at night and about 6 units at each meal. He felt generally much better although his loose stools had not completely eased. His treatment will need to be long-term but I would expect him to remain well. In such circumstances it is not realistic to expect him to be able to come off insulin completely.

There are some people who present for treatment with the early symptoms of diabetes mellitus but whose blood sugar is not dangerously high and there are no ketones. In such cases we may realistically expect that with holistic medical treatment, the condition will not deteriorate to the point where insulin is needed.

ADRENAL GLANDS

The adrenal glands (suprarenal glands) are situated on top of the kidney. They consist of an inner medulla and an outer cortex. The medulla has connections with the sympathetic nervous system and produces the hormones, adrenaline and noradrenaline. These are involved in the flight and fight response. Clinically recognisable disorders of this area are extremely rare and I will consider only disorders of the adrenal cortex.

The adrenal cortex produces several hormones with differing functions – Table 15.8. Each hormone has several effects but in each case, there is an emphasis of one particular aspect, e.g. cortisone primarily has a glucocorticoid action but also some mineralocorticoid and androgenic effects.

Cortisone and its relations have a primary glucocorticoid action. They have an effect that is opposite to that of insulin. It raises blood sugar by activating glycogen stores in the liver. It causes the breakdown of protein into carbohydrate, primarily sugar. This leads to depletion of protein structure such as the underlying substance of bone, collagen and connective tissue and muscle.

The anti-inflammatory effects are used clinically in diseases characterised by inflammation of non-infective origin. These include rheumatoid arthritis, Crohn's disease, ulcerative colitis, eczema, asthma, psoriasis and so forth.

Action	Effects	Example of hormone
Glucocorticoid	Opposite to insulin Anti-inflammatory Convert protein to sugar	Cortisone, cortisol (hydrocortisone), corticosterone[17]
Mineralocorticoid	Retains sodium Loses potassium	Aldosterone
Androgenic	Masculinising	Testosterone
Oestrogens	Feminising	Oestrogen[18]

Table 15.8: Hormones secreted by the adrenal gland and their functions

Overproduction of a particular hormone will lead to certain clinical features – Table 15.9.

Action	Effects	Symptoms
Glucocorticoid	Opposite to those of insulin Anti-inflammatory Converts protein to sugar[19]	Thirst, frequent urination, dehydration, increased susceptibility to infections[20] Risk of spreading infection and cell damage. Weakening of bone,[21] thinning of skin and mucous membranes, easy bruising, poor wound healing, ulceration of the stomach or duodenum
Mineralocorticoid	Retains sodium Loses potassium	Water retention manifesting as oedema and high blood pressure Muscle weakness, palpitations and tiredness
Androgenic	Masculinising	In men there may be aggressive and violent behaviour In women there is deepening of the voice, male distribution of hair on the face, temporal recession hair, hair along the central line of the abdomen, enlargement of the clitoris, reduction in breast size, disturbance of menstruation with scanty or absent periods
Oestrogens	Feminising	Leads to female distribution of fat, breast enlargement, reduction in size of penis in men

Table 15.9: Symptoms associated with overproduction of adrenal cortical hormones

Overactivity of the adrenal cortex

Cushing's syndrome

This is a syndrome due to excess corticosteroid production. It has many similarities with the clinical picture seen when corticosteroids are prescribed to treat disease. Cushing's syndrome itself may be due to overstimulation by adrenocorticotrophic hormone from the pituitary gland.

Symptoms

These are primarily due to an increased glucocorticoid action. There is central obesity – thin arms and legs with increased weight centrally on the trunk and face. The limbs are thin due to muscle wasting and the muscles are weak. There is oedema in the ankles or lower legs. The skin is thin and bruises easily. Injury to the skin easily results in tears, which are slow to heal. Infection is more likely and improves slowly. There is sugar in the urine. The bones become weaker due to osteoporosis and fractures may develop. High blood pressure is common and the complexion is ruddy. Skin infections are common. The skin is stretched and purple striae are seen. There is male pattern baldness with a masculine distribution of hair.

These symptoms are also seen with corticosteroid use for diseases such as rheumatoid arthritis but without the masculinising effects since synthetic hormones are used.

Holistic management
Corticosteroid use is discussed fully in Chapter 10 – Musculoskeletal system.

Underactivity of the adrenal cortex

Underactivity of the adrenal cortex is unusual in clinical practice but a useful condition to study, as its symptoms are similar to the effect of sudden withdrawal of corticosteroid drugs. With long-term corticosteroid use, the adrenal glands atrophy and decline in function. If the drugs are reduced suddenly, the adrenal glands cannot produce sufficient quantities and symptoms of underactivity are evident.

The disease state may be due to primary disease of the adrenal as in Addison's disease, congenital deficiency of enzymes required for the synthesis of adrenal hormones (congenital adrenal hyperplasia) or secondary to underactivity of the pituitary or hypothalamus.

Addison's disease

This is usually of an autoimmune nature. Occasionally, tuberculosis of the adrenal glands may lead to adrenal destruction. Women are affected twice as commonly as men. Antibodies to the adrenal gland are found in the blood. The adrenals are atrophied and smaller than normal. The onset can be acute or chronic. Frequently, there are associated autoimmune disorders such as thyrotoxicosis, Hashimoto's thyroiditis, pernicious anaemia and insulin-dependent diabetes mellitus.

Symptoms
There is weakness, weight loss, low blood pressure and gastrointestinal disorders including anorexia, nausea, constipation and diarrhoea. There is increasing mental and physical tiredness. Amenorrhoea is common in women. There is disturbance of pigmentation in long-standing cases with hyperpigmentation or vitiligo. The pigmentation disorder is often the first clinical sign. Increased melanin affects the area exposed to light and pressure and so is seen primarily on the face, neck, backs of hands, knuckles, elbows and knees. Scars present before the onset of symptoms are normal and those after become pigmented. Vitiligo develops in 10-20 per cent of people especially in dark-skinned races.

Treatment
This is by means of corticosteroids. The drugs usually given are cortisol with fludrocortisone.

Holistic management
Cases of corticosteroid withdrawal are described in Chapter 10 – Musculoskeletal system and Chapter 13 – Gastrointestinal system. In terms of Chinese medicine, too rapid a reduction of corticosteroids may lead to Collapse of Yang.

Case one
A woman of 30 years came for treatment. She had developed amenorrhoea some 12 months before attending the clinic. She had stopped the oral contraceptive and had had no periods since. She was feeling exhausted and tired with lots of cold feelings. Her hair was dry and falling out. She was thirsty and needed to get up to pass urine three times each night. Her blood pressure was low at 90/50 mm Hg. Her bowels were sluggish and she would miss days completely. She had abdominal bloating, wind and belching. She constantly desired sweet and salty food.

She had been diagnosed as suffering from pituitary failure. She had been started on hydrocortisone 10 mg daily but felt very swollen 'as if I am going to explode' and this was changed. Her current medication was:

- desmopressin nasal spray – anti-diuretic hormone to control nocturia
- prednisolone 2.5 mg at night, 5 mg morning – corticosteroid to replace adrenal hormones
- thyroxine 50 mcg one daily – to replace thyroid hormones.

I made a diagnosis of Yang collapse and gave her a Rescue Yang herbal formula. She was not keen to take her medication as they gave her side-effects but I impressed on her the importance of continuing them until she improved. She would also need monitoring of her hormone levels before any modification to the dosage of medication.

She responded well to treatment and felt much more energy and generally warmer. Her bowels were fine and she had no nocturia. After 1 month of treatment, she said she was feeling much better, 'brilliant' with few symptoms. Her tests at the hospital were normal and she decided to stop all her medication. She continued treatment with me over the next 12 months and remained well. Her hormone blood levels continued to be normal.

HOW TO RECOGNISE A SERIOUS CONDITION OF THE ENDOCRINE SYSTEM

Most people who come to the clinic with endocrine disease will already have a conventional diagnosis. In cases of underactivity of a particular endocrine gland, they will be taking hormone supplementation. In such situations it is merely necessary to be sure what would indicate an imbalance in their hormone control.

In those cases where diagnosis has not already been made, you can rely on symptoms as I have stated at the end of each Chapter dealing with a particular system. For example, in cases of diabetes mellitus with excessive urination you can refer to Chapter 9 – Urinary system. In cases of hyperthyroidism with palpitations you can refer to Chapter 7 – Cardiovascular system.

Disease	Situation of imbalance	Comments
Hyperthyroidism	Appearance of symptoms of overactivity	Review case. May be exacerbation due to too rapid drug withdrawal. Assess according to severity of symptoms
Hypothyroidism	Appearance of symptoms of underactivity	Review case. May be ineffective holistic treatment, too low a dosage of thyroxine
Diabetes insipidus	Excess urination, thirst	Is there too low a dosage of vasopressin?
Diabetes mellitus	Hyperglycaemia Hypoglycaemia	Check factors such as diet, recent reduction in exercise, increased stress levels, use of stimulant drugs, excessive reduction of hypoglycaemic agents, infection. Assess according to severity of symptoms. Check diet, recent increase in exercise, relaxation, cessation of stimulant drugs, failure to reduce dosage of hypoglycaemic agents. If frequent then must adjust hypoglycaemic drug dosage as a matter of urgency

Table 15.10: Diseases of endocrine system and states of imbalance

SUMMARY

Diseases of the endocrine system are increasing in incidence in the West. This mirrors the general increase in chronic disease.

People with endocrine disease will be seen in the clinic but not always because of their original disease.

Monitoring of endocrine function is important when dealing with such cases.

It is important to have an understanding of the factors affecting function of a particular endocrine gland.

Holistic treatment shortly after conventional diagnosis and treatment may have a realistic chance of removing the need for hormone therapy.

Holistic treatment after a long period of conventional treatment will generally lead to increased health and a reduced dosage of hormone replacement (hence the need for monitoring).

---

[1] By hormone replacement in this Chapter, I am referring to the prescription of a hormone in a deficiency disease. Hormone replacement therapy may be used to refer to oestrogen and progesterone supplements during or after the menopause. This is something quite different and is discussed in Chapter 18 – Women's Health. This phrase is somewhat of a misnomer since it is not a replacement. Menopause is not a disease state and low oestrogen levels at this time are not a deficiency disease.
[2] An end organ of the endocrine system is one that is stimulated by the pituitary gland to produce a hormone. The hormone has an effect on body tissues/metabolism.

3 'The three months of spring ... It is desirable to sleep at night, get up early in the morning, take a walk in the yard, to loosen up hair and relax the body ... The three months of summer ... It is desirable to sleep at night and get up early in the morning, to have no dislike of sunlight, possess no will of anger so that things will bloom beautifully and so that energy will move outward through perspiration as if in love with the outside world ...The three months of autumn ... It is desirable to sleep early and get up early with the crowing of the rooster, to maintain a peaceful will in order to slow down the killing effects of autumn, to constrict the energy of the spirits in order to calm down the energy of the autumn, to refrain from moving outward in order to clean up the energy of the lungs ... The three months of winter ... It is desirable to sleep early and get up late, to await the arrival of sunlight, so that the will remains dormant as if hiding or pretending, not unlike someone with private intentions, not unlike someone with all his desires already fulfilled.' *Neijing* Volume 1, Chapter 2. Translation by Henry Lu.

4 Lithium is used in the treatment of manic depression.

5 It can also be referred to as thyrotoxicosis. The term Grave's disease is reserved to describe hyperthyroidism of an autoimmune nature.

6 Goitre is a swelling of the neck due to thyroid gland enlargement.

7 This is thickening of the skin over the tibia. Confusingly, hypothyroidism may also be known as myxoedema.

8 This is described on Page 143.

9 In Chinese medicine, there are various types of seaweed available as herbal remedies. They have the effect of transforming Phlegm, which is considered to collect to form goitre.

10 This may be expressed as micrograms. The equivalent is 150 to 200 mcg per day.

11 There is an energetic connection between the neck and the pelvis, which explains why suppression of ovarian function may lead to thyroid enlargement. It is important to review all medication in cases of goitre.

12 Simple sugars, also known as monosaccharides, are single sugar molecules. Examples include glucose, fructose and galactose. More complex sugars are disaccharides that are made up of double sugar molecules. Examples include sucrose, maltose and lactose.

Starches are polysaccharides where many sugar molecules are joined together. They are an important form of carbohydrate in the diet. Glycogen is also a polysaccharide and is a source of carbohydrate stores within the body. It is the equivalent of starch.

13 There are many diets including Atkins, Pritikin and others that change blood sugar levels by advocating high protein, relatively low carbohydrate intakes. More healthy diets include the Hay diet (also known as food combining) that takes the strain off the digestion and allows blood sugar levels and other homeostatic mechanisms to be more balanced.

14 Sugar does not normally appear in the urine in health. It remains in the blood, as its level is not high enough to spill over the renal threshold. About 1 per cent of the population have a low renal threshold so that sugar appears in the urine. This is known as renal glycosuria and is an inherited trait. It is not associated with any disease in conventional medicine.

15 This is a sequence of blood sugar estimations performed over 2.5 hours to check their response to the intake of sugar. In health, there is a normal response as the pancreatic secretion of insulin can respond adequately. In borderline and overt diabetics, there is an abnormal response shown as an excessive rise in blood sugar levels. This may only occur an hour or so after meals and so would not be revealed by a random test. Some people may require a 5-hour glucose tolerance test to note any abnormality. For this reason, conventional practitioners may not recognise latent diabetes.

16 This corresponds to atherosclerosis and retinal damage that are common in treated diabetics.

17 The hormones used in clinical practice for their anti-inflammatory effects are betamethasone, prednisolone, prednisone, triamcinolone, cortisol (hydrocortisone) and dexamethasone.

18 This is discussed in detail in Chapter 18 – Women's Health.

19 The ability to breakdown protein reveals the strength of these chemicals.

20 These are the classical symptoms of raised blood sugar as described in the section on diabetes mellitus. There is a real possibility of this disease developing in such a circumstance.

21 Osteoporosis.

16 PSYCHOLOGICAL DISORDERS

INTRODUCTION

As discussed in Chapter 2 – Philosophy, conventional medicine concentrates on physical matters. In most cases this is to the exclusion of everything else. There *is* recognition that people have psychological symptoms but the conventional explanation is that they arise from a physical basis, usually the brain.

There is the added factor that such symptoms are frequently seen as being unimportant. There is a common thread throughout much of conventional medical practice where psychological symptoms are either ignored, minimised or seen as a secondary component of a 'real' or physical disease. In diseases where psychological symptoms predominate such as schizophrenia, there is an assumption that a physical basis will, at some time, be found. Research is directed either at biochemical abnormalities[1] within the central nervous system or attempts made to discover a genetic abnormality.

Dr Peter Breggin wrote the Foreword to *Reality Therapy in Action*[2] by William Glasser, M.D. saying: "Nothing has harmed the quality of individual life in modern society more than the misbegotten belief that human suffering is driven by biological and genetic causes and can be rectified by taking drugs or undergoing electroshock therapy. ...If I wanted to ruin someone's life, I would convince the person that biological psychiatry is right – that relationships mean nothing, that choice is impossible, and that the mechanics of a broken brain reign over our emotions and conduct. If I wanted to impair an individual's capacity to create empathetic, loving relationships, I would prescribe psychiatric drugs, all of which blunt our highest psychological and spiritual functions".

When an emphasis is placed on physical matters, people's psychological states are given little attention. People are dismissed as being neurotic.[3] They may be given chemicals in an attempt to 'rebalance' supposed chemical abnormalities in the substance of the brain. Surgical procedures are performed on the brain in an attempt to correct these abnormalities. In my experience, these are rarely of benefit and frequently lead to more problems. There is a fostering of the misunderstanding that psychological difficulties can only be remedied by external forces, either the doctor or medication prescribed by the doctor. There is little encouragement of self-help measures such as relaxation, yoga, Tai Chi or many other contemplative methods that have powerfully beneficial effects on the mind and emotions. As psychiatrist Thomas Szasz once said: "Trying to get rid of a so-called mental illness by having a psychiatrist work on your brain is like trying to get cigarette commercials off television by having a TV repairman work on your TV set".

In conjunction with a general increase in the number of chronic diseases in the West, it is more common to see psychological disorders. Homoeopaths report that remedies are used now to affect deep mental and emotional levels that would hardly, if ever, be used 100 years ago. In the UK there has been a 65 per cent increase in the number of children admitted to psychiatric wards in recent years. In the US, up to 1.5 per cent of children between 2 and 4 years of age are given stimulants, anti-depressants, or anti-psychotic drugs such as methyphenidate (Ritalin), fluoxetine (Prozac), and thioridazine.[4] The numbers of such prescriptions increased three times between 1991 and 1995 despite these drugs not being approved for children under the age of 6 years. This is particularly dangerous as this is at a time when the nervous system is developing and maturing.[5]

The cost to national health budgets is extreme. In the UK, some £100 million per year is spent on drugs to affect mood. This is 25 per cent of the national drug budget. There seems to be no end to this suffering and as each year passes, increasing numbers of people exhibit psychological symptoms. The use of conventional medical techniques merely deal with the symptoms – the effect – rather than the cause and so can only be suppressive. Conventional medical techniques become part of the problem rather than the solution. Are there other ways of viewing these situations?

Oriental medicine has always sought to see symptoms within the context of an integrated whole. This is true of many traditions including Chinese and Tibetan Buddhist[6] medicine. There are two aspects of mind[7] that it is helpful to consider. There is the mind that is discursive, distracted and always getting ourselves (and others) into difficulty and dissatisfaction. At the same time, there is Mind[8] that can be likened to the sky on a cloudless day – the unchanging aspect of ourselves that is beyond all suffering and discomfort.

The usual thoughts and emotions of our everyday experience can be likened to clouds that appear in the sky from time to time. They are not the sky itself but merely obscure it. They come and go. It is when we are attached to the clouds of our thoughts and emotions that we begin to experience suffering.

From a Buddhist point of view, all suffering originates from the Mind. It arises from our mental processes that see events, others and ourselves as fixed entities, unchanging and permanent. This is not the true nature of reality. All events are merely a manifestation of constantly changing causes and conditions. Nothing is static and permanent.

The level of Mind must be addressed in order to achieve any long-lasting change. Treatment, by whatever means, is particularly effective if people are encouraged to see their psychological processes for what they are – impermanent and constantly changing. They are not 'us', not our Mind, they are merely transitory. In this way, people become less attached to problems and suffering and can experience periods of comfort and ease. Approaches that directly deal with inner states are the most powerful methods of transformation. Visualisation and meditation are just some of the methods that can be used. Certainly, as practitioners, it is helpful to have a view of these two aspects. Unless we have this overall perspective or view, we tend to get stuck in the level of thoughts and emotions where problems circulate around and around with no progress.

Spiritual practice is another level of approach completely and it is important that we, as practitioners, are clear about our particular role. Guidance along a spiritual path can only be given by a qualified spiritual teacher and is of inestimable value in working with the fundamental level of Mind.

CLASSIFICATION OF PSYCHOLOGICAL DISORDERS

The conventional classification of psychological disorders is complex and allows for doctors to diagnose and treat people with psychological disorders. The categories tend to be fairly rigid as they are an ordered method of labelling. There are two main systems of classification used.

Fourth edition of the Diagnostic and Statistical Manual of the American Psychiatric Association (DSM-IV)
  I   Psychiatric syndrome, clinical syndromes
  II   Personality disorders, mental retardation
  III   Psychosocial and environmental problems
  V   Overall level of functioning.

International Classification of Diseases and Related Health Problems (ICD-10) published by the World Health Organisation
  Organic disorders (F00 – F09)
  Mental and behavioural disorders due to psychoactive substance use (F10 – F19)
  Schizophrenia and delusional disorders (F20 – F29)
  Mood (affective) disorders (F30 – F39)
  Neurotic, stress-related and somatoform disorders (F40 – F49)
  Behavioural syndromes (F50 – F59)
  Disorders of adult personality and behaviour (F60 – F69)
  Mental retardation (F70 – F79).

The emphasis here is on naming and it is of limited use for practitioners who do not use conventional methods of treatment. Another source of confusion is the use of the word, mental. In conventional medicine, this is applied loosely to any psychological disturbance.[9] I intend to use it as I did in Chapter 2 – Philosophy, where I applied it to thought, cognition and perception.[10] I use the term 'emotion' to describe mood, feeling or affect.[11] A further difficulty is the use of the term, organic.[12] This means that symptoms are associated with physical, structural changes, which are considered in conventional medicine to be the cause of all symptoms.

The holistic view of psychological symptoms is that they are part of the whole picture of a person. Schizophrenia, for example, would merely be a label applied to a disturbance that mainly manifests on the mental level. In terms of holistic medicine, the key is to assess where is the emphasis of the symptoms, on the mental or emotional levels. If symptoms arise primarily on the mental level, then one could say the person has a mental disturbance. In severe cases, this may be labelled as a psychosis. If the symptoms are primarily emotional in nature then an emotional disturbance can be diagnosed. The term, neurosis may be used here. The significance for the person's health of these manifestations is discussed in Chapter 2 – Philosophy. Clearly these divisions are not rigid since most people develop symptoms on all three levels, mental, emotional and physical. The important factor is which level is *mainly* affected. Therefore, a holistic classification of psychological disorders can be summarised as in Table 16.1 The point here, therefore, is not the particular 'name' of the disorder, but the manifestation of the symptoms.

Mild disease

Neuroses[13] – Disturbances of mood/emotion
Anxiety, phobias, depression, obsessions, hysteria

Psychoses[14] – Disturbances of thought/perception

Acute –   Delirium[15]

Chronic –   Eating disorders
             Manic depressive illness
             Schizophrenia
             Dementias

Severe disease

Table 16.1: Energetic classification of psychological disorders

Psychoses may be seen as being primarily disorders of thought whilst the neuroses are primarily disorders of emotion.

INVESTIGATION OF PSYCHOLOGICAL DISORDERS

Generally, a psychological disorder is clearly diagnosed by the symptoms. In individual cases investigations may be done if an underlying physical abnormality is suspected. The relevant investigations performed are detailed with the individual disorders.

DISORDERS OF THE EMOTIONAL LEVEL (neuroses)

A useful working definition of neurosis is to say that it is an exaggeration of a normal emotional state. We all have emotions such as anxiety, depression, sadness, anger and so forth. When these become excessive or unbalanced in some way, then it may be possible to say that a neurosis exists. In one sense we could all be considered neurotic.

In conventional medicine, a diagnosis of neurosis is made according to certain criteria. There must be one of the typical syndromes with a recent setback, e.g. disturbance in a relationship. This is in order to exclude a physical cause and underlines the rigid line of division between mental, emotional and physical aspects of the person in conventional medicine. The setback may not be gross but may trigger off an association from the distant past.

Anxiety neurosis

This is the most common form of neurosis and refers to a state of inner tension and anticipation that is perceived as unpleasant. There may also be feelings of fear and panic. Often there are accompanying physical symptoms. There are frequently symptoms in the immediate family. Some 15 per cent of parents and siblings are affected compared with 5 per cent of the general population. Women are diagnosed twice as commonly as men. There is often a past history of emotional disturbance and insecurity. Bereavement, disappointment, work problems or relationship difficulties may precipitate the overt symptoms.

Symptoms
The main emphasis may be either on the emotional state or the associated physical symptoms. There may be anxiety and nervousness, a feeling of apprehension, anticipation or panic. In some, there may be preoccupation with fear of physical illness such as cancer or heart disease. There is poor concentration, indecision, restlessness and agitation. Sleep may be disturbed, either by difficulty in getting off to sleep or by waking in the night. Shortness of breath with feelings of faintness may lead to a confusion with a heart attack or stroke. This latter presentation is usually termed 'hyperventilation'.

Accompanying physical symptoms include sweating, tremor and palpitations. Tiredness is common. Headache, frequent urination and loose stools may also be present.

Treatment
The mainstay of conventional treatment is by means of drugs. Those commonly used are the 'minor' tranquillisers, which are not to be confused with the 'major' tranquillisers used in the treatment of psychotic illnesses. Examples of 'minor'

tranquillisers include the benzodiazepines, e.g. diazepam, chlordiazepoxide, and the barbiturates. All these drugs have a propensity for being rapidly addictive and there are well-described withdrawal syndromes.

In recent years, there has been some recognition of this. However, this has, sadly, led to the increased prescription of 'major' tranquillisers, antidepressants or betablockers. People may be told that these other drugs are safer and non-addictive. This is nonsense. No drug is non-addictive and it is dangerous to assume so. The prescription of drugs such as betablockers or antidepressants to replace tranquillisers is *more* likely to cause difficulties since they are more powerful.

Treatment with 'minor' tranquillisers remains the most common approach with almost 16 million prescriptions for benzodiazepines in the UK in 1992. Side-effects[16] with all drugs given to alter mood are extremely common and although the incidence of these may vary no drug is exempt. Tiredness, fatigue and a generalised sense of numbness and detachment are common. Triazolam, a benzodiazepine, has been linked with paranoia and aggression. Side-effects include amnesia, anxiety, depression and, more seriously, aggressive behaviour. Between 1984 and 1991, some 3555 adverse reactions were filed with the Food and Drug Administration (FDA) in the US compared to 833 with flurazepam since 1970 and 318 for temazepam since 1981. The FDA had received reports of 49 'homicides and attempted homicides' connected to use of the drug.[17]

Holistic treatment

The general holistic management of the neuroses is summarised on Page 312. In terms of Chinese medicine, the benzodiazepines are cooling and primarily affect the Heart. They can be likened to the group of Chinese herbs that Calm the Spirit. There are three main consequences of using single substances particularly for a long period of time. Firstly, the Calming of the Spirit leads to depression. Secondly, long-term use damages other organs particularly the Spleen and Kidneys. Thirdly, in some people there is the generation of Heat as a result of their stagnating action and this manifests as violent outbursts, aggression and the like.

Withdrawal of these drugs leads to flaring up of Heart Fire such as anxiety, mania, hallucinations and, in severe cases, convulsions. Such withdrawal must be done slowly in conjunction with treatments that strengthen and support.

Case one

A woman of 20 years came for treatment with a feeling of 'butterflies in her chest' accompanied with an inability to relax. She would have many negative thoughts and palpitations. She had always been a light sleeper but recently had not been able to fall asleep for hours. These symptoms had begun some 3 months before her University examinations and had gradually worsened the closer she came to taking them. I made a diagnosis of Heart Blood Deficiency and treated her with acupuncture and herbs. Her symptoms quickly subsided and some 2 months later felt well. She had had one attack of palpitations in that time but her mood was good and the sensations in her chest had subsided.

Case two

A woman of 40 years came for treatment of her anxiety. She would get attacks of panic and palpitations with breathlessness, sweating and fear of dying. She had not been outside of her local town for the past 11 years because she was fearful that she would die of a heart attack. The symptoms had been there since the age of 5 when she had been hospitalised after a fall. Her family had not been allowed to visit her for the 4 weeks she was there as she was 'always upset when they did visit'. She could go a whole week without opening her bowels. She had frequent urination with nocturia twice and passing urine 20 times each day. I made a diagnosis of Blood and Qi Deficiency with underlying Kidney Yang Deficiency. Treatment was more complicated because of her medication:

- Anafranil 10 mg 2 at night
- Lexoton 3 mg 2 daily.

I treated her with acupuncture and herbs. She responded slowly but after 4 months was able to go out more and visited the nearest town. Since then, she has had holidays abroad (a major achievement as she has always been very frightened of travelling). Her conventional medication remains unchanged some 18 months later. I am hopeful that her progress will continue and at some point she will feel confident enough to reduce it. Her treatment continues.

Phobic neurosis

This is a fear of an object, situation or activity. It is conventionally described as 'irrational' although this merely reflects a lack of insight as to the cause since there is a reason for everything. The fear may be non-specific and generalised or it may be directed towards a specific situation. A common manifestation is fear of open spaces – agoraphobia. This may also be an inability to leave home or be in stressful situations. The person may avoid such situations entirely and live their life in a restricted manner. In less severe cases, the situation may be tolerated but with marked feelings of fear. The number and variety of foci for phobias are limitless and each case must be dealt with on an individual basis.

Symptoms

These are similar to those of anxiety neurosis described above. They are particularly severe when a specific trigger is present. Otherwise, there is a general feeling of tension and apprehension.

Treatment

This is frequently with antidepressants of which the imipramine (see tricyclic antidepressants on Page 310) is the most commonly used. Benzodiazepines, usually alprazolam, may also be employed. Drugs are less effective where the fear is non-specific.

Psychotherapy with or without behaviour therapy may also be used. Some people are treated by gradually increased exposure to the phobic situation as a means of desensitisation.

Hysterical neurosis

This is the production of physical symptoms as a result of a psychological disturbance. The appearance of the physical symptoms, e.g. paralysis, numbness, blackouts, memory loss, leads to relief of the psychological symptoms. Challenge and confrontation lead to a return of the psychological disturbance and the physical symptoms may improve or disappear only to return some time later.

This so-called 'conversion' hysteria is not common now. It may occasionally be associated with compensation awards after an accident. It is usually anatomically incorrect. Such symptoms may be viewed with disdain and there is often an unvoiced accusation that the person has deliberately and wilfully developed them.

The term 'dissociative' hysteria is used to describe a similar process, which manifests as altered states of awareness. These may be faints, fits or trances. The diagnosis is made by excluding physical disease whilst considering the actual symptom picture. There will be a precipitating event.

Treatment

This is seen to be difficult conventionally as the person finds some comfort with their situation.

Obsessional neurosis

This term is applied to people who perform activities on a repetitive and compulsive basis. There are constantly recurring thoughts or feelings but the person has insight and recognises these as their own. Some 1 per cent of the population is considered obsessive but the true incidence is certainly higher.

There is an element of anguish and people seek to perform repetitive actions as a way of relieving psychological discomfort. Resisting the urge to perform actions leads to exacerbation of these feelings.

It is important in the assessment of such people to determine whether the issue is *primarily* with thoughts or feelings. This distinction may not be made conventionally. However, for our purposes this would greatly affect the meaning. Obsessions of thought indicate a more serious disturbance than those of emotions. In some cases, it leads to a particular behaviour consequent upon the particular thought process and belief system. This would classify the disorder as being psychotic in nature. Other cases are where the compulsive action relieves a particular emotional state. This can be classified as being truly neurotic in nature.[18]

Symptoms

There are usually three forms of this condition. There may be merely ideas and thoughts in the mind. There may be impulses to perform a particular action or the fear that they may develop such an impulse. Lastly, there may be the constant churning of things over in the mind. The performance of an action relieves such symptoms. The thoughts are frequently of an aggressive or sexual nature. There may also be combinations of these three forms.

The effects may be so severe that they take over a person's life. Typical actions include hand washing or constantly checking that doors and windows are closed.

Treatment

This is notoriously difficult conventionally. Reassurance and behavioural therapy are employed. People are frequently treated with tricyclic antidepressants, usually the newer selective serotonin reuptake inhibitors (SSRIs) but at much higher doses than for treatment of depression. Psychosurgery is sometimes used for this condition.

Depressive neurosis

Depression is classified into 'major' or 'minor' types. 'Major' depression, so-called endogenous depression, is the type described under manic depressive illness. 'Minor' depression, so-called reactive depression, is the type discussed here.

It occurs after a personal setback, e.g. loss due to divorce or bereavement. There is not always a clear line between this and the depression described in manic depressive illness above. Depression, as a low mood, is a common feeling and all of us develop this from time to time. When it becomes excessive, it may be diagnosed as depression. It may develop at any age, with women twice as likely to be diagnosed than men. Around 10 per cent of people develop such symptoms at some time in their life. Recurrences are common although the first presentation is usually as a young adult.

Symptoms

The term depression is a loose one, which is often applied to mean low mood. It may be used to mean sadness, weeping, unhappiness, dissatisfaction and so forth. When clinically diagnosed there are several criteria to be fulfilled:

- personal setback
- pre-disposing situation of vulnerability or emotional difficulties
- fluctuating situation that responds to changes in the environment.

The distinction between this type and that of 'major' depressive illness is that the latter has more severe symptoms. There are strong feelings of negativity and self-blame along with associated physical symptoms. However, even in this 'minor' type there may be physical symptoms such as sleep disturbances, loss of libido and tiredness. Occasionally, suicidal thoughts or feelings may be seen in severe cases. Counselling and psychotherapy tend to be utilised more with this type of depression than with the 'major' type.

Treatment

This is commonly by means of prescribed drugs – the antidepressants.[19] They are commonly given and there were 8.5 million prescriptions for antidepressants in the UK in 1989. There are several groups of antidepressants.

The tricyclic antidepressants increase the stimulant actions of noradrenaline and serotonin thus leading to the main side-effects of constipation, tremor, palpitations, mania and restless sleep. Examples include imipramine, amitriptyline, nortriptyline, mianserin, lofepramine, clomipramine, doxepin and trazodone.

The monoamine oxidase inhibitors such as isocarboxazid, phenelzine and tranylcypromine block the enzymes monoamine oxidase A and B thereby leading to increased levels of noradrenaline and other stimulant chemicals. They produce high blood pressure with certain foods, e.g. cheese, yeast extract, some red wines.

Serotonin reuptake inhibitors (SSRIs) are newer antidepressants. They include fluoxetine hydrochloride (Prozac), fluvoxamine, sertraline and paroxetine. These are much in vogue at the moment. They are advertised as helping clinical states of depression as well as relieving some of the minor irritations and dissatisfactions of life. It is currently taken by 4.5 million Americans and 0.5 million Britons. Seventy per cent of users in the US are women.

They have many side-effects, which are shared by the other antidepressants. They include anorexia, weight loss,[20] anxiety, nervousness, mania, hypomania, insomnia, fatigue, tremor, dizziness, convulsions, reduced libido, excess sweating and rash. All the antidepressants have a similar action that is reminiscent of amphetamine (known colloquially as 'speed'). This lifts the mood of depression but, of course, does nothing to remedy the underlying cause.

These newer drugs are also marketed as more than antidepressants. The approach is similar to that taken with the tranquillisers, benzodiazepine, which were marketed as 'mother's little helpers'. The 'non-pathological' trend of prescribing is increasing as they are touted as the answer to all psychological ills. Doctors in the US may give Prozac, for example, to people who wish to overcome perceived personality deficiencies. There are people who take Prozac to boost their confidence for a job interview, to be more 'successful' with relationships and as a recreational drug to 'feel good'.

Many people, however, feel that the personality produced is not a real or useful one. It also has the effect of making people who take it develop the same personality, 'shiny, happy people' as Professor David Rothman[21] has described them. He sees 'a danger of it being used as a method of pharmacologically induced social control'. It would be more accurate to acknowledge that this is what is already happening.

Conventional psychiatric treatment is an example of how one group of the population seeks to remove or control the feelings, thoughts and experiences of another, more vulnerable, section of the population. It happened with the benzodiazepine tranquillisers, it happens daily with powerful anti-psychotic agents and electroconvulsive treatment and it is beginning to happen with Prozac. This is not to say that people with psychological disturbances do not have real problems. Of course they do. However, once one group of society starts to label such disturbances and prescribe mind-altering drugs, the result for the recipients can only be dependence and powerlessness.

Electroconvulsive treatment (ECT) is the administration of electric shocks to the brain. It is used to treat severe depression, mania, schizophrenia in cases where patients are suicidal, injures themselves, refuse to eat or drink, or 'cannot or will not take medication'. It is performed under general anaesthesia[22] and is related to earlier methods of inducing epileptic attacks as it was noted that schizophrenia was less common in people with epilepsy. An example was insulin shock treatment where doses of insulin were given to induce hypoglycaemic coma.[23] These and similar treatments are described in an interesting book based upon real-life experiences in the 1940s.[24]

Some 20,000 people in the UK have ECT each year. In the US this figure is given as 30,000 to 50,000 with some estimates suggesting 100,000 people in the US each year receiving ECT. A series of five treatments is usually given with follow-up administration of antidepressants. There are differences according to area as psychiatrists have different preferences. If you live in the west of England, for example, you are twice as likely to receive ECT than if you live in Oxford. At least 600 children have had ECT over the past decade, which is particularly worrying, as their development is still taking place. About 70 per cent of recipients of ECT are women. This is not surprising since depression is twice as likely to be diagnosed in women. ECT is relatively overused in people from ethnic minorities but this reflects the greater likelihood of a diagnosis of psychological disturbance in these groups.

It is claimed that improvement in depression can result from ECT.[25] Short-term side-effects include confusion, headache, disorientation, palpitations, muscle ache, physical weakness, dizziness and memory loss. Longer lasting side-effects, which may be permanent, include memory loss,[26] apathy, learning difficulties and loss of creative drive and energy. If people have such treatment as an outpatient they have to be taken to their house rather than dropped off at the end of the road. It may be that the confusion and loss of memory are the methods by which any perceived improvement is achieved. ECT advocate, Max Fink, ascribes the damaging effect to the substance of the brain as the reason for improvement. He states, 'It is similar to that of craniocerebral trauma or head injury'.[27] The person no longer knows or can remember how they feel![28]

In the US there is a group of 500 people who have experienced memory loss for up to 2 years after ECT. Psychiatrists reveal their innermost thoughts by their reactions to various groups. They state that the memory loss of ECT is temporary in relation to treating housewives but still express caution over treating 'patients whose occupation requires intellectual ability'.[29]

A further issue is that ECT, as with all conventional medical treatments, gives the message that psychological distress is a mechanical process. This denies a person's experience and feelings and is inherently depersonalising. It is also disempowering as it leaves the doctor with the responsibility for relief and fosters a continuing pattern of dependency. Compulsory treatment is clearly even more disempowering and may be experienced as a form of punishment[30] or torture. Psychologist Norman S. Sutherland points out in his book, *Breakdown*, that ECT 'was widely dreaded', and he says 'there are many reports from patients likening the atmosphere in hospital on days when ECT was to be administered to that of a prison on the day of an execution'.

A muscle relaxant is used during treatment to prevent muscle contraction due to the passage of electric current through the brain. It renders the person unable to breathe independently and necessitates respiratory support (essentially a general anaesthetic). This leads to further feelings of lack of control.

Despair and worthlessness frequently accompany depression. Any reinforcement of these by disempowering treatments can only be harmful. ECT is banned in California and Italy. There are restrictions on its use compulsorily in both Canada and the Netherlands. *Against Therapy*, published in 1988, by psychoanalyst Jeffrey Masson, Ph.D., asks: "Why do psychiatrists torture people and call it electroshock therapy?".

Holistic management

The holistic management of the neuroses is described on Page 312. In terms of Chinese medicine, the antidepressants are heating and primarily affect the Heart and Liver. They move the Qi by warming and dispersing. This causes weakening of Qi and damage to Blood and Yin. Long-term there will be syndromes of Heart and Liver Blood and Yin Deficiency with ultimately Kidney Yin Deficiency. Withdrawal of antidepressants leads to a flare-up of Yin that manifests as Stagnation syndromes such as Stagnant Liver Qi. There may be weeping and emotional releases, depression and so forth. Withdrawal of such drugs must be slow with appropriate support and treatment at the same time.

Case one

A woman of 42 years came for treatment. She had been taking Prozac for over 2 years after suffering from depression for some time. She was taking three tablets per week. She had been on courses of antidepressants in the past. She had low energy, frequent urination with leaking and lumbar pain. The diagnosis in terms of Chinese medicine was Kidney Yang Deficiency and Heart Blood Deficiency.

I treated her with herbs and acupuncture to primarily strengthen her Kidney Yang. Her energy slowly improved and her urinary symptoms lessened. It is important in such cases not to attempt a dosage reduction of such powerful drugs too early or too quickly.

After several months of treatment, we discussed the possibility of drug reduction. She decided that she would try to do so. She found that reducing the dose gradually made her feel quite ill and she decided to stop completely. She began to develop some depression with negative feelings, sensitivity and critical thoughts. This was not as severe as she had experienced previously. They began to subside after 2 to 3 weeks.

Her treatment continues but she finds that she is coping without the drug and not descending into depression. She was worried that this would happen as it had in the past. The point here is that people can change their responses when they have support. It is difficult to stop a drug without the help of balancing and curative health care. This time she had that help and the outcome was markedly different.

GENERAL COMMENTS ABOUT HOLISTIC MANAGEMENT OF THE NEUROSES

Holistic medicine does not seek to divide and separate the levels of a human being. Physical, emotional and mental aspects are considered as a whole. In terms of Chinese medicine, each of the five major organs, Liver, Heart, Kidney, Spleen and Lung have aspects that correspond to these three levels as well as their paired organs. Table 16.2 lists their mental and emotional aspects.

Organ	Mental aspect	Emotional aspect
Liver	Kindly and giving attitude, sharing	Anger, jealousy, assertiveness, resentment, guilt
Gall Bladder	Decision making	Timidity, lack of courage
Heart	Responsibility, gratitude, appreciation, politeness, humility	Joy, happiness
Small Intestine	Awareness, sensitivity, discernment	
Kidney	Intellect, intelligence, wisdom, insight, will power, ambition	Fear
Urinary Bladder		Jealousy, resentment
Spleen	Belief, faith, confidence, trust	Sympathy
Stomach	Endurance, stamina, ability to keep going	
Lung	Sensibility, compassion, attitude, sensitiveness, vulnerability	Grief, sadness
Large Intestine	Forgiveness, letting go	

Table 16.2: Mental and emotional aspects of organs[31]

It can be seen from this Table, that emotions such as depression may arise from several sources. It may be sadness and grief due to a Lung imbalance or a lack of joy from the Heart. It may be the apathy due to lack of ambition relating to the Kidney. There may be a lack of free flowing of Qi due to a Liver imbalance or a churning, rumination from the Spleen. It is essential, therefore, whatever the prime, presenting symptom, to individualise the case and give appropriate treatment. What is not helpful is to give every person the same thing as in conventional prescribing of tranquillisers or antidepressants.

It is helpful to summarise the help that can be offered people with psychological disorders. A specific treatment such as homoeopathy, acupuncture or herbs is of inestimable value in supporting people and correcting energetic imbalances. It is not enough, however, to think that this is the complete story. In the West, particularly, psychological disturbances are deep-seated. They frequently arise out of infancy and childhood. We are often brought up in environments that may be emotionally deprived and conflict ridden. These environments expose us to inappropriate influences often at an early age.

A common 'inappropriate' influence is abuse. This may be sexual and is frequently emotional. Twenty per cent of women who had been sexually abused as a child have mental health problems, as opposed to 6.3 per cent of the non-abused population. Almost half of psychiatric in-patients had histories of sexual/physical abuse.

These issues are not going to be completely remedied by treatment with holistic medicine over some weeks or even months. Although we all have witnessed remarkable success stories where genuine transformations have taken place rapidly, for most people, the process is more gradual.[32]

Psychological approaches are valuable in giving people extra help. My view is that this may be counterproductive if it is too cathartic, too confrontational, and too invasive. The mind is complex, its neuroses so rich and varied, we can dig forever and come up with a problem or difficulty to be analysed. This is not necessarily helpful. The important issue, in my view, is how to encourage people to recognise their own wisdom and clarity. As the Tibetans say, 'if the dung is dry, do not stir it.' Gentle methods of transformation are usually more helpful than constant identification with the problem. Identification with the solution is more beneficial. There are too many individual therapies to list here and it is, in any case, the approach of the therapist that is the key. 'It is not what you do but the way that you do it.' It is helpful for us as practitioners to know therapists in our area to whom we can refer people.

DISORDERS OF THE MENTAL LEVEL (psychoses)

Delirium

This is an acute disturbance of the mental level, which accompanies a physical disease. It may also be known as acute brain syndrome, acute confusional state, toxic psychosis or metabolic encephalopathy. It is seen in the following situations:

- drug intoxication, e.g. alcohol, LSD
- drug withdrawal
- infectious disease particularly when associated with a fever
- metabolic disturbances, e.g. liver failure, kidney failure, hypoglycaemia
- vitamin deficiency, e.g. Vitamin B_{12}
- lack of oxygen supply to the brain, e.g. pneumonia, chronic bronchitis, cardiac failure
- head injury.[33]

Symptoms
The onset is usually rapid with a speedy development of symptoms. There may be the symptoms of the associated physical disease together with disturbance on the mental level. These include mental restlessness, disorientation, poor memory, hallucinations (particularly visual, which may be fearful) and, eventually, confusion. Insomnia is common and agitation may be more marked at night. A particular syndrome is related to the withdrawal of excess alcohol intake. This is termed 'delirium tremens' (DTs).

Investigations
Those done will depend upon the suspected underlying disease and details of these are found in the relevant chapters.

Treatment
The treatment is of the preceding condition.

Holistic management
In terms of holistic medicine, the occurrence of mental symptoms in association with physical disease means that the imbalance on an energetic level has passed much deeper into the person. It necessarily indicates a more serious situation. Such situations are described at the end of relevant chapters dealing with symptoms. For example, the occurrence of breathlessness associated with confusion indicates a serious underlying condition – see Page 144. You may need to refer such people for acute medical care.

Dementia

This is a chronic situation that becomes more common with increasing age. There are considered to be around 1 in 20 cases at the age of 70 years and 1 in 5 at the age of 80 years. In conventional medical thought, it is considered to be secondary to a chronic disease of the brain. These include cerebrovascular disease and Alzheimer's disease.[34]

Symptoms
The age of first development of symptoms is variable and partially dependent upon the associated condition. For example, Alzheimer's disease may first develop when aged 40 years or so. Cerebrovascular disease manifests at later ages. A distinction is sometimes made at the age of 60 years. Onset before this is denoted presenile dementia whilst the later development of symptoms is called senile dementia.

The onset is slow as would be expected with a chronic disease. The symptoms depend upon the previous personality and emotional state of the person. There is interference with judgement and reasoning. Memory becomes poor, particularly for recent events. There may be emotional instability and the emotions may fluctuate from euphoria or mania to depression.

Eventually the person affected may have difficulty with personal hygiene, dressing, eating and so forth. There can be increasing agitation, particularly at night, insomnia and eventually confusion. In severe cases, there is loss of recognition of even close relatives and the only events remembered may be several decades previously. Consequently, this can be distressing for relatives who are involved with care. There is a large part to be played here by voluntary organisations or professional carers to help support the family.

In the most severe cases there is gradual deterioration until the person cannot leave the bed. At this stage there is a risk of respiratory problems and pneumonia may be the final life-threatening event.

Investigations
Routine investigations may be performed to exclude 'physical' causes of such a clinical picture. These include brain scan, thyroxine and Vitamin B_{12} levels. It is important to review medication, as there are many drugs that cause confusion.

Treatment
The conventional treatment of psychotic disorders in general is summarised below. Hydergine may be used in Alzheimer's disease and other dementias and can accelerate the progression of the disease.[35] The first drug approved for use in Alzheimer's disease is donepezil, which may produce slight improvements in mental function. Other medications that may be given include Vitamin E and selegiline, a monoamine oxidase inhibitor.

Holistic management
This is as described under schizophrenia.

Schizophrenia

This condition can be described as a disintegration of the personality leading to detachment from the social environment. It can affect any age group but usually first develops between the ages of 19 and 25. There are some 250,000 people with schizophrenia in the UK and 55 million worldwide. Schizophrenia affects 1 per cent of the world's population at any one time but in the UK, the diagnosis is 10 times more common in young Afro-Caribbean men. The Irish are also more likely to be so diagnosed. The reasons for these racial differences in *diagnosis* are discussed later. Some 50 per cent of psychiatric beds are occupied by people with schizophrenia.

Symptoms
Schizophrenia is primarily a disorder of thought. In the classical case, thoughts are rambling and disjointed. The emotions may be inappropriate. Actions, as a consequence, may be impulsive. Hallucinations are a characteristic feature. There may be threatening or unfriendly voices. Bizarre delusions are common. It is usual for people with this condition to consider their actions are controlled from the outside. This leads to ideas such as being controlled by aliens from another world. Delusions tend to be culturally specific. In the latter part of the 20th century in the West, it is common to see them related to space travel, electronics and computers. In a more religious age they tended to be linked to devils and spirits.

Another perception is that other people place thoughts in their mind – or that they remove them. Paranoia may be a feature where the person thinks others watch them and want to do them harm. This can lead to delusions that government agents are plotting against them. There is little insight with this condition although this varies from person to person and may change with time.

The person's ability to function declines with little capacity for work. Social relations are disrupted and self-care may be poor. Abrupt, inexplicable behaviour is seen which may be socially unacceptable to others. Compulsory hospital admission may be required in severely affected cases where there is disruption to the ability to care for oneself.

There may be worry about the safety of the person with schizophrenia or those who come into contact with them. This is frequently overstated and it is unusual that people need to be compulsorily admitted for their own or others 'good'.

Conventional treatment
Without treatment, many cases of schizophrenia improve spontaneously within 3-9 months after the flare-up of symptoms. This is more likely if the onset is acute and the symptoms are strong. A more chronic course is likely if the onset is slow with less prominent symptoms. Support for both the family and the patient are essential and directly affect the degree of success at managing patient's symptoms and allowing them to lead a normal life. Intensive psychotherapy is contraindicated and can

lead to exacerbations of the psychological state.

Conventional treatment is invariably with drugs, which suppress thoughts. They are essentially sedative in nature and are classified as the 'major' tranquillisers.[36] These are not to be confused with the 'minor' tranquillisers, which are used to treat simple anxiety. There were nearly 4.5 million prescriptions for antipsychotic drugs in the UK in 1987.

The main group of drugs is the phenothiazines of which chlorpromazine is a common example. Other phenothiazines are trifluoperazine, fluphenazine (injected weekly or less often), promazine and thioridazine. Other antipsychotic agents include the butyrophenones such as droperidol, haloperidol and benperidol and the dibenzoxazepines of clozapine[37] and loxapine. A newer type with fewer side-effects affecting the central nervous system is the benzisoxazole derivative, risperidone.

There are many side-effects with these groups of drugs but the most severe is tardive dyskinesia, a disorder similar to Parkinson's disease. It is a result of damage to the brain by prescribed drugs and is usually irreversible. Up to 65 per cent of long-term users of antipsychotic drugs develop tardive dyskinesia. Symptoms include tremor, slow movement, uncontrollable facial grimaces and lip smacking.

In acute situations, large doses of such drugs may be given and this can lead to fatal consequences. Professor Malcolm Lader, Professor of Clinical Psychopharmacology at the Institute of Psychiatry, estimates that one death per week in the UK occurs from reactions to antipsychotics. The cause of death may often be attributed to a disease rather than the drug and so accurate figures are difficult to obtain. There are, however, regular occurrences of deaths in psychiatric hospitals after the administration of large doses of antipsychotic drugs. A Channel 4 television programme, *Dispatches*, identified 52 cases in the UK in the period 1988-92.

The doses used may be in excess of those recommended in the literature. The drugs are used to immobilise people. Chlorpromazine (Trade name – Largactil) is known in prisons as the 'liquid cosh' for this reason. It is certainly a method of restricting activity and is quicker than more gentle methods, which may require more staff and care.

Electroconvulsive therapy is occasionally used in the treatment of acute schizophrenia with variable effectiveness.

Some people with psychotic illnesses are compulsorily admitted to hospital. There is much discussion about the need for and usefulness of such an action. Certainly, there have been notable critics of dealing with psychological problems in this way. Well known, at least in the UK, is R.D. Laing who questioned the right of any society to deem some of its members 'insane'.[38] Medical labels applied to groups of people may appear, on the surface, to be for the benefit of the patient. In reality, the reasons for such labels and subsequent treatment may be more to do with social control.[39]

High rates of psychiatric admission are found amongst people from central urban areas of low social class and a high concentration of immigrants. Although, in the UK, it may be true that West Indian immigrants are no more likely to become psychiatric in-patients, when they do so it is more likely to be on a compulsory basis. Those of West Indian origin are twice as likely as white people to have been admitted compulsorily. They were also more likely to be sent to hospital from prison or by police agencies with little GP involvement.[40]

In one survey, out of 286 patients admitted by police to a psychiatric hospital, an excess of black people was recorded. Black men were not only younger but also more likely to be given antipsychotic drugs and put on compulsory orders. They were also more likely to be given an outpatient appointment when discharged from hospital. In addition, more black men were given a diagnosis of schizophrenia or drug-induced psychosis.[41]

In the UK, the numbers of compulsory admissions have been falling over recent years. In 1964 this was 32,735 (21 per cent of total admissions). In 1977 this had fallen to 19,426 (10.5 per cent). There has been a general move in recent years away from hospital admission for psychiatric disturbances. It has been part of a much-advertised 'care in the community' scheme.[42] This is a euphemism for lack of care by the community and large numbers of vulnerable people have been left to fend for themselves. There has been some effort to replace hospital beds by sheltered housing or hostel accommodation. However, this has been generally inadequate and many people with severe mental problems live in the streets as best they can. Some have died as a result and others live a miserable existence.

In the UK, the Mental Health Act of 1983 regulates the compulsory admission and treatment of people with psychiatric illness. It is applied when a person has a named psychological disorder, their own or other's safety is at risk and they are unwilling to be hospitalised voluntarily. It clearly must not be applied without serious thought since the individual is deprived of their liberty and certain legal rights. The Act also deals with people's rights, appeals tribunals and the supervision of the use of compulsory powers. Despite these safeguards, many people find themselves in the difficult position of having to *prove* that they are sane within the meaning of conventional psychiatry. How many of us would find this easy or even possible! Therefore, it can be difficult for some people to obtain discharge from hospital or remove themselves from continual supervision.

Different sections of the Act deal with different situations. Table 16.3. is a summary.

Section	Details	Comments
2[43]	Valid for 28 days. Requires signatures of nearest relative or social worker plus two doctors one of whom must be an approved specialist psychiatrist	Used for assessment and treatment
3	Valid for 6 months. Requires signatures of nearest relative or social worker plus two doctors one of whom must be an approved specialist psychiatrist	Used for treatment
4	Valid for 72 hours. Requires signature of nearest relative or social worker plus one doctor	Emergency admission
5(2)	Valid for 72 hours. Requires signature of the doctor in charge of care	Emergency detention of person already in hospital
5(4)	Valid for 72 hours. Requires signature of registered mental nurse	Emergency detention of person already in hospital
136	Police officer	Assessment. Used in public places when person thought to be mentally ill and requiring place of safety

Table 16.3: Main sections of the Mental Health Act 1983

Operations on the brain, so-called psychosurgery, are not common but may be performed for a range of psychological conditions. Such treatment used to be more common for schizophrenia around 30 years ago but has reduced in popularity due to the use of drugs. Nowadays it is usually reserved for severe depression that is unresponsive to drugs, obsessional neurosis, anxiety neurosis and manic depressive illness. There were 27 operations in the UK in 1990 compared with 70 in 1979. Parts of the brain are surgically disconnected or destroyed by the implantation of radioactive materials. Those who perform such operations claim they are successful despite the fact that no trial of their usefulness has ever been performed. In addition, the understanding of the relationship between the emotions and the brain is tenuous to say the least. Noted effects include apathy, excessive weight gain, disinhibition and epilepsy. Psychosurgery has been used to reduce aggression and anti-social behaviour.

Holistic management

These disorders, in any terms, are difficult to manage. Disturbances of the mental level indicate some of the most severe disorders of health. A multiple approach is necessary, preferably involving people experienced in dealing with serious mental disorders. The more severe the problem, the more it seems necessary to take complete care of someone.[44] There are several groups who look after and treat mentally disturbed people without recourse to drugs and conventional treatment. It is helpful to have access to these for those few people who seek your help.

You must be aware that prescribed drugs are heavily suppressive of thought disorders. Their removal may result in an acute flare-up of symptoms including loss of insight. This may only develop some weeks after total cessation of the medication with little or no prior warning. This is the reason why several approaches are necessary with facilities for care. In the context of outpatient practice it is difficult to treat such people.

In terms of Chinese medicine, there are considered to be two main categories of schizophrenia although a similar diagnosis may be made in any similar mental disturbance. There is an active, manic (Yang) type where depression and anger transform to Fire in the Liver and Gall Bladder. This is accompanied by Phlegm, which disrupts the Spirit in the Heart.

The quiet, depressive (Yin) type is where excessive anxiety impedes the circulation of Qi and causes fluids to congeal and form Phlegm. When Phlegm rises, the senses become obscured and consciousness is disrupted.

Case one

A man of 17 years was brought by his family for treatment. He had been diagnosed 3 months previously with schizophrenia and had recently been discharged from hospital. His main symptom was sleepiness due to the medication he was taking. He still had symptoms of hearing voices, which tended to be abusive. He would be quite angry and distressed on hearing them but particularly if people around him tried to explain them away or say it was not happening. I made a diagnosis of Phlegm-heat Harrassing the Mind due to long-term Stagnation of Qi in the Lung and Heart. He had experienced several losses and changes in his life including the loss of a parent as well as changes of school and home. I treated him three times weekly with acupuncture to good effect. Each time after the treatment, he would feel more relaxed, be more out-going and be more energetic. His treatment continues. A difficulty in treating people with severe mental disorders is the amount and severity of the medication they are taking. It is possible to treat alongside the drug and I am strongly of the opinion that it is helpful to treat in all circumstances if possible. Long-term side-effects will be minimised and general health will improve. It is always tricky in any individual case to predict what will be the eventual outcome. However, treatment by means of holistic medicine will be supportive to the patient and their family.

Manic depressive disorder

There are several categories of mania and depression depending upon the particular manifestation. Classical manic depressive illness is a swing between the extremes of mania (elevated mood), and depression (depressed mood). Some people exhibit only mania whilst others seem to develop only depression. This type of depression may also be known by the term 'endogenous' depression. The milder, 'reactive' form of depression is described below under depressive neurosis.

The conventional view at the moment is that these disorders are due to imbalances of chemical transmitter substances within the brain. In mania, they are in excess. In depression, they are lacking. This is seen very much as a justification for chemical methods of control. Psychological and psychotherapeutic models are not given credence at this time. Consequently, treatment is invariably by means of drugs.

Symptoms
Mania is a persistent elevation in mood that may last for weeks or months. There is agitation, insomnia and restlessness. Thoughts arrive rapidly and usually involve grandiose yet unrealistic plans. The mood is essentially euphoric but with lack of insight. Resultant behaviour may be disruptive such as spending large amounts of money, travelling long distances and so forth. The person may become violent if their ideas are resisted. There may be associated hallucinations, delusions and other thought disorders resembling classical schizophrenia. Milder forms are known as hypomania.

Mania may alternate with depression. The use of the word depression is something of a misnomer. The term can mean many different things to different people. It may be used to described a low mood, a state of sadness or apathy. In this condition, it is a gloominess or despair and is severe.

It is not the feeling of lowness that many people have from time to time, which could be considered a variation of normal. It is the depths of a black despair where there may be severe associated symptoms of unworthiness, self blame, guilt and perhaps even suicidal thoughts or feelings. There may also be associated physical symptoms of constipation, poor appetite, weight loss, headaches, reduced libido and so forth. Suicide is a risk. In severe cases the feelings of guilt, self-blame and futility may attain delusional levels.

Some people seem to develop only mania or only depression.

Treatment
Compulsory hospitalisation may be necessary if symptoms are very strong. This usually involves sedation by means of antipsychotic medication (for details see treatment of schizophrenia).

To prevent relapse, lithium compounds are used.[45] The drug has severe effects and requires careful medical supervision as it can affect the thyroid, liver, kidney and central nervous system. It may also interfere with water and mineral homeostasis. There should be thyroid and kidney screening before prescription and lithium levels must be checked every 3 months. It has to be stopped before pregnancy because it can cause malformations of the cardiovascular system in the foetus.

Without treatment, manic depressive episodes may resolve over several months or a year or so. Treatment is often continued for life. Other treatments include electroconvulsive treatment and perhaps additional tranquillisation.

Holistic management
Manic depressive illness, in terms of Chinese medicine, corresponds to the syndromes listed under schizophrenia.

Case one
A man of 25 years came for treatment of recurrent symptoms of agitation and restlessness. These had started after he had taken Lariam, a malarial preventative, some 4 years before and caused increased anxiety and worrying over small things. His sleep was often disturbed due to his mind being busy. His energy was low. Every spring and autumn for the 2 years prior to attending for treatment he had become hyperactive and agitated. He would spend large amounts of money and find it impossible to sleep at all. Physically, he would often feel a 'knot' in his stomach and a feeling of 'butterflies'. He would have

palpitations when anxious. His bowels were generally normal but constipated when agitated. I made a diagnosis of Kidney and Heart Yin Deficiency with Empty Fire Flaring. The causes were the original prescription of Lariam together with overwork and worry whilst at University.

I treated him with both acupuncture and herbs for several months and then he moved away because of work commitments. During this time, he developed severe agitation and manic symptoms. He was admitted to hospital for 3 months and given haloperidol to sedate him.

I resumed treating him and recommended that he saw a counsellor to help resolve some long-standing emotional issues arising from the death of a relative some years before. He also commenced yoga classes. Over the course of the next 3 months, his medication was slowly withdrawn by the hospital with no relapses. He would sometimes develop restless and dream-disturbed sleep after a reduction in medication but this would settle. I have reason to believe that things would have progressed in this satisfactory manner except for a couple of important events. One was a tendency to socialise late at night and take mild stimulants. The other was a change in psychiatrist who was keen to prescribe lithium. The conventional view is that if there have been one or more relapses, lithium is the drug to balance the chemicals within the brain. He decided that lithium would offer more long-term stability. He has continued with acupuncture and herbal treatment, which I have modified slightly in view of his medication. I have encouraged him to continue with the counselling work and his treatment continues.

In treating people with conditions such as mania, it is important to take a long view. Such disturbances are deeply rooted in the psyche and there are many influences on people's lives. Progress will tend to be slow and there are many aspects of thought and feeling to unravel. It is helpful not to become over attached to progress or its perceived lack. There is a need for support and treatment over many months and years.

Eating disorders (anorexia nervosa/bulimia nervosa)

Anorexia and bulimia nervosa are eating disorders that are associated with disturbances in perception and for this reason may be realistically labelled psychoses. The perception is usually of being overweight or 'the wrong shape'. Anorexia is a desire to lose weight through controlling the appetite, whilst bulimia involves over-eating and bingeing on certain foods and is often followed by self-induced vomiting.

Ninety-five per cent of those who develop such disorders are female. Such conditions, therefore, cannot be separated from societal views of women and their shape. Women are bombarded from an early age with images of (supposedly) fit and healthy women. In my opinion, such images are the result of anorexic behaviour and certainly not to be considered a normal female shape. Females tend to be Yin, which manifests as a rounded shape. Angular forms are a sign of malnutrition.

Symptoms
There is a preoccupation with food. A variety of feelings and thoughts about appearance are invariable. The person frequently has feelings of disgust for food yet with uncontrollable urges to eat. There may be almost complete absence of desire for food. Eating to the point of vomiting or producing vomiting is common. Cathartics and laxatives may be taken in an effort to reduce weight.

There is a general lack of concern for any physical deterioration as weight, appearance, and food intake preoccupy the person. Extreme weight loss can be seen in some cases. Amenorrhoea is a common occurrence. Emotional and sexual immaturity is associated.

Treatment
This is notoriously difficult and some people may die as a result of anorexia nervosa. In-patient treatment may be required for severe cases where malnutrition is evident. The conventional medical approach is to combine regimes of forced feeding to achieve a certain rate of weight gain with behavioural approaches. A 'carrot and 'stick' method may be applied. 'Counselling' may also be used but is undermined by the punitive feeding regime. Various approaches are attempted to help alleviate the mental symptoms. Psychotherapy is the best option to help attain emotional maturation.

Holistic management
This is a condition that reflects a disturbance at deep levels. The person has difficulty in nourishing themselves. This is a consequence of a lack of nourishment on a mental and emotional level in the past. There are frequently disturbances in the family unit and these need to be addressed if possible. The desire for weight loss is an attempt to avoid growth and maturity. Common associated events are the disappearance of menstruation together with emotional and sexual immaturity. There may be sexual or emotional difficulties between the parents, which result in this particular manifestation in the child.

In terms of Chinese medicine, it is common to see Spleen Qi deficiency as a result of irregular eating together with Liver Qi Stagnation as a result of long-term emotional suppression. A psychological approach is helpful as well as treatment to strengthen the digestion.

Case one

A woman of 30 years came for treatment. She had had a reaction to a bowel cleansing formula of oils and herbs. She felt 'hung over', weak and emotionally upset. She had a history of episodes of over-eating alternating with fasting. In terms of Chinese medicine, her diagnosis was Spleen Qi Deficiency (of long-standing) exacerbated by a history of irregular eating together with Liver Qi Stagnation.

In my experience, this is not the origin of the problem as the irregular eating is the result of earlier disturbances. This condition arises early in childhood due to a lack of nourishment within the family. This may not be, and often is not, a lack of physical nourishment. It is more related to a deprivation of emotional care together with the development of messages of guilt and responsibility. Feelings and thoughts of disgust and a poor self-image are universal. The attempts of women to attain and maintain an 'ideal' shape are very destructive of their digestive health. A cycle of eating, fasting and excess exercise can only be depleting.

I treated her by strengthening her Spleen and recommending a regular diet of warm food. Over the course of the next few months, she experienced feelings and dreams that were unpleasant as old memories surfaced. Gradually she became more positive and after 6 months of treatment she would only occasionally revert to her old eating patterns. Even so, the associated emotions and thoughts were not as strong and she felt a greater sense of non-attachment. Interestingly, her weight increased in this time by some 10 pounds. This was of some concern to her but it is important to reassure people that this is healthy. Also, education about the nature of health and the importance of psychological health is needed. Physical changes occur secondary to changes in our mental and emotional levels and people may require patience to allow this process to develop. Any weight fluctuations will eventually settle although many women in this situation are underweight initially.

CLASSIFICATIONS OF THE PERSONALITY

The idea of personality groups arose from the view that a number of people do not conform to the prevailing norm. This has led to a recent recognition in conventional circles of personality disorders. It has been noted that certain personality types tended to develop particular patterns of behaviour and psychological states (e.g. obsessional neurosis in people with obsessional personality disorder). The precise classification and description depend upon the source.[46]

The concept of 'disordered personality' is a tricky one and certainly a source of potential abuse. It is difficult to see the rationale behind labelling some people as 'sick' whilst society at large is hardly 'sane'. This remains a dilemma for conventional psychiatry, which is usually not addressed.

It is more helpful to use personality classifications as a way of trying to understand how different people may respond to different situations. Eventually, it is for each individual to come to terms with their own 'neurosis' and find ways in which they can function most effectively. In the clinical setting, such issues arise because people are dissatisfied with themselves most of the time, there is a limitation to their everyday life and relationships or there is difficulty in achieving goals and ambitions.

Obsessional personality

This person has little regard for the emotional aspects of a situation. There is rigidity and attention to detail. Such people prefer order and predictability. They are methodical and punctual. There are psychological disturbances if routines are upset.

The desire for order and perfection may lead to interference with other aspects of life. The energy and emotions may suffer as a result. Blind faith and reliance on others in authority is common. There may be 'tightness' with money. It is difficult for such people to share with others or to delegate responsibility.

Schizoid personality

This type of person is solitary, detached and distant from other people. They may be the classic 'introvert'. They are frequently shy, solitary workers and have little empathy with other people. There may be strong emotions, which are hard to express. There may be suspiciousness and sensitivity.

There is a lack of lightness of mood. Vulnerability, warmth and the ability to relate to others' feelings are difficult. Such people may become fixated on matters that assume great importance. They may take up campaigns and crusades with fervour. It is considered by some that such traits arise because of an upbringing where anger is dominant, obvious and inappropriate.

Hysterical personality

This group is liable to excessive displays of emotion. They crave attention and seek to please and influence others. Such people are showy and histrionic in behaviour. Long-term relationships are difficult due to the lack of emotional maturity. This is frequently the result of emotional deprivation in childhood.

The extremes of emotion may be manifest quickly and fluctuate as easily. There may be a history of failed relationships.

Personality theorists have indicated that such a style stems from a dependency with associated feelings of inadequacy and lack of confidence. It is a type that tends to be overdiagnosed in women.[47]

Sociopathy

Such people are described as 'affectionless'. It is the most severe of all the personality disorders. There is a lack of conscience. They are loveless, indifferent and may be destructive. There is impulsive behaviour, which may be considered socially unacceptable, e.g. stealing, excessive gambling, and physical assaults. There is a noted lack of regard for the consequences of actions. There are frequently legal problems as a result and management is difficult.

HOW TO RECOGNISE A SERIOUS PSYCHOLOGICAL DISORDER

Psychological disorders are common and particularly so in the holistic medical clinic. They are frequently neurotic in nature and mild. Occasionally, they can be severe and limiting. Rarely, they may be psychotic in form. It is important for you to know the significance of psychotic symptoms and the differences in management between neurosis and psychosis. Table 16.4 lists symptoms indicating cause for concern. Such people may require hospitalisation or another place of safety.

Symptom	Cause for concern
Suicidal thoughts	Always
Suicidal feelings	Always
Hallucinations	Always
Delusions	Always
Thought disorders	If severe
Emotional symptoms, e.g. anxiety, fear, depression	If severe
Disturbance in body image	If associated with weight loss, amenorrhoea

Table 16.4: How to recognise a serious psychological disorder

SUMMARY

Psychological disorders are extremely common in the West.

It is important in your management of the case to be able to determine the emphasis of the symptoms – mental or emotional.

People with these disorders need help and support from several sources.

Counselling and psychotherapy, of an appropriate nature, can be extremely beneficial in helping people resolve psychological issues.

It is essential for the practitioner to understand the different aspect of mind and its functioning. This is so that the person's psychological state can be viewed within the whole perspective of human experience and its possibilities.

[1] In the words of psychiatrist David Kaiser: "Patients have been diagnosed with "chemical imbalances" despite the fact that no test exists to support such a claim, and ... there is no real conception of what a correct chemical balance would look like"

[2] *Reality Therapy in Action* by William Glasser, M.D. (HarperCollins, 2000).

[3] The common usage of neurosis and neurotic is invariably pejorative. They are applied more readily to women than men.

[4] Research carried out at University of Maryland School of Pharmacy, *Journal of the American Medical Association,* February 23, 2000.

[5] Dr Peter Breggin, M.D., psychiatrist and David Cohen, Ph.D., social work professor state: "There are no drugs that improve mental function, self-understanding, or human relations. Any drug that affects mental processes does so by impairing them." *Your Drug May Be Your Problem: How and Why to Stop Taking Psychiatric Drugs* by Breggin and Cohen, (Reading, Massachusetts: Perseus Books, 1999).

[6] For more details of the Tibetan medical approach, I would recommend *The Healing Buddha* by Raoul Birnbaum (Rider, 1980) and *The Diamond Healing – Tibetan Buddhist Medicine and Psychiatry* by Terry Clifford (Crucible, 1984).

[7] *The Tibetan Book of Living of Dying* by Sogyal Rinpoche (Rider, 1993) provides a clear discussion of Mind and its true nature. Chapters 4, 5 and 10 in particular deal with Mind.

[8] To differentiate the aspects of mind I have delineated here, I use 'mind' to denote the busy, chattering and discursive mind with which most of us are all too familiar, and 'Mind' to denote that aspect of ourselves that is beyond all suffering, that is spontaneously pure and perfect. This is called Mind in Tibetan Buddhism, God in Christianity, the Tao in Taoist thought, Allah in Islam, Krishna in Hinduism, etc.

[9] Psychosis is defined by conventional medicine as 'Severe mental illness in which the sufferer loses contact with reality. Delusions and hallucinations occur and so thought processes may be altered' – *Concise Medical Dictionary,* (OUP, 1998).

A neurosis is defined conventionally as 'a mental illness in which insight is retained but there is a maladapted way of behaving or thinking that causes suffering. A classification of neurosis is based on the symptoms which may be a pathological severe emotional state or physical complaints' – *Concise Medical Dictionary,* (OUP, 1998). Here we see the confusion of conventional medicine in that mental, emotional and physical are all included in the same definition.

[10] I restrict the term ' psychosis' to mean a disturbance of the mental level.

[11] I restrict the term 'neurosis' to mean a disturbance of the emotional level.

[12] Organic is another term for physical disturbance. It is a term which is frequently paired with functional which implies a non-physical, i.e. psychological, disturbance.

[13] These may be termed, 'minor' disorders to differentiate them from the 'major' disorders of the psychoses. They are frequently treated by means of 'minor' tranquillisers, e.g. benzodiazepines.

[14] These may be termed, 'major' disorders to differentiate them from the 'minor' disorders of the neuroses. They are frequently treated by means of 'major' tranquillisers, e.g. phenothiazines.

[15] This corresponds to subcategories of organic mental disorder in Table 16.1. It is the acute development of mental symptoms associated with other disease, e.g. respiratory or cardiac disease or with the use, abuse or withdrawal of intoxicating drugs.

[16] There are comprehensive descriptions of all drug groups including the benzodiazepines included in *The Prescribed Drug Guide – A Holistic Perspective* by Dr S Gascoigne (Jigme, 2001).

[17] Article in *The Independent* of Dec. 3rd, 1991.

[18] The differentiation in this paragraph into psychotic and neurotic is my own. You would not see such in conventional thought.

[19] 'Listening to Prozac but Hearing Placebo: A Meta-Analysis of Antidepressant Medication' is the title of a study of 2,318 patients by University of Connecticut psychologist Irving Kirsch, Ph.D., and Guy Sapirstein, Ph.D. They found that 75% of the effect of antidepressant drugs is a placebo effect and that the other 25% may be caused by the fact that 'most participants in studies of antidepressant mediation are able to deduce whether they have been assigned to the drug ... or the placebo' because those receiving the drug have symptoms such as dry mouth, dizziness and lightheadedness.

[20] For this reason, it may be used to 'treat' bulimia nervosa.

[21] Article in *The Guardian* newspaper of Dec. 4th, 1994.

[22] The death rate from ECT is similar to that from general anaesthesia.

[23] All these treatments (ECT, insulin shock treatment, drugs) have one thing in common. They produce brain damage. Post-mortem examinations reveal evidence of the death of nervous tissue. This is how they produce their effect.

[24] *Savage Sleep* by Millen Brand (Crown, 1968).

[25] Studies in the UK at Leicester, Northwick Park and Nottingham have revealed that ECT produces short term improvement in depression for some people but that this is not sustained beyond 4 weeks. In contradiction, Dr Richard Weiner, a psychiatrist who specialises in treating people with ECT at Duke University, puts the success rate at 75 per cent in people with complications and 80-90 per cent in those without. These are amazing claims, to say the least, for a complex condition such as depression. If I thought there were any truth in them I might consider ECT myself!

[26] It has been stated in one study that 'some husbands used their wives' memory loss to establish their own definitions of past situations in the marital relationship'. *Electroconvulsive Therapy, the Self and Family Relations* by C.A.B. Warren, 1988.

[27] Euphoria is common after any neurological damage and this could be the source of any lift in mood.

[28] 'It is easier to numb people and induce forgetfulness than to try to eradicate poverty, provide worthwhile jobs and deal with people's demands to be listened to, understood, loved and valued as part of the community.' See *ECT – Effective but for Whom?* by J Wallcraft.

[29] Herskovitz, 1943.

[30] Atonement was given as an explanation of how ECT worked. *Fifty Shock Therapy Theories* by L Gordon, Military Surgeon 1948; 103.

[31] These organs are energetic rather than the narrow physical understanding of conventional medicine.

[32] It is difficult, on occasions, to see the benefits of a particular course of action. This is particularly true when dealing with energetic matters. Our relatively gross minds may not be able to perceive subtle changes. This does not, of course, mean that there is no effect from a particular treatment or action. The following story was told by Christine Longaker at a workshop on death and dying at Rigpa Buddhist Centre, London in 1993. I have since heard a similar story told by Elisabeth Kübler-Ross. There was a multiple car pile-up on a motorway. A woman about 10 cars from the front of the crash was unhurt but couldn't get out of her car because of other vehicles. She knew that some people had probably been injured or killed and she began to pray. About a year later, a man came to see her at her home whom she had never met. He had been in the same crash on the motorway but had been seriously injured. He had an out-of-body experience which is not unusual as part of a near death experience. He remembered passing over smashed cars and injured people and then seeing a woman praying. He felt the powerful effects of this and felt drawn back towards his body. He spent some time in hospital but very much felt that the power of her prayers had an important influence on his recovery. He had managed to trace her through the number plates of her car which had seen during his out-of-body experience.

This story reveals that our actions can have effects in areas which we may not be aware of. This is important to remember when treating people as we may not see any short-term or obvious result.

[33] I have placed this here as head injury is an acute event although the resulting clinical picture has more in common with that of dementia described below.

[34] Be careful not to confuse physical changes and mental symptoms. In terms of the classification of a disease, it depends upon where the symptoms manifest. If symptoms are primarily mental in nature then the disease is classified as mental. It does not matter whether there are physical changes. It is only the conventional view that physical changes lead to mental symptoms.

[35] *New England Journal of Medicine,* Aug 16, 1990.

[36] In this text I use the terms 'major' tranquillisers, antipsychotics and neuroleptics interchangeably to indicate groups of drugs which suppress thought disorders.

[37] All the antipsychotics have powerful side-effects and I mention some in this book. For more details see, *The Prescribed Drugs Guide – A Holistic Perspective* by S. Gascoigne (Jigme Press, 2001).

In the case of clozapine, 2 per cent of users develop a potentially lethal blood disorder. People who take it require weekly blood tests for early signs of such a disturbance. The average yearly cost to prescribe and monitor clozapine is over £2000 per person.

[38] *The Divided Self* by R.D. Laing (Penguin, 1990) This was first published in 1960 and continues to be a radical holistic to the suppressive actions of people who cannot bear to face mental and emotional states. As he quotes in his preface, '....psychiatry can so easily be a technique of brainwashing, of inducing behaviour that is adjusted, by (preferably) non-injurious torture. In the best places, where straitjackets are abolished, doors are unlocked, leucotomies largely forgone, these can be replaced by more subtle lobotomies and tranquillisers that place the bars of Bedlam and the locked doors inside the patient. Thus I would wish to emphasise that our 'normal' 'adjusted' state is too often the abdication of ecstasy, the betrayal of our true potentialities, that many of us are only too successful in acquiring a false self to adapt to false realities.' Other books by Laing which pursue these themes are *The Politics of Experience, The Bird of Paradise, Sanity, Madness and the Family,* and with A. Esterson, *Self and Others.*

[39] There are excellent sociological analyses of the impact of modern medical techniques and the reasons behind their application (rather than the oft-quoted superficial one that they are 'for your own good'). These include *Medical Nemesis* by Ivan Illich (Bantam, 1976) and *The Mirage of Health: Utopian Progress and Biological Change* by Rene Dubos (Anchor, 1959).

[40] Psychiatric Hospital Admissions in Bristol. Ineichen, Harrison and Morgan: *British Journal of Psychiatry* 1984;145:600-611.

[41] Police Admissions to a Psychiatric Hospital. Dunn and Fahy: *British Journal of Psychiatry* 1990;156:373-378.

[42] Some 70,000 in-patient places have disappeared in the UK in the last 20 years.

[43] In 1989, there were 16,900 compulsory admissions to hospital, 56 per cent of these were under Section 2. In-patients formally detained under the Mental Health Act, 1984-90, Department of Health.

[44] 'In treating insanity, the physician should constantly stay with the patient....'. *Nei Ching and Nan Ching,* Volume III, 22.1. Translation by Henry Lu.

[45] Lithium was first described as a psychiatric drug in 1949 by an Australian psychiatrist, John Cade.

[46] There are many and varied ways of labelling personality. A clear description is contained in *Body Centred Psychotherapy: The Hakomi Method* by Ron Kurtz (Hakomi Institute, 1988). Also see *Personality Types – Jung's Model of Typology* by Daryl Sharp (Inner City Books, 1987).

[47] The word hysteria, is derived from *hysterus,* the Latin for womb. It was believed, and probably still is in many areas, that such states could only exist in women and hysterectomy would cure them.

17 PREGNANCY AND CHILDBIRTH

INTRODUCTION

Obstetrics is the management of women who are pregnant or giving birth. There is overlap with gynaecology – Chapter 18. Although the application of holistic medical techniques to pregnant women is not well advanced, this is changing as more women recognise they have choices in how and where they may give birth.

There are essentially two situations that may face pregnant women. The first is medical interference in normal processes,[1] which is sadly a common situation nowadays. The second is abnormalities within these normal processes. The usual way to classify disturbances of the normal processes of pregnancy and childbirth is according to the stage at which they occur – Table 17.1.

First trimester[2]
    Morning sickness
    Miscarriage
    Large-for-dates
Second trimester
Third trimester
    Pre-eclampsia
    Antepartum haemorrhage
        Abruptio placentae
        Placenta praevia
First stage of labour[3]
    Difficult labour
    Disproportion
    Malposition
    Malpresentation
    Multiple pregnancy
Second stage of labour
    Difficult labour
    Disproportion
    Malposition
    Malpresentation
    Multiple pregnancy
Third stage of labour
    Retained placenta
    Post-partum haemorrhage
Post-natal period

Table 17.1: Classification of obstetric situations

ANATOMY AND PHYSIOLOGY

The knowledge of anatomy and physiology that is useful for the study of gynaecology is also helpful here. This is the baseline from which any changes during pregnancy can be noted. Table 17.2 lists the information it is useful to know before studying pregnancy and childbirth. To study pregnancy and childbirth it would be helpful to be able to:

- list the structures that develop after fertilisation of the egg
- describe the subsequent changes in hormone release and control
- explain the changing anatomy and physiology of the pregnant woman divided into the three trimesters
- describe the process of labour
- list the stages that occur during childbirth
- describe the puerperium.[4]

In common with gynaecology, conventional medicine sees the processes of pregnancy and childbirth as being essentially mechanical. Abnormalities are considered to be inevitable if not inherent and attempts to manipulate function (by prescribed synthetic hormones) or structure (by physical interferences) are common during pregnancy and childbirth.

HOLISTIC VIEW OF PREGNANCY AND CHILDBIRTH

The ideas expressed here are gathered mainly from Chinese medicine texts and give an energetic explanation of the events that occur at conception and pregnancy. They are necessarily holistic in nature. They provide a model that can allow people to optimise their health and that of the baby.

According to Chinese philosophy, it is the interaction of Yin and Yang that provides the basis of all existence. A human being is one aspect of this. Immaterial Yin and Yang[5] transform into material Yin and Yang. One consequence is the formation of a new life, the baby.

Conception occurs when the Yang sperm meets the Yin egg. The optimum time is considered to be about the time of the first cockcrow – about 4 or 5 a.m. This is when the energies are balanced with the Yang energy beginning to flourish. The Yang energy, in this context, is the life force itself.

It is recognised by Oriental philosophies that life begins with conception. As the Yang of the father and the Yin of the mother come together, this provides the material basis for Mind to enter. Interference with life at this early stage has long-lasting effects, which may be detrimental to health – both physical and psychological. I would include in-vitro fertilisation, freezing of embryos, experimentation on embryos and termination of pregnancy.

Techniques of termination, for example, have consequences far beyond this life as they end the life of a sentient being. They also have effects *in* this life as they disrupt the intimate connection between the foetus and the mother, which may commonly lead to menstrual abnormalities, and psychological disturbances. They can be relieved by treatment, perhaps with the help of counselling, but need to be addressed if they are to be resolved. Meditation and spiritual practices are of inestimable value in transforming such effects.

Health arises from supporting, in a natural way, the processes of conception and foetal development. In the Orient, the tradition is that people take care of their children whilst they are still in an immaterial form and whilst they are still in the uterus. So, pre-conceptual and antenatal care are of paramount importance.

The material aspect develops into the foetus in the uterus. The uterus is known as the Envelope of Yin and is intimately connected with the three Yin organs of the Liver, Spleen and Kidney. The foetus develops from the Yin and Blood of the mother. In order for the foetus to remain in the uterus and develop there need to be several associated changes.

There has to be some degree of Liver Qi Stagnation[6] to prevent the energy moving and the foetus being lost. There has to be some degree of Spleen Qi Deficiency[7] to prevent the developing foetus being transformed and transported. There has to be some degree of Kidney Deficiency[8] to allow the development within the uterus. These statements explain why certain acupuncture points and herbs are proscribed during pregnancy. It is important not to move Liver Qi too strongly or tonify the Spleen or Kidney too much.

The foetus continues to develop throughout the 9 months of pregnancy (10 lunar months). At the end of this time, labour will begin as the energies begin to descend. This is a normal and natural process, which becomes abnormal either because of a specific energetic imbalance or because of outside interference.

The delivery of the baby is the culmination of the whole process of pregnancy. It is to be interfered with as little as possible to maximise the health of the baby. The baby can be taken directly to the breast for feeding or lain in close contact with the mother to allow an early connection to be made. Bright lights and loud noises are best avoided.

Delivery in water is increasingly common and of great effectiveness in reducing pain.[9] Labour goes more smoothly and is much enjoyed by mother, partner and baby. There is no danger with giving birth in water as the baby has been in water for 9 months already! The baby obtains oxygen through the umbilical cord and this continues to pulsate for several minutes after delivery. Whilst the baby is under water it does not breathe. It only breathes on first contact with air. I had the opportunity to observe a woman in labour who used a birthing pool and she found it a pleasurable, helpful experience. It was her first pregnancy and labour was prolonged over about 15 hours. She had chosen to deliver at home and had a supportive independent midwife. She delivered a healthy baby boy by face presentation,[10] which in hospital would have entailed an automatic Caesarean section.

The delivery of the placenta is the final stage of childbirth. The placenta is an integral part of the baby as it develops from the embryo. The mother may choose to eat it as it is an excellent preventative for post-natal depression. It is a rich source of Qi and Blood. It may be dried and powdered or turned into a jelly to be given to the child at major times of progress such as birthdays and attending school. It is strengthening on many levels.

The post-partum time is an opportunity for the body to cleanse itself and the lochial discharge is its manifestation. This is one of the reasons why women live longer than men. They have opportunities at childbirth and menstruation to remove toxins. It is better not to interfere and allow the process to complete normally. Care needs to be taken that the mother does not become overtired or exposed to extremes of climate. The Chinese texts state that the mother is best attending only to herself and the baby for the first 4 weeks after delivery.

HOW TO HAVE A HEALTHY PREGNANCY[11]

At the moment, the vast majority of women deliver in hospital (around 95 per cent). Pregnancy and particularly labour, are seen by the conventional profession as inherently dangerous and certainly life-threatening events. At all costs the mother and baby must be protected from these 'dreadful risks'. Intervention by highly trained professionals is conventionally seen as the only way to ensure a healthy live infant. Fortunately, the medical profession is moving, albeit slowly, towards a different viewpoint and some centres are very flexible about methods of delivery.

The current movement towards home deliveries and natural childbirth is a reflection of the desire to find other methods. Ancient texts of Chinese medicine describe pregnancy as a spiritual practice, which lasts for the nine months of childbearing. The mother is encouraged to spend time in prayer and contemplation surrounded by pleasant things – be they mental, emotional and physical. This is not only an opportunity for the mother to benefit from such actions but also for the baby to begin life with a solid foundation of spiritual education. There are direct connections between the mother's mind and that of the developing baby.[12]

If pregnancy is an opportunity for the development of spirituality and emotional well-being, I would suggest that delivery is of at least equal importance. Current practices of induction, inappropriate use of epidural anaesthesia and subsequent forceps delivery can cause difficulties. Anxious staff may rush the process unnecessarily as well as using the whole range of invasive techniques available in hospital.

There are, of course, some women for whom these techniques may be necessary. Vaginal delivery is not possible in every woman and it would be foolish to suggest otherwise. However, the vast majority of women could deliver at home given adequate support and preparation. Remember that 98 per cent of the people currently alive in the world were born at home – not in hospital. In Holland where more than two-thirds of deliveries are in the home there is no evidence of more problems and there may be less. Intervention leads to difficulties – ask any farmer or veterinary surgeon.

How can women prepare themselves for delivery at home in a safe environment? Intervention at the time of health problems is the crudest form of care and attention is better paid to prevention. In this way, difficulties are minimised or do not occur. The mother's diet needs to be well balanced and most people nowadays understand what this means. Regular gentle exercise moves the energy of the body and benefits mother and baby. Strenuous activity should be avoided in later months as the joints and ligaments start to loosen in preparation for childbirth. Specific yoga exercises are of benefit and if done regularly prepare the mother for the time of delivery.

Attention to psychological aspects is of supreme importance as the Chinese texts observe and relaxation techniques are a good grounding in this. A spiritual practice can play a larger part of the mother's life during the pregnancy but, at the least, relaxation sessions and an avoidance of unpleasant situations and stimulation would be of benefit. The Chinese classic, *Admonitions to Ladies* says: 'A pregnant woman carries with her the finest piece of jade. She should enjoy all things, look at fine pictures and be attended by handsome servants'. Whilst some of this advice may, sadly, not be possible the meaning is clear.

Drugs are harmful to life and should be avoided unless they are necessary to maintain or preserve the life of the mother or baby. Massage during pregnancy helps to prepare mother and baby for delivery. For the baby it can be one of the first contacts with the outside world. During delivery, massage can help with pain relief and the progress of labour.

It may be that, despite all these preparatory measures, a health problem arises. Perhaps this was a condition present before conception or a result of the pregnancy. Whatever the origin it is preferable to seek treatment perhaps with Chinese medicine or homoeopathy both of which have proven track records of safety and effectiveness.

Acupuncture is helpful at the end of the third and the sixth month to treat the mother's kidney energy and thereby strengthen the baby. Chinese medical treatments and homoeopathic medicine[13] exist to ease the pain of labour, regulate contractions and prevent problems such as retained placenta.
Essentially the choice for the mother will depend on what she wants. Whatever the mother's decision, this should be supported and conflict avoided. There is little benefit in creating argument since this only disturbs the mother and the baby.

If a home birth is chosen then conventional practitioners may put pressure on the mother. Avoidance of potential conflicts may be the wise option for the mother at this vulnerable time.

Despite all this discussion of what to do when pregnancy has arrived the ideal situation would be one of the woman and her partner planning and preparing themselves prior conception. Attention to diet, exercise, relaxation and any specific health condition at this stage will go a long way to minimising problems in pregnancy.

So, if pregnancy is anticipated or has already happened, think of a plan of action:

- pay attention to diet, exercise and relaxation to maximise health
- seek advice and information about place of delivery and when selected search out supportive help
- obtain treatment for specific health problems
- think about homoeopathic, Chinese medical or other options to minimise difficulties during delivery and afterwards
- who will you want at the actual birth? I would suggest a maximum of partner or helper, midwife and perhaps one other. You don't have to invite the whole neighbourhood or sell tickets!
- arrange for at least a month of rest and recuperation afterwards so that you can be involved solely with the new baby (or as far as possible given your home situation)
- relax and enjoy the experience. Pregnancy and delivery are normal, joyous human events.

INVESTIGATIONS

Most people were surprised when it was announced in 1978 by the US Office of Technology, when referring to conventional medicine in general, that: 'It has been estimated that only 10 to 20 percent of all procedures currently used in medical practice have been shown to be efficacious in controlled trial.' Subsequently, there have been many reassessments of long-established procedures since 1978. Unfortunately, it has also been noted that just because a procedure is overused, obsolete or useless it has little effect on the practice of medicine.

Two procedures commonly used in labour are included in the many medical techniques that are irrelevant to producing a healthy baby, if not downright dangerous. Electronic foetal monitoring leads to high rates of Caesarean section and surgically assisted childbirth. A new study has revealed that when premature infants are given such monitoring, the rate of cerebral palsy is increased by three times. In the case of episiotomy, no evidence could be found to support the various reasons that doctors give for performing the surgery.[14]

There are several investigations performed in pregnancy and these are listed in Table 17.2. Ultrasound, chorionic villus sampling, foetal blood sampling and amniocentesis are described in detail in Chapter 4 – Investigations. A medical practitioner usually requests a particular investigation for a different reason from the person having it. A doctor is looking for an abnormality whilst the mother will be looking for reassurance that all is well. This dichotomy is more important than it may appear since a doctor cannot possibly detect normality from an investigation, only the absence of an abnormality. This provides the basis for, at the very least, disappointment on the part of the mother.

There are several points to make here. Women may be put under intolerable pressure by hospital and medical staff to conform to a standard approach. They are made to feel that *they* have a problem if they decline such an approach. Women are not counselled about the management and treatment of abnormal results *before* an investigation. Hospitals and medical staff often rely upon persuading people to have investigations and treatment out of fear rather than a rational decision made in an informed way. The consequences of this are emotional difficulties for the mother and these will be passed to the baby.

Investigation	Comments	Invasiveness
Weight measurement	Done regularly for early detection of pre-eclampsia	1
Blood pressure	Done regularly for early detection of pre-eclampsia	1
Full blood count	Done regularly for early detection of anaemia	1
Urine test	Done regularly for early detection of pre-eclampsia	1
Maternal blood tests	Screening test for foetal abnormalities. May lead onto invasive procedures of amniocentesis and chorionic villus sampling	1
Ultrasound	Used at least once in most pregnancies. Best to delay to the third trimester	2
Amniocentesis	Threatens the life of the foetus. Only to be risked in those who are contemplating termination	3
Chorionic villus sampling	See comments for amniocentesis. Risk of foetal abnormalities	3
Foetal blood sampling	See comments for amniocentesis	3

Table 17.2: Investigations performed in pregnancy

DISORDERS IN THE FIRST TRIMESTER

General overview

The first trimester is considered to begin at conception and end at 12 weeks. Most of the disorders listed may occur during this time and some, e.g. morning sickness, may continue through to about 14 weeks or so. The first 3 months is the time of greatest foetal development. This is the time when the foetus is particularly vulnerable to the toxic effects of drugs, chemicals and ultrasound.

Morning sickness

This occurs in about a third of pregnancies. A pregnant woman may also develop other causes of nausea and vomiting which are considered in Chapter 13 – Gastrointestinal system. In terms of conventional medicine, morning sickness is associated with rising levels of chorionic gonadotrophin. These reduce at 12-14 weeks of pregnancy.

Symptoms
There is nausea and sometimes vomiting which begins at about the 6th week of pregnancy. It usually subsides at around the 14th week. It is frequently only present in the morning, hence its name, but may occur at any time of day.

In some women, the vomiting may be severe and continue beyond the 14th week of pregnancy. It may then be called hyperemesis gravidarum. Occasionally, dehydration may occur and require hospital care.

Treatment
This is by reassurance and simple dietary measures. Drug treatment with antihistamines such as promethazine may be used. If symptoms are severe and require hospitalisation, rehydration with intravenous fluids may be required.

Holistic management
In terms of Chinese medicine, there are several syndromes represented by morning sickness. Fire in the Stomach and Liver may pass upwards together with thickened fluids. Phlegm and Dampness may interfere with the normal descent of Stomach Qi so that it rises leading to nausea and vomiting. Other syndromes are Stomach Yin Deficiency, Stagnant Liver Qi Invading Stomach, Stomach Qi Deficiency, Heart Qi Deficiency and Heart Fire.

Specific treatment and dietary changes are generally effective. The general advice of dietary management discussed in Chapter 13 – Gastrointestinal system – is applicable here. It is clearly helpful to avoid cold, sweet and greasy food. Food is best taken at regular intervals throughout the day.

These symptoms can be considered from a psychological perspective. Nausea and vomiting are a result of an inability to 'stomach' a situation. The developing foetus is a new life within the mother and this may produce a state of conflict. Nausea may be the consequence as the mother tries to 'expel' the foetus. The strength of symptoms may be a reflection of the strength of the foetus. Some women have strong symptoms as a result of a strong life within them. This is not to say that absence of nausea or vomiting indicates a weak foetus! The symptoms subside as the mother becomes more comfortable with the situation.

Bleeding in the first trimester

This is always abnormal although relatively common. There are several causes:

- miscarriage[15]
- ectopic pregnancy
- gynaecological conditions.

I concentrate here on miscarriage, as the other conditions are discussed in Chapter 18 – Women's Health. The majority of cases of miscarriage are due to unknown causes. There are various theories but it is unusual for there to be a specific reason:

- foetal abnormality – over a third of miscarriages reveal chromosomal abnormality in the foetus
- immune system defect leading to maternal antibodies attacking the developing foetus
- structural abnormalities of the uterus (rare)
- maternal illness, e.g. fever, diabetes mellitus, kidney disease
- drugs, e.g. ergotamine, quinine, cancer chemotherapy agents, lead
- hormone deficiency.

Symptoms of miscarriage
There are several categories of miscarriage.

A threatened miscarriage subsides and results in continuation of the pregnancy. There is slight vaginal bleeding which is frequently brownish or dark red in colour. There may be backache and dragging pains in the lower abdomen.

An inevitable miscarriage is one that ends with death of the foetus. Vaginal bleeding occurs which is heavier than with a threatened miscarriage. It is often red in colour. Pain may be greater depending upon the duration of the pregnancy. After 10 weeks or so, cramping pains are marked. If the foetus and uterine contents are expelled, this is classified as a complete miscarriage.

An incomplete miscarriage is when placental tissue or foetal parts remains within the uterus. There is a danger of infection in these cases.

Investigations
These are only performed in more severe cases. Ultrasound will determine if the foetus is alive.

Complications

Complication	Symptoms to look for
Infection	Fever, offensive vaginal discharge, malaise
Toxic shock	Low blood pressure, rapid pulse rate, pallor, sweating
Missed miscarriage	Missed periods, slight vaginal bleeding, foetus dies but is not expelled, uterus does not enlarge, pregnancy tests may still be positive. Spontaneous labour is the rule.

Table 17.3: Complications of miscarriage

Treatment
Rest is essential for threatened miscarriage. This should be absolute until vaginal bleeding has stopped. Hormonal supplementation with progesterone may be given with little evidence that it makes any difference to the outcome. This is a routine prescription in cases of several miscarriages (habitual miscarriage).

Inevitable miscarriage is treated by administration of ergometrine to empty the uterus. Dilatation and curettage may be carried out to ensure that all tissue has been removed from the uterus.

Holistic management
Specific treatment is helpful in treating such symptoms. In terms of Chinese medicine, miscarriage is usually seen as part of a condition known as 'Motion of the Foetus' There are six categories:

- Qi Deficiency
- Blood Deficiency
- Kidney Deficiency
- Hot Blood
- Liver Qi Stagnation
- Injury or accident.

Treatment is beneficial to try to prevent miscarriage and afterwards when the bleeding has settled. This is important so that any underlying cause is addressed. If the miscarriage is complete, it is good to have treatment so that the women's health can be helped. She may wish for another pregnancy and treatment will help prepare for this.

Large-for-dates

This is the detection of a uterine size larger than expected for the duration of the pregnancy. It may be found at any stage of pregnancy but with early checks in pregnancy will be spotted relatively early. There are several reasons:

- multiple pregnancy
- excess amniotic fluid, e.g. foetal abnormality, unknown cause
- maternal diabetes mellitus – leads to large foetus and placenta.

Symptoms
There may be none at early stages of pregnancy but the unexpected uterine size may be detected at routine antenatal visit. After about the 30th week of pregnancy, the enlarged uterus may cause pressure symptoms such as abdominal discomfort and, in severe cases, breathlessness.

Pre-eclampsia is more common in cases of multiple pregnancy and symptoms of this may be present.

It is useful to know the normal stages of development in pregnancy so that comparisons can be made with women in the clinic. Before the 12th week, uterine size can only be determined by vaginal examination (or by ultrasound).

By the 13th week or so the uterus becomes palpable above the symphysis pubis. The top of the uterus (fundus) reaches the umbilicus by the 24th week and the xiphoid cartilage by the 36th. It may descend a little thereafter if the baby's head engages in the pelvis.

Foetal movements may be felt at 19 or 20 weeks if a first baby and at about 17 or 18 weeks in subsequent pregnancies. Foetal heart sounds may be heard with a stethoscope at about the 24th week.

Management
This lies in detecting the cause of being large-for-dates. The management of each condition is detailed in the relevant section.

DISORDERS IN THE SECOND TRIMESTER

It is unusual for women to have difficulties during the second trimester. Miscarriage may occur due to the reasons discussed above. The foetus gradually grows in size, most development having already taken place in the first trimester.

Monitoring is done of weight, blood pressure and urine as well as uterine enlargement. The aim is to detect early any evidence of pre-eclampsia (see below).

DISORDERS IN THE THIRD TRIMESTER
General overview

The third trimester is the final stage of pregnancy and when the body prepares for the labour to come. It is now that the benefits of any preparation will be experienced. The healthier the woman, the fewer difficulties she will have.

It is beneficial if the mother can sleep and rest with her legs straight on a small soft pillow as this helps the head of the baby to engage. The temperature of the room should be neither too hot nor too cold. Gentle walks after meals are helpful, as is avoiding hard or heavy work. It is important to avoid cold, raw food and emotional stress and worry. Emotional upsets deplete the Qi and Blood and may lead to difficulties during labour. Strengthening of Qi and Blood is very helpful from about 32 weeks as this helps to ensure that labour is easy and smooth.

Pre-eclampsia

This is the appearance of high blood pressure, oedema and proteinuria in the last 3 months of pregnancy. A small number of women progress to full-blown eclampsia with convulsions. It is also known as toxaemia of pregnancy.

It is differentiated from other causes of such symptoms, e.g. essential hypertension, glomerulonephritis, systemic lupus erythematosus. It is more common in teenage women, women over 35 years and in multiple pregnancies. The symptoms quickly resolve after delivery or if the foetus dies.

Symptoms
These usually only develop after the 28th week of pregnancy. The blood pressure rises with an increase of at least 20 mm Hg in the systolic and 10 mm Hg diastolic. Oedema, which may be slight in 'normal' pregnancy, is marked particularly in the ankles, face and hands. Weight increases normally in pregnancy but a gain of more than 1 kg (2 lb) per week may indicate the collection of oedema fluid. Proteinuria is found in severe cases.

Headaches and vomiting develop if the diastolic pressure rises to over 100 mm Hg. There may be blurred vision. Epigastric pain and jaundice arise in severe cases due to liver damage.
The problem with pre-eclampsia for the foetus is that placental function is diminished. The foetus is underweight and in severe cases may die in utero.

If the symptoms progress, eclampsia may supervene. This is the occurrence of repeated convulsions, unconsciousness and the development of spontaneous labour. Maternal and foetal death rates are high.

Investigations
These are performed to exclude other causes of these symptoms. Urinalysis reveals only proteinuria with no blood or casts. In pre-eclampsia there will be no evidence of bacterial infection. Blood tests reveal raised uric acid but normal urea and creatinine.

Treatment
Antenatal care is recommended for every pregnant woman as a means of early detection. There is no means of prevention according to conventional medicine. All women with such symptoms will be admitted to hospital for bed rest, observation and investigation. There is no specific treatment although tranquillisation may be used to reduce the blood pressure. When I worked on an obstetric unit, the antipsychotic promazine was frequently used to sedate women with pre-eclampsia. Diuretics may be given for the oedema. Hypotensive drugs such as hydralazine or methyldopa are used for high blood pressure.

The foetus is monitored by means of ultrasound and placental function tests.[16] Labour may be induced if symptoms are severe, foetal growth is greatly affected or the pregnancy is at or near term.

Eclampsia is an obstetric emergency, which is treated by anticonvulsants and hypotensive agents. If labour has not already begun, it is induced. Caesarean section is performed if labour may be prolonged for whatever reason. The urgency here is to deliver the baby as symptoms subside soon afterwards. In eclampsia, the maternal mortality rate may be 5 per cent. Foetal mortality in established pre-eclampsia is about 3 per cent but rises to 30 per cent in eclampsia.

Holistic management
The main issue for holistic medicine is to ensure that the health of the mother is as good as possible. Treatment before conception will minimise any risk of such a condition developing.

In terms of Chinese medicine, oedema in pregnancy is seen as being due to Spleen Deficiency, Kidney Deficiency or Qi Stagnation. Pre-eclampsia, specifically, often corresponds to Blood Deficiency, Heat in the Liver, Liver and Kidney Yin Deficiency with Liver Yang Rising, Spleen Deficiency with Liver Yang Rising and Phlegm or Wind-cold Invasion. Eclampsia can be usually be differentiated as Wind due to Blood Deficiency, Liver Wind or Phlegm-fire.

Bleeding in the third trimester

This is always abnormal and can indicate several possibilities. It should always be viewed seriously. If bleeding is seen after the 28th week of pregnancy, it is known as an antepartum haemorrhage. This term usually excludes non-pregnancy related causes of bleeding. There are several causes of vaginal bleeding in the third trimester which include:

- abruptio placentae

- placenta praevia
- gynaecological conditions, e.g. cervical erosion, cervical polyp, cervical cancer.

Abruptio placentae

This is bleeding from a normally situated placental site. It may (if 'revealed') or may not (if 'concealed') manifest as vaginal bleeding. The placenta partially separates from the uterine wall. The cause is not fully understood in conventional medicine. High blood pressure is seen in about a third of cases. It is more common in women whose diet and social conditions are poor. Occasionally, injury[17] may precipitate bleeding.

Symptoms
In a revealed haemorrhage, there is vaginal bleeding. There is pain and localised tenderness over the uterus. The uterus feels hard and may be distended. Labour may begin spontaneously. A concealed haemorrhage will only be evidenced by the abdominal symptoms.

Investigations
Vaginal examination is absolutely contraindicated in all cases of vaginal bleeding at this stage because of the possibility of placenta praevia. An ultrasound scan will show placental position and any blood clot due to the placental separation.

Complications

Complication	Symptoms to look for
Shock	Rapid pulse rate, low blood pressure, pale, sweating
Foetal death	Absent foetal movements, absent heart sounds

Table 17.4: Complications of abruptio placentae

Treatment
This is mainly supportive in hospital. Pain relief is given and blood transfusion may be required where blood loss is marked. Labour is induced or Caesarean section performed in severe cases. If the symptoms are mild and there is no evidence of placenta praevia on ultrasound examination, bed rest is the only thing that is necessary.

Holistic management
It is important that you understand the significance of bleeding in the third trimester (see also placenta praevia). Most women will be hospitalised, as this is an obstetric emergency.

Placenta praevia

This is a placenta that is situated over or near the cervix. It occurs in about 0.5 per cent of pregnancies. The placenta may overlie the internal opening of the cervix completely or be situated on the uterine wall nearby. For all practical purposes, these slightly different cases are dealt with in the same way.

Symptoms
There is vaginal bleeding that occurs late in pregnancy or in labour. Intercourse or vaginal examination may initiate it. The bleeding is painless and may be recurrent. The head of the foetus cannot engage[18] and so the presence of placenta praevia may be suspected. If bleeding is severe, there may be rapid pulse rate, low blood pressure, pallor and sweating.

Investigations
Vaginal examination is absolutely contraindicated in all cases of vaginal bleeding in the later months of pregnancy. If placenta praevia is present there is torrential haemorrhage as the examining fingers damage the placenta.

Ultrasound examination reveals the placental position.

Treatment
In cases of placenta praevia, there is clearly no treatment that can alter the placental position. Delivery by Caesarean section is the only option and this is done at about 39 weeks. If vaginal bleeding is heavy, an emergency section is performed with supportive treatment such as blood transfusion if necessary.

Holistic management
It is important that you understand the significance of bleeding in the third trimester (see also abruptio placentae). Most women will be hospitalised, as this is an obstetric emergency.

Premature labour

This is the onset of labour before 40 weeks. There are several associated circumstances and these include:

- multiple pregnancy
- excess amniotic fluid
- smoking
- urinary tract infection
- rupture of membranes, e.g. multiple pregnancy, excess amniotic fluid, weakened cervix
- foetal abnormality
- foetal death.

Symptoms
There is the onset of the symptoms of labour but before 40 weeks' gestation. The consequences for the foetus are directly dependent upon its maturity. Birth after 34 weeks suggests a good chance of survival although now premature babies who are even premature than this are living.

Treatment
It may be possible to stop some cases of premature labour with drugs that relax uterine muscle. These include isoxsuprine and salbutamol. Corticosteroids may be given, e.g. dexamethasone in an attempt to reduce the severity of respiratory distress syndrome.[19]

Postmaturity

This is prolongation of the pregnancy beyond the accepted normal of 40 weeks. About 10 per cent of pregnancies do not start until the 42nd week. There are some risks attached to this situation although they are often overstated. Placental insufficiency may develop leading to a reduced growth rate of the foetus. Also, the foetal head may not mould during labour so well and so prolong delivery.

A consideration is that the 40-week gestation may not be as fixed or 'normal' as we think. Some pregnancies last 40 weeks, some less and some more. In fact, a recent survey showed that the average gestation in the West has risen to 41 weeks. The conventional tendency is to induce if the pregnancy goes much over 40 weeks. This may lead to the delivery of a baby with immature lungs. This can occur at any stage of pregnancy although it is more a risk at earlier stages. I remember working in an obstetric unit where induction was performed on virtually all women who did not spontaneously begin labour at 40 weeks. There were a number of babies born with respiratory difficulties. In my opinion, it is preferable to wait until there is clear evidence of problems requiring induction. Routine procedures lead to routine difficulties.

LABOUR

Introduction

Labour is almost always a normal process with a healthy, normal baby at the end. Difficulties occur because of a health problem with the mother, a disproportion between the size of the baby and the size of the mother's pelvis or due to interference with this normal process. The latter case is common now as many women in the West deliver their babies in hospital. There are increasing moves towards technological management of birth. In the past few years, groups of women, midwives and health professionals have come together to offer help. Such methods, often labelled natural childbirth,[20] are gaining ground and increasing numbers of women are choosing to deliver at home or perhaps in hospital in a manner that suits them. It is still early days but as each year passes the movement of power shifts more towards women. This can only be beneficial and soon the days of passive childbirth and unnecessary intervention will be no more.

Intervention/investigation	When	Comments
Shaving pubic hair, enema	Before or at start of labour	Not common now. Unnecessary
Urine test	Before or at start of labour	Check for sugar or protein
Blood pressure	Before or at start of labour, regularly throughout	Check for pre-eclampsia
Surgical rupture of membranes	To induce labour	Via vaginal examination. Danger of placental separation, presentation of foetal hand or leg
Induction of labour	To induce labour	Dangerous if baby's lungs are not fully mature. Labour tends to be more painful and more likely to require intervention
Abdominal examination	Throughout labour	Check on engagement, strength and regularity of contractions
Foetal heart measurements	Throughout labour	Check on foetal heart rate – normal is 120-160 beats per minute. It may increase (or decrease) in cases of foetal distress[21]
Vaginal examination	Throughout labour – at least three hourly	Check on cervical dilatation, confirm presenting part of the baby. Frequently overused
Foetal scalp monitor	During first stage of labour	Electrode attached to scalp of baby. Painful and intrusive
Foetal blood sampling	During first stage of labour	Obtained from foetal scalp. Painful and intrusive
Pethidine injections	During first stage of labour	For pain relief. Suppresses the baby's respiration
Epidural anaesthesia	During first stage of labour	For pain relief. High risk of back pain for months afterwards
Forceps, Ventouse extraction	During second stage of labour	To assist delivery
Episiotomy	During second stage of labour	Cutting of the perineum to assist delivery. Can be prevented by adequate preparation and by experienced midwife
Oxytocin injection	At end of second stage of labour	To cause the uterus to contract in bid to prevent post-partum haemorrhage. Unnecessary in well-managed delivery where baby is put to breast immediately

Table 17.5: Interventions and investigations during labour

Stages of labour

Labour is divided into three stages. Painless contractions occur throughout pregnancy. When the first stage of labour begins, they become painful and the cervix starts to dilate as the baby is gradually advanced down the pelvic canal. When labour begins there may be a 'show'. This is the discharge of bloodstained mucus from the cervix. The membranes may rupture at this stage or later.

The duration of the first stage depends upon the individual. Conventional medicine frequently lays down quite rigid ideas about how long each stage and part of a stage should last. The degree of cervical dilatation is taken as the guide to progress. This is only a rigid labelling of a natural process and has no inherent truth of its own. Each case must be assessed on its own merits. It is helpful to consider factors such as the number and strength of contractions, condition of the mother and condition of the baby. The reliance on the state of the cervix subjects women to repeated vaginal examinations that may interrupt the natural rhythm of labour. This is unnecessary and invasive. If all is progressing, there is no need to interfere. Medical voyeurism is not a healthy aspect of pregnancy and labour.

Transition occurs as the first stage of labour gives way to the second stage. This is when the mother actively pushes the baby down the vaginal canal to help uterine contractions by 'bearing down'. The second stage begins when the cervix is fully dilated and ends with the delivery of the baby. The membranes usually rupture at this time.

The third stage ends when the placenta (afterbirth) is delivered. There is some bleeding as this occurs but eases as the uterus contracts. Putting the baby to the breast immediately after delivery stimulates contraction of the uterus.

The practice of shaving the pubic hair and giving women enemas in preparation for labour is, fortunately, dying out. There is no evidence of any need for these procedures.

In the vast majority of women, labour progresses normally with no requirement for the paraphernalia of modern hospital obstetrics. The use of foetal monitoring, epidural anaesthesia and so forth tend to delay labour and make it more painful.

Induction of labour due to some perceived difficulty about delay also leads to painful labour and an increased incidence of intervention later. There is no need for induction if the mother is healthy and the baby is active and growing. It may be helpful to check the placental function tests but use these only as a guide, not as an absolute indication of what to do.

Difficult labour

This is labour which progresses slowly or with difficulty. There are considered to be several causes in conventional medicine which include:

- foetus – malposition, malpresentation
- mother – small pelvis, pelvic tumours
- weak uterine action
- uncoordinated uterine action.

Symptoms
There will be a lack of cervical dilatation with continuing painful contractions of the uterus. The contractions may increase in strength and painfulness.

Treatment
This depends upon the cause and the condition of the mother and baby. If there is evidence of maternal exhaustion or foetal distress, obstetric intervention may be necessary. If the cervix is not fully dilated, a Caesarean section will be performed with either general anaesthesia or an epidural. If the cervix is fully dilated, it may be possible to use forceps to help deliver the baby. This is done with local anaesthesia or an epidural. An episiotomy is necessary.

Holistic management
In terms of Chinese medicine, there are two main situations of delayed labour. They are Deficiency of Qi and Blood and Stagnation of Qi and Blood. Deficient conditions can be prevented or minimised by strengthening treatments before and during pregnancy. Treatment can be instituted during labour by means of acupuncture, herbs, homoeopathic remedies or massage to help maintain uterine contractions and support the woman.

Malposition

Normally, the vertex of the head is the presenting part. That is, the part which enters the pelvis first and leads into the vaginal canal in the second stage of labour. The occiput is towards the front (respective to the mother). Any variation from this vertex presentation is known as malposition.

In 15 per cent of deliveries, the occiput is to the back (respective to the mother). This is known as occipito-posterior position. In about 1 in 4 of these cases there are difficulties in labour because the head does not flex to reduce the diameter of the presenting part. Labour is likely to be prolonged and perhaps more painful. Backache is common in such situations.

The management of malposition is included in that of difficult labour described above.

Malpresentation

Presentation of the head is the normal situation. Malpresentation is the presentation of any other part of the baby. All malpresentations tend to delay labour and the comments I made under difficult labour are relevant here.

The presentations that are possible are:

- face
- brow
- breech
- shoulder.

Caesarean section will be employed if labour is unduly difficult or delayed and in cases of foetal distress or maternal exhaustion. Most face, all brow and all shoulder presentations have to be delivered by this method. Breech delivery is possible vaginally with care and some now occur at home in well-selected cases.

It is possible to turn a foetus so that it presents correctly. This is termed external version. It is used in the case of a transverse foetus or a breech presentation. It is performed after the 35th week or the baby merely turns back. There is a risk of placental separation or premature labour and for this reason is not so favoured.

There is an excellent method available in Chinese medicine that has no side-effects and is virtually 100 per cent effective. The application of heat provided by burning moxa to the acupuncture point Urinary Bladder 67 would invert the foetus in almost every case. Merely warming this point is adequate. Homoeopathic remedies (e.g. Pulsatilla taken at week 36) can also be used effectively.

In terms of Chinese medicine, malpresentation indicates that the Qi of the Kidney and Spleen is chaotic.

Disproportion

This is the situation where the presenting part of the baby is too large for the size of the pelvis. It is a relative situation and depends on several factors such as movement of pelvic bones due to ligamentous softening in later pregnancy and moulding[22] of the baby's head. The size of the pelvis is assessed at about the 36th week of pregnancy although a previous delivery will be a definitive assessment of what is possible. Lack of engagement of the head may indicate a small pelvis. It normally engages at about 37 weeks in first pregnancies and not until labour in those who have previously delivered.

The results of assessment govern the management of these cases. In those situations where the outcome is unsure, a *trial labour* may be conducted. This is the monitoring of labour with preparation for Caesarean section if progress does not happen or stops.

If vaginal delivery seems to be impossible, an *elective* Caesarean section is performed at about 38 or 39 weeks. There is support amongst some obstetricians for such women to begin labour anyway, as there are psychological benefits. There is less chance of feelings of failure and women may prefer to attempt to give birth even if Caesarean section will be the option for delivery.

Multiple pregnancy

This is the occurrence of more than one foetus. Twins occur in 1 in 80 pregnancies, triplets in 1 in 1000 and quadruplets in 1 in 500,000. There is an increased chance of multiple pregnancy if there is a family history of it, if ovulation stimulants are used in the treatment of infertility and when pregnancy is the result of in vitro fertilisation (IVF) or gamete intrafallopian transfer (GIFT) treatment (as several fertilised ova are replaced together).

The diagnosis is suggested by the finding of a large-for-dates uterus. Ultrasound will confirm the diagnosis. When I worked in an obstetrics unit, a woman was expecting to deliver two babies, confirmed by ultrasound. Everyone was surprised when three appeared!

The symptoms of morning sickness are stronger with multiple pregnancy. Pre-eclampsia and premature labour are more likely. Most women are admitted to hospital routinely for rest from the 32nd week until delivery.

Induction of labour

This is the artificial initiation of labour by means of drugs or surgical procedures. It is commonly performed in some hospitals but less so than previously. Induction rates vary between 1 in 2 to 1 in 10 deliveries in the UK. It was originally employed as a way of preventing postmaturity but quickly became a way of trying to get all women to deliver between 9 a.m. and 5 p.m. on weekdays.

It tends to lead to more painful labour and is intimately connected with epidural anaesthesia and other aspects of technological obstetrics. Intervention with forceps and Caesarean section is also more common. This is either because labour is more problematic or because the woman, not surprisingly, finds it difficult to push a baby out when anaesthetised from the waist downwards.

The obstetric indications for induction include:

- hypertension
- chronic nephritis
- abruptio placentae
- unstable presentation
- postmaturity

- diabetes mellitus
- foetal abnormalities
- foetal death.

Induction is likely to fail if there is no engagement of the presenting part, if the cervix is long, firm and tightly closed and it is before the 36th week.

There are various methods of induction. Prostaglandin pessaries inserted into the vagina stimulate the uterus to begin contractions. If contractions do not begin, the membranes are ruptured surgically by means of a metal hook during vaginal examination. Intravenous infusion of synthetic oxytocin is either given at the same time or if contractions fail to begin. The rate of infusion must be closely monitored and adjusted according to the rate and strength of the contractions. Over vigorous contractions produced by this method may lead to foetal death or uterine rupture. Monitoring of the foetus by means of foetal scalp monitors, monitors to the mother's abdomen to measure foetal heart rate and contractions and epidural anaesthesia are, therefore, integral parts of induction.

The American College of Obstetricians and Gynaecologists concluded that, 'there is no clinical value to continuous electronic foetal monitoring.' Listening with a stethoscope is of the same effectiveness.

Delivery

This is the second stage where the woman pushes downward to aid the uterine contractions. It occurs when the cervix is fully dilated (10 cm) and the woman has the urge to push downwards. It lasts for up to 2 hours but most are much shorter than this. An hour with no progress during the second stage indicates a serious problem.

A relatively high percentage of deliveries are the subject of medical intervention. Such intervention is usually the culmination of a series of invasive procedures where there is interference with natural processes.

The standard method of delivery was invariably with the woman lying flat on her back. It is not physiologically desirable and may lead to more foetal distress as the pregnant uterus obstructs the circulation. More upright positions make use of that most natural of forces – gravity.

Nowadays, women are asking to be able to deliver in more comfortable and comfortable positions. The standard advice is changing slowly[23] but delivery at home with a sympathetic midwife[24] remains the best way to ensure the woman's wishes are respected.

There is ample evidence available to show that home delivery of the baby is at least as safe as that of hospital delivery.[25] Nothing is risk-free but it is helpful to consider how to ensure, as far as is possible, that a home delivery is problem-free.
- Good nutrition and adequate weight gain.
- Abstain from smoking, drinking alcohol.
- Getting good prenatal care and avoiding high blood pressure and other complications that can be helped through nutrition.
- Find a competent midwife who is skilled, confident and experienced in deliveries at home.
- Information through reading, classes, videos, and getting supplies together.
- Have homoeopathic or herbal remedies on standby.
- Ensure the baby presents head down – or that the midwife is skilled in breech deliveries, twins[26] and so on.
- Have adequate support during labour and postpartum.
- Have a plan for emergencies, have phone numbers easily available.
- Holistic medical practitioner to assist in case of specific difficulties.
- Make an informed (and stated) choice about whether you want to receive oxytocin or your baby to receive vitamin K.

The baby descends the birth canal with each contraction helped by voluntary efforts of the mother. The head (assuming a vertex presentation) is delivered first followed by the shoulders. Tearing of the perineum may occur if the delivery is rapid and episiotomy may be performed in an attempt to prevent this. This is the cutting of the perineum so that any tear will not pass posteriorly to affect the anal sphincter. This risk is much overstated and episiotomy is unnecessary in all uncomplicated deliveries. Competent midwifery and care of the perineum in pregnancy will prevent any problems.

Throughout North America, the episiotomy rate is about 70 to 80 per cent of first-time vaginal deliveries. It would seem that at least as effective and infinitely preferable is the use of pelvic floor exercises throughout pregnancy and perineal massage (with oil) before birth. Neither of these techniques, of course, involves doctors.

Episiotomy is, paradoxically, likely to make tearing worse. A study of 241 births in the Albert Einstein Hospital in New York found that this practice, especially if the woman had her legs in stirrups (lithotomy position), led to more harm.[27]

Researchers at the Jewish General Hospital and McGill University in Montreal, Canada studied women who had an episiotomy and compared them with a group who did not. There was no difference in the outcome as all had healthy babies. The second stage of labour was reduced in time by only 9 minutes on average. There was the risk of sexual difficulties after birth.[28]

In this study, 46 out of 47 women receiving episiotomies had the tear extend into the rectum, which is the most serious complication. Researchers noted that doctors are so programmed to perform surgery that those in the part of the study where women did not have episiotomies '... were unwilling or unable to reduce their episiotomy rate'.

Intramuscular oxytocin is routinely given in hospitals when the baby's shoulders are delivered to contract the uterus and minimise the risk of post-partum haemorrhage. This risk, again, is very much overstated and the immediate placing of the baby at the breast will produce natural secretion of oxytocin.

Vitamin K has been given to newborn babies since the 1940s and 1950s. It is given to prevent haemorrhagic disease of the newborn, which may present at about 10 weeks of age. Cerebral haemorrhage is a possibility, which may be fatal.

Babies are born with a slight vitamin K deficiency, which may be a protective mechanism. The injectable medication contains phenol as well as vitamin K. By 1958, about 5 per cent of babies received it, 25 per cent by 1970 and 98.5 per cent by 1977-87. In the UK at the current time, 58 per cent of babies have the injection form, 30 per cent the oral form, and 12 per cent nothing.

Two studies have shown a connection between vitamin K injection and the development of childhood cancer. The first was published in 1990 and the second in 1992.[29]

The risk of any child developing leukaemia by the age of 10 is about 1 in 1000 and that for all childhood cancers is about 1 in 500. The results of these studies reveal that vitamin K could increase this risk to about 1 in 200. Regarding Great Britain, there are about 700,000 births a year. The excess number of cancers caused by giving intramuscular vitamin K to all babies could range from 400 to 2000. By contrast, the risk of haemorrhagic disease of the new-born if no vitamin K is given is about 1 in 10000 which would work out as 70 cases a year in Britain. There was no association, however, between cancer and oral vitamin K.[30]

The cord can be left alone until it has stopped pulsating and then cut. Early clamping and cutting of the cord can lead to feelings of forced separation and loss. It is important to allow natural processes to run their course. In this way, long-term problems are minimised particularly on a psychological level.

The delivery of the baby ends the second stage of labour.

If there is a delay in labour, signs of maternal or foetal distress then delivery may be aided. Forceps delivery may be performed under local anaesthesia. It is more common in epidural anaesthesia as the woman cannot push so well and she has little or no sensation of her perineum. The complications of forceps include:

- death or brain injury of the foetus
- skull fractures
- facial paralysis – usually completely recovers
- vaginal or cervical lacerations.

An alternative to forceps delivery is the use of Ventouse extraction. This is the application of a metal cup to the head of the baby. It is attached to a vacuum pump so that the pressure exerted allows the cup to remain firmly fixed to the head. Traction on the cup can aid delivery. A large bruise develops over the site of the cup, which fades in the next few days. Application of the cup for over 30 minutes may lead to serious injury to the scalp.[31]

Epidural anaesthesia is commonly applied nowadays. It involves the passage of a tube into the epidural space in the lumbar spine. Local anaesthesia is injected so that there is numbness of the lower parts of the body. Complications include low blood pressure, temporary respiratory paralysis if the injection enters deeper layers lining the spinal cord, poor voluntary effort in the second stage leading to forceps or vacuum extraction.

The use of epidural anaesthesia during labour leads to the development of several long-term symptoms in women. These include backache, frequent headaches, neckache, pins and needles in the hands or fingers, numbness or tingling in the lower back, buttocks or legs. Backache is almost twice as common in women who have received epidural anaesthesia.[32-33]

Some cases of epidural anaesthesia are complicated by dural puncture. This is puncture of the dura mater and arachnoid mater, which are the membranes surrounding the spinal cord and brain. Dural headache often affects the neck and shoulders as well, and symptoms usually arise within two days of the procedure. The headache is typically frontal, severe, throbbing and better for laying flat. The discomfort frequently affects the neck and shoulders and may be associated with auditory or visual symptoms or nausea. The headache can last for up to six days. There may be muzziness of the head for another day or so.[34]

Caesarean section is the delivery of the baby through an abdominal incision. It may be performed under general or epidural anaesthesia. The indications for Caesarean section are similar to those of any aided delivery. That is, there has to be maternal or foetal distress usually with some degree of delayed labour. Elective Caesarean sections are performed in cases of known disproportion.

According to figures in 1993, about 25 per cent of births in the USA and nearly 20 per cent of those in Canada were by Caesarean section. This compared with 6-7 per cent in the Netherlands, Japan, Slovenia, and the former Czechoslovak Republic. Rates for other 'developed' countries range from 10 to 15 per cent. In the UK, it is difficult to obtain accurate figures. They seem to show an increase in the Caesarean section rate from 10 per cent in 1988-89 to 12 per cent in 1989-90 and 13 per cent in 1990-91.[35]

This operation has become increasingly common over the years as obstetricians become more interventionist.[36] The common justification is that of worry of litigation. It seems somewhat paradoxical that obstetricians will practise a *more* hazardous method of delivery just to prevent litigation. One would think that the most appropriate method of treatment is the one indicated rather than the one preferred by the medical defence company. Fear of litigation is considered to be the main reason why Caesarean rates are so high in the US. However, there are similar rates in Canada where litigation is not so widespread. Doctors rather than midwives supervise most deliveries in Canada and the US and this is more likely to be the explanation. Countries where midwives are mainly responsible for delivery have consistently low rates of Caesarean section delivery. High rates of Caesarean section are also observed where women receive private medical treatment.[37] Item-of-service payments also play a role here.[38]

The complications of Caesarean section are those of any anaesthesia and abdominal operation. These are outlined on Pages 38 and 39. In particular, there are problems with anaesthesia if applied in an emergency. Other complications include haemorrhage, infection, pulmonary embolism and rupture of the scar in a subsequent pregnancy or labour.

There is no evidence that elective operative delivery leads to a better outcome for term breech or for very small babies. Despite this, Caesarean rates for these indications have increased in 'developed' countries.[39]

A programme was developed with the intention of reducing the Caesarean delivery rate without harm to the mother or baby.[40] A target was set of between 11 and 12 per cent Caesarean section delivery rate after 2 years of the programme. At the end of the pregnancy, 70 per cent of women who had a previous section delivered vaginally. The reduction in Caesarean deliveries was not associated with a rise in forceps and other operative deliveries. The rate of forceps and vacuum extractions fell during the study, from 10.4 to 4.3 per cent. The proportion of spontaneous vaginal deliveries increased during the study. There were no changes to the health of the newborn baby or foetal and neonatal mortality rates

Retained placenta

This may occur with post-partum haemorrhage, which is described below. Frequently, there is no excessive bleeding and the placenta does not deliver. It may be due to abnormal adhesion to the uterine wall or spasm of the lower part of the uterus. This latter may be caused by the injection of oxytocin as the baby is delivered.

Symptoms
There will be no sign of placental delivery. It may have separated from the uterine wall. If so, this is evidenced by a hardness of the top of the uterus, mobility of this area from side to side, lengthening of the umbilical cord and a small gush of blood.

Treatment
Manual removal is performed under general anaesthesia if it cannot be removed by pulling on the umbilical cord.

Holistic management
In terms of Chinese medicine, this may be due to either Deficiency of Qi and Blood or to Cold Invasion leading to Stagnation of Blood. It is helpful to massage acupuncture points such as Gall Bladder 21, Urinary Bladder 60, Large Intestine 4 and Spleen 6. These descend the energy and help the uterus expel the placenta. Most cases will be alleviated by such methods. There are herbal and homoeopathic treatments also. In extreme cases with haemorrhage, surgical intervention may be necessary.

Post-partum haemorrhage

This is heavy blood loss after delivery of the baby. It may occur just after delivery or a day or so later. It is arbitrarily defined as blood loss in excess of 500 ml.

There are various causes that include:

- failure of uterus to contract adequately
- retention of placenta
- lacerations – due to delivery of the head and shoulders or to obstetric intervention.

Symptoms
The blood loss will be self-evident. In severe cases there will be pallor, rapid pulse rate, low blood pressure, sweating and light-headedness. Symptoms are more likely to occur in those women who were already anaemic.

Treatment
It is fear of this condition that has led to the practice of oxytocin injection as the baby is delivered. If the placenta has not been delivered, manual removal under general anaesthesia is done immediately. If the placenta has been delivered, an injection of ergometrine is given to cause the uterus to contract.

Replacement of blood by transfusion may be necessary. Later iron supplementation is given.

Holistic management
The treatment of women before and during pregnancy will go a long way to reducing the risk of such a complication. There are emergency acupuncture, herbal and homoeopathic treatments available. The stimulation of oxytocin production naturally by breast-feeding is helpful in prevention.

POST-NATAL CARE

The main issue in the post-natal period is the replenishing of Blood and care of the mother and baby. Supportive helpers to minimise the amount of work and worry are invaluable. It is preferable to have assistance of this kind for 4 weeks after delivery. This may be an ideal that cannot be attained but perhaps it is something at which to aim.

Breast milk is a product of Yin and Blood and this places further demand upon the mother. Therefore, diet needs to be nutritious and similar to that described at the beginning of Chapter 13 – Gastrointestinal system. Cold food is depleting of digestive energy and may lead to the appearance of symptoms due to Cold in those with low energy.

The lochia is the loss from the uterus after delivery. It is red for the first few days and becomes pinker and less heavy with time. It is excessive if placental tissue remains in the uterus. It is offensive in cases of infection.

Care of the breasts is important to minimise problems with breast-feeding. Engorgement or even overt mastitis may occur from about the 4th day as breast milk secretion increases. It is preferable to allow the baby to control the number and amount of feeds rather than keep to a rigid schedule. In this way, the baby is happy and there will be more harmony between baby and mother.

In terms of Chinese medicine, no lactation is due to Qi Stagnation in the Middle Jiao or to Qi and Blood Deficiency. Milk leaking continuously from the breasts is due to Kidney and Spleen Qi Deficiency so the milk is not held. Mastitis is due to weakness of the Ren and Chong channels, Damp-heat Accumulation in the channels or disharmony of the Liver and Stomach with underlying Blood Deficiency. There are effective treatments available in homoeopathy and herbal medicine.

Breast-feeding is more likely to be successful when the mother is in a supportive environment. The most preferred is at home. Hospitals can directly reduce the number of women who breast-feed successfully with their policies of providing commercial milk formulae at discharge.[41]

Post-natal exercises are helpful, particularly those which strengthen the pelvic floor. These can help reduce the frequency of urinary problems later.

There is a routine post-natal examination performed at 6 weeks after delivery. A cervical smear may be performed at the same time. Cervical erosions are commonly seen and do not require conventional treatment. Most resolve of their own accord.

HOW TO RECOGNISE A SERIOUS CONDITION IN PREGNANCY OR CHILDBIRTH

Most pregnancies are normal and those that are not rarely reach the stage of seriousness. It is important, however, to recognise those symptoms that may indicate a potentially serious problem for mother or baby.

Symptom	Comments
Bleeding	Always
Uterine pain	Always unless at normal time for labour
Vaginal discharge	Heavy, blood-stained
Vomiting	Severe, prolonged, evidence of dehydration
High blood pressure	If severe especially if associated with oedema and proteinuria
Oedema	If severe and especially if associated with high blood pressure and proteinuria
Proteinuria	With dysuria and backache, with high blood pressure and proteinuria
Delayed onset to labour	If more than two weeks overdue
Prolonged labour	If cervix not dilating, with exhaustion, with changes to foetal heart rate
Bleeding after delivery	If heavy
Retention of placenta	If with heavy bleeding, if prolonged (over an hour)

Table 17.6: How to recognise a serious condition of pregnancy and childbirth

SUMMARY

Pregnancy and childbirth are normal processes.

Difficulties appear either because of problems with mother and baby or because of inappropriate medical intervention.

You should know the symptoms that would indicate a potentially serious condition of pregnancy and childbirth.

Ensure you have treatment options that can be used when pregnancy or labour does not follow the normal processes.

Appropriate treatment of women in pregnancy, during labour and of the baby at delivery will greatly help future generations to regain their health.[42]

---

[1] *A Savage Enquiry* by Wendy Savage (Virago, 1986) is an account of attempts to suspend a woman gynaecologist who tries to offer choices in childbirth. *The American Way of Birth* by Jessica Mitford (Gollancz, 1992) is an excellent account of the pressures of conventional obstetrics.

[2] Trimester is a three-monthly stage of pregnancy.

[3] Labour is defined as 'the sequence of actions by which a baby and afterbirth are expelled from the uterus at childbirth. In normal obstetric practice, the definition may be made of regular uterine contractions with progressive cervical dilatation. This can lead to fixed ideas of what is the normal duration of labour and the need for frequent vaginal examinations.

[4] The period up to 6 weeks after childbirth.

[5] All material aspects must arise from the immaterial. This is a fundamental principle of all energetic philosophies.

6 The energetic functions of the Liver are described in Chapter 14 – Central Nervous System. It has several functions but the important one of relevance here is its role in the free flowing of Qi.

7 The energetic functions of the Spleen are described in Chapter 13 – Gastrointestinal System. It has several functions but the important one of relevance here is its role in transforming and transporting. This usually refers to food but not exclusively.

8 The energetic functions of the Kidney are described in Chapter 9 – Urinary System. It has several functions but the important one of relevance here is its role in governing the function of the pelvic area.

9 *Water birth* by Janet Balaskas and Yehudi Gordon (Unwin, 1990 and Thorsons, 1992).

10 Presentation is that part of the baby which is lowermost during labour. A face presentation is difficult to deliver because the presenting part is of a large diameter. A further discussion of presentations, normal and abnormal, can be found later in this Chapter.

11 An excellent book, *The Path of Pregnancy* by Bob Flaws (Blue Poppy Press, 1993) outlines the Chinese philosophical view of pregnancy. This was my main source text for this section.

12 The Chong channel. See discussion in *The Path of Pregnancy* by Bob Flaws (Blue Poppy Press, 1993).

13 *Homeopathy for Pregnancy, Birth, and Your Baby's First Year* by Miranda Castro (St Martin's Press, 1993) is an excellent resource for women and their partners. Also, there are homoeopathic treatment kits on the market. Contact Helios Homeopathic Pharamacy in Tunbridge Wells, UK or look on the Internet at www.homeopathykits.com.

14 *HealthFacts,* 1990;15(135):1(2).

15 Abortion is a medical term meaning loss of the foetus from the uterus up to 28 weeks of pregnancy. I use the term miscarriage in this text as, colloquially, abortion is used to indicate termination of pregnancy.

16 Placental function tests are blood tests that give some indication of its efficiency. Serum oestriol measurement is the prime example of these.

17 External version (i.e. attempting to turn the baby mechanically by the hands on the abdominal wall) in a breech presentation may be such a cause.

18 The presenting part of the foetus is said to have engaged when its widest diameter has entered the brim of the pelvis.

19 This is a condition due to immaturity of the lungs where a sticky secretion may obstruct the smaller airways. In severe cases there is cyanosis and breathlessness.

20 Natural childbirth and active childbirth are two terms in common usage. They are gaining in popularity due to the benefit they offer to mother and baby. Excellent source books include *Active Birth* by Janet Balaskas (Harvard Common Press, 1994), *New Active Birth* by Janet Balaskas (Thorson's, 1991), *The Active Birth Partners Handbook* by Janet Balaskas (Sidgewick and Jackson, 1986), *The Encyclopaedia of Pregnancy and Birth* by Janet Balaskas and Yehudi Gordon (Little, Brown, 1992) and *Preparing for Birth with Yoga* by Janet Balaskas (Element, 1994).

21 Foetal distress is the oft-quoted reason for intervention in labour. You should not forget that 'obstetrician's distress' may also be a reason for such intervention.

22 This occurs because of the pressures exerted during delivery. It is a normal event and allows for easier passage during labour.

23 The conventional attitude can be ascertained from the following quote. The italics are mine. "There are a few patients who *demand* to be delivered in 'natural' positions, standing, crouching, or on their hands and knees. While their right of choice cannot be denied, it must be explained to them that there is a danger to the child if the foetal heart rate is not regularly observed, and that care of the perineum is hardly possible in such positions." *Obstetrics and Gynaecology* by Clayton and Newton (Churchill Livingstone, 1988).

24 There are several groups of midwifes in the UK who now offer holistics to obstetric interventions in hospital. They work in the community and are known as independent or radical midwives.

25 *British Medical Journal* 1991;303:1517.

26 The delivery of twins at home after a previous Caesarean section may also be possible with care. An account of such an event is an article by Cronk, Mary: *Nursing Times,* 1992;88(47):54(2).

27 Twenty-eight per cent of those who had episiotomy and lithotomy had serious vaginal tearing. This rate dropped to 19 percent for women who had just the episiotomy and 1 per cent of those who had neither. *The Edell Health Letter,* 1989;8(6):6(1).

28 *Mothering,* Spring 1993;66:28(1).

29 The conclusions of this study may be summarised. The figures relate to the UK. If no one received any vitamin K then there would be about 30-60 cases of late haemorrhagic disease and no extra cancers. If all received oral vitamin K there would be about 10 cases of late haemorrhagic disease and no extra cancers. If all received intramuscular vitamin K there would be one case of late haemorrhagic disease and 980 extra cancers. Golding, Jean *et al British Medical Journal,* 1992;305(6849):341(6).

30 Kingman, Sharon. *British Medical Journal,* 1992;304(6837):1264(2).

31 Cranial osteopathic treatment is invaluable for dealing with problems experienced after operative delivery. It is to be considered in any newborn or young baby with symptoms attributable to delivery.

32 MacArthur, C. *et al. British Medical Journal* 1992;304(6837):1279(4).

33 MacArthur C. *et al. British Medical Journal* 1990;301:9-12.

34 MacArthur, C. *et al. British Medical Journal* 1993;306(6882):883(3).

35 Macfarlane, Alison *et al. The Lancet* 1993;342(8878):1005(2).

36 Some 1 in 8 babies in the UK are born by Caesarean section, which means the rate has doubled in the last 15 years. In some parts of South America, 80 per cent of babies are delivered by this method.

37 Macfarlane AJ. *British Medical Journal* 1988;297:852.

38 Stafford RS. Caesarean section use and source of payment: an analysis of Canadian hospital discharge abstracts. *Am J Publ Health* 1990;80:313-15.

39 Enkin MW. *et al* (eds) *Pregnancy and childbirth module.* Cochrane database of systematic reviews published through Cochrane updates on disk. (Oxford: Update Software, 1993).

40 *American Family Physician* 1989;39(6):258(1).

41 "Commercial discharge pack studies indicated that the packs had a negative effect on total breast-feeding at one month and any breast feeding at one and four months. The packs were linked to poor lactation among women during their first delivery and poor women in developing countries. Rooming-in accompanied by breast-feeding guidance had a greater positive effect on lactation success than did either procedure alone. Other programs including early mother-infant contact after birth, breast-feeding on demand and removal of in-hospital commercial formula supplementation had significant beneficial effects on breast-feeding." Perez-Escamilla, Rafael. *et al. The American Journal of Public Health* 1994;84(1):89(9).

42 In my opinion, the major contributions to disease in this century have been mass vaccination, routine use of antibiotics and the medicalisation of normal processes.

18 WOMEN'S HEALTH

INTRODUCTION

This Chapter deals with the health of women. In conventional medicine, the speciality of gynaecology – the study of women – is concerned with specific disorders of the female reproductive system. This tends to continue the narrow, departmentalised view of the human being. In addition, there are many negative associations with the word 'gynaecology'. There may be feelings associated with the treatment of women both in society at large and in the doctor's consulting room. Feelings of violation, disempowerment, resentment and frustration are all too commonly the result of the conventional medical treatment of women. This is an emotionally charged subject and it is important to bear in mind when you are treating a woman that there may be a whole history of conventional gynaecological treatment to be considered in addition to the original complaint. Such treatment, besides clouding the original symptoms, adds another dimension to be addressed.

In my opinion, the treatment of women by gynaecologists mirrors current attitudes towards women in Western society. The sexist attitudes in society are reflected in the gynaecology clinic. Most gynaecologists are men and female gynaecologists frequently display the same male-centred attitudes. There is an underlying agenda that there is something inherently dysfunctional about female physiology. This idea is prevalent in Western society as a result of various religious and social ideas about women.

It is a Judaeo-Christian belief that woman, in the form of Eve is responsible for the initiation of a 'fall from grace'. Since menstruation symbolises being female, it is viewed as a pathological discharge which is inherently abnormal or unclean. Women themselves take on this belief. Colloquially, there are terms for menstruation such as 'the curse'. There are negative associations with the pre-menstrual and menstrual times, with sexual activity, with pregnancy and childbirth. These are deeply ingrained and cover the whole treatment of women both in gynaecology and in obstetrics.[1]

Certainly female physiology is poorly understood and this may be because Western philosophical thought regards physical matters as all-important. Women are considered to be mechanical objects and the use of female sex hormones, oral contraception and hormone replacement therapy is a crude attempt to manipulate hormonal states in order to control menstruation and ovulation. The word 'manipulate', of course, can be used on many levels and I do not think that these drugs are used solely for their physical effects. A study of the side effects of these hormones makes it difficult to see the justification for taking such drugs. There is a often a subconscious view that as women are abnormal to begin with it is reasonable to take any means to try and 'make them better'.

Women just before, at and after the menopause are given large doses of female sex hormones in an attempt to treat the 'disease of menopause'. There is no end to the 'need' for treatment according to these views of conventional medicine. Women grow up, manifest symptoms and receive treatment in an atmosphere of negativity that teaches women not to express their thoughts and feelings. This suppression means the flow of energy becomes blocked. Pathology then arises in the neck and throat leading to thyroid dysfunction or in the pelvis giving rise to menstrual symptoms. Normal events such as menstruation, ovulation and the menopause are frequently seen as abnormal and requiring treatment. Symptoms are viewed negatively and removed by chemicals or surgery. Women's negativity about themselves creates feelings of shame, resentment, guilt, excessive responsibility and so forth.

The holistic view of women's health is somewhat different and necessarily more positive. Chinese medicine, for example, is based upon an energetic anatomy and physiology and describes the importance of energetic channels in women. There is an energetic channel that directly connects the uterus with the heart.[2] The Heart in Chinese medicine, if I can remind you of Chapter 7 – Cardiovascular system, is considered to house the Mind. This direct connection is important in that it explains why psychological factors frequently affect menstruation and why gynaecological interference can have such a dramatic effect on the psyche. It is of relevance in pregnancy since this allows for a direct connection between the mind of the baby and the mind of the mother. Some authors have named the uterus, 'the second heart' and it is clearly an important organ. In conventional medicine, the uterus is seen as being unnecessary after women have their quota of children and hysterectomy is frequently performed. The indications for hysterectomy in these situations may be slight indeed. It can be seen from this energetic connection that such treatment can lead to emotional and mental disturbances. In addition, the prescription of female sex hormones can themselves disturb mental and emotional states.

In Chinese medicine it is considered that in healthy females, menstruation begins on a regular monthly cycle at around the age of 14. This is because females go through cycles of 7 years.[3] The menstrual cycle continues regularly until the age of menopause which normally occurs at the age of 49 years. The menstrual cycle, which in health is 28 days in length, corresponds with the lunar cycle.

Everything can be divided into Yin and Yang. The first half of the cycle, beginning with menstruation, is related to Yin and ends at ovulation. Ovulation is the time when conception may occur, the reception of the sperm coinciding with the most receptive time of the month. It corresponds to the new moon, which is the most Yin time of the lunar cycle – the moon is hidden or difficult to see, or is hidden and there is a dark sky. At ovulation, the Yang phase of the cycle begins. The energy gathers to push the blood out at the time of menstruation. This occurs, ideally, at the full moon which is the time of greatest flow, both in terms of menstruation but also in terms of ocean tides.

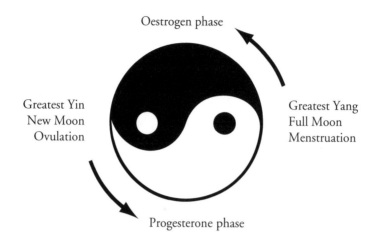

Figure 18.1: Diagram of Yin-Yang symbol related to menstrual cycle

As there are changes physically, there are also changes mentally and emotionally. We live in a society where it is considered normal to have a routine and not to take account of natural cycles. Nevertheless, it is clear to most women that they feel differently through the month and menstruation gives clear external evidence of such changes. Men are Yang in relation to the Yin of nature and the earth. Generally they are not as sensitive as women to natural cycles.

The Yang phase, the second half of the cycle, is where the energy gathers to push out the Blood. At this time, the energy may stagnate which is why pre-menstrual symptoms of painful breasts, headaches, bloating, irritability and anger may manifest. As menstruation begins, the changeover to the Yin part of the cycle starts, the energy moves down and out as evidenced by menstrual flow and the whole cycle begins again.

Frequently, at or around the time of menstruation, women may have feelings of wanting to be quiet and separate. Historically, and in traditional cultures, this is a time when women in the community withdraw and spent time by themselves rather than taking part in the hurly-burly of community life. It is a time when women perhaps feel more in touch with spiritual matters, their artistic, receptive side and so more connected to the power of being female. This, of course, is the reason why menstruation in modern society is regarded so negatively since recognition of this power would place women on an equal basis with men. Most trends in the modern world are designed to undermine women so there is a vested interest in undermining menstruation.

The absolute definition of normal menstruation I take from Chinese views of physiology. The normal cycle is of 28 days. This includes 5 days of menstruation. In health, the discharge of blood during menstruation is not too heavy or too light, it is painless with no clots, it begins clearly with a red flow, being heavier for the first day or so and then tailing off and it ends clearly. I would consider any cycle less than 26 days or more than 30 days as a symptom to be included in the case. If menstruation lasts less than 4 days or more than 6 days, this also indicates an imbalance. Pre-menstrually, women may notice changes in their psychological state. Symptoms such as irritability, depression, tiredness and headache indicate an imbalance to be considered as part of the case.

As can be seen from this description, symptoms are very common at or around menstruation. Unfortunately, there is an acceptance by many people that these symptoms are 'normal'. Education by the practitioner is clearly an important part of our work in women regaining their health.

The menopause which normally occurs around the age of 49 years is also a normal event and is associated with the cessation of menstruation. The commonest occurrence is the gradual increase in the interval between periods with decreasing loss at each menstrual period. Sometimes menstruation stops suddenly. Marked emotional changes, heavy periods, intermittent bleeding, sweats and hot flushes are abnormal although common in Western society, where women are considered to be of less value after the child-bearing years. This is a reason why female sex hormones will be given after the menopause since this continues the occurrence of bleeding every month, together with feelings of attractiveness. This illusion, or indeed delusion, is a major driving force in the prescription of hormone replacement treatment.

ANATOMY AND PHYSIOLOGY

It is important to have an understanding of the structure and function of the female reproductive system. To study women's health it would be helpful to be able to:

- identify the structures of the female reproductive system
- describe the functions of these structures
- explain the connections between the female reproductive system and the endocrine system
- describe the phases of the menstrual cycle
- describe the changes in the female reproductive system which occur at puberty and menopause
- describe the function of the breast and its relationship to the female sex hormones.

It can be seen from a knowledge of anatomy and physiology that there are certain common symptoms which arise from disturbances:

- no periods (amenorrhoea)
- irregular periods
- late periods
- early periods
- heavy periods
- painful periods (dysmenorrhoea)
- abnormal vaginal bleeding
- vaginal discharge
- abdominal pain
- infertility.

CLASSIFICATION OF GYNAECOLOGICAL DISORDERS

The most useful classification is to follow the pattern I have set throughout the book. That is, to take account of acuteness and level within the body. Such a classification is shown in Table 18.1. The conventional classification mainly centres on pathological processes, e.g. infective, inflammatory, tumours, hormonal.

Mild disease

Dysmenorrhoea
Pre-menstrual syndrome
Vaginal discharge
Pelvic inflammatory disease
Menstrual abnormalities
Endometriosis
Cancer of the cervix of the uterus
Cancer of the body of the uterus

Severe disease

Table 18.1: Energetic classification of gynaecological disorders

GYNAECOLOGICAL DISORDERS

Introduction

Most of the conditions in this Chapter are those Chinese medicine lists for study. These are 14 in number and may be divided into gynaecological and obstetric problems. They are mainly symptoms rather than conventional disease labels. They are discussed in detail in this Chapter in one form or another. The gynaecological disorders are:

- irregular menstruation
- amenorrhoea
- dysmenorrhoea
- infertility
- pre-menstrual syndrome
- abnormal vaginal bleeding
- leucorrhoea (this means vaginal discharge)
- menopausal symptoms
- uterine prolapse.

The obstetric disorders are discussed in Chapter 17 – Pregnancy and Childbirth and they complete the 14 listed in Chinese medicine. These are:

- morning sickness
- malposition of the foetus
- threatened miscarriage
- post maturity and/or difficult and painful labour
- insufficient lactation.

VAGINAL DISCHARGE

Vaginal discharge can be an important pointer to gynaecological health. In all cases, it is important to specifically enquire about this. Sometimes a vaginal discharge is normal, particularly in the second half of the cycle. It is important to enquire about the heaviness of the discharge, time of day, changes with menstrual cycle, colour of the discharge and any associated symptoms. It is also essential to enquire about the use of douches, tampons, sprays and drugs, particularly the contraceptive pill and antibiotics.

In Chinese medicine, the categorisation of vaginal discharges is in terms of colour. These are white, red, yellow, black, green and five-coloured. I use this terminology here as a basis for discussion

Black and five-coloured vaginal discharges are uncommon, particularly in out-patient practice. They usually occur in association with advanced cancer.

White vaginal discharge

White discharge is known as leucorrhoea although in some Chinese medical textbooks the term is used to indicate any vaginal discharge. This is a misconception as the prefix 'leuco-' means white.

Not all white vaginal discharges are abnormal. You should consider situations of pregnancy, sexual stimulation, ovulation, pre-menstrually and post-partum times associated with a normal white discharge. It is normal when it is not heavy and there is no associated smell, itching or discomfort.

In terms of conventional medicine, white vaginal discharge may be associated with several disorders including:

- cervical erosion
- cervical polyp
- fungal infection – *Candida albicans* (also known as thrush or monilia)

Symptoms

Classically, fungal infection causes profuse vaginal discharge of a thick or curdy nature where patches of white are seen on the vulva or vagina. Scraping of the white patches reveals a raw, bleeding surface. This accounts for the symptoms of severe itching, soreness and discomfort. It commonly occurs after treatment with the oral contraceptive or antibiotics since these drugs alter the normal bacterial and fungal content of the body. After antibiotics, 80 per cent of women have evidence of Candida whilst around one-third of those will have symptoms.

In women who have not received treatment with antibiotics, up to 60 per cent have evidence of Candida. The appearance of symptoms is associated with various factors. These include:

- pregnancy
- sugar intake, tight clothes, synthetic materials, allergic reactions,
- prescribed drugs, e.g. antibiotics, corticosteroids, female sex hormones, immunosuppressant drugs
- diabetes mellitus, AIDS, herpes simplex.

Some 50 per cent of cases have no such factors.

Treatment

Treatment of white vaginal discharge is usually considered unnecessary by conventional medicine unless there is evidence of thrush. This is invariably with anti-fungal agents which may be locally or systemically given. Systemic anti-fungal agents have a predilection for causing liver disease such as hepatitis. Up to 20 per cent of women treated develop recurrent vaginal symptoms, which can be a major difficulty.

Holistic management

In terms of Chinese medicine, white vaginal discharge infers deficiency of Spleen energy with the abnormal passage downwards of Dampness (mucus). There are mainly four variants seen which are Kidney deficiency, Spleen deficiency, Phlegm-dampness and Damp-heat.

The main point for holistic practitioners is that the occurrence of an abnormal white discharge implies an internal organ imbalance. This is not merely a disturbance of the vagina. It is important to enquire about any precipitating or maintaining cause such as those listed above. Of particular importance are the oral contraceptive, antibiotics and the use of irritant sprays and douches, which frequently cause allergic reactions. If these are avoided and constitutional treatment begun, then improvement can be expected.

Case

A woman of 45 years came for treatment. Her main complaint was constipation. She would open her bowels daily for several days and then miss up to 5 days. She had leaking urine which was worse on exercise and straining. This was despite a surgical repair for prolapse some years earlier. She also had a vaginal discharge which had been continued from childhood. It was white and heavy but with no itching or smell. Other symptoms included tiredness, low back ache and general cold feelings.

Her diagnosis in terms of Chinese medicine was Kidney Yang Deficiency. I treated her with acupuncture and herbs. I gave her advice about eating warm food with ginger and cinnamon to increase her Yang energy. Within a few weeks of beginning treatment her energy had improved. Her urinary symptoms lessened and her vaginal discharge had disappeared.

In this type of case, the discharge, and indeed the urinary symptoms, are examples of fluids leaking because the energy is weak. Strengthening the energy will lead to retention of the fluids. Her constipation improved as she became stronger and her intestines were more efficient.

She continued to improve with treatment and was well after 6 months.. Towards the end of the course of treatment, she had mild flare-ups of some symptoms that she had as a child. This 'return of old symptoms' is a curative response and reflected her increased levels of health.

Yellow vaginal discharge

In conventional medicine, the appearance of any yellow or green vaginal discharge is considered to reveal the existence of bacterial infection. The causes of such a discharge are considered to be inflammation of the cervix (cervicitis), retained pessary, inflammation of the vagina or endometrium and pelvic inflammatory disease. Cervicitis is the term used to describe an inflammation of the cervix. It may be, but not necessarily, of infective origin, Any yellow discharge will automatically be treated with antibiotics.

Symptoms

The precise symptoms associated with yellow vaginal discharge are dependent upon the site of the condition. In the case of vaginitis (vaginal inflammation) there will be soreness and discomfort in the vagina. Cervicitis is associated with frequency of urination, tenderness of the cervix on pressure and painful intercourse. The symptoms of pelvic inflammatory disease are discussed in detail below.

Treatment

As stated above, this condition is invariably treated with antibiotics that lead to further problems with vaginal discharge (see above information on white vaginal discharge). If there is disease of the cervix such as cervicitis or an associated condition, cervical erosion, then there may be cauterisation by heat or lasers.

Cervical erosion is considered to be secondary to cervical discharge in conventional medicine. Despite its name it is not in itself a primary inflammatory condition, nor is it an ulcer. This can lead to confusion and women can be worried about the term unless it is properly explained. It is the growth of cells from inside the cervical canal over the surface of the cervix.

Cervical erosion is seen as a bright red velvety area extending from the external opening of the cervix over the vaginal surface. The surface bleeds easily, especially on contact and post-coital bleeding is a common symptom. Erosions are common in women on the pill. They commonly occur in pregnancy and in the post-natal period and usually disappear with no treatment. They seem to be related to high hormone levels.

Holistic Management

In terms of Chinese medicine, yellow vaginal discharge is again due to Dampness, as is white vaginal discharge. There is associated Heat causing the yellow colour. This usually implies some Stagnation of Liver energy.

Case

A woman of 33 years came for treatment because she had not been well since glandular fever some 4 years previously. She had particularly been ill for the past 6 months. Her main complaints were extreme fatigue, occasional fever with sore throat. She had diarrhoea four or five times each day with undigested food in the stools, nausea, palpitations and general muscle weakness.

In terms of conventional medicine, this could be diagnosed as myalgic encephalomyelitis (ME) although no-one had ever made that diagnosis. In terms of Chinese medicine, this was a case of Heart Blood Deficiency and Spleen Yang Deficiency with Damp Accumulation.

After some weeks of treatment, her bowels became normal and she began to feel more energetic. Her treatment continued for some 5 months. At the end of this time, she felt generally well with good energy. She then developed a vaginal discharge with lower abdominal pain. It was yellow in colour and occasionally blood-streaked. It was particularly heavy after menstruation.

She had had a history of inflammation of the cervix which had been discovered by cervical smear investigation. She was somewhat worried about her symptoms and had a repeat cervical smear. This showed normal cells. A vaginal swab showed evidence of 'thrush'. Despite this, her doctor gave her antibiotics.

During and after the course of antibiotics she felt tired and depressed with diarrhoea and a bloated abdomen. The Cold and Damp qualities of the antibiotics in the presence of her weak Spleen energy caused a recurrence of her original symptoms. If she had had further courses of antibiotics, these would have worsened and she would develop a clinical picture similar to that of ME discussed on Page 55.

Her vaginal discharge was the passage of mucus out of the body and, in that sense, was a curative response. Mucus collects in the intestines and this may be evident in the stools or, in women, as vaginal discharge as the uterus is often also involved. The mucus had begun to move out of her body as her energy had been improving.

It is important in such cases to continue the process so that the movement towards health can be maintained.

Green vaginal discharge

This is a more severe condition than yellow vaginal discharge and in conventional medicine is usually associated with infection by *Trichomonas vaginalis*. This is an organism classified as a protozoon. A related organism is Giardia which is associated with bowel symptoms.

Symptoms

There is the appearance of a green vaginal discharge containing tiny bubbles. There may be small red erosions over the surface of the vagina with severe inflammation. There is marked pain and discomfort in the area. There is frequently evidence of the organism in sexual partners and so sexual transmission is an issue in this condition.

Treatment

This is by means of the antiprotozoal agent, metronidazole, for around 7 days and the sexual partner is treated in the same way. Sexual intercourse should be abstained from during this time.

Holistic Management

This is a more severe type of yellow vaginal discharge and therefore in terms of Chinese medicine there is much more Heat, as evidenced by the green colour and the degree of pain. There are similarities energetically between this condition and the description of cystitis in Chapter 9 – Urinary system.

Red vaginal discharge

Clearly this is bleeding and must always be taken seriously. In terms of conventional medicine it may occur as a result of:

- cervical erosion
- tumour, benign or malignant of uterine cervix or uterine body
- inflammation of the vagina
- inflammation of the endometrium[4]
- retained pessary
- associated with pregnancy.

The latter case is considered in Chapter 17 – Pregnancy and Childbirth.

Such bleeding from the vagina, other than around the time of the menses, may be of serious significance. In the case of cervical cancer there may be an association with intercourse and in cases of uterine cancer there may be intermenstrual bleeding.

Holistic Management

It is important to bear in mind what conventional medicine sees as a possible underlying cause. In Chinese medicine, red discharge is seen as a consequence of Damp-heat or Blood and Yin deficiency where there may be signs of Deficient Heat.

PELVIC INFLAMMATORY DISEASE

This is a term that indicates inflammation in the pelvis usually involving the fallopian tubes and ovaries. It may also be known as salpingitis or salpingo-oophoritis. It is considered to be associated with infection. This used to be more commonly of the gonococcal type but is now usually associated with organisms such as chlamydia. The relationship between these two organisms was discussed in Chapter 9 – Urinary system – Page 150.

Symptoms

There are a wide variety of presentations but in the severe acute case there may be confusion with other causes of acute abdominal pain. The differential diagnosis of acute lower abdominal pain is shown in Table 18.2.

Disease	Symptoms	Comments
Appendicitis	Pain central abdomen that migrates to right iliac fossa. Vomiting, fever	Classical cause of pain in right iliac fossa. Short history
Ectopic pregnancy	History of amenorrhoea in the sexually active, vaginal bleeding usually brownish or dark	Symptoms worsen over days and possibly weeks. Surgical emergency
Pyelonephritis	Dysuria, haematuria, loin pain, fever	Pain mainly in the loin but may be referred down the ureter on the affected side to give iliac fossa pain
Torsion[5] of ovarian cyst	Pain in the iliac fossa, vomiting, rapid pulse and low blood pressure if severe, slight fever, uterine bleeding (occasionally)	More likely during pregnancy or after childbirth
Ruptured ovarian cyst	Severe abdominal pain but of short duration	

Table 18.2: Differential diagnosis of acute lower abdominal pain

In the case of pelvic inflammatory disease, there is sharp, lower abdominal pain which is usually felt in both iliac fossae. If the pain is only on the right side, the possibility of appendicitis must be considered. There is disturbance of menstruation with spotting around the period, and heavy, painful periods. There is a yellowish discharge and frequent urination. There may be associated nausea and vomiting. Painful intercourse is common. There is a fever of around 39°C (102°F) with lower abdominal tenderness and guarding.

Pelvic inflammatory disease is more common when there is vaginal douching and frequent sexual intercourse particularly with different partners. With any vaginal discharge it is helpful to think about whether there are associated symptoms developing in pelvic inflammatory disease. It is useful to enquire of previous medical history that may reveal:

- gonorrhoea
- non-specific urethritis
- genital herpes
- genital warts
- trichomonal infection
- recent change of sexual partner
- urethral symptoms in a partner
- use of intra-uterine contraceptive device (the 'coil')
- gynaecological or pelvic surgery.

Chronic pelvic inflammatory disease is usually characterised by recurrent attacks of lesser severity than the acute picture. There is persisting pelvic pain and back ache. Painful periods are common and intercourse may also be painful. Periods may be heavy. There is an associated yellow vaginal discharge. The recurrence of continuing pain, discomfort and heavy menstruation may cause general symptoms of ill health. Blockage of the fallopian tubes causes infertility. Fever may be absent.

Investigations

This is by means of vaginal swabs to isolate any organism associated with the symptoms. Green vaginal discharge may occur in several situations. Table 18.3 itemises how to differentiate its causes.

Symptom	Vaginitis	Cervicitis	Pelvic inflammatory disease
Vaginal discharge	green	green	green
Menstrual abnormalities	no	no	yes
Painful intercourse	superficial	deep	deep
Frequent urination	no	yes	yes
Fever	no	no	yes

Table 18.3: Comparison of conditions associated with green vaginal discharge

Treatment

Conventionally this is with a combination of several antibiotics such as metronidazole and tetracycline. Non-steroidal anti-inflammatory agents may also be prescribed but the condition often becomes chronic.

Holistic management

It may be considered as a more internal problem than the causes of vaginal discharges we have considered above, particularly the white and yellow types. This comparison can be seen in Table 18.3.

There have been increasing numbers of women with these symptoms over the past few decades. It is almost certainly related to changes in sexual habits together with the increasing use of drugs such as female sex hormones and antibiotics.

In terms of Chinese medicine, the usual diagnoses include Damp-heat in the Lower Jiao, Stagnation of Blood in the Lower Jiao and Deficiency of Spleen and Kidney Qi. The occurrence of the symptoms indicates a chronic constitutional imbalance and treatment may need to be prolonged. Complicating factors such as the use of antibiotics or female sexual hormones need to be stopped. Advice about stress, sexual activity and diet is helpful. These factors were discussed on Page 156 in relation to cystitis.

MENSTRUAL ABNORMALITIES

Before considering whether a particular pattern of menstruation is normal or abnormal, I would refer you to Page 344 of this chapter where a definition of normal menstruation is outlined. Any variation from this implies abnormality.

Dysmenorrhoea

This is painful menstruation. It is generally considered that about 5 per cent of women have sufficient pain to seek treatment but this is probably an underestimate. The number of women who have painful periods is far in excess of this figure. It is stated that about half of these women are too ill to work when symptoms are present.

Symptoms

The pain may begin before menstruation, at the onset of menstruation or towards the end of the period. These are important questions to ask together with information about the menstrual loss and associated symptoms.

In terms of conventional medicine, painful menstruation is divided into two categories. So-called primary dysmenorrhoea usually starts after puberty. There are colicky pains in the lower abdomen due to uterine contractions (spasmodic dysmenorrhoea). It may cease after childbirth, hence the old advice 'to have a baby'.

Secondary dysmenorrhoea is the appearance of menstrual pain after several years of painless periods. This is considered to be due to the development of conditions such as uterine fibroids, endometriosis or pelvic inflammatory disease. The pain tends to be prolonged throughout the period of perhaps a dragging quality. There may also be menstrual abnormalities.

Treatment

There are several treatment options for primary dysmenorrhoea. These are listed in Table 18.4. Treatment of secondary dysmenorrhoea will be of the primary condition.

Treatment (mildest to strongest)	Comments
Analgesics, usually non-steroidal anti-inflammatory drugs	These are described in detail in Chapter 10 – Musculoskeletal System
Oral contraceptive	Suppresses menstruation and ovulation
Dilatation of the cervix	This requires a general anaesthetic and reduces symptoms in about one third. May damage cervix leading to premature labour in pregnancy

Table 18.4: Conventional treatment of primary dysmenorrhoea

Holistic Management

In terms of Chinese medicine, the common pattern seen is Stagnation of Liver Qi, which is commonly associated with emotional disturbances. In this type there will be associated symptoms of pre-menstrual syndrome with perhaps painful breasts, irritability, headache.

Another pattern is exposure to Cold and Damp that lodge in the uterus usually associated with Deficiency of Kidney Yang. Here, pain at the beginning of menstruation will be associated with perhaps diarrhoea, cold and faint feelings.

Further patterns include Deficiency of Qi and Blood due to Deficiency of Liver and Kidneys, Stasis of Blood and Damp-heat. Some cases of Liver Qi Stagnation may lead to Flaring of Liver Fire.

It is important to take each case individually and treat accordingly. Emotional factors, sexual activity and diet are all important here. In China, it is well known that the ingestion of cold foods or drinks during menstruation may stop the menstrual flow and so cause pain. This may be the origin, in the West, of recommendations not to wash your hair or have a bath during a period. These are not simply 'old wives' tales' or superstition but have a basis in truth. This should not be misconstrued as saying that women are inherently weak and need to avoid certain activities. It is merely recognition of the changes that occur during menstruation.

The treatment of painful menstruation by holistic medicine is usually successful but clearly the underlying disturbances are of importance. It is more difficult to treat if structural abnormalities are present such as endometriosis.

Endometriosis

This is the existence of endometrium in situations where it is not usually present. The usual sites, in decreasing order of frequency, are ovaries, uterus, fallopian tubes, general pelvic area, umbilicus and lower abdominal scars particularly after hysterectomy. The endometrium bleeds at menstruation and so these areas also bleed. However, the blood cannot escape as it can from within the uterus. There are symptoms of lower abdominal pain which may be severe in nature. There may be the occurrence of intestinal symptoms, such as adhesions and scarring of pelvic masses may interfere with intestinal function. Eventually, quite large collections of old blood develop in the areas affected, these are known as 'chocolate cysts' as they are full of dark sticky material.

The cause in conventional medicine is not well understood. There seems to be a correlation with the use of tampons, intercourse during menstruation and the use of the intra-uterine contraceptive device (the 'coil'). It is more common in women who have had few or no children.

Symptoms
Twenty or so years ago it was unusual to see this condition in anyone below the age of 30 years. Nowadays it is more common to see endometriosis in younger age groups. The main clinical feature is pain on menstruation – dysmenorrhoea. Menstrual irregularities such as heavy periods and irregular bleeding are common. Infertility is an association since the existence of inflammation, scar tissue and adhesions in the pelvis may obstruct the passage of ova along the fallopian tube.

Typically, the pain is severe beginning before the menstruation and continuing almost to the end. There may be associated symptoms of diarrhoea and vomiting. Fainting may occur in some. In extreme cases where disease is widespread there may be the development of intestinal obstruction.

Complications

Complication	Symptoms to look for
Infertility	Inability to become pregnant
Intestinal obstruction	Abdominal distension, constipation, colicky abdominal pain

Table 18.5: Complications of endometriosis

Diagnosis
This is primarily by means of the clinical history. Confirmation is usually obtained by laparoscopy.

Treatment
The conventional treatment of endometriosis is not particularly successful and the cause is ill understood. The main aim is to produce a state of 'pseudo pregnancy' where menstruation is halted. In this way cyclical endometrial bleeding is prevented and any areas of endometrium outside the uterus may have an opportunity to recede.

There are two main drugs used. Danazol affects the release of hormones by the pituitary gland and thereby inhibits ovulation and the normal hormonal cyclical change. It also affects adrenal gland function. Common side-effects include masculinisation such as deepening of the voice, reduction in breast size, oily skin and acne, development of hair in a male distribution and occasionally enlargement of the clitoris. It is a powerful drug as can be estimated by its side-effects and by the deep site of its action, the pituitary gland.

The other drug that may be used is a progesterone compound, norethisterone. This is given continuously in an effort to suppress ovulation and prevent menstruation. The side-effects are those of the progesterone group in general.

Holistic management

At menstruation the blood should normally flow down and out and endometriosis would seem to suggest that the opposite is happening. The associations mentioned above of tampon use, intercourse during menstruation and the use of the intra-uterine contraceptive device (IUD) are all associated with energy and blood flowing upwards rather than downwards. Tampons block the normal downward flow of menstrual blood.[6] Intercourse leads to energy flowing upwards and the 'coil' is also associated with a backward flow in the reproductive organs. Peristalsis along the fallopian tube is often reversed and ectopic pregnancy (pregnancy developing in a fallopian tube) is much more common where an IUD is present. In terms of prevention, certain measures may be helpful. The use of sanitary towels rather than tampons, abstinence from intercourse during menstruation and the use of holistic methods of contraception may go a long way to reducing the incidence of endometriosis.[7]

As for treatment of the condition once it has developed, it is important to consider the underlying energetic diagnosis. In terms of Chinese medicine, endometriosis usually corresponds to Stagnation of Blood in the Lower Jiao.

Amenorrhoea

This is absence of menstrual periods. The importance of amenorrhoea is that it does not always denote disease. There are times when the absence of periods is normal. The commonest cause of amenorrhoea between the ages of 15 and 45 years is pregnancy. This may seem obvious but when practitioners see people with various symptoms the first thing to jump to mind often is a pathological situation. Normal absence of periods is also seen before puberty, during pregnancy and lactation and after the menopause.

Conventionally amenorrhoea is divided into two types. The primary type is where the woman has never menstruated. This is unusual and usually associated with rare endocrine disturbances. Secondary amenorrhoea is where menstruation has occurred previously and then stopped. Women with this seek help in the clinic and holistic practitioners quite commonly see such cases.

Investigations

I would repeat again that pregnancy is the commonest cause of amenorrhoea in the fertile years and this should always be remembered. Stopping the contraceptive pill is another common cause and may result in no periods for a variable length of time. The oral contraceptive actually stops menstruation as its primary action and bleeding only occurs because it is not taken for seven days each month. Therefore, when it is finally removed, it takes the body some time to recover and for normal menstruation to resume.

General health and psychological factors also need to be taken into account as part of the general case-taking. Menstruation is commonly connected to nutritional state, emotions or may be disturbed in association with chronic diseases. Hormone estimations may be done by means of blood test but most cases reveal no abnormality. The majority of cases of secondary amenorrhoea are temporary and recover with no conventional treatment.

Two specific conditions to mention here are anorexia nervosa and polycystic ovarian disease. Anorexia nervosa is described in Chapter 16 – Psychological disorders. Amenorrhoea is a feature of severe cases where weight loss is present. There are strong mental symptoms of disordered perception where the woman thinks or perceives herself as being overweight.

Polycystic ovarian disease, sometimes known as Stein-Leventhal syndrome, is a particular group of symptoms that include amenorrhoea. There is also hair growth on the face and in a male distribution up the central line of the lower abdomen as well as cysts on the ovaries. It is treated conventionally by surgical resection of part of the ovary or by hormonal suppression of ovulation.

Holistic management

In terms of Chinese medicine, amenorrhoea usually corresponds to one of several possible syndromes. There may be Blood Stagnation where the Blood does not move. This is usually due either to Qi stagnation or exposure to cold. The most common situation is Blood Deficiency associated with Spleen or Kidney deficiency. This is seen in athletes particularly those who are vegetarian. It is an indication of the weakness that may result in the Blood as a result of over-exercise. This connection was discussed in Chapter 10 – Musculoskeletal system, in relation to joint disorders. Some cases of amenorrhoea are due to Phlegm obstruction.

Other menstrual symptoms

There are several types of menstrual disturbances including heavy or light periods, early or late periods, and irregular periods.[8]

In conventional medicine, the aim is always to distinguish between those causes of menstrual abnormality that are physical in nature and those that are not. The term, dysfunctional uterine bleeding is used to describe those cases of abnormal bleeding which are not due to complications of pregnancy or structural disease of the uterus or ovaries.

In terms of dysfunctional uterine bleeding, the assumption is that there is a degree of endometrial abnormality associated with a hormone imbalance. This is usually an excess of oestrogen in relation to progesterone. In practice, investigations show normal hormonal levels in the majority of cases. It is true to say that conventional medicine finds this group of diseases difficult to classify. It is therefore grouped according to age of onset of symptoms.

Pubertal cases

The first menstrual cycles are usually not associated with ovulation and consequently no progesterone is produced. The endometrium becomes thickened and overactive leading to heavy and perhaps painful periods. This situation is extremely common in young women just after the onset of periods and it frequently settles with no treatment. The conventional approach is either to wait and see or to give progesterone supplements in the second half of the menstrual cycle. A frequent prescription is the oral contraceptive pill in an attempt 'to regulate the menses'. This is clearly impossible using the oral contraceptive pill since this suppresses ovarian function and stops periods completely. The only reason why women bleed when they take the pill is because they stop taking it for seven days so this is more accurately termed 'withdrawal bleeding'.

During the reproductive period

During this age group, irregular or cyclical excessive bleeding may occur. It is treated in a similar way to the pubertal cases. Either progesterone is given in the latter half of the menstrual cycle or the oral contraceptive pill is used. It is very difficult in conventional terms to determine a cause of these symptoms in most cases. Some women have normal hormone estimations (by far the commonest finding), some have reduced progesterone levels and yet others have a lack of ovulation. There is no consistent finding and an empirical approach is taken.

Dilatation and curettage (D & C) is a surgical procedure where the cervix is dilated and the inside of the uterus is scraped to remove endometrium. This may be done as a diagnostic procedure to determine the state of the endometrium but is more commonly performed, at least at this age, in an attempt to prevent heavy periods. It has been noted that heavy menstruation may be moderated after such an operation. The rationale behind this is difficult to determine. Perhaps it is akin to kicking the television set when it does not work. Certainly repeated D & Cs may lead to permanent damage of the endometrial lining of the uterus. It is a considerably invasive procedure that is probably only ever indicated if cancer of the body of the uterus is suspected or in cases of incomplete miscarriage. The operation is performed under general anaesthesia.

In some hospitals, a small plastic tube may be inserted through the cervix to obtain samples of endometrium without any anaesthesia. The effects of this are similar to surgery on the cervix of the uterus, the consequences of which are discussed later in this Chapter.

In many cases of heavy menstrual bleeding a hysterectomy may be performed where the woman has had children and there is no desire for more. There were 20,000 hysterectomies in the United Kingdom in 1985. Most are performed for irregularities in menstruation. Up to 45 per cent of women develop infections of the wound or urinary tract in the post-operative period. Even if the ovaries are left alone, the woman is likely to pass through the menopause 4 years earlier than normal.

It is important to remember that the uterus is not useless just because childbirth has finished. Hysterectomy disrupts the energetic connection between the Heart and the uterus and may lead to mental and emotional disturbances. If a hysterectomy is performed for heavy bleeding, the woman will feel somewhat better after the operation since the cause of the blood loss has been removed. However, this may well turn out to be a short-term effect as the energetic imbalance at a deeper level still remains.

A more recent technique is that of endometrial ablation. In the UK there are between 8000 and 12,000 performed each year. A tube is inserted into the uterus and an electrically heated loop or laser is used to burn the endometrium. A general anaesthetic is necessary but women stay in hospital for only one or two days. There is concern about the risks of such a procedure particularly if it is performed by inexperienced surgeons. At the time of writing at least four women have died as a result of this operation.[9]

Pre-menopausal cases

Around the time of the menopause, ovulation and thence progesterone production ceases. For a time, oestrogens are still produced. Their unopposed action may over-stimulate the endometrium leading to irregular or heavy periods. This imbalance is usually for a short time only, although blood loss can be severe. The main issue conventionally is that cancer of the body of the uterus becomes more common at this age. Dilatation and curettage is used to investigate such cases. In the absence of cancer, the use of hysterectomy is relatively common in an attempt to merely remove the symptoms. Hormone replacement therapy is a common prescription at this time.

Investigations

Most cases are treated with investigation on the assumption that a 'hormonal imbalance' is the cause. Routine investigations which may be performed are:

- full blood count – to check for anaemia
- hormone level estimations – pituitary hormones, oestrogen, progesterone
- dilatation and curettage – particularly around the time of the menopause (this is an example of investigation and treatment combined).

Holistic management

The four main situations of vaginal bleeding which may indicate a serious underlying condition are:

- pre-pubertal bleeding
- inter-menstrual bleeding
- post-coital bleeding
- post-menopausal bleeding.

Pre-pubertal bleeding is rare and, in these days of increased awareness of child sexual abuse, this is always considered first as a possibility.

Inter-menstrual bleeding is relatively common and may be part of the supposed hormonal imbalance and so included in the category of dysfunctional uterine bleeding listed above. I would refer you to the details of each in the relevant sections. Usually, if inter-menstrual bleeding is persistent or recurrent, investigation will be performed to exclude structural diseases. These include examination of the cervix, cervical smear, dilatation and curettage.

Bleeding after the menopause (post-menopausal bleeding) is relatively uncommon and may arise from the uterus, cervix, vagina or vulva. At this age, cancer is a more common diagnosis and this is always the underlying physical problem that conventional practitioners seek to exclude. Inflammation is relatively common since the reduction in oestrogen secretion leads, in some cases, to marked degeneration of the mucous membranes and the endometrium. Inflammation may develop in these areas as a consequence. Investigation of this age group is similar to that described above for abnormal bleeding during the reproductive years.

In terms of Chinese medicine, there are three main syndromes associated with menstrual disturbances. These are Heat in the Blood leading to reckless bleeding, injury to the Chong and Ren channels or Deficiency of Qi (inability to hold blood in the circulation). The actual pattern of symptoms and associated symptoms can lead to a differentiation between these three conditions.

Patterns due to Heat are usually associated with early menstruation, excessive menstruation of a bright red nature and perhaps symptoms of general heat in the body such as constipation, restlessness and anxiety.

Deficiency of Qi may lead to difficulty holding Blood in the circulation. It is usually associated with pale menstrual loss which can on occasion be heavy. There may be flooding. Spotting is common and there may be associated symptoms of Qi deficiency such as tiredness, pallor, poor appetite, diarrhoea, and uterine prolapse.

It is important to bear in mind that a more serious situation may be present in some cases. This is more likely with symptoms that occur in older women or if the symptoms are persistent or recurrent. In these cases, it is important to consider that the underlying physical abnormality may be serious and that further investigation may be warranted. This is something that needs to be raised with women that you are treating. Please see the comments made in Chapter 6 – Cancer.

Extra-uterine pregnancy (ectopic pregnancy)

This is the presence of a fertilised egg in a site other than the endometrium of the uterus, usually a fallopian tube. The cause in conventional medicine is not well understood except to say that the passage of the fertilised egg is clearly delayed along the fallopian tube. The two main situations that are associated are the use of the intra-uterine contraceptive device and pelvic inflammatory disease. The ovum embeds in the wall of the fallopian tube and starts to develop. There is no endometrium here and the thin wall of the tube is eventually eroded and ruptured by the developing embryo.

Symptoms

The last menstrual period is some 6–8 weeks previously and there may be a positive pregnancy test or symptoms of early pregnancy. The woman presents with lower abdominal pain and the loss of dark blood from the uterus. This may be mistaken for a late period and further confusion may result from negative pregnancy tests.[10] It is important to have a high awareness of the possibility of such a condition in women where pregnancy is a possibility. Eventually the bleeding continues with increasing lower abdominal pain. There is then rupture of the fallopian tube with death of the embryo and possible death of the mother.

Complications

Complication	Symptoms to look for
Rupture of fallopian tube into abdominal cavity	Severe lower abdominal pain, guarding, rigidity, immobility, low blood pressure, rapid pulse, sweating, pallor
Miscarriage – rupture into lumen of fallopian tube	Lower abdominal pain but less than the above. Uterine blood loss, pallor, slight fever. There may be retention of urine

Table 18.6: Complications of ectopic pregnancy

Treatment

Unless the embryo dies before rupture the only treatment that is possible is surgical removal. This condition is considered to be a gynaecological emergency as rupture may lead to death of the mother due to massive blood loss. The embryo and fallopian tube on the affected side are removed. Ectopic pregnancy is more likely after any surgery to the pelvis so a subsequent ectopic pregnancy is a possibility. Ultrasound is helpful in diagnosis.

Holistic management

This is a condition where surgical treatment is inevitable and there must be no delay in instituting it. Holistic medicine will centre on treatment after the necessary surgery has been performed. Blood loss may occur unless diagnosis is made early and so anaemia will be seen. Also, loss of a baby has taken place and issues around bereavement need be addressed. The after-care of such a case is described on Page 113.

OVARIAN CYST

A cyst is an example of a tumour. It is defined as an abnormal sac or closed cavity lined with epithelium and filled with liquid or semisolid matter.[11] There are many different types but essentially the distinction is made, conventionally, between benign and malignant. Ovarian cysts are not particularly common but occasionally women seek treatment in the holistic medicine clinic. The symptoms depend upon the size of the cyst and whether or not it secretes hormones.

Symptoms

Frequently, cysts are asymptomatic and only found on examination for some other reason.

Cysts that produce oestrogens may become evident through abnormal uterine bleeding. There may be post-menopausal bleeding, amenorrhoea or irregular bleeding.

Cysts that become markedly enlarged produce symptoms due to pressure within the pelvis. Abdominal swelling is the first thing to be noticed and eventually abdominal discomfort. Frequency of urination and even retention may develop with large cysts.

Pain can also be experienced with relatively small cysts due to the underlying energetic diagnosis which is described below.

A specific situation is that of Stein-Leventhal syndrome. This is the development of amenorrhoea with hairiness on the face. There are multiple cysts on both ovaries (polycystic ovaries). Treatment for this condition is by means of clomiphene or gonadotrophins. I have known some women to be given the oral contraceptive for this syndrome.

Investigations

Ultrasound scans and laparoscopy are commonly used to diagnose ovarian cysts.

Treatment

All cysts larger than 5 cm in diameter tend to be surgically removed. This is because of the possibility of malignancy. The whole ovary is usually removed. A small section of the ovary may be left if the cyst is benign. In women over 45 years, both ovaries may be removed if there is any evidence of abnormality in them.

In the case of malignancy, the ovaries, uterus and fallopian tubes are removed. Radiotherapy and chemotherapy are routinely used afterwards. Cisplatin, based upon platinum, is commonly given as a form of chemotherapy. It has many toxic side-effects but is an example of conventional medicine stumbling across the appropriate energetic remedy by chance. Platinum, in its homoeopathic provings, produces ovarian tumours. Unfortunately, in conventional medicine, high doses are used causing toxicity.

Holistic management

In terms of Chinese medicine, ovarian cysts usually correspond to Stagnation of Liver Qi, Retention of Food and Phlegm, Stasis of Blood, Stagnation of Qi and Blood. They are relatively easy to treat at an early stage where they are usually Stagnation of Qi. You need to bear in mind the underlying cause of the Stagnation in your diagnosis and treatment plan. The case is more difficult when Stagnation of Blood is apparent. It is valid to treat by means of holistic medicine and monitor progress of the cyst by means of ultrasound scans every 6 months. There is not likely to be much change in the size of the cyst in a shorter time.

Women with such syndromes may have evidence of other Stagnations in the body such as breast lumps, pre-menstrual syndrome symptoms and so forth. There may also be factors in the medical history that indicate the cause of such Stagnations. Common ones include emotional stress and frustration, surgery to the pelvic area (particularly termination of pregnancy) and the use of female sex hormones such as the oral contraceptive and treatments for infertility.

Case one

A young woman of 18 years came for treatment. She had had a long history of (continuing) dysmenorrhoea. A few months earlier she had had two cysts removed from her left ovary. Since then she had had no energy. Now she had similar pains alternating between the left and right hand side of her abdomen. Her breasts throbbed for 2 weeks prior to her period.

She had become increasingly withdrawn and wouldn't speak to teachers or students at school. She felt stupid when she spoke to anyone and scared to say anything. She said several times that she believed people were laughing at her behind her back. She felt like crying.

She was prescribed Lac caninum (a single dose of 1M), as a keynote of the remedy is pains at alternate sides. It also fitted her mental state well.

Her first period after the remedy was more painful, but her energy had greatly improved and she said she didn't 'notice the pain as much'. She didn't worry about people laughing about her and was talking to people a bit more. She felt more confident. After 3 months her physical symptoms all resolved and she was feeling very good mentally and emotionally. She repeated the remedy if her symptoms returned.

Case two

A woman of 35 years of age came for treatment of adhesions that were the result of an appendicectomy 14 years before. She had also been diagnosed with two cysts on the left ovary. She had had severe abdominal cramping pain for 4 weeks, with a sensation of her insides being pulled downwards. She also had stitching pain on the right hand side.

She had a horror of children and said she would kill herself if she became pregnant. She used violent language.

Since she was in great pain, she was immediately prescribed Thiosinaminum 7x, which is a specific for the treatment of adhesions, whilst a constitutional remedy was chosen. Thiosinaminum eased the cramps, but did not change any other symptoms.

Platina 30c was prescribed, which fitted both her physical and mental symptoms well.

After taking it she had excruciating pain, but then she said she could feel the cyst getting better everyday for 3 weeks. The pulling down sensation also went and returned three weeks later. Her mental state seemed calmer. She said: 'I'd been hobbling around like an invalid when I saw you, but I got better and was perfect until a week ago'. I repeated the remedy.

FIBROIDS

These are an example of a benign tumour and are known as fibromyomas. The cause of their development is unknown in conventional medicine. They are unusual before the age of 30 years and do not begin to develop after the menopause. They are commoner in women who have not had children.

Symptoms

Most fibroids are asymptomatic and may only be found at routine examination, operation or post-mortem.

Heavy menstrual bleeding is the classic symptom associated with fibroids. The period is prolonged and the cycle may be shortened. Pain is unusual with the fibroid itself although the heaviness of the menstruation may be associated with discomfort.

Large fibroids may be felt on abdominal examination. Smaller tumours are detected by vaginal examination.

Investigations

Ultrasound scan will reveal the presence of fibroids.

Treatment

Small, asymptomatic fibroids are not treated conventionally. Large ones are removed surgically by means of hysterectomy. Occasionally, a myomectomy is performed where the fibroid alone is removed from the wall of the uterus. This is to be favoured in those women who wish to have children. Fibroids may recur later.

Holistic management

In terms of Chinese medicine, fibroids usually correspond to Stagnation of Damp-phlegm, Qi or Blood. The causes are considered to be emotional stagnation, over consumption of dairy products, sexual intercourse at too early an age[12] and emotional imbalance especially in the teenage years.

CANCER OF THE UTERUS

There are two types as the uterus has a body and cervix (neck). They differ in their symptoms and the most common age of presentation and so are considered separately.

Cancer of the body of the uterus

This is not common before the menopausal period. The main incidence is between the ages of 50 and 65 years. It occurs more often in women who have had no children. There is no evidence that fibroids predispose to cancer. The cancer spreads locally through the wall of the uterus and there is frequently involvement of ovaries and other organs at the time of diagnosis. Cancers of this type spread locally within the pelvis via the lymphatic system.

Symptoms

The classic appearance is of post-menopausal bleeding. At first, this may be fairly nondescript and infrequent but becomes commoner and heavier with time. Eventually the haemorrhage can be severe. If the woman is still pre-menopausal then inter-menstrual bleeding is seen. Pain is late and signifies advanced disease.

Diagnosis

This is confirmed by dilatation of the cervix and curettage of the endometrium (D & C).

Treatment

The main treatment, if the cancer has not spread too far, is by surgery. The usual operation is hysterectomy with oophorectomy and removal of lymph glands within the pelvis. There may be a post-operative course of hormonal treatment with progesterone. The latter may be the only treatment given in cases not suitable for surgery.

Radiotherapy may also be applied if surgery is not possible. The five-year survival rate is 60 per cent.

Holistic management

The main issue for a holistic practitioner is to recognise the importance of post-menopausal bleeding as an early symptom of cancer. In terms of treatment, please see the comments made in Chapter 6 – Cancer.

Cancer of the cervix of the uterus

This disease provides a classical example of the principle of staging by the conventional profession. Conventional thought is that the cells on the outside surface of the cervix begin a change towards abnormality that eventually may become malignant after several years. Each stage that the cells pass through is designated a number. The classification currently used is CIN.[13] There have been several classifications used in the past and the current one is:

- normal or subcategory of normal such as 'inflamed', 'signs of infection'
- probably normal but recheck regularly because of mild changes
- precancerous changes
- superficial or early cancer
- invasive cancer.

The condition of the cervix is discovered by means of a cervical ('Pap') smear. This is recommended to be performed every 3 years or so. This is the vital prerequisite to conventional management and treatment. The current belief is that these stages lead onto each other in a progressive way and treatment early will stop development.

The most common age at presentation with cancer of the cervix is between 40 and 50 years. However, increasing numbers are seen in younger women. Ninety-five per cent of women have had children. There is a relationship with the frequency of intercourse and number of partners. It is rare in nuns and more common in women who have had intercourse from a relatively early age and with different partners. It is suspected that there may be a male factor as it is very rare in Jewish women – the great majority of Jewish men are, of course, circumcised. The virus of genital herpes is associated with the cancer although the significance of this is not known.

The cancer spreads by various means. These include local spread to vagina and uterus, by the lymphatic system to the glands of the pelvis, by blood spread (late in the disease) and by implantation of malignant cells further down the vagina.

Conventionally, there is held to be a need for routine cervical smears every 3 years or so although this time span keeps changing. Some women have a normal smear and then quite advanced disease 1 or 2 years later. It was always considered that there were at least 5 years between each stage and that the development of actual carcinoma would therefore take about 15-20 years. This now seems to be very much an overestimate.

Symptoms
Once ulceration of the cervix has occurred there is slight irregular bleeding especially on examination or intercourse and diagnosis can be made at this stage by examination or earlier by cervical smears. Pain is a late symptom and is due to inflammation or to extensive spread of the growth.

Treatment
The main aim of conventional treatment is to remove abnormal cells and surgery is the considered choice. For cancer itself, the preferred operation is hysterectomy with removal of ovaries. Radiotherapy may be used with the insertion of radioactive rods into the cervical canal and the upper vagina.

In the case of dysplasia, treatment depends upon the particular stage and the preferences of the gynaecologist. There are wide variations in approach. Generally, early changes may be left alone and checked every 3 or 6 months. If there are signs of inflammation, antibiotics may be given on the assumption that bacterial infection is present. Later stages are treated surgically. This is either with lasers to remove the affected surface cells or by means of cone biopsy.

Laser treatment is performed in the out-patient clinic with no anaesthesia. The conventional belief is that the cervix has no pain sensation. This is not the experience of women who undergo these procedures. Any such treatment to the cervix is decidedly painful and certainly traumatic. Such expressions of discomfort are not dealt with seriously in most cases. Bleeding after such procedures and longer term menstrual irregularities are common.

Cone biopsy is, as its name suggests, the removal of a cone of tissue from the cervix. It is performed under general anaesthesia. This necessitates a stay in hospital of several days. Long-term problems include menstrual abnormalities and a weakened cervix which may make miscarriage more likely.

Holistic management
One important consideration is to separate the issues of cancer and of dysplasia. Dysplasia is not necessarily cancer and does not mean that cancer is an inevitable result. The whole process frightens women and words like 'cancer smear', 'smear' and 'abnormal cells' only serve to magnify this. Reassurance is helpful along with help in dealing with their current state of health.

In terms of Chinese medicine the abnormalities detected at the surface of the cervix usually correspond to Stagnation of Qi or a combination of Stagnant Qi and Blood, according to the stage of diagnosis. Holistic medicine is successful in treating stages 1 and 2 and smears return to normal usually in 3 to 6 months. Later stages can also be treated but it takes longer for the smear to show improvement. Certainly, the more abnormal the stage, the more severe the imbalance in the immune system.

PRE-MENSTRUAL SYNDROME

This is extremely common and affects women at any age during their menstrual life. It means many different things to different people. It has only been in recent years that the conventional medical profession has largely accepted its existence.

Symptoms

There are several symptom pictures and different women may have a different clinical picture. The symptoms tend to get worse before the period for a variable amount of time which in severe cases could be from the onset of ovulation. It is more common about 1 week to 10 days before menstruation.

Emotional symptoms include irritability and depression. In severe cases, there may be personality changes which can include aggressive behaviour. Physical symptoms include breast discomfort, headaches, weight gain, desire for sweet food and lower abdominal discomfort. Lower back pain may also be a feature. Some women gain immediate relief when the period starts. With others, the symptoms gradually diminish over the course of the first 2 days or so of the period.

Treatment

Treatment (mildest to strongest)	Comments
Supplements such as Vitamin B$_6$, evening primrose oil	These may be suppressive in that symptoms return when they are stopped. They may not remedy the underlying energetic imbalance
Diuretics	These remove fluid retention but damage the kidneys if taken regularly
Antidepressants, tranquillisers	These are completely inappropriate since they rapidly lead to addiction, deny the experience of women and maintain the myth that doctors can relieve uncomfortable feelings
Female sex hormones	This acts by suppressing hormonal function and the menstrual cycle. Paradoxically, in some women it may worsen the symptoms for reasons discussed later

Table 18.7: Conventional treatment of pre-menstrual syndrome

Holistic management

In Chinese medicine, this condition is usually associated with Liver Qi Stagnation. There may also be evidence of Spleen Qi Deficiency. It is important to consider two main aspects in dealing with women who have such symptoms.

Firstly, the Stagnation of Liver energy leads to depression, frustration, irritability, breast discomfort, headaches and so forth. One of the main factors that may be involved with this is an irregular life-style not in keeping with natural cycles. There is a 28-day menstrual cycle in health, which is affected by the weather, climate, phases of the moon and so forth. Sadly, in our society, these influences are often dismissed as being non-existent. People tend to live each week in the same way despite changes in their physiology. In the case of pre-menstrual tension, I have found that advising women to pay attention to these cycles can go a long way to relieving the symptoms. It is as if the tension is a resistance to a life-style that may be out of harmony. The same things happen with men but it is not so obvious. Men do not find it so easy to be in touch with their emotions and there is not the clear evidence of menstruation revealing the presence of these physiological cycles.

Secondly, diet is important because of Spleen Qi Deficiency. This is outlined in more detail in Chapter 13 – Gastrointestinal system.

INFERTILITY

Although this term is in common usage it is sometimes labelled sub fertility or impaired fertility which perhaps does not have so many negative associations. It is defined as inability to conceive (or in the case of the man, to induce conception). It is becoming more common in the Western world with around 1 in 8 couples having difficulty conceiving. In the US infertility affects over 7 per cent or 2.8 million couples.

There are many causes – both male and female. It is rare to find solely a male or a female problem. In the majority of cases, around 95 per cent, it is the woman alone who will be investigated and treated conventionally.

Male factors include impotence, premature ejaculation and abnormalities in the number or quality of sperm.[14] Impotence and premature ejaculation are described in Chapter 9 – Urinary system. Abnormal or few sperm are usually considered to be due to congenital factors, mumps, irradiation or poor general health. However, in most cases of abnormal sperm count, no significant cause is determined. There is often an assumption that a normal sperm count is equivalent to normality.

Female factors include lack of ovulation, blocked fallopian tubes, endometrial dysfunction and disease of the vagina or cervix. Most investigations are normal because most women ovulate, have patent fallopian tubes with little or no sign of uterine dysfunction.

Conventional medicine divides cases into primary infertility where there have been no children and secondary where children have been born but there is a difficulty in subsequent conception. In women who have had no children but have had a miscarriage, this is still classed as primary infertility.

Symptoms

Apart from the obvious lack of pregnancy there may be no abnormal signs or symptoms although clearly if there is an associated condition, this will be noted by conventional practitioners. Careful case-taking frequently reveals symptoms such as menstrual irregularities and abnormal menstrual flow, which are difficult to classify conventionally. This is because they do not fall into one or other of the gross disease labels.

Investigations

Investigation of infertility is now quite complex. It involves intricate technology and there are several investigations that may be performed.

In the case of the male, a sperm count and estimation of their normality are done. This may not be done if it is a case of secondary infertility and the woman's partner is the father of her children. This assumes a certain permanence of testicular function and it is always wise to have a recent seminal examination. Certain religious groups, e.g. orthodox Jews, may be prohibited from masturbating to produce a sample of sperm and testing is done by means of a post-coital examination. The remaining investigations are all performed on the woman.

Blood tests on the woman include hormone levels of oestrogen and progesterone as well as thyroid, prolactin and androgen. Ovulation can be checked in several ways. At ovulation there is a slight fall in body temperature and followed by a persistent rise. The basal body temperature (BBT) in the second half of the cycle is 0.5°C higher than that in the first half of the cycle. This simple and effective method is less popular these days and more invasive investigations are usually performed.

Dilatation and curettage in the second half of the menstrual cycle obtains a sample of endometrium. Ovulation must have occurred if it has been affected by progesterone. Endometrial biopsy as an outpatient procedure is available in some centres. Direct ovarian examination by laparoscope around ovulation may reveal the presence of an egg about to be released. Blood levels of progesterone taken in the second half of the cycle will determine the amount of progesterone secreted and are an indication whether ovulation has occurred.

Post-coital tests are performed within a few hours of intercourse to check on the condition of sperm in the vagina. In some situations, sperm die off relatively quickly and cannot make it past the vagina through the cervix. This situation which is often known by the term 'hostile vagina' is relatively uncommon. The mere labelling infers a certain sexual bias as I have never seen the term 'wimpy sperm' used, for example.

Investigations are performed to ensure that the fallopian tubes are not blocked. There are two methods. Dye may be injected through the cervix at the time of laparoscopy to see whether it comes through the abdominal end of the fallopian tubes. Otherwise, hysterosalpingogram is performed which is the injection of radio-opaque dye through the cervix. No anaesthetic is used. Subsequent pelvic X-rays can also reveal the same. Neither of these investigations are infallible since mere spasm of the fallopian tube may prevent the passage of dye. Therefore, the failure of dye to pass does not necessarily mean scarring by pelvic inflammatory disease or another permanent situation. A hysterosalpingogram is clearly much less invasive than a laparoscopy although lower abdominal cramps are common after this procedure. Laparoscopy is described in detail in Chapter 4 – Investigations.

Check for	Investigation	Degree of invasiveness[15]
Ovulation	Temperature chart	1
	Progesterone blood test	1 (more than above)
	Dilatation and curettage	3
	Laparoscopy	3
Sperm function	Sperm count	1
	Post-coital test	1 (more than above)
Fallopian tube blockage	Hysterosalpingogram	2
	Laparoscopy	3

Table 18.8: Investigation of infertility

Question to ask	Comments
Previous pregnancies	Pregnancy is possible. Sperm count, endometrium, fallopian tubes and ovulation satisfactory at least at that time. Check for subsequent changes in health
Previous pelvic surgery,[16] ectopic pregnancy, intra-uterine contraceptive device, pelvic inflammatory disease	Possibility of blocked fallopian tubes

Table 18.9: Important questions to ask in cases of infertility

Treatment

This may be given to women who fail to conceive although in most cases there is little evidence of abnormality. This is one of the reasons why treatment failures are common since it is difficult to treat rationally if the causes are unknown. In 10 per cent of cases there is no discernible abnormality at all.

A specific abnormality such as lack of ovulation or reduced progesterone levels in the second half of the cycle is treated directly. Ovulation can be induced by drugs (including clomiphene, tamoxifen and pituitary hormones) that stimulate the ovary. These are powerful agents that force which force the ovary to produce several eggs at once. One side-effect is multiple pregnancies. All drugs which are used to alter hormonal balances may have powerful psychological effects. Lack of libido is common. Anxiety and depression are almost universal. It is true to say that these are rarely addressed conventionally and are an added factor to deal with.

Progesterone may be given in the second half of the cycle if there is evidence of deficiency. A similar situation may occur here as with dysfunctional uterine bleeding. That is, progesterone may be given even with normal hormone estimations just because it is considered to be 'a good thing'. It is literally believed to be pro-gestation.

Blockage of the fallopian tubes by scar tissue after ectopic pregnancy, pelvic inflammatory disease and so on may be corrected surgically. The success rate is relatively low.

Artificial insemination has been available since the early 1900s and may be done using either the sperm of the sexual partner or a donor. Ovulation stimulants (see below) are frequently given also. This procedure is the exchange of body fluids and I do wonder about the risk of infection. There are also ethical issues in the case of artificial insemination by donor since the child invariably is unaware of their biological father. The success rate in terms of pregnancy is between 5 and 25 per cent. There is no data available on the number of live births from this procedure. The cost of the treatment if using the partner's sperm is $200 to $500 per treatment.

Ovulation stimulants or the so-called fertility drugs are commonly used either alone or as part of other treatments. The two most commonly used are clomiphene (oral) and human menopausal gonadotrophin (injected). Clomiphene works by stimulating the pituitary to produce more follicle-stimulating hormone (FSH) that then stimulates the ovaries to produce eggs. Human menopausal gonadotrophin consists of purified FSH and directly stimulates the ovaries itself. After up to 12 days of injections, the woman is given an injection of human chorionic gonadotrophin (hCG) which tells the ovaries to release the egg(s). Such stimulation of the ovaries is associated with an increased rate of multiple births.

Donor eggs and embryos are used in over 70 per cent of women who seek treatment for infertility. In the US, there are 1200 babies born each year using these methods. Donor eggs from a relative, friend or provided anonymously are used if the woman herself cannot ovulate. Donor embryos from known or anonymous donors are used if her partner's sperm is not available or healthy. The woman undergoing infertility treatment and the woman donating the egg will both be given female sex hormones such as the oral contraceptive so that their cycles are synchronised. The egg donor will also be given ovarian stimulants to prepare the eggs. These are harvested and standard in-vitro fertilisation (see below) is done. There may be legal difficulties with who owns the sperm or eggs but generally the donor signs away any rights they may have to these. Success rates are a 43 per cent chance of getting pregnant and a 36 per cent chance of having a live child. The cost for each treatment cycle is $10,000 to $15,000.

In-vitro fertilisation (IVF) is by far the most common high-tech treatment for infertility. This is bringing the egg and sperm together in a test tube, allowing fertilisation to take place and at some later stage implanting the embryo into the uterus. It accounts for more than 70 per cent of all infertility treatments. The first baby born by such a technique was in 1978 in the UK. There have been 45,000 babies born in the US since its start there in 1981. It involves the stimulation of ovulation since several eggs are removed and fertilised. A number such as two to four, depending upon the clinic, is placed into a fallopian tube. In up to one third of women, more than one embryo implants. Progesterone supplements may be given in an attempt to maintain the pregnancy. Several fertilised eggs may be held in reserve for later insertion. These embryos are frozen awaiting later use.

The overall success rate of in-vitro fertilisation, in terms of how many women leave the programme with a live baby, is variable. Overall, it is in the order of around 22 per cent, with some centres having a lower success rate and some higher. There is an increased risk of foetal abnormality, miscarriage and stillbirth. In-vitro fertilisation is merely the first stage in a whole series of invasive medical techniques throughout pregnancy. Since several embryos are implanted together, multiple pregnancy is a risk. The chance of ectopic pregnancy is increased with IVF and the use of ovarian stimulants in general has been connected to uterine and ovarian cancer. The cost is $10,000 per treatment cycle.

Clearly this whole area raises ethical and moral issues, very few of which are addressed by the medical profession. They are certainly important issues for couples with religious or moral beliefs, particularly Catholics and Buddhists, who believe that life begins at conception. Medical practices such as multiple fertilisation, freezing of embryos, medical experimentation on embryos and selective termination of implanted embryos may be viewed as unacceptable. Some doctors recommend termination if the foetuses will be lost anyway. This is an increasingly important issue in medicine as more people are offered such treatments.

Surrogacy is more common in the US where it hit the headlines in 1985 when a surrogate mother went to court to keep her child. The New Jersey Supreme Court ruled that the surrogacy contract was invalid and she won custody with her partner. Surrogacy is fraught with pitfalls, not all of them legal, and it is illegal in many countries and in some states in the US. Some estimates state that there have been up to 10,000 babies born to surrogate mothers since 1976 but it is difficult if not impossible to quantify. Costs vary widely but arranging surrogacy through a recognised agency may cost around $35,000.

Intracytoplasmic sperm injection was introduced in 1992 and is used to treat male infertility. About 2,000 babies have been born in the US by this method. The woman is given ovarian stimulants to develop several eggs for fertilisation. Sperm is obtained from the man by means of needle aspiration or testicular biopsy. Individual eggs gathered from the woman are injected with individual sperm. Subsequent treatment is the same as with IVF. Success rates are a 24 per cent chance of pregnancy and 23 per cent chance of a live baby. Each treatment cycle costs between $8,000 and $10,000. There are some concerns about this technique as it bypasses the natural processes whereby weak and feeble sperm do not get to fertilise the egg. One study recently showed that children born by such a method develop slower mentally when compared with those born by IVF.

Gamete intra-fallopian transfer (GIFT) is the placing of an egg and sperm into the fallopian tube without prior fertilisation in the hope that getting them together in the same place will aid conception. Otherwise, it is identical to IVF treatment. This is not always any more successful than the normal procedure of attempted conception. A possible practical reason would be if the fallopian tubes are obstructed and the sperm cannot physically make contact with the egg. The cost is $8,000 to $10,000 per treatment cycle.

ZIFT or Zygote intra-fallopian transfer is more invasive and surgery is required to implant the fertilised eggs (zygotes) into the fallopian tubes. Otherwise the techniques used are as with IVF. It is used in less than 2 per cent of infertility treatments. Some 260 babies are born by this method each year in the US. There is a 29 per cent chance of pregnancy and a 28 per cent chance of live birth. The cost is $8,000 to $10,000 per treatment cycle.

Holistic management
In Chinese medicine, infertility is a complex issue. It is not made any easier by the great anxiety surrounding the problem or by the efforts of conventional medicine in attempting to obtain fertilisation. The usual conditions seen in women are Kidney Deficiency, Cold uterus, Blood Deficiency, Liver Qi Stagnation, Stagnant Heat and Phlegm-dampness. Most cases are due to either Kidney Deficiency or Liver Qi Stagnation.

It is important to consider the timing of intercourse, which needs to be adjusted to the optimum moment. Ovulation conventionally always occurs 14 days before the menstrual period but in real life this is not so certain. I have known women who have regular 28-day cycles and consistently ovulate at around 11 days of their cycle. This is seen as being impossible conventionally. I treated a woman who always ovulated at 11 days, some 17 days before her period, but the hospital always insisted on artificial insemination at 14 days.

Constitutional treatment for both partners is the most beneficial course of action although it may be difficult to persuade a couple that the man may also require attention. Normal sperm counts may be taken by the man as indicating that there is no problem to be addressed. Certainly a joint approach is much more helpful since issues around fertility are joint ones.

Psychological factors are very important to bear in mind. I have treated several couples for infertility where the woman had a previous termination or miscarriage and there is clearly still some energetic blockage in the pelvis. Whilst this remains there is little possibility of another conception taking place. These issues need to be resolved perhaps with psychological counselling or support as well as whatever constitutional treatment is undertaken.

CONTRACEPTION

This is the prevention of conception. Although, conventionally, methods such as oral contraception and the intra-uterine contraceptive device are included in this as they mainly act by preventing implantation of the fertilised embryo. It would be more accurate, therefore, to describe them as abortifacients. This has moral implications for those who believe that life begins at conception.

Those methods used are assessed according to a failure rate that is expressed as the number of pregnancies per 100 women using the method for the year. In the case of oral contraception, this is 0.1, the intra-uterine device 2, diaphragm with spermicide 6, condom with spermicide 8 and spermicide foam 24.

Oral contraception has many side-effects although it seems to be one of the most effective ways of preventing pregnancy. It is as if the greater the effect in preventing pregnancy, then the more hazardous it will be to the woman. Although the oral contraceptive in use today is known as the low dose pill, this is relative to the doses used in the 60's and 70's. It does not mean that there are few side effects. I discuss the side-effects of contraception more fully with hormone replacement therapy since these chemicals are the same.

As an aside, I see many people who take a prescribed drug and tell me that they are taking a low dose of a particular chemical. It is important to remember that a low dose is not the same thing as a mild effect. Low doses of some chemicals can be very hazardous.

Oral contraception is either by means of a combined pill (oestrogen and progesterone) or the so-called mini pill (progesterone only). The use of the oral contraceptive is an attempt to prevent ovulation. The administration of female sex hormones will interfere with the negative feedback mechanism mentioned in Chapter 15 – Endocrine system. Ovarian function is suppressed and so ovulation does not occur. However, with oral contraceptives of recent years where dosages are much lower and certainly with the progesterone-only pill, ovulation does still occur in some cases. It may be that pregnancy is prevented not merely by the suppression of ovulation but more usually by the prevention of implantation of the fertilised ovum. In the latter situation, oral contraception is as likely to be a method of termination as a method of contraception. It is difficult to know how many women still ovulate whilst using the oral contraceptive. It is almost certainly more common than generally realised.

The intra-uterine contraceptive device (the 'coil') is a metallic or plastic device placed inside the uterine cavity. It acts as an irritant and prevents implantation of the fertilised embryo. Common complications include heavy periods, infection leading to pelvic inflammatory disease and ectopic pregnancy. It is more commonly used in women who have already had children. Sterilisation is a permanent method of preventing pregnancy by surgical means. Few can be reversed although this may be attempted. In women, this means an abdominal operation under general anaesthesia of tying of the fallopian tubes (also known as tubal ligation). This necessitates a short stay in hospital and is clearly more invasive than any equivalent operation on the male. There is an association with heavy periods after this operation although this connection is rarely seen in conventional textbooks. A significant number of women will then go on to have treatment for heavy periods and some may require hysterectomy.

Vasectomy in men is tying of the sperm ducts. Psychological difficulties may manifest as loss of libido or impotence. There seems to be an association with an increased risk of other health problems.[17] Certainly in terms of Chinese medicine, the operation will lead to Stagnation of Liver Qi, which can lead to tumours.

Barrier methods of contraception are relatively common since they carry fewer moral objections. The methods available are vaginal diaphragm (the 'cap'), condom and spermicidal foam. Local allergic reactions can occur. Barrier methods can be messy and certainly not as effective as oral contraception. However, with correct use I feel that the success rates are far higher than those in the conventional data quoted above.

The rhythm method and related methods[18] use information about natural cycles. They work best for those women who have regular menstrual cycles but can be used by anyone and there are teachers who will instruct couples in their correct application. They are of varying efficiency and clearly depend upon co-operation between the couple and abstinence from intercourse around ovulation.

Retention of semen by various practices is a useful method to consider. It is cheap, has no side effects and is 100 per cent effective. It has to be taught by a qualified teacher and belongs to the tradition that includes Qi Gong (Chi Kung) and other Qi exercises.[19]

BREAST DISEASE

Disorders of the female breast are common. Any woman who has lumps or discomfort in the breast is also worried about the risk of breast cancer. With anatomy and physiology, you should certainly know the normal lymphatic drainage of the breast. I would remind you that the lateral part of the breast drains to the axilla whilst the medial side drains internally. Therefore, enlarged lymph glands in the axilla may be due to lumps in the lateral half of the breast. This area of the lymphatic system also drains the pectoral region of the upper abdominal area and the upper back.

Lump in the breast

This is a common condition and 95 per cent of cases will either be cancer (see Chapter 6 – Cancer) or a benign tumour such as fibroadenoma or chronic mastitis. Lumps (tumours) may be either benign or malignant. It is difficult in the early stages to determine, definitively, whether a lump is cancerous or not. This leads to anxiety for doctors and for women. Emphasis is placed on detecting the presence of lumps that are malignant. This leads to screening programmes such as routine mammography. The consequence, for an individual woman, can be traumatic and stressful. This, in itself, can generate disease.

The type of tumour a person has, the degree of its abnormality (and malignancy), its rate of growth and its propensity to spread are all a direct result of the condition of the person's immune system. They are not dependent upon time. The emphasis for any system of medicine that is curative, therefore, must be on the immune system rather than the precise presenting symptom.

Sadly, conventional medicine is obsessed by lumps and their histological type. It directs its energies at removing the lump itself without addressing its cause. This approach has the effect of further magnifying any anxiety. It depersonalises people's symptoms, denies inner processes and necessarily produces brutal and brutalising treatments to remove symptoms *at any price*.

In practical terms, it is possible to gain some idea about whether a lump is serious or not. Most lumps in the breast are found by self-examination or by accident. Ask questions about its size, shape, mobility, regularity and whether it is painful. Malignant lumps tend to be hard, irregular, fixed and non-tender but in the early stages are indistinguishable from benign ones. If the lump changes with the menstrual cycle, it is more likely to be benign. If it remains the same throughout the month, this increases the likelihood of malignancy.

A mammogram may give a little more information about the nature of the lump but there are several reasons to be careful about mammography and its interpretation.

All women with a breast lump have to make a decision about their course of action. There are many possibilities and some of them are covered later when I detail some case histories. Conventionally, lumps in the breast, and certainly cancer, are treated as surgical emergencies. In my opinion, women can gather information over some weeks and months whilst formulating their decision. It is wise not to make decisions in a state of shock. A time of appraisal may be helpful and allows some calming of the situation. In my experience, this panic and urgency is a reflection of the fear which *doctors* experience rather than the fear which women experience. It is not usually beneficial to decide upon a course of treatment because of the emotional state of the practitioner.

Cancer of the breast

This is common, leading to 10,000 deaths per year in England and Wales. It is rare in men and unusual before the age of 30 years. There seems to be a rapidly increasing incidence of breast cancer and this may be related to the widespread use over the past 30 years or so of female sexual hormones. The cancer may involve the skin where it can cause dimpling and tethering. It spreads by the lymph system to glands in the axilla and by blood to the lung, liver and bone, as well as skin.

Cancer in older women in the US is 40 per cent more common than in the UK and this may reflect different rates of hormone replacement treatment (HRT). In the US, about half of women take HRT whilst it is around 1 in 20 in the UK. Breast cancer in England and Wales increased by 36.8 per cent in the years 1962-84. There was a sharp increase in the 25-54 year olds. There was an increase of some 35-45 per cent in the 1970s. It is clear from several sources, that the use of female sex hormones directly increases the risk of breast cancer – see discussion on Page 370.

In the US today a woman is twice as likely to develop breast cancer than she was in 1940. Breast cancer is the most common cancer in women living in the US, causing about 44,300 deaths in 1990.

According to conventional medicine, only 30 per cent of breast cancer cases are linked to identifiable causes and most of these have to do with diet or constitutional factors. There have been two recent studies, one from Israel and the other from Vermont, suggesting that women with breast cancer may have been exposed to more toxic chemicals than cancer-free controls. A common toxic chemical, of course, is the use of prescribed female sex hormones.

Symptoms

There may only be a lump found, usually on bathing or self examination. There may be prickling sensations or occasionally breast pain which may pre-date the appearance of a lump.

Depending upon the extent of growth of the cancer there may be nipple retraction of recent history, fixation to overlying skin or fixation to an underlying muscle. As stated in Chapter 6 – Cancer, these types of lumps tend to be hard, fixed and irregular in nature. It is important to acknowledge that the early detection of a lump may find it at a stage where this has not yet occurred. Discharge from the nipple of blood-strained appearance may indicate cancer.

Investigations

It is usually diagnosed by a combination of clinical examination and mammography and aspiration or biopsy. Mammography is an X-ray of the breast. It is uncomfortable and requires exposure to significant amounts of radiation. This is an issue particularly for those women who have repeated examinations and screening.

It is interesting to note the historical development of mammography services.[20] In 1973 the National Cancer Institute in the US and the American Cancer Society began a national screening programme. There was no evidence of benefit to screening women under the age of 50. Despite this all women aged over 35 years were encouraged to take part.

In 1973, John C. Bailar, III, M.D., then deputy associate director for cancer control in the National Cancer Institute, expressed concern that the inclusion of women under the age of 50 in the screening project could cause more cancers than were being detected. His concern was based on several factors. The breast has a known sensitivity to radiation's cancer-causing effect. There is a relatively high radiation dose used. The effect of radiation damage is cumulative. Mammography has a known inaccuracy in finding cancer in the denser breast tissue of younger women. The *Annals of Internal Medicine* in 1976 published Dr. Bailar's analysis showing more risks than benefit to screening young women.

In 1977 the Health Research Group made a Freedom of Information Act request for the inspection reports from the 27 cancer centres participating in the screening project. Sixteen of the mammography machines were found to be exposing women to unacceptable levels of radiation.

In the same year there were reports in the US of 48 women whose tumours were mistakenly diagnosed as cancer as a result of the screening project. The cell types were re-examined, read by an independent panel of pathologists which deemed them 'not classified as cancer.' Sadly, 30 of these women have already had a mastectomy.

In 1991 the National Cancer Institute issued a press release showing the breast cancer rate has risen steadily over the years. They stated that the rise was consistent with the increasing use of mammography. It was noted at the same time that the incidence of cancer-in-situ[21] has increased three times in the last 10 years. Many conventional medical practitioners are doubtful that cancer-in-situ is true cancer but women are still treated with mastectomy.

Also in 1991, a US General Accounting Office report found *no* progress in reducing the rate of breast cancer deaths since the 'war on cancer' was begun some 20 years earlier. Despite this, women are continually told of the various percentage rates of success they can expect from mammography, surgery, chemotherapy and radiotherapy.[22] Conventional statistics are presented as a competition with the prizes only available to those who have conventional treatment.

The use of mammography is definitely helpful for women who have a breast lump. It can provide information about the likely pathological process, but is not infallible. It should be used as one of several methods of assessment. It is, however, less invasive than biopsy or needle aspiration. Of course, any damage to the lump may lead to an increased risk of spread. There is also the issue of traumatic and stressful investigations and their effect on the immune system. These are all things to be taken into account before deciding upon a course of action.

Mammography screening, particularly in those under the age of 50 years is not only wasteful[23] it is positively harmful. Only 15 per cent of breast cancers arise in those under the age of 50 years. The widespread use of screening exposes these women to three times the number of biopsies[24] and investigations as older women.[25]

Dr Shapiro of Johns Hopkins University, said on May 5, 1992 that he had reviewed data from a controversial large Canadian study about to be published. This found that women in their 40's who had annual mammograms were *more* likely to die of breast cancer than those who had only physical examination.

The Canadian researchers speculated that the squeezing of the breast in the mammography machine might force cancer cells from tiny tumours into the blood stream, speeding their spread. This is also the danger with biopsy of breast lumps. The traumatic injury to the breast may lead to increased risk of spread.[26]

There are hazards from the use of radiation with one cancer caused per 25,000 mammograms. The difficulty is, of course, that no individual woman can possibly foretell if she is going to be the susceptible one.

A mammography examination of both breasts exposes a woman to a dose of radiation 20 to 25 times greater than that of a typical chest X-ray. The American Cancer Society guidelines recommend a mammogram at age 35, followed by others once or twice each year between the ages of 40 to 50, and a yearly examination after age 50. If these guidelines were followed, a woman would be absorbing significant doses of radiation. The breast is considered to be extremely sensitive to the effect of radiation. Before a mammogram, a 35-year-old woman has a statistical risk of 1 in 4999 of developing breast cancer. After mammography it increases to 1 in 660.[27]

An international workshop in February 1993 indicated that for every 1000 women under 50 years of age screened with mammography, 700 would require some sort of diagnostic procedure to detect fewer than 15 tumours. Seven tumours would be missed completely.

Before a cancer is detectable by a mammogram, it has been present and growing in the breast for 8 to 10 years. Statistics show that up to one in four breast lumps may not even be detected on the X-ray film. Misdiagnosis of lumps may also occur, with an average of one in three benign conditions identified as malignant.[28]

Current imaging technology may also not be the best method for young women because of the density of their breast tissue. It is a relatively new technique with the difficulties associated with interpreting any new method. The American Board of Radiology has included questions on mammography in the past three examinations only. In 1993, the US Congress passed the National Mammography Standards Quality Assurance Act following reports that over half of clinics and operators failed to meet minimal quality assurance standards. Another serious flaw in the use of mammography is the lack of proper training for those administering the tests. Only 20 States require that an X-ray operator be certified by the American Registry of Radiological Technologists, through a two year training program.[29]

In many southern states of the US, less than a third of radiology centres complies with the American College of Radiology guidelines for safety and effectiveness. An assessment of screening films in one practice found that false images[30] accounted for more than half of cases recommended for biopsy.[31]

It has been said about the mammography debate, '...if our society had been oriented towards finding out whether new technology is efficacious as soon as possible after its introduction there would not be much left to debate more than 30 years later....'[32]

The investigations carried out on a woman with a breast lump are shown in Table 18.10.

Investigation	Degree of invasiveness
Clinical examination	1
Mammography	2
Aspiration	2
Biopsy	3 (general anaesthesia)

Table 18.10: Investigation of breast lumps

Treatment[33-35]

The majority of cases of breast cancer are treated by surgery. The lump is removed at more progressive centres using the most recent conventional treatments or by mastectomy (removal of the breast) in other centres or if the disease is more widespread. The mastectomy performed nowadays is usually a simple mastectomy where merely the breast and axillary lymphatic glands are removed. In previous years, operations such as a radical mastectomy and super-radical mastectomy were used which remove underlying muscle and even part of the rib. There has never been any difference in outcome between any of the surgical procedures so now conventional surgeons tend to take a more conservative approach.[36] Even in lumpectomy, some axillary lymph glands will be removed for examination. If cancer has spread to any of these, clearance of lymph glands from the axilla will be performed. This commonly leads to severe oedema of the arm.

Fortunately, the practice of frozen sections is becoming less favoured by surgeons. This is the situation where a woman goes to the operating theatre and the lump or part of it is removed. A 'frozen section' of this is sent for examination. If the result shows cancer, the surgeon would remove the breast and whatever lymph glands they considered necessary. The woman, therefore, would not know whether she would wake up from the anaesthetic with her breast removed.

Following surgery radiotherapy and/or chemotherapy is offered routinely. Most women are advised to have these in sequence. The side-effects of both can be extreme but particularly with chemotherapy.[37-38]

The standard conventional belief is that chemotherapy and radiotherapy improve survival rates. There is conflicting evidence for this[39-41] although women themselves will only be told one side of the story.[42] One clinical trial published in 1976 showed that combination chemotherapy benefited women with pre-menopausal breast cancer and evidence of spread to lymph nodes in the axilla. The findings drew rapid acceptance and, by the end of 1976, the percentage of women receiving chemotherapy for this type of breast cancer had almost doubled. Usage continued to increase steadily until 1982. By then, the survival rate should have reflected the benefit shown in the clinical trial but, in fact, no improvement was found. This was determined in a report by the US General Accounting Office.

Such treatment would be expected to increase death rates as they severely damage the immune system. There is some evidence to suggest that this is true.[43]

It is common for women to be given tamoxifen, which blocks the effect of oestrogen. Tamoxifen was originally developed as a contraceptive but found to be unsatisfactory. The rationale of such treatment is that as the breast is under the influence of oestrogen the cancer may also be stimulated by oestrogen. Tamoxifen interferes with the effects of oestrogen and so the cancer will not be stimulated.

It is a very powerful drug although there has been no long-term follow-up to check for side-effects.[44] It is known to produce symptoms of tiredness, heat in the body, flushing and restless legs. It may also cause damage to the eyes,[45] hepatitis[46] and pre-cancerous conditions of the uterus.[47-48]

In terms of holistic medicine, it should be viewed as similar to chemotherapy as it has a heating effect in burning the Blood. More recently it has been suggested that it can be given to healthy women in an attempt to prevent the development of breast cancer.

Holistic management

There are several categories of Chinese medical syndrome seen in connection with breast disease manifesting as lumps. The immediate cause of the symptoms is Liver Qi Stagnation. This is very much related to emotional states and is common in the West. This may be particularly true around the menopause when women may have difficulties with feeling unappreciated. Society tends to undervalue women unless they are of child-bearing years. The conflicting emotions that can occur during this transitional phase in life may lead to such conditions. The underlying diagnosis may be Spleen Deficiency, Kidney Deficiency, Blood Deficiency, Liver Qi Stagnation affecting the Chong and Ren channels and Fire Flaring.

Chapter 6 outlines the multiple approaches to take with a specific treatment, counselling,[49] dietary therapy and meditation or visualisation. I describe cases below to illustrate this approach.

Case one

A woman of 28 years came for treatment. She had developed a breast lump after administration of a homoeopathic remedy. This had also brought into consciousness traumatic emotional events from her childhood. The lump was over 4 cm in diameter and rubbery in consistency. This could, conceivably, have been cancer but she knew that she did not want conventional diagnosis or treatment. We discussed her options and she decided to treat the lump as if it were cancer. In this way there would be no harmful, invasive investigations or depleting treatments. Over the course of several months when she had some further homoeopathic treatment, the lump disappeared. She has remained well and continues in her efforts to resolve remaining psychological issues.

Case two

A woman of 80 years came for treatment. She had been diagnosed as having a malignant breast lump after biopsy some 4 weeks previously. She was taking tamoxifen regularly. She was having follow-ups at the hospital, where they had suggested that she might need further surgery to remove the lump entirely.

She had few other symptoms and her general health was good. In the elderly, breast lumps are typically slow growing and can persist for years with little or no progression. I treated her with acupuncture and herbs after making a diagnosis of Yin Deficiency with Phlegm Stagnation.

She felt generally better after some months of treatment and the lump reduced in size. Each visit to hospital would be accompanied by renewed comments about the risk of the lump enlarging, spreading or ulcerating. She had declined further surgery. She has a strong spirit and she continues to take herbs and has a long-standing Buddhist meditation practice.

Some 2 years later, she was well, her lump unchanged in size or shape and she was able to make a long distance trip to see relatives and friends. Her quality of life was good and she was happy.

Case three

A woman of 33 years had a lump in the breast removed that was diagnosed as cancer. She had some glands removed from her axilla that revealed two to be involved. She decided to undergo the full course of radiotherapy and chemotherapy but declined intravenous chemotherapy at the time of the operation.

She was concerned about possible conflict between holistic medicine and conventional treatment. Some people decide to have both treatments and it is important to support them so that any adverse effects are minimised. She started herbal treatment before the radiotherapy and chemotherapy so that she was as strong as possible. Her diagnosis in terms of Chinese medicine was Blood Deficiency.

She did surprising well with few side-effects of toxicity. The main problem was with generalised aches and pains in the muscles and lymphatic glands. This arose as her Blood became weakened by the effects of the conventional treatment.

She also received healing each week and practised visualisation. She had regular psychotherapy as the cancer had developed about 18 months after emotional traumas. She recognised the relationship between these and her illness and the fact they reflected certain underlying psychological patterns.

She continues to have 'maintenance' treatments each month or so and is generally healthy about 2 years after the initial diagnosis.

Chronic mastitis

This is equivalent to fibroadenosis and the cause is not known in conventional medicine.

Symptoms

There is a discrete lump (fibroadenoma) or general lumpiness in the breast with discomfort, which is worse pre-menstrually. There may be a discharge from the nipple. It is important to check the axillary area for lymphatic gland enlargement since the differential diagnosis is with cancer. Some enlargement is common which tends to vary with the menstrual cycle. Conventional treatment is either to excise the specific lump or to merely observe the patient.

Holistic Management

In terms of Chinese medicine this condition is very much associated with Liver Qi Stagnation.

Discharge from the nipple

There are a variety of possible discharges from the nipple. Bloody discharge means either cancer or chronic mastitis. Watery discharge is seen in early pregnancy and a yellowish or greenish discharge is due to chronic mastitis. Milky discharge is known as galactorrhoea and occurs in lactation and is a side-effect of some drugs.

Chinese medicine sees it as being due to Spleen and Stomach Qi Deficiency or Liver Fire.

Pain in the breast

This is common and may be due to several conditions. It is usually benign in nature but may herald the development of breast cancer in the future. In conventional medicine, there may be breast abscess, mastitis or cancer. Occasionally musculoskeletal disorders affecting the chest wall may be confused with pain in the breast.

USE OF FEMALE SEX HORMONES

Oestrogen and progesterone, the female sex hormones, are produced by the ovary. They have been utilised by conventional medicine for many years. They suppress the function of the ovary and may be used to prevent pregnancy. Since they consequently suppress menstruation, they are used in the treatment of a wide range of menstrual disorders such as dysmenorrhoea, heavy menstruation, irregular menstruation and even amenorrhoea. They are commonly said to 'regulate the periods'. This is clearly not the case since they prevent true menstruation.[50] Bleeding only occurs due to the withdrawal of the artificial hormone for 7 days each month. The term 'withdrawal bleeding' is therefore a more accurate one.

They may also be used to increase oestrogen levels around the time of the menopause when they are normally falling. This is an attempt to alleviate symptoms sometimes associated with the menopausal period as well as preventing or delaying the onset of osteoporosis.[51-52] Osteoporosis is a thinning and weakening of bone, which may lead to fractures after relatively minor injuries. It is more common after the menopause and it is thought to be partly due to a reduction in circulating oestrogen.

As I discussed in the Introduction to this Chapter, the male-oriented medical profession tends to see women as inherently imperfect. The menopause is considered to be an illustration of this. I have heard gynaecologists express the view that the female menopause is 'a design fault of God'. The use of female sex hormones at this time is, by implication, the rectifying of this mistake by those who wish to assume 'his' mantle.

The menopause is not a disease state. Nor is any normal physiological stage of life be it birth, puberty, pregnancy or even death. They do not, therefore, have to be prevented through 'treatment', or medicalisation.

In this discussion, I shall concentrate on the use of oestrogen and progesterone for contraception and hormone replacement treatment. In terms of Chinese medicine, the time of the menopause is when Blood and Yin Deficiency with Empty Heat symptoms may develop. These lead to hot flushes, sweating, emotional imbalances, palpitations and the like. The treatment principle is to nourish the Yin and root the Empty Heat. The use of female sex hormones at this time may change the symptoms but that does not mean such drugs are nourishing.

The energetic qualities of these drugs may be deduced from the energetic changes which occur during pregnancy. These were described in Chapter 17 – Pregnancy and Childbirth. Essentially, the female sex hormones are Yin in nature. They are Cold, therefore. They have the effect of increasing Yin although I do not think this a tonifying effect. They draw on reserves of Jing from the Kidney to increase Yin and Blood to other organs, particularly the Heart and Liver. This results in cooling of the heat symptoms sometimes associated with the menopause and reducing the degree of anxiety.

The problem with increasing Yin but making no attempt made to support the Yang is that Stagnation is likely. This is why side effects of such drugs lead to thrombosis,[53] migraine headaches, high blood pressure, breast cancer,[54-66] uterine cancer,[67] increase in weight and so on.[68] The extra Yin can swamp the Yang and lead to serious consequences. These will be more severe in those women who are already Yang Deficient. Yin Deficient women will feel better in the short-term but as the drugs draw upon reserves of Yin within the Kidney, the long-term effects can only be harmful. It is an almost invariable finding that women who take female sex hormones have a deep and thready Kidney Yin pulse.

The flooding of the Heart with Yin may lead to heart attack. On an emotional level it may lead to the alleviation of anxiety or the development of depression. On a mental level, it tends to produce a state of euphoria. This may be extreme and lead to psychotic features. 'Steroid psychosis' is a well-recognised complication of all the drugs whose basic make-up is the steroid molecule.[69] More commonly, a general perception of well-being exists where the woman believes she is extremely well. This is particularly hazardous as there is a lack of awareness as to the damaging qualities of these drugs.

There are also other effects as the Yang is depleted. The main one is on the Spleen. Weight gain, oedema and desire for sweet foods are common as the digestive energy is damaged by the Cold nature of the female sex hormones.

The use of such drugs for contraception is to suppress ovarian function and thereby ovulation. There is some evidence to suggest that ovulation may still occur in some women. Pregnancy may be avoided because the drugs prevent implantation. This would suggest that oral contraceptives might act as abortifacients rather than contraceptives.

Interestingly, mung bean powder is used in China as contraception. It is effective because it is Cold in nature and has an affinity for the Kidneys and lower parts of the body. It produces a Cold Uterus so that conception is impossible. It would seem that the oral contraceptive works in a similar way. Essentially, it produces a state of infertility. This 'freezing' may continue for some time after the oral contraceptive is stopped so that amenorrhoea and infertility are well-known after effects of taking 'the pill'.

There are conventionally several contraindications to the use of female sex hormones. These are:

- liver disease
- severe heart or kidney disease
- history of thrombosis
- tumours of the uterus or breast
- undiagnosed abnormal vaginal bleeding
- otosclerosis.[70]

In my opinion, no woman should be given female sex hormones without at least several checks being made. I would consider the minimum to be:

- no contraindications to their use
- annual checks must be made. These will include vaginal examination, blood pressure and breast examination
- pre-selection for the prevention of osteoporosis. Only about 25 per cent of women will develop problems. These tend to be those who smoke, are thin and slightly-built
- a full discussion of side-effects to take place before the consideration of treatment
- oestrogens must never be prescribed without progesterone because of the greatly increased risk of cancer of the uterus. Hysterectomy obviously removes this requirement.

What can we do as holistic practitioners? We have an important role to play in education as many women are simply not aware of the problems posed by such drugs. The prevalence of well-women clinics with mammography, cervical smears and advice about the menopause and contraception are too often connected with sponsorship by pharmaceutical companies who manufacture female sex hormones. A neutral source of information is of benefit to women who are interested in taking control of their health.

Holistic medicine has an important message for women at many stages of their lives. It provides the philosophical basis and effective tools with which to regain health and maintain vitality. With access to these tools, women can make a proper, well-informed choice as to whether they need to take prescribed chemicals.[71]

HOW TO RECOGNISE A SERIOUS CONDITION IN GYNAECOLOGY

Gynaecological symptoms are common in our society and the symptoms listed below are extremely frequent. It is important to know how to recognise if a symptom arises from a serious situation. You can use Table 18.11 as a guide to refer to when faced with a person who has one or more of these symptoms. I do not mention disease labels in the column on the right as I would not expect you to be able to diagnose conventionally. Seriousness can be assessed merely by reference to symptom pictures. However, you will be able to recognise that there are clinical appearances that would be diagnosed as a particular disease. For example, if you look at vaginal bleeding and its seriousness, you will see that these are the appearances of diseases such as cancer of the uterus.

Symptoms	Cause for concern
Post-menopausal bleeding	Always – unless taking HRT
Pre-pubertal bleeding	Always – consider sexual abuse
Inter-menstrual bleeding	Persistent particularly around the menopause
Post-coital bleeding[72]	Persistent
Heavy periods	Persistent, with pallor, tiredness

Table 18.11: How to recognise serious conditions in gynaecology

SUMMARY

Gynaecological symptoms are common in Western society.

The medical treatment of women cannot be separated from the society in which it takes place.

Conventional treatment frequently exacerbates any imbalances.

As a holistic practitioner, you need to be aware of the original imbalance and any overlying mental, emotional or physical problems caused by conventional investigations and treatment.

The holistic medical treatment of gynaecological disorders is extremely effective.

Effective healing can only occur when the woman concerned can harmonise her inner energies. This is not dependent upon changes in the outer world but can be attained through inner processes.

---

[1] There are numerous books dealing with these issues. I mention *Changing of the Gods* by Naomi Goldenberg (Beacon Press, 1979), *Goddesses in Every Woman* by Jean Shinoda Bolen (Harper and Row, 1985), *The Paradise Papers* by Merlin Stone (Virago, 1976) and *The Whole Woman* by Germaine Greer (Anchor, 2000).

[2] The Chong channel. See discussion in *The Path of Pregnancy* by Bob Flaws (Blue Poppy Press, 1982) on Page 12.

[3] *Essentials of Chinese Acupuncture* compiled by Colleges of Traditional Chinese Medicine in People's Republic of China (Beijing, Foreign Languages Press; 1980).

[4] Inflammation of the vagina and endometrium may occur at or after the menopause due to the reduction in oestrogen secretion.

[5] This is twisting of a cyst on its stalk.

[6] This may be the genesis of toxic shock syndrome. This is an unusual occurrence of high fever and the development of shock which may be fatal. It has been related to the use of tampons. In terms of Chinese medicine, stagnation of the flow of Qi or Blood may lead to the generation of heat manifesting as fever.

[7] There are many sources of information about natural birth control and the use of barrier methods of contraception. All are much safer for the women's health. For example, see *Natural Birth Control* by Katia and Jonathan Drake (Thorson's, 1984).

[8] Menorrhagia is heavy periods. Metrorrhagia is uterine bleeding but not at menstruation. Epimenorrhoea is a shortened menstrual cycle.

[9] *New Scientist,* 7 November 1992.

[10] A negative test does not, of course, mean that pregnancy does not exist.

[11] *Concise Medical Dictionary* (OUP, 1998).

[12] In Chinese medical thought this is considered to be before the energies are mature at around the age of 18 years.

[13] This is pronounced 'sin' which reflects Western philosophical views of the origin of women and their symptoms.

[14] The sperm count that is considered to be normal has fallen over the past 40 years. Formerly it was 60 million per ml and now is 20 million.

[15] These criteria are discussed in Chapter 4 – Investigations.

16 Pelvic surgery is any surgery to the lower abdomen and pelvis. It would include appendicectomy.

17 There is an increased risk of prostate cancer. Giovannucci E, *et al. JAMA* 1993;269:873-877 and Giovannucci E, *et al. JAMA* 1993;269:878-882.

Letters to the Journal later revealed the way in which conventional practitioners dismiss data they do not agree with. 'Concern about recent studies linking vasectomy and prostate cancer has been tempered by the absence of any clear biologic rationale for the association'. Daniel W. Cramer, MD, ScD, Brigham and Women's Hospital, Boston, Mass. USA.

18 *Natural Birth Control* by Katia and Jonathan Drake (Thorson's, 1984).

19 *Taoist Secrets of Love – Cultivating Male Sexual Energy* by Mantak Chia (Aurora, 1984)

20 *HealthFacts* 1992;17(157):5(1).

21 There are various stages of cancer that are dependent upon its 'aggressiveness'. Cancer-in-situ is a type that remains in its site and does not spread. This indicates that the immune system is relatively strong and can maintain the cancer in that local area.

22 At a news conference a group of scientists and physicians released a statement condemning the US National Cancer Institute (NCI) for ignoring or trivialising evidence of how carcinogens in air, food, water and workplaces are major factors in the cancer epidemic in America.

In addition, Dr Samuel Epstein, professor at the University of Illinois School of Public Health, presented data indicating significant cancer risks in mammograms and their lack of effectiveness for pre-menopausal women. He also accused the American College of Radiology (ACR) with misrepresenting data on mammography risks. *Cancer Weekly,* Feb 17, 1992:2(4).

23 'Women under 50 years of age may not benefit from mammographic screening for breast cancer, despite screening recommendations'. Davis, Devra Lee; Love, Susan M. *JAMA* 1994;271(2):152(2).

24 Ninety per cent of biopsies are not malignant and these women are subjected to the stress and worry of invasive investigations.

25 *The Journal of the American Medical Association,* 1994;271(2):152(2)

26 *Special Delivery* 1992;15(3):12(1).

27 *Special Delivery* 1993;16(3):11(1).

28 *Special Delivery* 1993;16(3):11(1).

29 *Special Delivery* 1993;16(3):11(1).

30 These are known in medical parlance as 'imaginomas'.

31 Gillian Newstead, MD, director of Breast Imaging, New York University Medical Center, August 6, 1993.

32 Chalmers TC. 'Mammography after 30 years'. Online *J Curr Clin Trials.* May 28, 1993.

33 Although annual mammograms improve the chances that breast cancer will be detected, early detection and treatment do not decrease the mortality rate for women under 50 years old. The Canadian National Breast Screening Study tested 90,000 Canadian women, ages 40 to 59. The major finding of the first 7 years of the study is that no reduction in mortality in the 40-49 age group can be attributed to mammography screening. "There is no evidence, either from this study or other studies, that mammograms save lives in women under the age of 50," said study chief Dr Anthony Miller, chairman of the Department of Preventive Medicine at the University of Toronto.

More women from the mammogram group died of cancer after seven years. *Cancer Weekly,* Nov 23, 1992:2(2).

34 The National Cancer Institute in the US has spent more than $1 billion on breast cancer alone over the past two decades. According to their figures, 26.9 women out of every 100,000 died of breast cancer in 1973; by 1988, the number had grown to 27.5 per 100,000, and the trend seems to be heading upwards.

The National Cancer Institute has spent $22 billion in the past two decades with remarkably few results. Overall death rates from many common cancers remain stubbornly unchanged – or even higher than before the NCI much-advertised 'war on cancer'. Only a few years ago, NCI leaders were setting optimistic goals, such as aiming to reduce the cancer death rate within the next decade by 50 per cent. Any targets have now been dropped from NCI literature. Marshall, E. *Science* 1991;254(5039):1719(2).

35 The number of women diagnosed with breast cancer has risen steadily, and the death rate has remained virtually unchanged. A 15 year review of cases of breast cancer have revealed there is no benefit from early diagnosis or changing conventional treatment.

There were was a peak of breast cancers diagnosed in the US in 1974. This was the year when the wives of the President of the US and his vice-president were both diagnosed. A large number of these were followed-up for 15 years but show no decline in the breast cancer death rate in the US. *HealthFacts* 1991;16(148):3(2).

36 In the last 40 years, there has been only slight improvement in breast cancer survival rates, according to a 1987 GAO report. At a 1980 cancer conference, George Crile, Jr., M.D., of the Cleveland Clinic, was asked to name the advances in breast cancer treatment. "The major advances in the treatment of breast cancer have actually been retreats," he responded. Physicians are performing less aggressive surgical treatments and finding the survival rates unaltered or sometimes improved. *HealthFacts* 1990;15(131):1(2).

37 Many patients receiving cancer chemotherapy develop infections and/or ulcerations of the mouth. The combination of mouth ulceration and infection is not only distressing for the patient but can also be life-threatening. G.M. McCarthy, *et al Cancer Weekly,* April 22,1991:5(2).

[38] There is an increased frequency of second tumours, mainly leukaemias, in women treated with chemotherapy. Rosner F, et al – *Am F Hematol* 1978;4:151-72, Geller RB, *et al* – *Cancer* 1989;64:629-34 and Kaldor J *Acta Oncol* 1990;29:647-55. It may also lead to an increased frequency of cancer of the oesophagus. *Cancer Weekly* 1991:4(1).

[39] 'The relative efficacies of cytotoxic chemotherapy regimens in the treatment of advanced breast cancer are generally assessed by comparing response rates achieved in randomised trials. Treatment ideally prolongs survival as well as achieving successful palliation. Trials rarely demonstrate a statistically significant survival advantage'. Ebbs, S.R. *et al, NCI Cancer Weekly,* 1989:16(1).

[40] A conference of cancer specialists in the US in 1990 failed to show that chemotherapy gives any benefit to women with breast cancer. *HealthFacts* 1990;15(135):6(1).

They agreed that for most women the lumpectomy plus radiation therapy is preferable to mastectomy for early-stage cancer because it preserves the breast without jeopardising a woman's chances of survival.

[41] Until 1988, either mastectomy or lumpectomy and radiation constituted the complete treatment for women with cancer confined to the breast. Despite such treatment about 30 percent of all such women will suffer a recurrence and die of their disease. The prescription of chemotherapy or hormone drugs for these women would mean that the vast majority will endure side effects without benefit.

For the past 15 years, postoperative chemotherapy has been used to treat pre-menopausal women with cancer that has spread to the lymph nodes by the time of diagnosis and treatment. There has never been a subsequent study performed, which makes the basic assumption questionable. A review of five studies was conducted. There is now evidence that challenges the original conclusion that pre-menopausal women with affected lymph nodes should undergo chemotherapy. The authors suggest that the recommendation of chemotherapy as the standard treatment for these women should be seriously reconsidered and most probably be withdrawn. Mueller, C. et al – *Annals of Surgery* 1991;214(3):206(7).

[42] Virtually all women with breast cancer will at least have some discussion with their physicians regarding the wisdom of taking chemotherapy or the anti-oestrogen drug tamoxifen. Many have received inappropriate recommendations to undergo chemotherapy. See 'Women and Cancer Conference' *Health Facts,* December 1985.

[43] Although postoperative radiotherapy is widely used to reduce the rate of local recurrence after treatment for early breast cancer, no significant increase in rates of survival have been shown in those who undergo the procedure.

An overview (Cuzick *et al., Cancer Treatment Report,* 1987;71:15-29) of 10 randomised trials studying surgery with radiotherapy versus surgery alone showed radiotherapy had no significant effect on survival up to 10 years after treatment. There was, however, a significantly increased mortality amongst those who had received radiotherapy by the time of 10 years after treatment. A total of 1,376 of the women had simple mastectomies followed by post-operative radiotherapy. Another 1,424 had simple mastectomies with no post-surgical irradiation. The authors confirmed the Cuzick et al. finding that mortality increased slightly in the irradiated patients roughly a decade after treatment. They found that this was due to an excess of deaths from causes other than breast cancer. The most frequent cause of excess mortality was due to other cancer and cardiac disease.

In the total follow-up period (up to 1988) of the Cancer Research Campaign trial 65.9 percent (783/1376) of the irradiated group died, compared with 55.5 percent (791/1424) of the group allocated to a wait-and-see policy. Haybittle *et al, NCI Cancer Weekly,* July 24, 1989:18(1).

[44] In one study, 75 per cent of women taking tamoxifen were not told of the possibility of side effects.

[45] Low-dose tamoxifen treatment can induce ocular toxicity. Pavlidis, NA, *et al* – *Cancer,* 1992;69(12):2961(4).

[46] It has been linked with the formation of liver cancer in animals and there is currently a fierce debate as to the risks or benefits of giving it to healthy women.

[47] The authors of a study recommended that routine periodic endometrial sampling be performed on all post-menopausal patients receiving tamoxifen. In those women receiving tamoxifen in this study who had examination of their endometrium, 100 per cent had evidence of endometrial abnormality. Cohen, I *et al, British Journal of Obstetrics and Gynecology* 1993;100(6):567-570.

Women taking tamoxifen developed cancer of the body of the uterus at a rate of over 6 per thousand. Women on placebo developed no such cancers. This has implications for trials giving tamoxifen to healthy women. *Cancer Researcher Weekly* 1994:4(1).

[48] Women who had used tamoxifen for more than 2 years had more than twice the risk of endometrial cancer than those who had never taken the drug. Vanleeuwen, F.E. *et al* – *Cancer Researcher Weekly* 1994:23(1). Also see summary in *American Family Physician* 1994;49:2.

[49] Researchers at the Stanford University School of Medicine and the University of California, Berkeley, found that breast cancer patients survived an average of 18 months longer if they participated in a psychological support group. 'I was quite stunned, since it was so contrary to what we expected to find,' says David Spiegel of Stanford. This comment reveals the stunning ignorance of conventional medicine.

The study reviewed 86 women whose breast cancer had spread to other parts of their bodies. Fifty of the women were given the opportunity to participate in a weekly support group for one year. Survival times of the two groups were compared ten years later, and the rate for women offered support was 36.6 months, compared to 18.9 months for the other women. *NCI Cancer Weekly* 1989:3(1).

[50] The suppression of any discharge from the body may have serious implications for health. Homoeopathic repertories provide many remedies for the treatment of disease caused by such a suppression.

[51] The extreme focus of chemical medicine on issues such as the menopause and osteoporosis leads to increases in anxiety and fear. 'The promotion of hormone replacement therapy and oestrogen replacement therapy for osteoporosis and heart disease treatment is premature and being applied too generally. Research shows these therapies have serious risks that may outweigh the benefits, especially for low-risk women, but patients are rarely given the risk-benefit analysis and high-risk groups are not targeted.' Worcester, N. *et al – Feminist Review* 1992;41:1(26)

[52] A recent study suggested it might be best for women with intermediate decreases in bone density to follow an exercise-calcium regime. Exercise with oestrogen is better to be reserved for those with low bone density. Prince, RL *et al – The New England Journal of Medicine* 1991;325(17):1189(7).

[53] The most serious of those include an increased risk of heart attack, stroke, or blood clots – all of which are relatively rare conditions in women of childbearing age. *Consumer Reports* 1989;54(8):498(3).

[54] The connection between oestrogen, progesterone and breast cancer is hotly debated in conventional circles. It is often stated that there is little hard evidence of such a connection. This is despite the presence of numerous trials stating that such a causal relationship exists. See the footnotes below. The following comment, however, is typical.
Dr. Bruce Stadel, Chief of the Epidemiology Branch at the US Food and Drug Administration and a co-author of a study looking at the link between female sex hormones and breast cancer "likens the recent findings to 'blips' on an otherwise clear radar screen". These 'blips' of course represent women with severe life-threatening disease!

[55] An increase in risk of 1.8. Armstrong BK – *Med J Aust* 1988;148:213-214.

[56] *Hunt K. et al – Br J Obstet Gynaecol* 1987;94:620-635 showed an increase of 1.6. This was later confirmed – Hunt, K. *et al – Br J Obstet Gynecol*, 1990;97(12):1080(7).

[57] Ewertz M – *Int J Cancer* 1988;42:832-838 showed an increased risk of 2.3.

[58] Brinton LA, *et al – Br J Cancer* 1986;54:825-832 gave an increased risk of 1.5.

[59] There is an increased risk following the long-term use of injectable hormones. Hulka BS, Chambless LE, Deubner DC, *Am J Obstet Gynecol* 1982;143:638-644.

[60] Two studies have shown an increase in the risk of breast cancer for women with the largest number of recorded prescriptions. Hoover R, Glass A, Finkle WD, *et al – JNCI* 1981;67:815-820 and Hiatt RA, *et al – Cancer* 1984;54:139-144.

[61] Scientist finds new connection between oestrogen and cancer. Liehr, JG. – *Cancer Researcher Weekly,* 1994;13(2).

[62] An increased risk of 1.5. Brinton LA, *et al, Cancer* 1981;47:2517-2522.

[63] An increased risk of 1.4. Ross RK, *et al, JAMA* 1980;243:1635-1639.

[64] A doubling in risk. Hoover R, *et al, N Engl J Med* 1976;295:401-405.

[65] Since the 1980s, there have been reports of an increased risk of breast cancer in women who received hormone replacement therapy. Hulka, Barbara S., Ca-A *Cancer Journal for Clinicians* 1990;40(5):289.

[66] A study by a group of Massachusetts' researchers indicated that long-term oral contraceptive use may quadruple the risk of breast cancer in women below the age of 45. Miller, D.R. et al, *NCI Cancer Weekly* 1989;12(2).

[67] There is a strong association between cancer of the body of the uterus and prescribed female sex hormones. Smith DC, *et al – N Engl J Med 1975*;293:1164-1167 and Ziel HK, et al – *NEJM* 1975;293:1167-1170.

[68] There is a detailed discussion of female sex hormone side effects in *'The Prescribed Drugs Guide – A Holistic Perspective'* by Dr S Gascoigne (Jigme, 2001).

[69] This can be deduced from the common root of progesterone, oestrogen and testosterone. They are derived from cholesterol and reveal the close relationship between these drugs, the liver and fat metabolism.

[70] There is fusion of the bones in the middle ear. It is rare in blacks and occurs to some extent in 10 per cent of Caucasians. Only 0.5-1 per cent will have symptoms. Females are twice as likely to be affected as men. Symptoms of impaired hearing that is progressive begin in late teens and early twenties. Surgical treatment is helpful with 85 per cent having excellent results and some improvement in 14 per cent. 1 per cent after the operation are totally deaf. The administration of oestrogen causes rapid, irreversible worsening of otosclerosis.

[71] *The Bitter Pill* by Dr Ellen Grant, *Premenopause – What Your Doctor May Not Tell You* by Dr. John Lee (Time Warner, 1999), *What Your Doctor May Not Tell You About Menopause* by Dr John Lee (Time Warner, 1996) are excellent sources of information about adverse effects of hormone replacement treatment.

[72] I know of a woman who had several invasive investigations for post-coital bleeding only to discover later that her partner had blood-streaked semen.

19 CHILDREN'S HEALTH

INTRODUCTION

The treatment of children can be a complex affair and is more difficult than treating adults. In Chinese medicine, it is known as the 'treatment of mutes' since they may not be able to relate their symptoms. It is said that it is 10 times easier to treat a man than a woman. It is 10 times easier to treat a woman than an elderly person and it is 10 times easier to treat an elderly person than a child.

Disorders may arise in childhood for several reasons. There may be a problem that is only with the child leading to the development of symptoms or symptoms may arise because of disharmonies and imbalances within the home and with family relationships. In most cases, there is a combination of these two factors. It is beyond the scope of this book to explore all the psychological issues that are important in childhood, but there are some excellent books available on the subject.[1]

The health of the child is strongest when the mother's health is good. The care of the woman through pregnancy, delivery and the post-natal period has important effects on the health of the developing child. An added factor to take into account in the modern world is that disease can arise from medical interference. The monitoring of children through regular health checks is of benefit in detecting abnormality early. However, the indiscriminate use of conventional treatments such as vaccination and antibiotics can be particularly damaging.

In this Chapter, I concentrate on those disorders that are specific to childhood and not mentioned elsewhere.

GROWTH AND DEVELOPMENT

In conventional medical practice, it is common to assess the progress of growth and development. In the UK, it is recommended that children be seen by a doctor at 6 weeks, between 2 to 3 years and between 4 to 5 years. Health visitors see the child at 7-8 months and 18 months. Measurements are taken of height and weight. Note is made of the attainment of developmental stages. It is also an opportunity to discuss feeding and other issues. Sadly, it may be used as an opportunity to pressurise mothers into vaccination.

Charts of 'normal' growth are used to check that increases in height and weight are in line with a perceived norm. As with most measurements, they can only be used as a guide because there are many variations in a healthy population. Allowance has to be made for the height of the parents, for example. Such measurements can only be one aspect of the child.

Milestones are the times at which most children have attained a certain stage of development. They are useful to know so that when you are faced with a child, you can have a good idea as to its progress. Table 19.1 is a list of the normal milestones of childhood.

AGE	MILESTONE
Birth	Normal heart rate 140 per minute
6 weeks	Normal heart rate 135 per minute Head control begins to develop Moves arms and legs like swimming Neonatal reflexes present Smiles, alert
4-8 weeks	Posterior fontanelle closes
4 months	Head control
6 months	First tooth

7-8 months	No head lag
	Sits alone for a few seconds
	Beginning to move around, usually by rolling
	Neonatal reflexes disappeared
	Steady and accurate reach of hand
	Secure grasping in palm of hand
	May be interested in objects which disappear from view
	Able to localise sound at ear level
	Tuneful babbling
8-9 months	Begins to crawl
10-18 months	Anterior fontanelle closes
12 months	Normal heart rate 115 per minute
	May begin to walk
18 months	Able to walk alone
	Balance momentarily on one leg
	Walk upstairs
	Crawls backward downstairs
	Accurate reaching for objects
	Mature voluntary reach and grasp
	No mouthing of toys and drooling
	No deliberate throwing of toys in a repetitive manner – gone by 15 months
	Tuneful jargon, occasionally two words together
	Drinking from a cup and using a spoon depend upon their degree of practice
2½-3 years	Runs well in straight line
	Goes up and downstairs two feet to a step
	Can jump and climb
	Hand preference but can use other hand for assistance
	Visual screening possible as child can co-operate with tester
	Understands pictures and plays meaningfully with objects
	Vocabulary of at least 200 words
	Sentences used in speech
	Persistent questions such as 'What?', 'Where?' and so on are common
	Can skilfully feed, wash and dress
	Most are dry in the day and some are dry at night
4½-5 years	Normal heart rate 100 per minute
	Motor skills can reveal a degree of 'clumsiness'. Only a problem if severe and accompanied by other symptoms
	Holds pencil maturely
	Can copy shapes
	Can draw people
	Audiogram testing of hearing possible[2]
	Speech is clear, fluent and easily understood
	Independent in feeding, washing, toileting
5 years	20 milk teeth
5-6 years	Permanent teeth begin to erupt
10 years	Normal heart rate 90 per minute
13-15 years	28 permanent teeth
25 years	Wisdom teeth

Table 19.1: Major milestones of childhood

CONVENTIONAL MEDICINE AND THE TREATMENT OF CHILDREN

General medical practitioners rather than paediatricians deal with most diseases in childhood. Further investigation and treatment is given in hospital for more severe or difficult problems. This only occurs in around 5 per cent of consultations.

The conditions with which children present to general practitioners in the UK are summarised in Table 19.2.

Reason for consultation	Per cent
Respiratory disease	28
Non-specific symptoms	13
Infectious disease	11
Skin diseases	10
Reputedly preventative procedures (includes vaccination)	10
Accidents	10

Table 19.2: Main reasons for children presenting to general practitioners[3]

There are several areas of work for the general practitioner. They are the recognition and treatment of episodic illness, the diagnosis of rare yet serious disease,[4] disease prevention[5] and dealing with the long-term consequences of chronic disease.

RECOMMENDATIONS FOR HEALTHY BABIES AND CHILDREN

It is helpful to discuss how babies and children can be given the best opportunity for health. These ideas are obtained from Chinese medical sources[6] and may be at variance with what is normally considered to be healthy in the West. I can only say that the methods of Chinese medicine have been proven over several thousand years, whilst advice given in the West frequently fluctuates with fashion and may not always be health-enhancing.

Babies, in terms of Chinese medicine, are immature Yang and immature Yin. This means that they are vulnerable to influences that may affect such immaturity. The immature Yang must be protected from the application of excessive coldness. Treatment techniques in Chinese medicine such as clearing heat, and this is the effect of antibiotics, are injurious to the Qi and Yang. Treatment is usually directed at supporting the Yin and Blood.

Attention must be paid to diet as described in Chapter 13 – Gastrointestinal system. Many illnesses in childhood are the result of diet and cold food or food that produces mucus has a greater effect before the Yang energy has fully matured. Fevers flare-up quickly in children because of this immaturity of the Fire aspect. The immaturity of the Yin means that children tend to produce fluid discharges such as mucus. There are several recommendations about diet that can be given to parents of babies and children:

- at birth use a decoction of licorice to clean the tongue. This helps the energy of the Stomach. The baby cries at birth because the Stomach Qi flares up. The baby may be quiet and relaxed if the birth is trouble-free and relaxed
- breast-feed if possible
- breast-feed when relaxed
- do not breast-feed directly after working hard or sexual intercourse
- begin solid food with soaking rice and toast it until swollen. Powder it and add to boiling water
- start mixed feeding at about 6 months and certainly not before 3 months. The baby will let you know when they want to start solids
- avoid raw foods including raw fruit
- well-cooked grains and warmly cooked vegetables are the mainstay of a healthy diet
- do not introduce more than one new food per day and then allow the child to become accustomed to the new taste
- avoid junk food, processed food, and tinned food
- avoid cold, greasy and excessively sweet tastes (this means sugar and foods which have sugar added).

For babies, there is a serious health risk from pesticides in drinking water particularly if feeds are made up with tap water. Children ingest four times the amount that adults take when considered on a weight-for-weight basis.[7]

Children usually respond well to treatment with holistic medicine, as their energy is relatively strong. They generally have less emotional turmoil than adults do. Chinese medicine, homoeopathy, cranial osteopathy and *tuina*[8] all have an important role to play in gaining and maintaining health in childhood. Parents can be encouraged to nurture their children in the ways of health by recommending that they:

- do not expose them to extremes of cold or heat
- do not carry the child all the time – lack of contact with the earth leads to shyness and fear
- do not overdress them when playing
- keep their back and stomach warm to protect Stomach and Kidney energy
- keep hands and feet warm to protect Heart and Lung
- do not let their child play with dangerous toys
- do not let their child watch films that are horrific, violent or pornographic
- remove some of their clothes if the back of neck feels hot or they may get a fever the next day
- massage the child regularly
- pay attention to their diet
- do not over bathe – once weekly is fine
- do not let children be exposed to adult stress or arguments
- give appropriate treatment only.[9]

SPECIFIC DISORDERS OF CHILDHOOD

Children may suffer from similar diseases to adults and these are discussed in their relevant sections. For example, asthma and upper respiratory tract infections may be found in Chapter 8 – Respiratory System, epilepsy is discussed in Chapter 14 – Central Nervous System, glue ear and otitis media are found in Chapter 12 – Special Senses.

Cot death

This is also known as sudden infant death syndrome (SIDS). It is the sudden death of a baby, due to an unidentifiable cause, usually occurring overnight whilst in its cot. It can occur from a few days old up to 2 years. Most deaths occur between the ages of 2 and 4 months. Cot death is more common if social conditions are poor and less likely if the baby is breast-fed.

On post-mortem examination, there may be evidence of an upper respiratory tract infection, pneumonia or gastro-enteritis. In about a third of cases there are minimal signs of disease and some 10 per cent of cot deaths have no abnormal post-mortem findings.

There may be symptoms immediately before the cot death and these include skin rashes, vomiting, diarrhoea, and shortness of breath and coughing.

Conventional medicine has little understanding of the mechanism of cot death. Recent advice has included laying the baby on its back following a study that suggested that this might lead to a reduction in deaths. Interestingly, in Chinese medicine the back is Yang (related to heaven) but in young babies it is Yin. It becomes Yang later. The front is Yang in babies. It would be healthier, therefore, for babies to be placed face down so that their Yang front faces the Yin of the Earth. The observations of the conventional study may be a result of greater attention given to the baby.

There are two issues to consider when discussing cot death. The first is vaccination, which usually begins at about 2 or 3 months of age. There is ample evidence to connect vaccination to minor symptoms such as skin rash, vomiting, diarrhoea, crying, irritability and upper respiratory tract symptoms. In addition, breathing abnormalities are definitely triggered by vaccinations. This is thoroughly researched and described in Viera Schreibner's seminal work on vaccination.[10]

The second issue is that of separation of the baby from its mother. In Western cultures, this may be done at a very early age. It is helpful to consider the benefit of the baby sleeping with the mother for some months so that early and forced separation is avoided. The Lungs are considered in Chinese medicine to be affected by loss and separation. It is easy to see how breathing may be affected by placing a baby of a few days or weeks old in a cot away from its mother.[11]

Failure to thrive

There is no formally agreed definition of failure to thrive. It is a general term that is applied to those children who grow and develop at a slower rate than normal. It may be noticed when the child has routine monitoring of height and developmental milestones. General practitioners and health visitors are the people most likely to diagnose such a situation.

Growth of the child is connected to many factors including family history and constitution. The size of the child must also be assessed considering their birth weight. Most children catch up with their peers and the length it takes to do so depends upon their original weight. In severe cases, the child may always be smaller than normal.

As a rule, if the child is happy and healthy there is nothing to worry about. If the child is small but miserable and unhealthy, further investigation may be necessary.

There are several causes of failure to thrive. The most common include chronic digestive or bowel disturbances, low grade infection, poor nutrition and chronic illness, e.g. asthma.

Febrile convulsion

This is a convulsion that occurs between the ages of 6 months and 6 years in association with a fever. It is an arbitrary definition and excludes known causes of convulsions such as meningitis, encephalitis, brain damage or epilepsy. It occurs in up to 5 per cent of all children.

The cause in conventional medicine is not known but fever due to any cause may precipitate the convulsion. Common situations, therefore, are upper respiratory tract and urinary infections. An attack is more likely if one or both parents had febrile convulsions as a child. This increases the risk by a factor of 50 per cent. Boys are affected twice as often as girls.

The convulsion occurs because of the rate of rise in temperature as well as the height of the temperature. Of the two, however, the risk has lessened somewhat by the time the height of the fever has been reached.

Febrile convulsions often occur more than once. Half of affected children have more than one attack whilst 20 per cent have four. Up to 10 per cent of them go on to develop epilepsy.

Symptoms
There is a short lasting convulsion of the grand mal type. Occasionally it may last for 30 minutes. The child typically sleeps after the attack.

Treatment
The main treatment, conventionally, is aimed at reducing the fever. This is by means of paracetamol as aspirin is prohibited for use in children. Undressing the child and tepid sponging may also be used.

Anticonvulsants are given if the convulsion is prolonged and if they are recurrent. An EEG may be performed before treatment. The duration of treatment varies from doctor to doctor. It is usually for at least a year after the last fit.

Most children grow up and have no further attacks and seem to be no worse for the experience. A minority continues to have problems and are then diagnosed as epileptic.

Undescended testis

The testes are originally an abdominal organ and they descend into the scrotum at about the eighth month of pregnancy. About 3 per cent of male babies have undescended testes. This figure rises to 21 per cent in the case of premature births. Virtually all testes descend within the first 9 months of life.

Symptoms
The undescended testis cannot be felt in the scrotum. It is important to distinguish this from the situation of retraction which occurs in the cold and if nervous. Occasionally the testis may be congenitally absent.

Complications
There are various complications of undescended testis. It is more likely to twist (torsion of the testis), has an increased risk of becoming malignant at some later stage (even if the testis is brought down by surgery) and fertility of the affected testis will be impaired. There may be cosmetic problems later as a result of only one testis in the scrotum (or none if both are undescended).

Treatment
Surgical treatment is performed certainly before the age of 5 and perhaps around the first birthday. The testis is brought down and fixed into the scrotum.

Holistic management

In terms of Chinese medicine, this condition is related to the function of the Liver as this channel crosses the external genitalia. It is treatable by means of holistic medicine and is certainly worth delaying any operation until there has been a fair trial of treatment. Surgery can easily be postponed until the age of 5 years with no risks.

Infantile phlegmy

This is a term from Chinese medicine and has no direct counterpart in conventional medicine. It is the appearance of mucus in the child that is frequently manifest as loose stools with runny nose. In severe cases, hearing may be affected and there may be specific symptoms in the upper respiratory tract such as sore throat and cough.

The cause is weak digestive energy that cannot transform food completely. This leads to the generation of mucus that passes up to the Lungs. Avoidance of factors that cause further weakening of the digestion is essential. Repeated vaccination and antibiotic use are the two medical procedures that commonly damage the digestion. It is also helpful to take dietary habits and emotional stresses within the family into account. Symptoms may appear at times such as when teething. If simple measures such as dietary changes do not effect an improvement, consider the application of homoeopathic remedies, herbs or *tuina*.

Colic

This is commonly seen in babies between the ages of 2 and 6 months. The baby begins to cry in the early evening and is frequently inconsolable. The duration of the crying is variable but may be for several hours. There may be difficulty getting off to sleep and repeated waking during the night.

In terms of Chinese medicine, there are two main syndromes that lead to colic. There may be Heat in the Heart or Spleen Qi Deficiency. Effective treatments exist in homoeopathy, herbal medicine and *tuina*.

Some mothers are advised to stop breast-feeding in the mistaken belief that the milk is of 'poor quality'. Switching the infant to cow's milk formulas may lead to a lessening of symptoms but this is because cow's milk, particularly the pasteurised variety, is heavy and hard to digest. There is a degree of sedation as a consequence. The baby is then more likely to develop Infantile Phlegmy.

Attention deficit and hyperactivity disorder (ADHD)

This is one of several labels applied to children with behavioural difficulties, poor concentration and attention and difficulty learning. Other symptoms include agitation and hyperactivity. This condition is related to Attention Deficit Disorder (ADD) and may also be known as Hyperkinetic Disorder[12]. Almost 2 per cent of the UK population are considered to suffer from such disorders with males more commonly affected than females. The cause is unknown in conventional medicine and there are various theories put forward including birth trauma, psychological factors and genetic influences. Certainly, from my experience of treating children a common association is with vaccination, reactions to certain foods and psychological factors within the family.

Symptoms
Formal diagnosis is based upon the presence of a minimum number of symptoms of lack of attention, hyperactivity and impulsive behaviour. Such symptoms require to have been present for at least six months taking account of the child's age and intelligence. Symptoms include lack of attention or inability to maintain attention, easily distracted, poor memory for day-to-day activities, restlessness and agitation.

Diagnosis
This is based upon the history and clearly so-called 'normal' children exhibit such behaviour and this can vary with time and situation. Careful assessment of the child must be done and the diagnosis is usually made by a child psychologist or psychiatrist preferably with experience of such children. The condition should be differentiated from other disorders such as autism, anxiety, depression and the like which may all manifest in related ways.

Treatment
This is difficult in many cases as the cause cannot be identified. A variety of methods may be advised including psychological advice for the parents of how to create a daily routine, giving clear instructions to the child, setting and maintaining boundaries, avoiding disturbing influences and rewarding so-called positive behaviour.

In clinical practice, medication is frequently used such as stimulants such as methylphenidate (Ritalin®). Antidepressants of the tricyclic types may be given as may anti-psychotics. Methylphenidate and its relatives are amphetamine-like in their action and cause addiction as well as anxiety, insomnia and increased activity.

Case

A boy of 3 years was brought by his parents with a chesty cough. He was taking corticosteroid and bronchodilator inhalers. His appetite was poor and he would only eat small amounts of meat. The most striking symptom, however, was overactivity. He did not sit still during the consultation and it was impossible to take his pulse or look at this tongue. He tried to climb over all the furniture in the consulting room and ran out of the room at one point and ran upstairs. His mother had to prise him off the banisters in order to get him back into the room. I made a diagnosis of Phlegm Accumulation with underlying Yin Deficiency. This is a common diagnosis in children particularly as a result of vaccination and recurrent antibiotic use. This boy had received over 12 doses of antibiotics already.

Over the course of the next 5 months, his chest improved with markedly less mucus and a reduced cough. His appetite improved and he started to eat more food and more varied types of food. He was able to slowly reduce and stop his inhalers. Twelve months later his chest was fine and gave him no problems. He went through the winter with only one attack of a chesty cough after an air flight. This settled quickly. He was much more content and happy.

HOW TO RECOGNISE A SERIOUS CONDITION IN CHILDREN

In Chinese medicine, there are two sayings about children that are relevant here.[13] 'Children get illness easily, illness quickly becomes serious.' '*Zang, qi, jing, ling* (spirit) – easily ill, easily cured.' The dilemma for the practitioner is judging the situation with each child.

The help of the mother is invaluable here since she usually knows the child best and is aware of what is and what is not normal. You must remember that the mother is also probably anxious about the welfare of her child and this may colour her opinion. However, you neglect a mother's concern at your peril.

The essential issue about treating children is the importance of monitoring. See the child frequently, every day if necessary and maintain contact over the phone. This will provide reassurance for the family and allow you to know about the progress of symptoms more easily.

Individual symptoms are dealt with in their relevant chapter. See Appendix Three for an alphabetical list of all symptoms.

SUMMARY

Symptoms in children are common due to their immature energies.

Most conditions in childhood are minor and self-limiting.

Know the symptoms that may indicate a serious underlying condition.

Symptoms in children can change rapidly. Regular checking and monitoring are valuable. It enables you to observe the case closely and is reassuring for the family.

---

1 *Childhood and Society* by Erikson (Vintage, 1995), *Families and How to Survive Them* by Skynner and Cleese (Arrow, 1994), *The Inner World of Childhood* by Frances G Wickes (Coventure, 1977), *Thou Shalt Not be Aware: Society's Betrayal of the Child* by Alice Miller (Pluto Press, 1998) and *For Your Own Good: Roots of Violence in Child Rearing* by Alice Miller (Virago, 1987).

2 The proportion of children with speech problems has doubled in the last 6 years. This may possibly be due to excessive sound levels, e.g. television, hi-fi. Hearing problems can occur very early with babies not responding to sound. This is of relevance in special care baby units or wards in hospitals where excessive noise may affect young babies.

3 Source *Child Health: A Textbook for the DCH* by Harvey and Kovar (Churchill and Livingstone, 1985).

4 These are primarily meningococcal meningitis, tuberculosis, diabetes mellitus and malaria.

5 Vaccination and developmental screening. Screening of the newborn is performed for phenylketonuria by means of heel-prick blood test. This is a rare disease where brain damage is the result of a congenital inability to metabolise certain proteins. A simple clinical examination will detect congenital dislocation of the hip. Failure to spot it before the child walks may lead to severe hip problems in later life.

6 There are several books that provide further information about children's health and Chinese medicine. *Acupuncture in the treatment of children* by Julian Scott (Eastland, 1999), *Turtle Tail and Other Tender Mercies* by Bob Flaws (Blue Poppy Press, 1985). Information was also obtained from lecture notes of Chinese Herbal Medicine course of Tinh Thong Nguyen, London Academy of Oriental Medicine.

The classical book concerning children's health and medical treatment is *How to Raise a Healthy Child.... In Spite of Your Doctor* by Robert Mendelsohn (Ballantine Books, 1987).

7 Report by US National Research Council, 1993.

8 *Tuina* is a type of remedial massage originating from China. It is simple, safe and painless. It can be used to treat a wide range of disorders in children. See *Infantile Tuina Therapy* by Luan Changye (Shandong Science and Technology Press, 1993), *Chinese Bodywork* Edited by Sun Chengnan (Pacific View Press, 1993) and *Chinese Massage and Acupressure* (Bergh, 1991).

9 It should be clear by now that I do not classify conventional medicine as 'appropriate'. It should be reserved for life-threatening disease.

10 Viera Schreibner's book, *Vaccination – A Medical Assault on the Immune System* (V. Schreibner,1997).

11 *Continuum Concept* by Jean Liedboff (Penguin, 1986 and Arkana, 1989) is an excellent discussion of separation in infancy, its consequences and the benefits of prolonged contact between mother and baby. Also see *Three in a Bed – The Benefits of Sleeping with your Baby* by Deborah Jackson (Bloomsbury, 1999).

12 The cover story in the November 30, 1998 issue of *Time* magazine, titled 'The Age of Ritalin' says "Production of Ritalin has increased more than sevenfold in the past eight years, and 90% of it is consumed in the U.S." The article says Ritalin, used for a nebulous "illness" called Attention Deficit Hyperactivity Disorder (ADHD) works "but in ways and for reasons that are still not entirely clear. ...not enough is known about the risks and benefits of long-term Ritalin use... Given the explosion in ADHD diagnoses and Ritalin use over the past decade, the disorder is surprisingly ill defined. No one is sure that it's a neurochemical imbalance ... There is no blood test, no PET scan, no physical exam that can determine who has it and who does not. ...For a drug that's been used for more than a half-century, we know surprisingly little about how Ritalin acts on the brain... ADHD is still something of a mystery to doctors, who speak of it sometimes as if it were a single condition and sometimes as if it were a broad range of problems. ...the latest research raises more questions than it answers. ...no studies have run long enough to see if it has a lasting effect on academic performance or social behavior. ...A positive response to Ritalin doesn't automatically mean a child suffers from ADHD. Stimulants can temporarily sharpen almost anyone's focus."

13 *Acupuncture in the Treatment of Children* by Julian Scott (Eastland, 1999).

BIBLIOGRAPHY

Vitalistic philosophy

Highly recommended:
Quantum Healing by Deepak Chopra (Bantam, 1989)
This is a very clear account of energetic medicine written by one of the foremost authors and practitioners of holistic medicine.

The Creation of Health by Caroline Myss, Norman Shealy, M.D., Bernie Siegel, M.D. (Stillpoint, 1988)
Electromagnetic Man by Cyril Smith and Simon Best (JM Dent)
The Presence of the Past: Morphic Resonance and the Habits of Nature by Rupert Sheldrake (Inner Traditions, 2000)
Subtle Energy by John Davidson (CW Daniel, 1987)
The Tao of Physics by Fritjof Capra (Flamingo, 1992)
The Turning Point by Fritjof Capra (Flamingo, 1983)

Homoeopathy

Highly recommended:
The Homoeopathy Workshop by Dr T Cook (Crowood, 2000)
This is an excellent introduction to homoeopathy. It gives readers a sound philosophical basis to understand its effects and breadth of application.

The Chronic Diseases by Samuel Hahnemann (Homeopathic Book Service, 1998)
The Complete Homeopathy Handbook : A Guide to Everyday Health Care by Miranda Castro (Pan, 1996)
Concordant Materia Medica by Frans Vermeulan (Merlijn Publishers, 1997)
A History of the Schism in Medical Thought by Harris L Coulter (North Atlantic Books, 1993)
Homeopathic Science and Modern Medicine by Harris Coulter (North Atlantic Books, 1980)
Homeopathy for Pregnancy, Birth and Your Baby's First Year by Miranda Castro (St. Martin's Press, 1993)
The Science of Homeopathy by George Vithoulkas (Grove, 1980)

Chinese medicine – general

Highly recommended:
The Chinese Way to Health by Dr S Gascoigne (Connections, 2000)
This book gives a comprehensive introduction to the underlying principles of Chinese medicine. There is an overview of the eight methods of treatment of Chinese medicine with information about massage, Qi Gong exercises, dietary therapy and herbal self-help remedies. It explains how to use them in your everyday life.

Between Heaven and Earth by Beinfield and Korngold (Ballantine, 1992)
Principles of Chinese Herbal Medicine by John Hicks (Thorsons, 1996)
Principles of Chinese Medicine by Angela Hicks (Thorsons, 1996)
Qi Gong for Health and Vitality by Michael Tse (Piatkus, 1995)

Chinese medicine – textbooks

Highly recommended:
The Web That Has No Weaver by Ted Kaptchuk (Contemporary Books, 2000)
This has been described as 'a bible for those interested in traditional Chinese medicine'. Ted Kaptchuk clearly explains the underlying principles of Chinese medicine and their application to the understanding and treatment of disease.

Acupuncture in the Treatment of Children by Julian Scott (Eastland, 1999)
Acupuncture: A Comprehensive Text by Shanghai College of Traditional Medicine. Translated by O'Connor and Bensky (Eastland Press, 1981)
Blue Poppy Essays by Bob Flaws *et al.* (Blue Poppy Press, 1988)
BodyMind Energetics by Mark Seem with Joan Kaplan (Healing Art Press , 1989)

Dragon Rises, Red Bird Flies by Leon Hammer (Station Hill Press, 1991)
Essentials of Traditional Chinese Paediatrics compiled by Cao Jiming *et al*, (Foreign Languages Press, 1990)
The Foundations of Chinese Medicine by Giovanni Maciocia (Churchill Livingstone, 1989)
Fundamentals of Chinese Medicine by Wiseman and Ellis (Paradigm, 1997)
A Handbook of Traditional Chinese Dermatology by Liang Jian-Hui. Translated by Zhang Ting-Liang and Bob Flaws (Blue Poppy Press)
Mental Dysfunction as treated by Traditional Chinese Medicine compiled by Cheung *et al.* (American College of Traditional Chinese Medicine, 1985)
Something Old, Something New by Bob Flaws (Blue Poppy Press)
The Path of Pregnancy by Bob Flaws (Blue Poppy Press, 1993)
Traditional Acupuncture: The Law of the Five Elements by Dianne Connelly (Traditional Acupuncture Institute, 1994)
The Treatment of Cancer by Integrated Chinese and Western Medicine by Zhang Dai-Zhao (Blue Poppy Press, 1993)
Turtle Tail and Other Tender Mercies by Bob Flaws (Blue Poppy Press)
The Yellow Emperor's Classic of Internal Medicine (known as the Neijing) Translation by Henry Lu
Zang Fu Syndromes by John McDonald (New South Wales College of Natural Therapies)

Dietary therapy

Highly recommended:

Recipes for Self-Healing by Daverick Leggett (Meridian Press, 1999)
Over 100 recipes are given in this book that also explains the traditional Chinese medicine rationale behind applying diet to treat disease and prevent ill-health. There are great (and tasty!) ideas here for healthy eating.

Chinese System of Food Cures by Henry Lu (Ward Locke, 1986)
The Chopra Centre Cookbook by Gina Bragg, David Simon and Deepak Chopra (Rider, 2000)
Eat Yourself Slim – and Stay Slim! by Michel Montignac (Montignac Publishing, 1999)
Prince Wen Hui's Cook: Chinese Dietary Therapy by Bob Flaws and Honora Wolfe (Churchill Livingstone, 1993)
The Saccharine Disease by Cleave (Wright, 1974)

Birth

Highly recommended:

Active Birth by Janet Balaskas (Harvard Common Press, 1992)
This book deals with the postures and exercises that can facilitate and ease the process of delivery. It presents this information in a simple way without resorting to criticising conventional approaches. Very accessible and practical.

The Active Birth Partners Handbook by Janet Balaskas (Sidgewick and Jackson)
The American Way of Birth by Jessica Mitford (Plume, 1993)
The Encyclopaedia of Pregnancy and Birth by Janet Balaskas and Yehudi Gordon (Little, Brown, 1992)
Homeopathy for Pregnancy, Birth and Your Baby's First Year by Miranda Castro (St. Martin's Press, 1993)
Preparing for Birth with Yoga by Janet Balaskas (Element, 1993)
Waterbirth: The Concise Guide to Using Water During Pregnancy, Birth, and Infancy by Janet Balaskas and Yehudi Gordon (Unwin)

Children's health

Highly recommended:

How to Raise a Healthy Child .... In Spite of Your Doctor by Robert Mendelsohn (Ballantine, 1987)
Robert Mendelsohn, American M.D. and paediatrician, gives clear and appropriate advice to parents about children's illnesses. He presents an exceptionally sane view of how to deal with acute illnesses and is passionate in his belief that the use of vaccinations and the overuse of prescribed medication is a significant cause of ill-health. He stresses the importance of parental observation and clearly states when it is appropriate to seek medical help. This book has been described as a 'true gift'.

Banished Knowledge – Facing Childhood Injuries by Alice Miller (Virago, 1990)
Childhood and Society by Erikson (Vintage, 1995)
Chinese Massage for Infants and Children: Traditional Techniques for Alleviating Colic, Colds, Earaches, and Other Common Childhood Conditions by Kyle Cline (Inner Traditions International, 1999)

Chinese Pediatric Massage Therapy: A Parent's and Practitioner's Guide to the Treatment and Prevention of Childhood Disease by Fan Ya-Li (Blue Poppy Press, 1994)
Continuum Concept by Jean Liedboff (Arkana, 1989)
For Your Own Good: Roots of Violence in Child Rearing by Alice Miller (Virago, 1987)
Hanging Charts of Infantile Tuina Therapy by Luan Changye (Shandong Science & Technology, 1993)
Reflexology for Children by Kevin and Barbara Kunz (Thorson's, 1996)
The Inner World of Childhood by Frances G Wickes (Coventure)
Thou Shalt Not Be Aware: Society's Betrayal of the Child by Alice Miller (Pluto, 1990)
Three in a Bed – Why you should Sleep with your Baby by Deborah Jackson (Bloomsbury, 1999)
Infantile Tuina Therapy by Luan Changye (Shandong Science and Technology Press, 1993)

Better Eyesight Without Glasses by W.H. Bates (Thorson's, 1995)
Help Your Child to Better Eyesight Without Glasses by Janet Goodrich (Sally Milner Publishing, 1997)
Improve Your Eyesight by Jonathan Barnes (Souvenir Press, 1999)

Vaccination

Highly recommended:
Dispelling Vaccine Myths by Alan Phillips and Chris Beaton (Prometheus, 1999)
A small booklet covering the essential issues surrounding vaccination. It is ideal to give to parents who are seeking access to wider information about vaccination and its effects.

Immunisation, The Reality Behind the Myth by W James (Bergin and Garvey, 1995)
Immunization Theory Vs Reality: Exposure on Vaccinations by Neil Z Miller (New Atlantean Press, 1996)
Immunizations: The People Speak! Questions, Comments and Concerns about Vaccinations by Neil Z Miller (New Atlantean Press, 1996)
Mass Immunisation – A Point in Question by Trevor Gunn (Cutting Edge Publications, 1992)
A Shot In The Dark by Harris Coulter and Barbara Loe Fisher (Avery, 1991)
Vaccination by W James and R Mendelsohn (Bergin and Garvey, 1995)
Vaccination & Immunisation by Leon Chaitow (C.W. Daniel, 1987)
Vaccination – A Medical Assault on the Immune System by Viera Schreibner, Ph.D. (V Schreibner, 1997)
Vaccination, Social Violence and Criminality by Harris L Coulter (North Atlantic Books, 1990)
The Vaccine Guide – Making an Informed Choice by Randall Newstaeder (North Atlantic Books, 1996)
Vaccines: Are They Really Safe and Effective? by Neil Z Miller (New Atlantean Books, 1992)
The Vaccination Bible, Edited by Lynne McTaggart (What Doctors Don't Tell You, 2000)

Women's health

The Change – Women, Ageing and the Menopause by Germaine Greer (Penguin, 1992)
Menopause – The Commonsense Approach to by Ruth Appleby (Newleaf, 1998)
Natural Birth Control by Katia and Jonathan Drake (Thorson's, 1984)
Passage to Power by Leslie Kenton (Ebury, 1995)
Premenopause – What Your Doctor May Not Tell You by Dr John Lee (Time Warner, 1999)
Sex and Destiny by Germaine Greer (Secker and Warburg)
What Your Doctor May Not Tell You About Menopause by Dr John Lee (Time Warner, 1996)
The Whole Woman by Germaine Greer (Anchor, 2000)

Death and dying

Highly recommended:
The Tibetan Book of Living and Dying by Sogyal Rinpoche (Rider, 1998)
This book provides a complete vision of life and death and is written by one of the foremost spiritual teachers of this generation. Although rooted in the Tibetan Buddhist tradition, it is accessible to people of all spiritual traditions, or none, and provides a context to understanding the meaning of life and death as well as practical guidance that can be applied on a daily basis. I frequently recommend this book to patients and practitioners.

Facing Death and Finding Hope by Christine Longaker (Century, 1997)
Healing into Life and Death by Stephen Levine (Gateway, 1989)

Intimate Death by Marie de Hennezel (Warner, 1998)
Meetings at the Edge by Stephen Levine (Gateway, 1992)
The Natural Death Handbook, edited by Nicholas Albery, Gil Elliot and Joseph Elliot (Rider, 1997)
On Death and Dying by Elisabeth Kubler-Ross (Routledge, 1990)

Cancer

Highly recommended:

The Holistic Approach to Cancer by Ian B. Pearce (C.W. Daniel, 1995)
A common-sense approach to cancer and this book is eminently suitable for someone first diagnosed with cancer. It is written clearly and without overloading people with information or philosophical views.

Bristol Cancer Help Centre – Living with Cancer by Rosy Daniel (Constable Robinson, 2000)
Cancer and Leukaemia – An Alternative Approach by Jan De Vries (Mainstream, 1994)
Cancer – The Alternative Method of Treatment by I.Bryant (Saffron Walden, 1995)
A Cancer Therapy – Results of Fifty Cases by Max Gerson (Gerson Institute, 1999)
An End to Cancer? by Leon Chaitow (Thorson's, 1978)
Laetrile – Nutritional Control for Cancer by Glenn Kittler (Royal, 1978)
The Bristol Diet by Alec Forbes (Century, 1984)
The Cancer Cure that Worked!: Fifty Years of Suppression by Barry Lynes (Marcus, 1987)
The Healing of Cancer by Barry Lynes (Marcus)
Your Life in Your Hands by Jane Plant (Virgin Publishing, 2000)
Politics of Cancer by Epstein (Sierra, 1978)

Mind-Body connection

Highly recommended:

The Healing Power of Illness by Dethlefsen, T. and D, Rudiger (Element, 1990)
A revelatory book that seeks to understand the meaning of symptoms. The basic tenet of the book is that true healing can only occur when we are aware of what is behind the symptom. The authors explore the underlying mental and emotional issues that give rise to symptoms and suggest new ways of considering them in the search for healing.

Body Centred Psychotherapy: The Hakomi Method by Ron Kurtz (Life Rhythm, 1990)
The Diamond Healing – Tibetan Buddhist Medicine and Psychiatry by Terry Clifford (Samuel Weiser, 1990)
Full Catastrophe Living by Jon Kabat-Zinn (Piatkus, 1996)
Getting Well Again by Simonton, Creighton and Matthews (Bantam, 1992)
The Healing Buddha by Raoul Birnbaum and John Blofeld (Shambhala, 1989)
Love Your Disease: It's Keeping You Healthy by John Harrison (Hay, 1988)
Love, Medicine and Miracles by Bernie Siegel (Rider, 1999)
Mind as Healer, Mind as Slayer by K Pelletier and S Locke (Delta, 1992)
Personality Types – Jung's Model of Typology by Daryl Sharp (Inner City Books, 1987)
Rainbow of Liberated Energy by Ngakpa Chögyam (Element, 1986)
Will To Be Well by Neville Hodgkinson (Rider)
Reality Therapy in Action by William Glassner, MD (Harper Collins, 2000)
Savage Sleep by Millen Brand (Crown, 1968)
Families and How to Survive Them by Skynner and Cleese (Mandarin, 1990)

Conventional medicine

Highly recommended:

Concise Medical Dictionary (OUP, 1998)
Understanding Disease by John Ball and Misha Norland (C W Daniel, 1990)
There are many medical dictionaries and they are all good sources of conventional medical information. Understanding Disease by John Ball explains how diseases start, what the main symptoms are and how they may affect us. It is written in plain English and a useful starter book for the study of pathology and disease.
The Body at War by John Dwyer (Unwin, 1989)
Cecil's Textbook of Medicine, edited by Wyngaarden and Smith (WB Saunders, 2000)
Clinical Medicine – Fourth Edition – edited by Kumar and Clark (W B Saunders, 1998)

Davidson's Principle and Practice of Medicine, edited by Christopher Haslett (Churchill Livingstone, 1999)

Davies's Textbook of Adverse Drug Reactions, edited by DM Davies (Edward Arnold, 1998)

Dorland's Illustrated Medical Dictionary by Dorland (WB Saunders, 2000)

The Merck Manual of Medical Information: Home Edition by Robert Berkow (Mark H. Beers (Editor), Andrew J. Fletcher (Editor) (Pocket Books, 1999)

Stedman's Medical Dictionary by Stedman (Lippincott Williams and Wilkins, 2000)

Textbook of Medicine by Souhami and Moxham (Churchill Livingstone, 1994)

Pharmacology

The Prescribed Drugs Guide – A Holistic Perspective by Dr S Gascoigne (Jigme Press, 2001)

This book, originally published in 1992, has been completely revised and updated. It provides a method of categorising prescribed drugs so that holistic practitioners can safely and appropriately manage patients who take such medications. There is an analysis of the energetic effects of prescribed drugs. There are many cases describing how to manage patients who take prescribed drugs. It is supported by up-to-date information on Dr Gascoigne's website: www.drgascoigne.com.

Cured to Death by Arabella Melville and Colin Johnson (NEL)

Drugs and Pharmacology for Nurses by SJ Hopkins (Churchill Livingstone, 1999)

Critiques of conventional medicine

Highly recommended:

Confessions of a Medical Heretic by Robert Mendelsohn (Contemporary Books, 1997)

An inspiring account of Robert Mendelsohn's transition from orthodox trained paediatrician to 'medical heretic'. An essential read for all medically trained practitioners to show that there are other methods that can be used to treat illness. It is also revealing for holistic practitioners as it shows that over-reliance on conventional medicine is generally not helpful if healing is to occur.

Alternative Medicine by Robert Eagle (Futura, 1978)

And They Call It Help: The Psychiatric Policing of America's Children by Louise Armstrong (Addison-Wesley Pub. Co., 1993)

The Politics of Experience and The Bird of Paradise by Laing (Penguin, 1990)

Blaming the Brain: The Truth About Drugs and Mental Health by Elliot S. Valenstein, Ph.D. (Free Press, 1998)

The Controlled Clinical Trial: An Analysis by Harris L Coulter (Batus, 1991)

Dirty Medicine by Martin Walker (Gateway, 1995)

The Divided Self by R D Laing (Penguin, 1990)

Electroshock: Its Brain-Disabling Effects by Peter R. Breggin, M.D. (Springer Pub. Co. , 1979)

Health Shock by Martin Weitz (Hamlyn, 1982)

How to Survive Medical Treatment by Stephen Fulder (C W Daniel, 1995)

Law, Liberty, and Psychiatry by Thomas S. Szasz, M.D. (Syracuse Univ. Press, 1989)

Medical Nemesis by Ivan Illich (Penguin, 1995)

The Mirage of Health: Utopian Progress and Biological Change by Rene Dubos (Rutgers University Press, 1987)

Natural Medicine by Brian Inglis (Fontana)

The Persecution and Trial of Gaston Naessens by Christopher Bird (HJ Kramer, 1991)

Psychiatric Drugs: Hazards to the Brain by Peter R. Breggin, M.D. (Springer Pub. Co. , 1983)

Sanity, Madness and the Family by Laing with E Esteron (Penguin, 1990)

Self and Others by Laing (Routledge, 1998)

Toxic Psychiatry by Peter R. Breggin, M.D. (HarperCollins, 1993)

LIAISON WITH OTHER PRACTITIONERS

Liaison with other practitioners is an essential part of medical practice. There are several reasons for asking another professional about the person you are treating. You may wish to refer the person you have seen because you cannot treat the particular presenting problem. It may be because several treatment options are necessary and working with other practitioners is part of an overall management plan for that person. Perhaps you would like a degree of supervision from the other practitioner. Whatever the reason, it is helpful to know how to go about the practical matter of liaison.

It is much more helpful if you know the practitioner. A resource list is invaluable where you know people in your locality such as a homoeopath, osteopath, acupuncturist, herbalist, counsellor and so on. If you have had contact with them previously, any dealings now will be smoother.

The standard way of liaising professionally is by means of referral letter. This may not be necessary if you know the practitioner concerned and the case is not too involved. It is preferable to communicate by letter, at least initially, for other situations and particularly when dealing with conventional practitioners who you do not know. It is often helpful to have written records of such communications for inclusion in the case notes.

Below is a sample letter that may be of guidance. Always type such a letter on professional notepaper. The main points to bring out are:

- state the main issue to be dealt with
- say what you are intending to do about it
- describe what help or assistance you require
- offer to discuss the case further
- enclose literature about your therapy if necessary.

The Clinic of Chinese Medicine
Clonakilty
Co. Cork
Ireland

Tel No.

Date

Dear

Re: Mr A.N.Other, 14 Any Street, Anywhere

This man came to see me recently for help with his symptoms of anxiety and depression. As you know, he was diagnosed with a minor depressive illness some years ago. His main difficulties at the moment are disturbed sleep, palpitations, sweating, together with feelings of apprehension, anxiety and nervousness. When his symptoms are particularly strong he finds his work difficult to cope with. This is the type of condition that can respond to acupuncture and Chinese herbal medicine and I have arranged to see him for a course of treatment.

I would envisage that his improvement will be slow and that he would require help from other sources including counselling. I have given him a list of people who would be able to help.

He also wishes help in reducing his medication that currently consists of:

Anafranil 25 mg three times daily
Nitrazepam one at night
Diazepam 5 mg three times daily

I would appreciate your help later when it is appropriate to deal with these. In the meantime I shall keep in touch about his progress.

If you would like to discuss this case I can be contacted at the above address. I also enclose a leaflet giving information about acupuncture and Chinese herbal medicine.

Yours sincerely

Stephen Gascoigne

HOW TO RECOGNISE SERIOUS SYMPTOMS

In this book I have brought your attention to the question of serious conditions and how to recognise them. A list of symptoms that would indicate a serious situation is included at the end of most chapters. By a serious condition, I mean a situation where life may be threatened or a severe degree of limitation exists. If you understand the significance of a particular symptom, you can have confidence in your practice and know your limitations.

The seriousness of a symptom is dependent upon the degree of limitation of the person's activity or functioning. If health can be defined as freedom from limitation then disease or a symptom is a limiting factor. A serious symptom, therefore, would be one that is severely limiting, life threatening or indicative of a worsening situation, i.e. progressive over a short period of time.

What do you do in a situation where a symptom may indicate a serious condition? The answer to this depends upon the degree of your experience and expertise. It is important to recognise your limitations as to what is and is not possible. You may be able to deal with such symptoms. On the other hand, you may need to refer the person to someone else. There may be a need for emergency hospitalisation. This is true in acute life-threatening conditions.

If the case is not so severe, there may be time to refer to someone who may be of help. This could be a conventional practitioner or possibly a holistic practitioner. Whatever the situation, it is essential to discuss the issues with the person who has come to see you for help. You may be able to help later for the underlying problems whilst current circumstances require a different approach in the short-term.

The Table below is a summary of all the symptoms I have mentioned in the text and how to recognise if they indicate a serious underlying condition.

Symptom	Cause for concern
Anorexia	Severe, progressive, with mental symptoms of distorted body image
Anuria	Always
Appetite, increased	With weight loss, with mental symptoms of distorted body image
Belching	Not serious
Bleeding enlargement	Severe, persistent, recurrent, with pallor, sore throat and lymphatic gland
Bleeding, vaginal, inter-menstrual	Persistent particularly around the menopause
Bleeding, vaginal, post-coital[1]	Persistent
Bleeding, vaginal, post-menopausal	Always – unless taking hormone replacement treatment
Bleeding, vaginal, pre-pubertal	Always – consider sexual abuse
Bleeding, vaginal, after childbirth	If heavy
Bloating, abdomen	Progressive
Body image disturbance	If associated with weight loss, amenorrhoea
Breathlessness	Severe, acute, progressive, with confusion, with cyanosis, pulse rate > 120 per minute, paroxysmal attacks occurring at night
Bruising	Severe, spontaneous
Bullae	Large
Constipation	Severe, progressive, with blood, alternates with diarrhoea
Convulsions	Always
Cough	Persistent, with blood, with breathlessness
Cyanosis	Always unless cold weather only involving lips/extremities

Deafness	Short history, progressive
Dehydration	This may result from loss of fluids, e.g. diarrhoea and vomiting or lack of intake. In babies look for dry skin/lips, decreased skin elasticity, strong urine, scanty urine or even dry nappy, sleepy, lack of responsiveness. In older people there will be reported thirst also
Delusions	Always
Diarrhoea	Severe, persistent, progressive, in the very young or old, with blood, with mucus, alternates with constipation
Dizziness	Severe, progressive
Ear, deformity	Severe
Ear, discharge	Long duration
Emotional symptoms, e.g. anxiety, fear, depression	If severe, with mental symptoms
Enuresis	Severe especially if with incontinence in the day
Eye, discharge	Not if alone. Of concern if severe, prolonged and with pain in the eye
Eye, redness	Circumcorneal, with visual disturbance
Eye, soreness	Not if mild. Of concern if *pain* rather than soreness especially with circumcorneal redness
Facial weakness	With history of ear pain
Fainting	With exercise
Fever, mild	Perhaps 99°F – may indicate mild disease but could be the beginning of severe disease in a weak patient, i.e. vital energy too weak to generate fever
Fever, prolonged	Most fevers last a day or so. If several days have elapsed then this is of concern that the patient is not strong enough to throw off the problem
Fever, very high	103°F and above. This indicates potentially severe disease. There is strong vital energy but the process may damage the patient
Finger clubbing	Always
Flatulence	Not serious
Haematuria	Painless
Haemoptysis	Recurrent, older patient, smoker
Hallucinations	Always
Headache	Progressive, severe with short history, with other central nervous system symptoms
High blood pressure	If severe especially if associated with oedema and proteinuria
Hoarseness	Persistent (more than three weeks)
Jaundice	Unless mild in new-born
Labour, delayed onset	If more than 2 weeks overdue (this is flexible because it is dependent upon the mother and the baby)
Labour, prolonged	If cervix not dilating, with exhaustion, with changes to foetal heart rate
Loss of consciousness	With exercise, not if short duration with specific trigger (see Page 94)
Lumps, around or on the ear	Severe, if with redness, pain and deafness
Lumps, general	Short history, progressive
Lumps,, nodules in the skin	Short history, recent change, progressive, bleeding
Lymphatic gland enlargement	With pallor, bleeding and sore throat, progressive, moderately enlarged

Nausea	Severe
Numbness	Severe, progressive
Oedema symptoms	Acute, unilateral, severe, progressive, with cardiac symptoms, with renal
Pain	Severe
Pain, abdominal	Severe, with abdominal rigidity, with guarding, with rebound tenderness
Pain, chest	Severe, at rest, with vomiting, with rapid pulse and low blood pressure, long duration, increasing frequency of attacks, constant and dull
Pain, ear	Severe, with fever
Pain, eye	With visual disturbance
Pain, loin	Severe
Pain, urethra	Not serious
Pallor	Severe, with fainting, with marked light-headedness or dizziness
Palpitations	Pulse > 120 or < 50, with chest pain, oedema or loss of consciousness
Paralysis	Always
Periods, heavy	Persistent, frequent, with pallor and tiredness
Placental retention	If with heavy bleeding, if prolonged (over an hour)
Pregnancy, uterine pain	Always unless at normal time for labour
Pregnancy, vaginal bleeding	Always
Proteinuria	With dysuria and backache, with high blood pressure and proteinuria
Pulse diagnosis (Chinese medicine) in acute fevers	If you treat a patient with an External Pathogenic Factor (EPF) and the pulse is superficial, floating and even overflowing you would expect the pulse to moderate after treatment. If this does not occur it indicates that the EPF may be stronger than the upright Qi. Careful assessment of the case is then necessary as treatment is likely to be difficult. The next thing to happen may be collapse of the person
Skin, redness or weeping	Severe, large areas of skin surface
Sputum	Copious, green/yellow, blood stained, frothy
Stiffness	Severe
Stridor	Always
Suicidal feelings	Always
Suicidal thoughts	Always
Symptom, severity	The stronger the symptoms, e.g. lots of diarrhoea, lots of vomiting then the more likely they are to be potentially serious. However be careful since weak patients have weak symptoms, e.g. pneumonia in the elderly or patients with AIDS may present only with breathlessness – no cough and no fever. It is important to assess each case carefully.
Symptoms, progression	Assess the direction of the pathology. By this I mean is it moving to internal organs or becoming more superficial? It is of concern if symptoms start to appear indicating pathology at a deeper level, e.g. in the case of the respiratory system this would be illustrated by sore throat with fever, cough, breathlessness and finally confusion – an effect on the deepest level (mental)
Symptoms, site	Are these in the superficial levels of the body or involving internal organs? If symptoms occur indicating pathology in the lung, kidney, liver, heart or central nervous system then these are clearly more worrying. In terms of Chinese medicine, worry more if the symptoms are at deeper levels of the Taiyin, Shaoyin and Jueyin

Tendency to catch colds	Not serious (but indicates a weakened immune system)
Thought disorders	If severe
Tingling	Severe, progressive
Tinnitus	Progressive
Tremor	Severe, progressive
Urgency	Severe, short history
Urination, dribbling	Severe, short history
Urination, frequent	Severe, short history
Vaginal discharge	Heavy, blood-stained
Veins, distended	In an abnormal site, e.g. neck when sitting up, over the chest or abdominal wall
Vertigo	Severe
Vesicles	Haemorrhagic
Vision, blurring	Progressive
Vision, double	Short history
Vision, spots or floaters	If localised area of blurring
Visual disturbance	Short history, progressive, with pain, with redness
Vomiting	Severe, persistent, progressive, in the very young or old, with blood, with food eaten days before, projectile, evidence of dehydration
Weight loss	Progressive, unexplained, with mental symptoms of distorted body image
Wheezing	If accompanied by breathlessness

---

[1] Do not forget that it takes two to indulge in sexual intercourse. I know of a woman who had several invasive investigations for post-coital bleeding only to discover later that her partner had blood-streaked semen.

Distance Learning Course

written by Dr Stephen Gascoigne

A distance learning course has been written to accompany this text. This guides you through the book step by step with additional clarification and numerous practical self-assessment questions with valuable model answers. The course follows the structure of the book, but is divided into four study units with various topic-related sections to help you through the material. In addition to the main study, there are assignment questions at the end of each section, which will add further life to the subjects discussed, and will involve you in practical research of later benefit to you as a practitioner. Full marking of these assignments can be provided, with expert tutor feedback and support, and a certificate on completion.

Entitled **Pathology and Disease for Alternative Practitioners**, this thorough course will be of great help in developing your understanding of this complex subject. It is used extensively by colleges teaching a wide range of holistic therapies in the UK, USA and Ireland. Students world-wide have found the course to be an essential part of training in holistic medicine.

A preparatory course **Anatomy and Physiology for Alternative Practitioners** as well as **Nutrition for Alternative Practitioners** are also available. For details of these professional courses, contact:

Alternative Training
Orchard House
Merthyr Road
Llanfoist
Abergavenny
NP7 9LN
UK

Tel: (+0044/0) 1873 856872
Fax: (+0044/0) 1873 858962
Email: info@alternative-training.com
Website: www.alternative-training.com

PHARMACOLOGY

Throughout this book, I have made references to Chinese medicine. I have attempted to translate conventional medical labels into the syndromes of Traditional Chinese Medicine. There is always a risk when citing a treatment given in a particular case that Chinese medicine or homoeopathy may be over simplified and lead to the use of acupuncture, herbs or homoeopathic medicine based solely on a conventional diagnostic term. This is not my intention and such simplification will lead to the degeneration of holistic medicine.

The usefulness of considering energetic syndromes is that you can understand conventional disease terms through your knowledge of holistic medicine. This is your chosen field of practice and is the starting point. There is no benefit in merely learning conventional medicine for its own sake. It has to be translated and interpreted into a dynamic format.

At the same time, I have also provided some information about the energetic qualities of conventional drugs. This can help practitioners of Chinese medicine decide how a particular medication may affect the case. It can change the pulse, tongue and symptoms. This can be confusing unless you understand all the influences at work in a particular case. The information about energetic qualities of drugs is mainly my own work. I do not claim them to be the final word – merely a beginning.

How is it possible to gain information about conventional medicines and explain them in terms of Chinese medicine? There are several possibilities. Homoeopaths learn about the actions of substances through 'provings', that is, they gather information about symptoms produced when people take a particular substance. The information regarding the actions of Chinese herbs was gathered in a similar way. Experts in Qi Gong and Chinese medicine would take a herb and know its taste, quality and actions from the effects they experienced.

Further information may be gathered from texts on the side-effects of drugs. Unfortunately, conventional medicines are only studied on the basis of the effect they have on one symptom rather than being based on the totality of their actions. For this reason they should be considered a helpful, yet incomplete, guide.

Observation of people who come for treatment is invaluable in ascertaining the effect of drugs. This is particularly true if you already know, or can deduce, the original energetic diagnosis. Any changes due to the drug can then be more easily assessed.

The summary of the energetic actions of drugs given below is based on known side-effects and my clinical experience. Personal testing remains the most accurate means of assessing drugs and hopefully this can be done at some time in the future.

Summary of energetic qualities of drugs discussed in this text

Drug	Energetic action	Organs mainly affected
Anti-Parkinsonian drugs	Hot	Liver, Heart
Antibiotics (except sulphonamides)	Cold, damp	Lung, Spleen
Antidepressants	Hot	Heart, Liver
Antifungal	Hot	Spleen, Liver
Aspirin	Warm, dispersing	Lung, Blood
AZT	Hot	Liver, Kidney
Betablockers	Cold	Heart, Lung, Liver, Kidney, Spleen
Bronchodilators	Warm, dispersing	Lung
Cancer chemotherapy	Hot	Liver, Stomach, Blood
Codeine	Hot	Heart, Lungs, Large Intestine
Corticosteroids	Hot	Lung, Spleen, Kidney
Digoxin	Warm	Heart, Kidney
Diuretics	Cold	Kidney

Female sex hormones	Cold	Kidney, Liver, Heart, Spleen
Insulin	Cold	Spleen, Lung, Kidney
Nitrates	Hot	Heart, Liver
Non-steroidal anti-inflammatory drugs	Warm, dispersing	Lung, Liver, Kidney
Sulphasalazine	Warm, dispersing	Lung, Kidney
Sulphonamide	Warm, dispersing	Lung, Kidney
Tranquillisers	Cold	Heart, Liver

POURQUOI ETUDIEZ -VOUS LA MÉDECINE CONVENTIONELLE?[1]

'Why study conventional medicine?' is a question that has troubled students and colleges of alternative medicine for a long time. Why, when the aims of the course are to produce a homoeopath, i.e. one who prescribes homoeopathic remedies, should Western medical sciences be included at all? After all, homoeopaths do not investigate conventionally, they do not diagnose conventionally and certainly do not treat conventionally. So what is the point? Wouldn't it be better to spend this valuable time doing something more useful or more enjoyable or both!

It may be helpful here to relate a story as an illustration. One day whilst out walking with her children, mother mouse was confronted by a fierce cat that was about to leap on the young family. Standing her ground, the mother mouse drew herself up to her full 4 cm in height and barked ferociously. At this the cat, clearly frightened, jumped back and ran away. Turning to her children she said, 'There you are children. That shows the advantage of learning another language.'

So it is with conventional medicine. There may be some value in learning its language. However, unless you intend to be a medical practitioner there is no need to become fluent. A visit to France is more enjoyable if we know how to ask for bread, cheese and wine, but you needn't study French for 5 years. A phrase book is fine. Similarly the study of conventional medicine does not have to lead to fluency. The ONLY requirement is to learn aspects (phrases) that are relevant to the needs of the homoeopath.

What is necessary for the homoeopath? Ideally this needs to be defined by practising homoeopaths of experience since they deal with cases daily and know what is useful and what is not. However, as a non-homoeopath I shall be presumptuous enough to make a few suggestions.

The essence is to be practical, to know that which is useful in clinical practice. Principles are more important than facts as most information is available in textbooks and can be looked up.

I would suggest that the general aims would be to increase the skill of the homoeopath in dealing with cases complicated by conventional investigation, diagnosis and treatment.

Specifically this could include:

- warning signs – when a symptom indicates a serious condition which may necessitate urgent intervention
- legal restrictions on practice
- how to liase with medical staff
- how to understand medical terms
- how to understand conventional disease labels in terms of levels of health, hierarchies and direction of the pathology
- how to minimise and possibly overcome or prevent the effects of conventional investigation and treatment
- how to manage people who take prescribed drugs and eventually reduce or withdraw them
- learn diagnostic skills useful in the management of cases, e.g. auriscope, sphygmomanometer.

I make no mention here of increasing confidence. I strongly believe that confidence as a homoeopath arises out of your skill and competence at homoeopathy. Conventional medicine deals with fear and limitations not with health and freedom. Therefore, the study of conventional medicine can only ever be an adjunct to your practice, never a replacement.

If you learn conventional medicine to this level, I am sure you will have an appropriate perspective on its usefulness. It is helpful to tread a middle path between the extremes of over-reliance (involving expenditure of large amounts of study, time or energy) and outright rejection. Use conventional medicine for your practice as you need it – much the same as you would use a phrase book in the Dordogne.

Bonne chance!

---

[1] This is an article I was asked to write for the newsletter of a homoeopathic college. I know that many students feel overwhelmed by conventional medical information. This article outlines my ideas about the aims of learning such a subject and the general approach which must flow from this if students are to be inspired rather than 'expired'!

THE INTERNET

In the past few years, there has been an explosion both in the number of people who have access to the Internet and the amount of information available there. A major consideration for anyone searching for information is the need for discrimination – what is helpful and what is not?

Many patients are specifically told by their doctors not to look for information on the Internet. Partly this arises from a desire that patients are not confused by a bewildering mass of detailed information. Another, less positive, motivation for this advice may be that doctors, on occasion, become apprehensive when patients seek access to information in order to make informed decisions about their own treatment.

The world of medicine is rapidly changing. People are generally more questioning of their health-care practitioners and as more information becomes widely available, this can be of great benefit in the search for relief from illness and enhanced health. However, there is a need for clearly presented sources of information that are easily accessible and can be used by anyone to assess their own particular situation.

With this in mind, I have created a new and innovative website that provides information and support to health-care practitioners and to the general public. There are several aspects to the website that will be of interest to practitioners.

- Medical information based upon *The Clinical Medicine Guide – A Holistic Perspective*
- Information on prescribed drugs that supports the prescribed drug reference book: *The Prescribed Guide – A Holistic Perspective*
- Cases showing people treated with Chinese medicine or with homoeopathy
- Supervision and support service for holistic practitioners
- Support for the Study Guide that accompanies *The Clinical Medicine Guide – A Holistic Perspective*
- An 'Ask me' section for students and practitioners of holistic medicine
- Handy suggestion sheets on diet, relaxation, exercise, childbirth, etc.

Dr Stephen Gascoigne
The Clinic of Chinese Medicine
Glebe House
Ardfield
Clonakilty
Co. Cork
Ireland

Tel: +3530(0)23 40986
Fax: +353 (0)23 40985
Email: info@drgascoigne.com
Website: www.drgascoigne.com

INDEX

Main entries are in **bold** type
Entries followed by the letter 'n' refer to notes

A

B

C

D

F

G

H

I

O

Q

R

s

T

U

V

Y

Yang, 316, 347
    in childbirth, 324
    and childhood, 379, 380
    Collapse of, 103, 302
    Deficiency, 85, 101, 107, 163, 181, 370–1
        with Water Overflowing, 181
    excess, 169, 281
    and menstrual cycle, 344
    oedema, 24
    principle, 7, 16, 17n, 265, 287
    Rescue, 181, 302
    root of, 148
Yangming channels, 195
yellow fever, 47, 250
Yin, 316, 318, 339
    in childbirth, 324
    and childhood, 379, 380
    Deficiency, 56, 85, 86, 108, 130, 169, 281, 311, 369, 383
    Envelope, 324
    and female sex hormones, 370
    Heat Damaging, 299
    and menstrual cycle, 344
    oedema, 24
    principle, 16, 17n, 181, 265, 287
    root of, 148
    Stagnation, 370

Z

zalcitabine (DDC), 59
zidovudine (AZT), 59
Zygote intra-fallopian transfer (ZIFT), 363